W0050566

Contemporary Perspectives in Neurosurgery

Series Editor: Robert N.N. Holtzman

Contemporary Perspectives in Neurosurgery

Series Editor: Robert N.N. Holtzman

Surgery of the Spinal Cord: Potential for Regeneration and Recovery, Robert N.N. Holtzman and Bennett M. Stein, Editors

Spinal Instability, Robert N.N. Holtzman, Paul C. McCormick, Jean-Pierre C. Farcy, Editors

Endovascular Interventional Neuroradiology, Robert N.N. Holtzman and Bennett M. Stein, Editors

Robert N.N. Holtzman Paul C. McCormick
Jean-Pierre C. Farcy

Editors

Heidi Winston
Associate Editor

Spinal Instability

With 181 Figures in 399 Parts

Springer Science+Business Media, LLC

Robert N.N. Holtzman, MD
Assistant Clinical Professor of Neurological Surgery, College of Physicians and Surgeons of Columbia University; Associate Neurosurgeon, Lenox Hill Hospital, New York, NY 10021, USA

Paul C. McCormick, MD
Assistant Professor of Clinical Neurological Surgery, College of Physicians and Surgeons of Columbia University; Assistant Attending, Department of Neurological Surgery, The New York Neurological Institute, New York, NY 10032, USA

Jean-Pierre C. Farcy, MD
Associate Clinical Professor of Orthopedics, College of Physicians and Surgeons of Columbia University; Associate Attending, Department of Orthopedics, Columbia–Presbyterian Medical Center, New York, NY 10032, USA

Heidi Winston
The Harry Winston Research Foundation, 718 Fifth Avenue, New York, NY 10019, USA

Library of Congress Cataloging-in-Publication Data
Stonwin Conference (8th: 1991: Stonwin Estate)
Spinal instability/Robert N.N. Holtzman, Paul C. McCormick, Jean-Pierre C. Farcy, editors, with Heidi Winston, associate editor; Stonwin Medical Conference; [sponsored by] Harry Winston Medical Foundation, Inc.
p. cm.—(Contemporary perspectives in neurosurgery)
Includes bibliographical references and index.

1. Spine—Instability—Congresses. I. Holtzman, Robert N.N. II. McCormick, Paul. III. Farcy, Jean-Pierre C. IV. Harry Winston Medical Foundation. V. Title. VI. Series.
[DNLM: 1. Joint Instability—surgery—congresses. 2. Laminectomy—congresses. 3. Spinal Cord Injuries—surgery—congresses. 4. Spinal Diseases—surgery—congresses. 5. Spinal Fusion—congresses. WE 725 S881s 1991]
RD771.I58S86 1991
617.3′75—dc20
DNLM/DLC 92-48680

© 1993 Springer Science+Business Media New York

Originally published by Springer-Verlag New York, Inc. in 1993
Softcover reprint of the hardcover 1st edition 1993

All rights reserved. This work may not be translated or copied in whole or in part without the written permission of the publisher (Springer Science+Business Media, LLC), except for brief excerpts in connection with reviews of scholarly analysis. Use in connection with any form of information storage and retrieval, electronic adaptation, computer software, or by similar or dissimilar methodology now known or hereafter developed is forbidden.
The use of general descriptive names, trade names, trademarks, etc., in this publication, even if the former are not especially identified, is not to be taken as a sign that such names, as understood by the Trade Marks and Merchandise Marks Act, may accordingly be used freely by anyone.
While the advice and information in this book is believed to be true and accurate at the date of going to press, neither the authors nor the editors nor the publisher can accept any legal responsibility for any errors or omissions that may be made. The publisher makes no warranty, express or implied, with respect to the material contained herein.

Production managed by Natalie Johnson; manufacturing supervised by Jacqui Ashri.
Typeset by Asco Trade Typesetting Ltd., Hong Kong.

9 8 7 6 5 4 3 2 1

ISBN 978-1-4613-9328-3 ISBN 978-1-4613-9326-9 (eBook)
DOI 10.1007/978-1-4613-9326-9

This volume is dedicated to

My twin sister, Elizabeth Holtzman, the present comptroller of New York City
—RNNH—

My wife, Doris, and my son, Paul Jr.
—PCMcC—

My wife, Pommy, and my children, Frederick, David, and Sarah
—J-PCF—

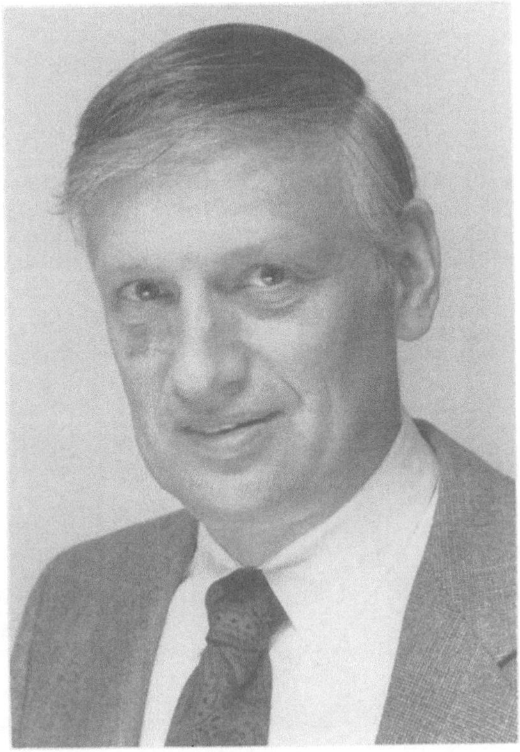

Guest of Honor:

John P. Kostuik, MD
President, North American Back Society
Professor of Orthopedic Surgery, Department of Orthopedic Surgery
Johns Hopkins Outpatient Center

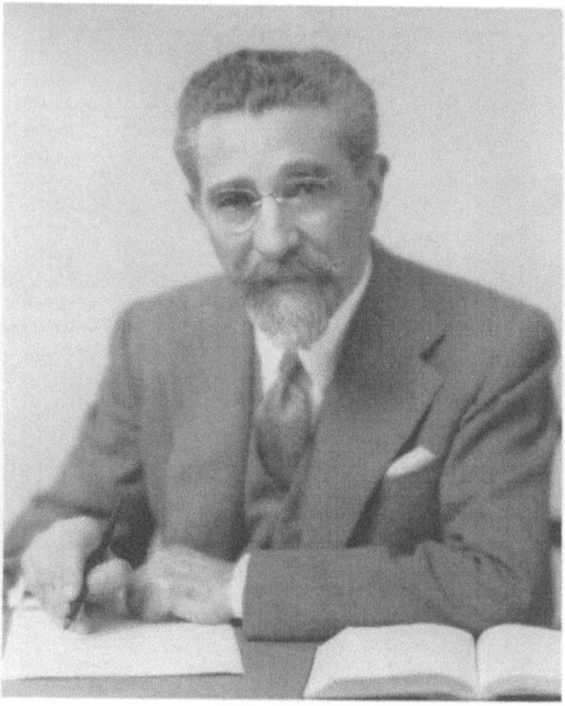

Henry Fleishmann, MD

Foreword

The Eighth Stonwin Medical Conference provided a unique forum for both orthopedic spine surgeons and spinal neurosurgeons who gathered together in the music room of the Stonwin Estate under the portrait of Edna Winston. There they exchanged views on the nature of spinal instability and the possible means of correcting that instability so as to preserve spinal mechanical function and to protect the neural tissues housed in its vertebral compartments.

The conference represented one of the first of such exchanges where orthopedists and neurosurgeons have formally met to discuss spinal instability and to consider the evolution of a new category of surgeon—the spine surgeon. It was both controversial and stimulating, and it will serve as a basis for collaborative efforts in the near future.

This could not have happened without the generosity of Ronald H. Winston, the son of Harry and Edna Winston, who has unswervingly given support to the exchange of scientific and medical ideas, in part from the influence of his maternal grandfather, Henry Fleishmann, a physician, and in part from his own scientific interests. We are deeply indebted to him for supporting and promoting these conferences as we believe they represent efforts to explore in depth problems on the frontiers of medicine and surgery.

HENRY B. ROBERTS, JR.
Publishing and Editorial Consultant
Stonwin Medical Conference

Preface

The definition of spinal instability centers on the interrelationships, disposition, and alignment of the vertebrae in both static and dynamic phases. The integrity of these relationships is structurally maintained by the intervertebral cartilaginous joints—the discs with their annulus fibrosis and nucleus pulposus; the zygapophyseal synovial joints; the anterior and posterior spinal ligaments, and to a lesser extent, the intertransverse ligaments, the interspinous ligaments, and the ligamentum flavum. A very important role is played in inertial loading by the paraspinal musculature.

The spinal cord and its roots, ganglia, rami, and their individual investing membranes generally become involved in the definition by signaling vertebral instability with focal or radicular pain, muscular spasms, or frank neurological symptoms. It is essential to consider these elements along with radiographically documented abnormal motion or position to derive a working definition of spinal instability.

The problem is that the definition is not perfectly stated for all instances. Therefore, judgments about instability are often made on a clinical basis without definitive radiographic correlation. Viewing the spine during the aging process discloses a variety of radiographic appearances that demonstrate vertebral motion but do not reflect true instability. These include the escalator-like steps in a child's flexed cervical spine, the more fixed dynamic lordotic and kyphotic curves in adulthood, and the pseudospondolytic slip of the aged. When there is "clear-cut" abnormal motion in pathological settings of tumor, infection, trauma, and the postoperative state seen on flexion-extension radiographs, which demonstrate varying degrees of vertebral displacement from 1 to 3 mm, most spine surgeons will concur on the presence of spinal instability and recommend internal fixation and fusion. On the other hand, when a patient has back pain with spinal stenosis or spondylolisthesis without radiographic evidence of abnormal translational or rotational motion, some spine surgeons will claim that instability exists and will perform extensive fusions whereas others will not, rather opting for decompression of the roots and thecal sac—keeping the fusion as a backup procedure and achieving equivalent clinical outcomes though perhaps more frequent residual low back pain in the unfused group. Another approach now offered by Dr. Arthur White is to encourage such patients to embark upon a specific spine stabilization training program.

It is these less-explicit situations relating to a numerical value of permissible vertebral motion, the presence or absence of pain with such motion, and the strict radiographic documentation of abnormal motion that in some instances necessitates examination under general anesthesia, that demand our attention in arriving at a formal definition of spinal instability. Evolving technology in the form of real-time magnetic resonance imaging (MRI) capable of performing kinetic imaging of the spine may ultimately be able to prove or disprove stability.

At the present time, fusion procedures and fusion technology are rapidly evolving. Despite the sophistication of the instrumentation, achieving a solid fusion always requires bone grafts as well as metallic constructs via highly complex combined anterior and posterior approaches. Primarily because of this, some guidelines are offered by Dr. Michael Neuwirth, namely, that the ultimate aim of internal fixation be to restore normal function, not to eliminate it with fusion, and when fusion must be performed under present circumstances it should preserve normal bony and neurologic anatomy while eliminating motion in the shortest segment possible. Of great importance in this regard is further knowledge concerning the *osteointegration* of foreign materials to insure the best bony-metallic interface possible and the strongest adherence of a given implant to bone.

The chapters of this volume address these matters in great detail. Structural integrity of the spine depends on bone growth, bone repair, and ligamentous integrity. Vertebral integrity may be dependent on a glucocorticoid and prostaglandin availability as was suggested from the recent work of the Columbia astronaut, Dr. Millie Hughes-Fulford. Osteoporotic, weakened bone is subject to fracture and it is precisely this susceptibility with ongoing microtrauma and incomplete healing that may be strongly implicated in the progressive instability or pseudospondylolisthesis of aging.

Initially the spine may be conceptualized as a structure with five basic motions: forward flexion, backward extension, lateral flexion, rotation, and elongation. Lesser motions include forward and backward wedging of the intervertebral discs and the shearing slippage of one vertebra on another. These basic motions are translated into static and dynamic axial and transverse stability. *Axial* stability is provided in two columns at C1-C2 and three columns from C2 to the sacrum according to Prof. René Louis. The anterior column is formed by the vertebrae and discs and the two posterior columns formed by the two zygapophyseal joints. *Transverse* stability of one motion segment-level is provided by bony buttresses consisting of end plates and facets and ligamentous brakes. Further stabilization is provided by the paraspinal muscles and the neuromuscular control system, which computes and sets the dynamic spine for varying inertial loads in all directions. In addition specific terminology relating to specific types of instability is being used: *longitudinal* for instability associated with disc space collapse and discogenic sclerosis, *translational* for spondylolisthesis, *angular* for kyphosis, *rotational* for scoliosis, and *complex* for varying combinations of the above.

Instability between adjacent or successive vertebrae causes mechanical deformation of intraspinal neural tissue. Compressive deformation of nerve roots and ganglia leads to alteration of their microcirculation and edema formation, which has been documented in the pig model by extravasation of labeled serum albumin. Edema is probably accompanied by an intraneural inflammatory reaction and demyelination. Painful ganglionitis and radiculitis may also result from chemical or autoimmune mechanisms from the adjacent degenerating disc or bleeding from traction on adjacent epidural veins leading to perineural fibrosis and varying degrees of root tethering. The combination of these events with disruption and inflammation of the richly innervated ligamentous systems may explain the associated clinical symptomatology.

The management of children with progressive scoliosis, intraspinal tumors, and trauma differs from that of adults in light of the need to preserve normal growth patterns and avoid deformities. Significant deformities accompanied multilevel laminectomies and removal of both facet joints at a single level. The incidence of these was substantially reduced by a team approach of neurosurgeons and orthopedic spine surgeons using Cotrel-Dubousset instrumentation, laminotomy instead of laminectomy, and bony fusion, reserving cast immobilization for cases where no other technique can be utilized. These stabilizing techniques should be performed at the time of initial neurosurgical intervention.

Trauma has special implications in children since there is greater elasticity in the "discovertebroligamentous complex" than in the adult, and, in some instances, greater vertebral column elasticity than the elastic tolerances of the spinal cord such that there may be significant neurological damage without evident vertebral injury.

Special emphasis is given in separate chapters to the varying aspects of vertebral injury and instability categorized as *axial compression*, *axial distraction*, *flexion*, *flexion compression*, *flexion distraction*, *extension rotation*, and *shear* as well as to specific spinal problems including occipitocervical and atlantoaxial instability; thoracic spine instability with tumors, trauma, and infection; lumbar spine instability with scoliosis, spondylolisthesis, degenerative disc disease, spinal stenosis, and the postdiscectomy and postlaminectomy syndromes; and lastly, sacral spine instability. The surgical treatment of failures of laminectomy and revision surgery in late spine instability are addressed as is the nonoperative management of cervical spine instability.

One chapter is exclusively devoted to the lateral extracavitary approach to the thoracolumbar spine. This novel approach may become extremely important in vertebral surgical exposures.

In summary, the subject of spinal instability is presented in detail with regard to its precise identification, surgical and nonsurgical management, and the outcomes of these therapies. Serious consideration is given to the creation of the new subspecialty—the spine surgeon.

New York

Robert N.N. Holtzman, MD
Paul C. McCormick, MD
Jean-Pierre C. Farcy, MD

Acknowledgments

The Stonwin Medical Conference has taken place over the past eight years with the generous help of a number of individuals whose concern with its success has taken precedence over other matters of importance. Their names are mentioned here with great respect and appreciation.

Dr. Sanford P. Antin, consultant neuroradiologist

Dr. Joseph Bossum, scientific consultant

Mrs. Ophelia Davidova, coordinator of the Exchange Program and all matters related to the Stonwin Conference in Professor A.N. Konovalov's office at the N.N. Burdenko Neurosurgical Institute

Dr. Thomas Q. Garvey III, archivist

Harvard Club House Committee, for permission to use the Harvard Club facilities

Ms. Carol A. Denko, organizer and coordinator; Ms. Adrienne Fischier, librarian; Mr. Jim Foley, concierge; Mr. Alan Lerner, pianist; Mr. Niall McGovern, concessionaire

Ms. Ioana F. Metianu, coordinator of all matters pertaining to the Stonwin Conference in Mr. Ronald H. Winston's office

Ms. Nancy McMenemy, coordinator of all matters pertaining to the Stonwin Conference in Dr. Robert N.N. Holtzman's office

Mr. Henry B. Roberts, Jr., publishing and editorial consultant

Mrs. Evelyn Smith, coordinator of all matters pertaining to the Stonwin Conference and the Exchange Program in Dr. Bennett M. Stein's office at the New York Neurological Institute

Professor Lionel Tsao, Department of Chinese Studies, Hunter College, New York

Mrs. Susan Weiler, transcriber of the manuscript

Mrs. Ruth Winston, coordinator of the travel arrangements

Leonid A. Yudin, MD Ph.D, Deputy Rector, Sechenov Medical Academy, Moscow, Russia

Acknowledgments

Contents

Contributors

The Eighth Annual Stonwin Medical Conference

Cochairman:

Bennett M. Stein, MD
Byron Stookey Professor of Neurological Surgery, College of Physicians and Surgeons of Columbia University; Chairman of the Department of Neurological Surgery, The New York Neurological Institute, New York, NY 10032, USA

Cochairman and Coeditor:

Robert N.N. Holtzman, MD
Assistant Clinical Professor of Neurological Surgery, College of Physicians and Surgeons of Columbia University; Associate Neurosurgeon, Lenox Hill Medical Center, New York, NY 10021, USA

Coeditor:

Paul C. McCormick, MD
Assistant Professor of Clinical Neurological Surgery, College of Physicians and Surgeons of Columbia University; Assistant Attending, Department of Neurological Surgery, The New York Neurological Institute, New York, NY 10032, USA

Coeditor:

Jean-Pierre C. Farcy, MD, FACS(C)
Associate Clinical Professor of Orthopedics, College of Physicians and Surgeons of Columbia University; Associate Attending, Department of Orthopedics, Columbia-Presbyterian Medical Center, New York, NY 10032, USA

Guest of Honor:

JOHN P. KOSTUIK, MD, FRCS(C)
President, North American Back Society; Professor of Orthopedic Surgery, Department of Orthopedic Surgery, Johns Hopkins Outpatient Center, Baltimore, MD 21287-0882, USA

Contributors:

GREGORY J. BENNETT, MD
Assistant Professor of Neurosurgery, Department of Neurosurgery, State University of New York at Buffalo, Buffalo, NY 14209, USA

GERARD BOLLINI, MD
Départment de Chirugie Orthopédique Pédiatrique, Hôpital de la Timoine, 13385 CEDEX 5, Marseille, France

J. COTTALORDA
Hôpital de la Timoine, 13385 CEDEX 5, Marseille, France

HAROLD M. DICK, MD
Chairman, Department of Orthopedics, Columbia-Presbyterian Medical Center, New York, NY 10032, USA

CURTIS A. DICKMAN, MD
Division of Neurological Surgery, Barrow Neurological Institute, Phoenix, AZ 85013, USA

JEAN DUBOUSSET, MD
Hôpital St. Vincent de Paul, Chirugie Orthopédique Infantile, 75674 CEDEX 14, Paris, France

JEAN-PIERRE C. FARCY, MD, FACS(C)
Associate Clinical Professor of Orthopedics, College of Physicians and Surgeons of Columbia University; Associate Attending, Department of Orthopedics, Columbia-Presbyterian Medical Center, New York, NY 10032, USA

YIZHAR FLOMAN, MD
Professor of Orthopedic Surgery, Department of Orthopedic Surgery, Hadassah University Hospital, Jerusalem 91120, Israel

ALLEYNE B. FRASER, MD
Department of Neurosurgery, Mount Sinai Hospital and Medical Center, New York, NY 10029, USA

JOSEPH GRANT, MD
San Francisco Spine Institute, Daly City, CA 94015, USA

ROBERT N.N. HOLTZMAN, MD
Assistant Clinical Professor of Neurological Surgery, College of Physicians and Surgeons of Columbia University; Associate Neurosurgeon, Lenox Hill Medical Center, New York, NY 10021, USA

JAMES E.O. HUGHES, MD
Assistant Clinical Professor of Neurological Surgery, College of Physicians and Surgeons of Columbia University; Associate Attending Neurosurgeon, St. Luke's–Roosevelt Hospital Center; Chief of Neurosurgery, Harlem Hospital Center, New York, NY 10037, USA

MILLIE HUGHES-FULFORD, PhD
Department of Research, Laboratory of Cell Growth and Differentiation, Department of Veterans' Affairs Medical Center; Department of Medicine, University of California at San Francisco, San Francisco, CA 94121, USA

J.L. JOUVE, MD
Hôpital de la Timoine, 13385 CEDEX 5, Marseille, France

JOHN P. KOSTUIK, MD, FRCS(C)
President, North American Back Society; Professor of Orthopedic Surgery, Department of Orthopedic Surgery, Johns Hopkins Outpatient Center, Baltimore, MD 21287-0882, USA

GEORGE KROL, MD
Department of Neurosurgery, Mount Sinai Hospital and Medical Center, New York, NY 10029, USA

SANFORD J. LARSON, MD
Chairman, Department of Neurosurgery, Medical College of Wisconsin, Milwaukee, WI 53226, USA

RENÉ LOUIS, MD
Professor de Clinique Orthopédique, Chirurgie de la Colome Vertébrale, L'Hôpital de la Conception à Marseille, 13005 Marseille, France

JOSEPH Y. MARGULIES
Hospital for Joint Diseases, Orthopedic Institute, New York, NY 10003, USA

PAUL C. MCCORMICK, MD
Assistant Professor of Clinical Neurological Surgery, College of Physicians and Surgeons of Columbia University; Assistant Attending, Department of Neurological Surgery, The New York Neurological Institute, New York, NY 10032, USA

MICHAEL G. NEUWIRTH, MD
Chief, Spine Services, Hospital for Joint Diseases, Orthopedic Institute, New York, NY 10003, USA

Patrick F. O'Leary, MD
Assistant Clinical Professor of Orthopedics, Mount Sinai School of Medicine; Chief, Spine Section, Hospital for Special Surgery; Associate Director, Department of Orthopedics, Lenox Hill Hospital, New York, NY 10021, USA

Kjell Olmarker, MD, PhD
Assistant Research Professor, Department of Orthopaedics, University of Göteborg; Sahlgren Hospital, S-413 45 Göteborg, Sweden

Manohar M. Panjabi, PhD
Professor of Orthopaedics and Rehabilitation and Mechanical Engineering, Director of Biomechanics Research, Yale University School of Medicine, New Haven, CT 06510, USA

James B. Reynolds, MD
San Francisco Spine Institute, Daly City, CA 94015, USA

Björn L. Rydevik, MD, PhD
Associate Professor of Orthopaedic Surgery, University of Göteborg; Shalgren Hospital, S-41345 Göteborg, Sweden

Volker K.H. Sonntag, MD
Professor of Surgery, University of Arizona, Tucson, AZ; Vice-Chairman, Department of Neurosurgery, Barrow Neurological Institute, Phoenix, AZ 85013, USA

Narayan Sundaresan, MD
Chief of Neuro-Oncology, St. Luke's-Roosevelt Hospital Center; Associate Professor of Neurosurgery, Mount Sinai School of Medicine, New York, NY 10029, USA

Arthur H. White, MD
Medical Director, San Francisco Spine Institute, Daly City, CA 94015, USA

I. BASIC SCIENCE

CHAPTER 1

Growth and Repair of Mineralized Osteoblasts

Millie Hughes-Fulford

One of the most serious health hazards in long-term manned space flight is the continuous and progressive loss of calcium and weight-bearing bone. Skeletal changes and loss of total body calcium have been observed in both human and animals who have flown from 1 week to more than 237 days. During the Apollo and Skylab missions, photon absorptiometry was used to assess pre- and postflight bone mineral mass. For the 12 crew members of Gemini 4, 5, and 7 and Apollo 7 and 8, the average postflight loss from the os calcis was 3.2% over an average of 8.5 days (11,12,28).

Greatest losses were observed in the longer Skylab 4 mission, where the crew routinely exercised to prevent bone loss. Even with this countermeasure, they lost an average of 4% of bone over the 84-day period (18). It was not determined in these Skylab studies whether the loss of mineral was primarily from weight-bearing bone. However, some evidence provided by Soviet space flight measurements showed that mineral loss was determined to be from the tubercle and plantar areas of the os calcis, predominantly from compact bone. Bone loss seemed to increase in general proportion to the duration of the space flight from 0.9% to 19.8% over 75 to 184 days (20).

The loss of bone in the Cosmonauts occurred despite the countermeasure of 2 to 4 hours of exercise in every day flight. Both compact and trabecular bone is lost from the heel (os calcis). Calcaneal mineral recovery is gradual and appears to take about the same length of time as loss (27). This measured recovery was incomplete in at least one Skylab 4 astronaut; only half of his bone loss was replaced by 90 days postflight. Although the Soviets suggest that calcaneal recovery is complete, spine mineral loss was observed in cosmonauts (using an x-ray computerized tomography technique) throughout 6 months postflight (4). These findings have serious implications for long-term inhabitants of space stations and for future space exploration. The consequences of bone loss in space that are of major concern include (a) the possibility of irreversible bone loss in astronauts after long-term (>1 year) flight; (b) the potential toxic effects of high serum levels of calcium and phosphate with the possibility of renal stone formation in long-term flight; and (c) the normal functional hazard of a diminished skeleton, which could result in later bone damage. Consequently, it is paramount to define the mechanism of bone formation in microgravity in order to discover new countermeasures to prevent bone loss during spaceflight.

To date, all countermeasures used to stop bone demineralization during spaceflight or bed rest have had limited success. Exercise, dietary supplementation with calcium or phosphorus, and pharmacological treatment with salmon calcitonin and diphosphonates have been tried either in flight or in bed rest studies. The most promising countermeasures are exercise and diphosphonate treatment. However, exercise is only effective in bed rest studies when there is activity of 4 hours' duration, and diphosphonates have side effects that include a potential for causing tumors. The newer diphosphonate compounds show promise and may be useful in future flights.

The physiological control of bone growth and remodeling is complicated and not yet well defined. We do know that growth and remodeling are influenced by systemic hormones such as calcitonin, parathyroid hormone, vitamin D, and glucocorticoids. Measurements of parathyroid hormone, vitamin D, calcitonin, and glucocorticoids are currently being made on samples taken from crew members of STS-40, NASA's first dedicated biomedical mission. In June of 1991 I was a scientist-astronaut on NASA's first dedicated biomedical mission Spacelab Life Sciences-1 also known as STS-40. Pre-, during, and postflight samples from myself and my fellow STS-40 crew members (Spaceship Columbia, launching June 5 and landing June 14, 1991) will help define the underlying mechanism of bone loss. The analysis of our blood and urine samples are not yet completed as of this writing. Analyses of in-flight urine, fecal, and plasma samples from Skylab crew members revealed changes in a number of biochemical parameters. Urinary output of hydroxyproline gradually increased, indicating degradation of the collagenous matrix substance of weight-bearing bones. Output of nitrogen, reflecting muscle atrophy, also increased. Increased concentrations of urinary calcium has been noted in astronauts starting within the first days of flight and in many of the astronauts remaining at elevated levels throughout the period of space flight.

Various lines of evidence from human and animal studies suggest that the loss of bone in space flight is due to a decrease in bone formation. Studies of animals flown on board the Cosmos biosatellites and Spacelab have also revealed changes in bone mineral content. Spacelab 3 rat studies, as well as previous animal studies flown on the Cosmos biosatellites, showed significant skeletal changes even on the short flights. The changes in skeleton in rats exposed to as little as 7 days of flight included decreased bone growth, decreased mineralization, decreased bending strength, and decreased weight of the lumbar (L3) spines (5,29). Flight rats after 18.5 days of microgravity showed a 30% decrease in mechanical bending strength (6) as compared to a 28% reduction after 7 days on board Spacelab 3 (3). No changes have been noted in rat kidney calcitriol receptors, suggesting an absence of causal roles of this system in regulating renal calcium loss (13). These and other studies suggest that the loss of bone mineral in space is primarily due to an inhibited bone formation, rather than an increased bone resorption (14,30). It is not known if the decrease in bone formation is due directly to the lack of gravity or to systemic hormonal changes, or to a combination of these factors.

In our investigation of the possible systemic causes of bone loss in spaceflight, we have been studying the role of the glucocorticoids and prostaglandins in bone growth. Mounting evidence points to prostaglandin E_2 (PGE_2) as a local bone growth regulator. Animals treated with prostaglandin E have been noted to have proliferation of their long bones (15). Moreover, infants with cyanotic congenital heart disease treated with prostaglandins to close the ductus, have been observed to have cortical proliferation of long bones (25,26). In contrast to parathyroid hormone, calcitonin and osteoclast activating factor (PGE_2) do not inhibit bone collagen synthesis (16). Prostaglandins have also been shown to cause an increase in the incorporation of proline into collagen and noncollagen proteins in chick bone (2). Prostaglandins are produced by osteoblasts and are prime candidates for local bone regulating hormones. In vitro stimulation of cultured bone cells can enhance prostaglandin production (17,22–24). Direct mechanical stimulation of cat bone tissue has been shown to increase the synthesis of PGE_2 in vivo (19). Recently Jee (8) has demonstrated that PGE_2 stimulates trabecular bone formation in vivo by 120% over a 21-day period.

One systemic factor that may regulate the prostaglandin effect on bone growth is the glucocorticoid, cortisol. Clinical observations show that increases of endogenous cortisol (two- to fivefold over normal levels) as seen in Cushing's syndrome is associated with bone loss and osteoporosis. Numerous investigations have shown that bone mass is subnormal in both Cushing's syndrome patients and patients treated with steroids for asthma and rheumatoid arthritis (1); however, the underlying cause of glucocorticoid-induced bone loss is still under debate. Treatments of patients with asthma and rheumatoid arthritis demonstrate the deleterious effects of glucocorticoids on bone formation; this bone loss involves trabecular bone and examination of these patients treated with the synthetic glucocorticoid, prednisone, show a reduction in bone formation that was postulated to be due to a direct effect of the glucocorticoid on osteoblast bone formation (1). Glucocorticoid-induced osteoporosis primarily involves decreased width of trabecular bone, suggesting a reduction of trabecular osteoblast proliferation (1). The inhibitory effect of glucocorticoids on bone formation was also observed in vivo in the rat, where cortisone inhibited new trabecular bone formation (10). Since glucocorticoids inhibit the synthesis of PGE_2, decreased synthesis of PGE_2 may be the mechanism by which glucocorticoids inhibit bone formation.

Glucocorticoids may well play a role in the loss of bone in space flight. Urinary analysis of nine Skylab astronauts showed that cortisol increased from 54 ± 4 to 94 ± 5 μg/total volume in-flight (10). In individual crew members, urinary cortisols increase from 1.2-fold preflight to 2.8-fold during flight (7). Many of these increased concentrations of cortisol are comparable to the increased levels seen in Cushing's syndrome, suggesting that the increased glucocorticoids occurring during spaceflight may contribute to loss of bone in astronauts.

Bone formation is a complicated process that consists of two distinct development stages at the cellular level—osteoblast proliferation and osteoblast mineralization. To help us understand this complicated process, we have used the cloned osteoblast cell line MC3T3-E1 as a model for examining the cellular and molecular effects of the glucocorticoids on osteoblast cell growth and mineralization. The glucocorticoids are known to enter the cell nucleus and cause the synthesis of a class of proteins called lipocortins. The lipocortins in turn inactivate phospholipase A_2. With decreased cellular phospholipase A_2, reduced amounts of membrane arachidonic acid (AA) are released into the cell, thereby reducing the synthesis of endogenous prostaglandins and other eicosanoids. This relationship is shown in the schematic of the synthetic pathway in Fig. 1.1.

Although the direct cause of glucocorticoid-induced osteoporosis is not known, one possible explanation is that a systemic increase in glucocorticoid causes a decrease in synthesis of the local growth factor PGE_2 by the mechanism shown in Fig. 1.1. The reduced PGE_2 synthesis would then result in lowered osteocyte proliferation and synthesis of collagen matrix. We have found, using our bone model, that exogenous glucocorticoid concentrations equivalent to the increases seen in spaceflight and Cushing's syndrome caused a significant decrease of PGE_2 synthesis, to less than half when compared with the untreated osteoblasts; this decrease in endogenous prostaglandin synthesis was accompanied by a decrease in bone growth as measured in milligrams of protein present in the culture (Table 1.1).

To test whether the decrease in growth and protein synthesis was directly related to reduced DNA synthesis in the osteoblasts caused by the glucocorticoid-induced decrease of synthesis of prostaglandin E_2, we designed experiments to test the ability of exogenous prostaglandin E_2 to reverse the effects of glucocorticoids on DNA synthesis. As seen in Table 1.2 addition of 100 nM dexamethasone caused a 75% decrease in the incorporation of tritiated thymidine into DNA. The addition of 5 μg/ml of prostaglandin E_2 caused a 50% increase in DNA synthesis of the glucocorticoid-treated cells. These data suggest that at least a portion of the effect of dexamethasone and other glucocorticoids is due to the inhibition of the specific eicosanoid, prostaglandin E_2. The failure of a 100% reversal of the glucocorticoid effect may be due to the inability of the added

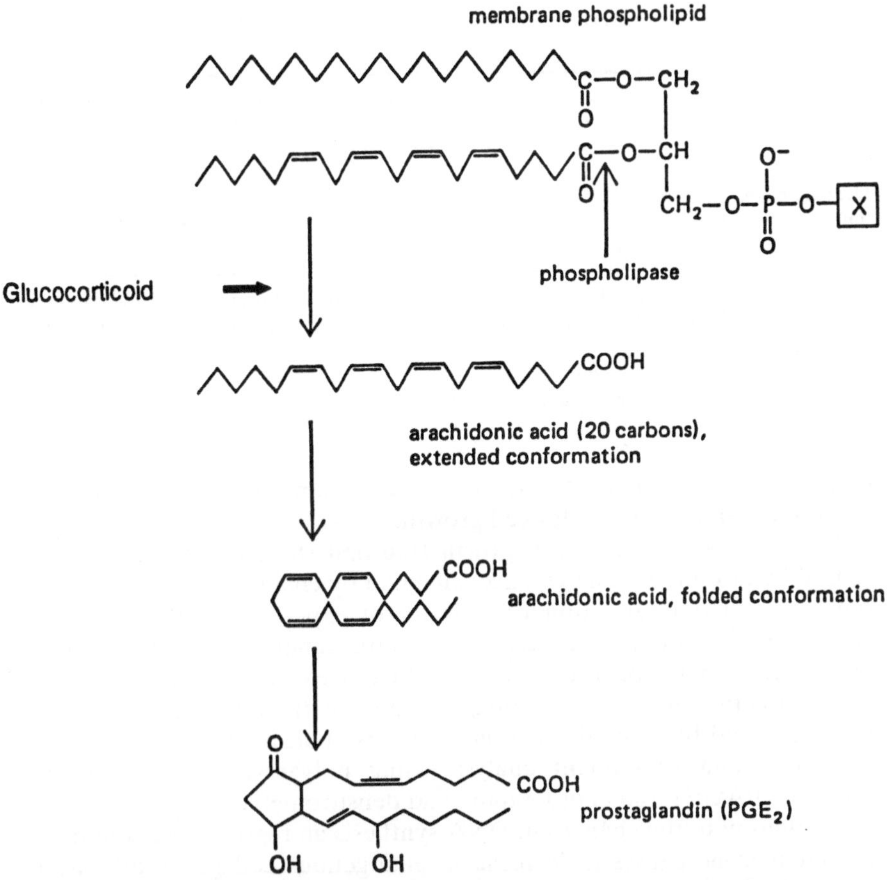

Figure 1.1. Metabolic pathway for prostaglandin synthesis. Prostaglandins are derived from arachidonic acid stored in the cell membrane phospholipid. Glucocorticoids inhibit phospholipase A_2 through a lipocortin-mediated pathway, thereby inhibiting synthesis of endogenous prostaglandin.

Table 1.1. Effects of dexamethasone on protein, DNA and prostaglandin E_2 syntheses.

Treatment	Protein (μg)	Percent of control	PGE_2 (pg)	Percent of control
Control	242 ± 11		500 ± 16	
Dexamethasone	201 ± 6[a]	83 ± 2	230 ± 3[a]	46 ± 1.2

MC3T3-E1 cells were grown as described in methods. The osteoblast cells were initially seeded at 1×10^6 cells/dish, then treated for 24 hours with dexamethasone before analysis.
[a] Significantly different from control, $p < .001$.

Table 1.2. Partial reversal of dexamethasone inhibition of osteoblast growth by $dmPGE_2$.

Treatment	Percent incorporation of [^{3}H]-Tdr (dpm/μg protein)
Control	100 ± 6.2
Dexamethasone (100 nM)	21.5 ± 6[a]
$dmPGE_2$ (5μg/ml) + dexamethasone (100 nM)	50.7 ± 2[a,b]

MC3T3-E1 cells were seeded at 0.5×10^6 cells/well and were allowed to grow overnight before treatment. Dexamethasone and/or $dmPGE_2$ were added and cells were incubated for 24 hours before analysis.
[a] Significantly different from control, $p < .001$.
[b] Significantly different from dexamethasone-treated cells, $p < .001$.

prostaglandin to fully enter the proper cell compartment or the requirement of other eicosanoids for cell growth.

The decrease in osteoblast growth (the first stage of bone formation) caused by dexamethasone was accompanied by changes in the mineralization stage of differentiation. In this set of experiments, the osteoblast cells were grown over a 20-day period, with mineralization beginning to occur after confluence (around 8 days of culture). One measure of mineralization is the production of collagen type I by the osteoblasts. Collagen was measured by prior incubation of the osteoblast with ^{14}C-proline for 20 hours, and subsequent analysis using polyacrylamide gel electrophoresis (PAGE), radioautography, and densitrometry analysis.

In addition to the changes in DNA synthesis and growth, we found that dexamethasone causes a decrease in endogenous collagen synthesis. In the early stages of mineralization, this decrease is due to the reduced capacity of the cell to make procollagen, followed by the inhibition of converting the newly synthesized procollagen into collagen in the cell (Table 1.3). This change in the synthesis and processing of collagen type I in the osteoblast was also examined using epifluorscence and an affinity-purified collagen type I antibody. The cells were first processed using von Kossa's staining technique to visualize mineralization, with the mineral appearing as dark areas in the photomicrograph. The cell was then treated using a double antibody method to visualize the collagen type I in the cell. The resulting photomicrographs are paired, showing the phase contract photo (von Kossa–stained mineral) and collagen type I matrix deposit. The control cells grow in parallel layers with the deposit of mineral showing as darkened grains in the phase contrast photomicrograph (Fig. 1.2A); in Fig. 1.2B, the light areas of the photograph are collagen matrix deposits visualized with immunofluorescent photomicrography. The osteoblast cultures treated with dexamethasone show mineralization around irregular-shaped cells (Fig. 1.2C), and the uneven

Table 1.3. Effects of dexamethasone on collagen type I synthesis.

Day of growth	Treatment	Total collagen type I percent of ^{14}C-proline–labelled protein	Total procollagen percent of total collagen type I unprocessed
8	Control	49.7	50.3
	Dexamethasone	39.3	60.7
11	Control	43.5	56.5
	Dexamethasone	36.3	63.7
13	Control	49.5	50.5
	Dexamethasone	39.4	60.6

collagen matrix caused by the dexamethasone is visualized by the light areas of Fig. 1.2D. Some of the collagen appears to remain inside the cell, supporting the chemical data that showed a higher percentage of procollagen in the dexamethasone-treated cell.

What do these data mean in relation to bone formation and the loss of bone during spaceflight or disease states that are associated with increased glucocorticoid serum concentrations? First, our findings demonstrate that new growth of bone osteoblasts is inhibited by conditions that lead to superphysiological levels of glucocorticoids. These increased glucocorticoid levels accompanied by decreased osteoblast replication correlate well with clinical findings of decreased bone mass in astronauts, Cushing's syndrome patients, and glucocorticoid-treated asthma patients, all of whom have superphysiological levels of glucocorticoids. Second, glucocorticoids are known to inhibit synthesis of arachidonic acid and its products; the addition of one of the products, PGE_2, can restore over 50% of the growth in osteoblasts. These data point to the pivotal role of prostaglandin in osteoblast growth and mineralization. Third, the increased concentration of glucocorticoids in osteoblasts also changes shape and causes an uneven formation of the collagen matrix, which in turn leads to a defect in the structure in the mineralized osteoblasts. This correlates well with the known decrease in flexibility and strength in bones of glucocorticoid-treated patients and in rats flown in space for as little as 7 days (1,29).

These cloned mouse osteoblasts, originally isolated by Kodama et al. (9), retain specific functions of differentiated bone cells, such as production of alkaline phosphatase, collagen, and osteocalcin, and the ability to synthesize a mineralized protein matrix reflecting intramembranous bone formation (21). Although the behavior of isolated cells in culture may not reflect all the properties of osteoblasts in their complex in vivo environment, which normally involves cell-to-cell interaction and mechanical loading of the tissue, the ability of these cultures to synthesize tissue-specific products suggests that a specific cell model system like this is a potentially useful model for osteoblast function. Even with these

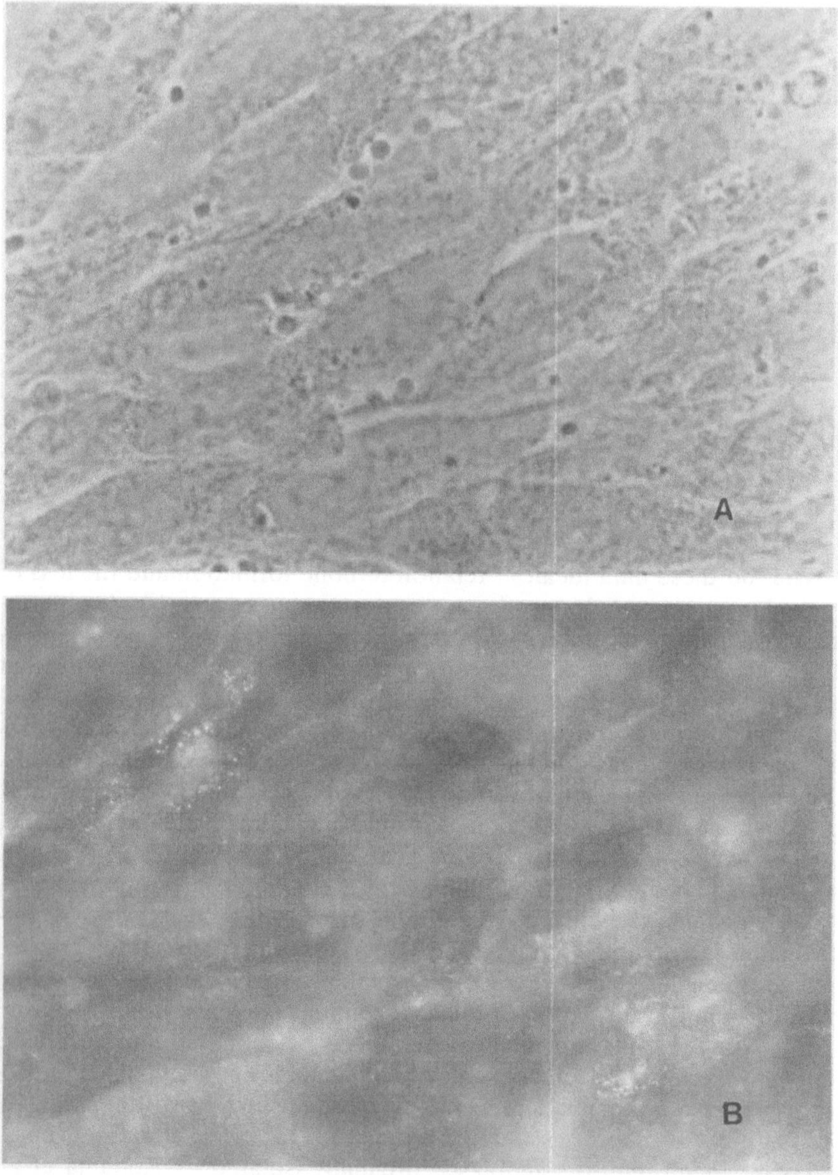

Figure 1.2. Normal osteoblast cell morphology in cell culture. A: The mineralizing control osteoblast under phase contrast, stained with von Kossa stain; the darkened nodules are calcium deposits in the mineralizing osteoblast. Osteoblasts grow in parallel and form classic octagon-shaped cells. B: The same osteoblast field using epifluorescence double-labeled affinity-purified collagen type I antibody. The white areas are the uniform extracellular matrix containing collagen type I. C and D: Dexamethasone-treated osteoblast cell morphology in cell cul-

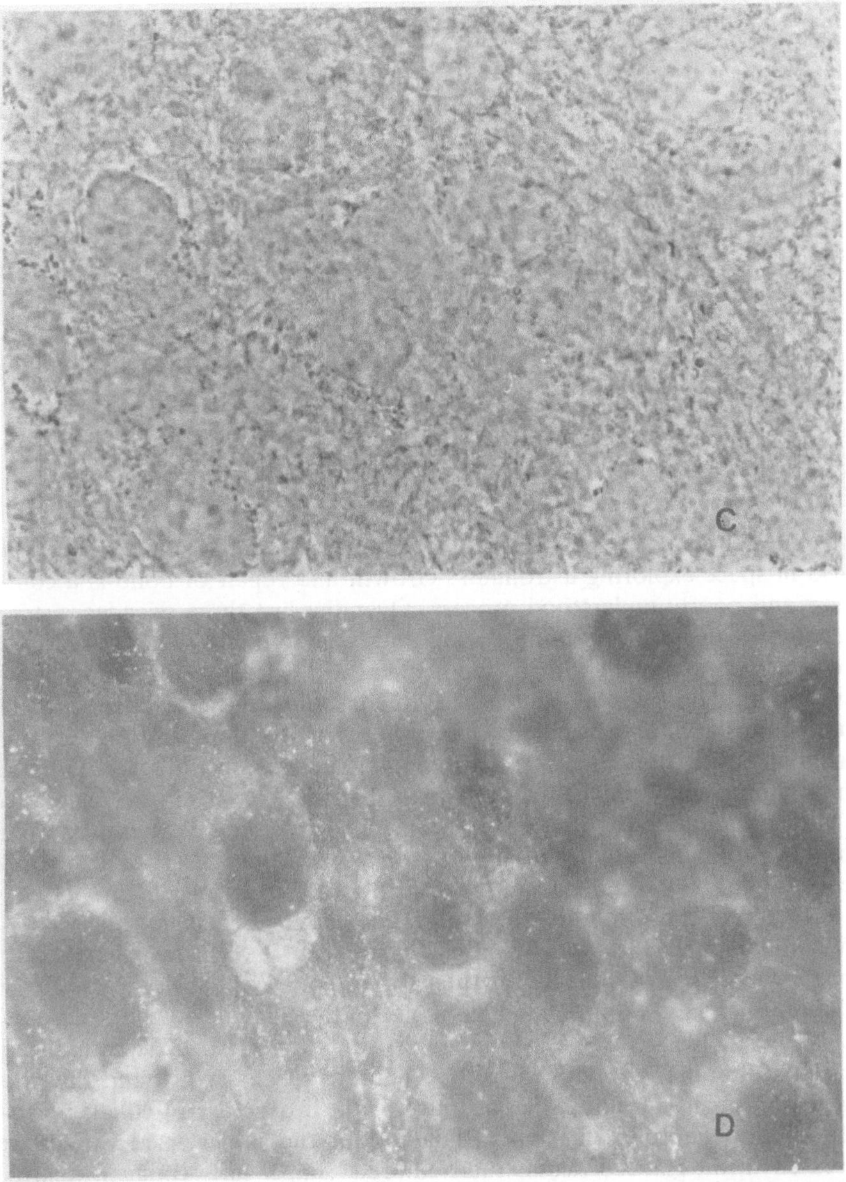

ture. **C:** The mineralizing dexamethasone-treated osteoblast under phase contrast, stained with von Kossa stain, the darkened nodules are calcium deposits in the mineralizing osteoblast. The glucocorticoid-treated osteoblasts grow in an irregular, larger form when compared to the control in **A**. **D:** The same glucocorticoid-treated osteoblast field using epifluorescence double-labeled affinity-purified collagen type I antibody. The white areas are the extracellular matrix with collagen type I with irregular matrix formation.

limitations, this model may provide insight into the cellular and molecular mechanisms by which glucocorticoids or spaceflight causes impeded growth of new bone.

Studies on tissue-specific cells like these will add to our basic knowledge of bone formation in spaceflight, and, it is hoped, help us to distinguish the difference between the systemic effects of spaceflight and the direct effects of microgravity on bone formation. Beyond the long-term benefits to space exploration, newfound knowledge of basic bone physiology using bone models directed toward finding the cause and treatment of decreased bone formation in microgravity can be applied to earthbound problems of bone repair.

Summary

The growth and repair of bone is important not oniy in spinal injury but also in space-exploring astronauts. Growth and repair of bone is a complex and poorly understood process. Over the last three decades, astronauts have been losing bone during microgravity flight. The mechanism by which bone growth is regulated is unknown; however, clinical observations have demonstrated that increased concentrations of cortisol as seen in Cushing's syndrome and glucocorticoid-treated asthma and rheumatoid arthritis patients are associated with bone loss and osteoporosis. Evidence from animal and human studies suggest that the loss of bone is related to the reduction of new bone growth. The glucocorticoid levels in the serum of the astronauts is elevated almost twofold, which suggests that the glucocorticoids may play a role in the loss of bone during spaceflight.

The direct cause of glucocorticoid-induced bone loss is not known and full understanding of the relationship between the glucocorticoids and prostaglandins in bone cell growth and differentiation has been slowed by the complex nature of mammalian bone. In these studies, we have used a cloned osteoblast cell line as a model to study the glucocorticoid-induced cellular alterations in growing and mineralizing cells. We found that the glucocorticoids caused a decrease in growth, a decrease in collagen synthesis, and altered cell shape. In addition, the mineralized osteoblast treated with glucocorticoids had altered shape and collagen matrix assembly.

The model for repair is the nonconfluent growing osteoblast. When glucocorticoids are added to the growing cells, there is a significant decrease in the growth of the bone cells. Glucocorticoids are known to inhibit the synthesis of prostaglandins, in this model, we found that the treated osteoblasts had reduced synthesis of prostaglandin E_2. When prostaglandin was added back to the culture, the growth was increased by 50%. Since prostaglandin is able to partially reverse the glucocorticoid growth inhibition, it is possible that prostaglandin plays a pivotal role in bone growth, and medications that disrupt prostaglandin synthesis could modulate bone growth and structure.

Acknowledgments. This work was supported by NASA grant NAGW 1244 and a grant from the Department of Veterans' Affairs. I greatly appreciate the fine technical assistance of Janis Schmidt and Renissance Appel, and the excellent editorial assistance of Pat Little.

References

1. Adinoff A, Hollister R. Steroid-induced fractures and bone loss in patients with asthma. *N Engl J Med.* 1983;309:265–268.
2. Blumenfrantz N, Sondergaard J. Effect of prostaglandins E_2 and F_{2a} on biosynthesis of collagen. Nature [*New Biol*]. 1972:239–246.
3. Buckendahl PE, Cann CE, Grindeland RE, Martin RB, Mechanic G, Arnaud SB. Osteocalcin as an indicator of bone metabolism during space flight. *Physiologist.* 1985;28(4):379.
4. Cann C. *Determination of Spine Mineral Density Using Computerized Tomography: A Report.* XII US/USSR Joint Working Group Meeting on Space Biology and Medicine, Washington, DC, November 9–22, 1981.
5. Duke J, Janer L, Cambell M. Microprobe analysis of epiphyseal plates from Spacelab 3 rats. *Physiologist.* 1985;28(4):379.
6. Gazenko OG, Il'om YeA, Genin AM, Kotovskaya AR, Korol'kov Vl, Tigranyan RA, Portugalov VV. Principal results of physiological experiments with mammals aboard the Cosmos-936 biosatellite. *Space Biol Aerospace Med.* 1980;14(2):33–37.
7. Hughes-Fulford M. Unpublished analysis of Skylab data.
8. Jee W, Ueno K, Deng Y, Woodbury DM. The effects of prostaglandin E_2 in growing rats: increased metaphyseal hard tissue and cortico-endosteal bone formation. *Calcif Tissue Int.* 1985;37:148–157.
9. Kodama H, Amagai Y, Sudo H, Kasai S, Yamamoto S. Establishment of clonal osteogenic cell line from newborn mouse calvaria. *Jpn J Oral Biol.* 1985;23:899–901.
10. Leach C, Rambaut P. Biochemical responses of Skylab crewmen: an overview. In: *Biomedical Results from Skylab.* Washington, DC: NASA;1977: 04–216.
11. Mack P. Bone density changes in a *Macaca nemestrina* monkey during the biosatellite II project. *Aerospace Med.* 1971;42:828–833.
12. Mack P, Vogt FB. Roentgenographic bone density changes during representative Apollo space flight. *Am J Roentgenol.* 1971;113:621–623.
13. Mangelsdorf DJ, Marion SL, Pike JW, Haussler MR. 1,25-Dihydroxy-vitamin D3 receptors in space-flown vs. grounded control rat kidneys. *Physiologist.* 1985;28(4):379.
14. Morey ER, Baylink DJ. Inhibition of bone formation during space flight. *Science.* 1978;201:1138.

15. *Physicians' Desk Reference*. Oradell, NJ: Medical Economics; 1986:834–836, 2065–2066.
16. Raisz L, Kream B. Regulation of bone formation. *N Engl J Med.* 1983:29–35.
17. Raisz LG, Sandberg AL, Goodson JM, et al. Complement-dependent stimulation of prostaglandin synthesis and bone resorption. *Science*. 1974; 185:789–791.
18. Rambaut P, Johnston R.S. Prolonged weightlessness and calcium loss in man, *Acta Astronautica*, 1979, 6:1113–1122.
19. Shanfeld JL, Lally EL, Kanese R, Davidovitch Z. Osteoblastic and fibroblastic PGE_2: in vivo effect of indomethacin and mechanical force. *Progress in Clinical and Biological Research.* 1985;187:331–342.
20. Stupakov GP, Kaziykin VS, Kozlovskiy AP, Korolev VV. Evaluation of changes in human axial skeletal bone structures during long-term space flights. *Kosm Biol Aviakosm Med.* 1984;18(2):33–37.
21. Sudo H, Kodama H, Amagai YI, Yamamoto S, Kasai S. In vitro differentiation and calcification in a new clonal osteogenic cell line derived from newborn mouse calvaria. *J Cell Biol.* 1983;96:191–198.
22. Tashjian AH Jr, Hohmann EL, Antoniades HN, Levine L. Platlet-derived growth factor stimulates bone resorption via a prostaglandin-mediated mechanism. *Endocrinology*. 1982;111:118–124.
23. Tashjian AH Jr, Ivey JL, Delcios B, Levine L. Stimulation of prostaglandin production in bone by phorbol esters and melittin. *Prostaglandins*. 1978; 16:221–232.
24. Tashjian AH Jr, Levine D. Epidermal growth factor stimulates prostaglandin production and bond resorption. Biochem Biophys Res Commun. 1978;85:966–975.
25. Ueno K, Kimmel D, Haba T, Jee SS. Increased metaphyseal hard tissue mass in growing long bone prostaglandin E_2 administration. In: *Endocrine Control of Bone and Calcium Metabolism*. New York: Elsevier Science; Cohn DC, et al., eds. 1984:151–154.
26. Ueda K, Saito A, Nakano H, et al. Cortical hyperostosis following long-term administration of prostaglandin E_1 in infants with cyanotic congenital heart disease. *J Pediatr*. 1980;97:834–836.
27. Vogel JM, Whittle MW. Bone mineral changes: The second manned Skylab mission. *Aviat Space Environ Med.* 1976;47:396–400.
28. Vose G. Review of roentgenographic bone demineralization studies of the Gemini space flights. *Am J Roentgenol.* 1975;121:1–4.
29. Wronski TJ, Morey-Holton ER, Maeses AC, Walsh CC. Spacelab 3: Histomorphometric analysis of the rat skeleton. *Physiologist*. 1985;28(4):376.
30. Yagodovsky VS, Trifaranidi LA, Goroklova GP. Spaceflight effects on skeletal bones of rats. *Aviat Space Environ Med*. 1976;47;734–738.

Discussion

Anti-Inflammatory Medications and Bone Loss

Dr. Neuwirth inquired about the effect of the anti-inflammatory medications on bone death as to whether the same effect was seen with all anti-inflammatory medications or just specific ones? Dr. Hughes-Fulford responded that most of them are implicated in bone deterioration. Some work was done in the rat demonstrating as much as a 50% loss of new ingrowth of bone when they were treated with anti-inflammatories.

Dr. Kostuik inquired if Dr. Hughes-Fulford would he against the use of anti-inflammatory medications for aches and pains and arthritic conditions in the post-menopausal female. She responded by saying that when she suffered an olecranon fracture she did not take aspirin, but rather acetaminophen.

Dexamethasone and the Unicameral Bone Cyst

Dr. Harold Dick mentioned the startling history of bone repair in unicameral cysts with the use of dexamethasone. Dr. Hughes-Fulford responded that if the levels of dexamethasone in cell cultures are not kept uniformly high but are allowed to fluctuate, then the cell cultures tend to have increased numbers of mineralizing nodules. This suggests that the effect may reflect duration of exposure as well as concentration. In some cases individuals on high-dose dexamethasone for long periods of time would be better served if the dosages were cycled. In addition there may be a rebound from the glucocorticoid dose reduction.

Fractures and the Release of Bone Growth Factors

Dr. Farcy raised the question concerning the liberation of a growth factor from a wounded or fractured culture. Dr. Hughes-Fulford responded: The only thing we have done so far is to take the media from a wounded culture and put it onto a confluent culture and we did indeed get some increase in growth. There is a new thought that perhaps a compound is released from the matrix. We have been grinding up bone and adding back the solution to see if there is an effect of something coming out of the matrix that stimulates bone growth, but the results have been uncertain. In the future we plan to wound large cultures, collect the media, and fractionate out the proteins to see if we can find out what is causing the increase in growth in the wounded culture. I reviewed the literature and tried to find examples of where people thought they had found these growth factors in bone. What needs to be done is to investigate in situ localization of the growth factors in bone by observing the changes in morphology that might suggest that these were sites of local growth factor release and therefore sites of certain types of bone formation. In addition it is necessary to be able to cut into the bone and actually take the antibodies to growth factor in order to do hybridization and determine if there are different regions that have a richer potential for each of the growth factors.

Dr. Kostuik noted that the work Dr. Hughes-Fulford is doing has tremendous theoretical and clinical implications. One of the major problems in orthopedics and spinal surgery is bone healing. How far away are we from the creation of an effective artificial bone? Dr. Hughes-Fulford responded that she had been contacted by the Baxter Company which has an artificial bone program to begin a collaboration to determine if we can augment artificial bone with growth factors or similar compounds to promote the faster ingrowth of osteoblasts and therefore faster healing.

Dr. Kostuik inquired further: Is there any danger if you promote more rapid growth, more rapid cellular growth of developing cancer? Dr. Hughes-Fulford responded: You are asking if we are going to get an increase in oncogene expression in these cells? We have done some probing and some messenger RNA analyses for the prostaglandin E_2 and indeed prostaglandin E_2 is stimulating an oncogene, about fourfold. The stimulation subsides with the removal of the prostaglandin. It is a fairly rapid onset and decline. Whether or not you would turn on an oncogene forever is probably a function of the lifetime of the mitotic compound you are adding. My thought would be if you attached it to the porous material that it actually would stimulate one or two rounds of mitosis, just enough to get the ingrowth. You would have to keep the compound on the osteoblast.

Dr. Kostuik noted that this would be adding it to an open wound rather than through some sort of induction or via intravenous injection. Dr. Hughes-Fulford replied: I think the more directly you added it, the more localized the effect, and I think that is what is really wanted. In case of a fracture itself, if there would be some way to deliver the compound to the fracture, that would be the best way of handling it, rather than via injection where you might be turning on a lot of other systems.

Magnetic Fields and Growth Factors

Dr. Farcy inquired if a local magnetic field can trigger one of these growing factors? Dr. Hughes-Fulford responded: I don't know. A lot of work has been done with electrical fields and it may be working. Would you say its working or not? Dr. Kostuik replied: I would say probably not.

Dr. Dick indicated that there is some work actually taking place in observing the effect of the combination of electrical stimulation along with prostaglandins. Brighton may have started an investigation in that area. I believe that they have shown in their preliminary studies that there is an effect of the electrical stimulation on prostaglandins. Dr. Hughes-Fulford commented: That would be of interest to me. Murray's group in Cambridge published a report about a year ago concerning the placement of a known torque onto bone cells and they actually saw the release of prostaglandin E_2 in those cells. This may go along with our experience during space flight. In space you are not putting any pressure on your legs so that you may be suffering the twofold effect of excessive serum cortisol and insufficient local prostaglandin E_2 in bones not receiving any direct pressure.

The Effect of Environmental Pressure on Calcium Entry into Bone

Dr. Holtzman asked: Could part of the problem with bone loss during spaceflight be due to the diminished environmental pressure affecting the equilibriun between serum calciun and that deposited in bone? Dr. Hughes-Fulford responded that the answer was not entirely clear. You have increased pressure on the upper part of the body and your legs are losing that 1 liter of volume. In effect the legs take on what is called the "chicken leg" syndrome during spaceflight. One of the members of the crew, Dr. Drew Gaffney, a cardiologist, wore a central venous catheter into flight and found that the central venous pressure was about 2 mm as compared to the average of 6 mm on the ground. The theory was that central venous pressure would rise, but in fact it decreased.

Dr. Holtzman inquired if there was any experience of treating fractures in hyperbaric chambers. Dr. Kostuik answered, Only infections. Dr. Farcy added that there is some work on treating compound fractures with infection in hyperbaric chambers, but it did not appear to have any action on the bone. Dr. Neuwirth added that there are simple noninvasive means of checking compartment pressures in the extremities. Fracture surgeons do that all the time and it might be a simple thing to add to the experimental protocol during spaceflight. Dr. Hughes-Fulford replied: That is probably well worth doing because the dogma was that in flight we would experience body fluid shifts and that we would have a diuresis within hours of reaching orbit. In practice we had a machine called the Urine Monitoring System (UMS) that collected urine. It calculated the total volume of the void and utilized a 20-cc sample for analysis. These tests were conducted for 32 days before the flight, in flight, and postflight to determine changes in calcium. The diuresis did not really occur until the fourth day continuing through the sixth, and it correlated with the lower back pain we were experiencing. Three of us had low back pain during the first four days of the flight and thereafter it disappeared. The commander Bryan O'Connor also had back pain that did not remit during his first flight, since that lasted only five days. During this nine-day flight his pain remitted coincident with the diuresis.

The Columbia Spaceflight, June 1991

Dr. Hughes-Fulford reported that the scientist-astronaut was chosen from a group of nominees. These individuals were medically screened and taken to Houston for interviews to determine interpersonal compatibility with other crew members and the like. Four were chosen from the group of 50 and of the four, two had an opportunity to fly. My exercise regimen is similar to 30 minutes of ergometers: 2 miles on the treadmill, 15 minutes with weights at least 5 times per week. In space we had an exercise protocol that lasted 45 minutes each day.

The trip began on June 5, 1991. We took off from Cape Canaveral and had a real rocket ride. At the very top of the ride we were going 18,500 miles an hour. We pulled about 3g during the maximum g force and once we were in orbit we saw a sunrise and sunset every 45 minutes. We were going Mach 25 during the flight. Our crew consisted of Drew Gaffney, a cardiologist at the University of Texas in Dallas; our commander Bryan O'Connor who is a Marine Corps colonel and flew harrier jets for many years; Tammy Jernigan, from Stanford; Sid Gutierrez, our pilot; Rhea Seddon and Jim Bagian, two career astronaut–medical doctors, and myself. We lived, worked, and played together for 9 days in the area of the middeck. It looks fairly large, but in fact is a compartment $4\frac{1}{2}$ feet by $10\frac{1}{2}$ feet, so it was crowded. Once we were in orbit we studied and worked in the space lab. The flight deck was for the commander and pilot. The mid-deck was for eating

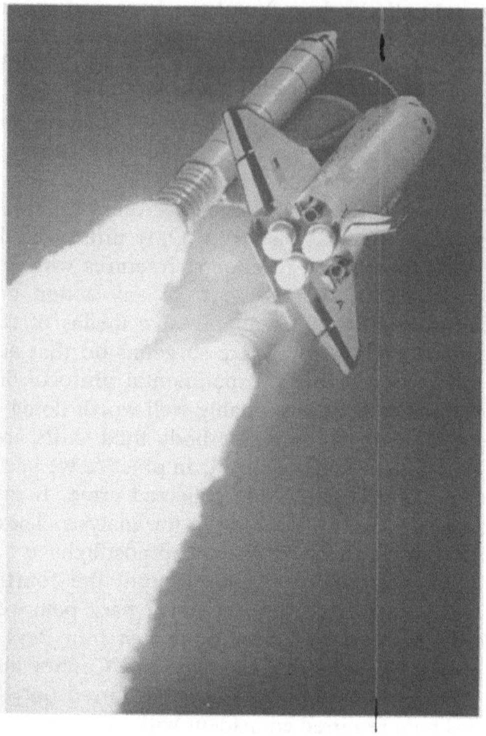

and sleeping, and that is where the bathroom was located. There was a long tunnel connecting to the space lab where we spent most of our day and ended up calling it "slave quarters." Our work included taking blood samples, looking at the changes in blood hormones to try to determine why we were losing bone during space flight.

The body undergoes a number of changes in space. The first is a fluid shift from the lower to upper body of about a liter. There is a loss of electrolytes, space motion sickness, and a drop in the heart rate—in my case from 75 to 58. In addition there is a loss of lean muscle mass calculated from animals to be approximately 20% during a 10-day flight. In a 2-week period 10% of the red blood cells are lost and the immune system changes. Most significantly there was a loss of calcium and bone, which the Russians have seen and which may amount to 12% during a 1-year period even when exercising 2 to 4 hours per day.

In space we all adopted a certain posture that was characteristic for floating. This consisted of holding the arms flexed in front of the body with the wrists in volar flexion, the body slightly flexed at the umbilicus, and the knees bent. The shifting of the center of gravity forward may have had the effect of preventing the tendency to tumble backward.

At the end of the day we took out our sleeping bags made of denim and just zipped up in them. They were hung across the space lab like hammocks and it was very easy to fall asleep in space because you were so tired. There were also head restraints to prevent bobbing during sleep. The fatigue was physical more than mental, since we felt fairly relaxed the entire time. One became accustomed to barely pushing off to go across the cabin. It did not take very much energy to do anything. The day was an 18-hour day, with the major effort being trying to concentrate in a three-dimensional world. We had to be very careful not to make mistakes. Our exercise regimen included bicycling and we were able to raise our heart rate to fairly high levels. Usually in orbit the body is not working that strenuously and therefore the heart rate slows.

The hard part for me occurred in the first 10 minutes, which was about the time it took to get into orbit. Once in orbit everything starts to float up, all the dust that is on the floor, all the bags that are tied down and I got sick immediately. I was one of the 70% of people that got sick, but I did not wait. Most astronauts wait an hour or two, not me. I fought it for about 2 hours and then I took some Phenergan, which cured everything instantly. After I got over the motion sickness I truly enjoyed it. The ability to look out at the planet, to understand that you are not on the planet any more, made one feel separated from it and this gave a different perspective of what life is all about, and I was most impressed by the fact that I could not see country boundaries; I just saw continents and oceans and it made one want to become philosophical and ask why we are always fighting down there, because it's one planet. We went over Kuwait and saw the fires and saw the smoke. The smoke was going over into China, it is affecting China. It made one very sad that a single person could do that much damage to an entire planet. Africa had some dust storms and we saw the dust as far over as Cuba. It makes one understand that we are living on a very small planet and that what one person does indeed can affect hundreds and thousands and millions of other people. I don't think we are there mentally yet. I mean, we are scientifically very progressive and very forward-thinking, but I don't think we have come far at all as far as human relationships and understanding other people and caring about the environment that we all live in. That's what impressed me the most.

The other thing that impressed me about the Earth was just looking at it. There is an Earth-glow that goes into the atmosphere. It is a blue irridescent color that does not show up on the film that we bring back. Looking at it reminded me of looking at my growing cells that also had this irridescence under the microscope. The colors were the same. It was the same type of phenomenon and it impressed me that the planet was definitely alive.

CHAPTER 2

Spinal Stability and Instability as Defined by the Louis Three-Column Spine Concept

René Louis

Stability of the spine is that quality by which the vertebral structures maintain their cohesion in all physiological positions of the spine. Instability, or loss of stability, is a pathological process that can lead to displacement of vertebrae beyond their normal physiological limits.

As compared with limb anatomy, spinal anatomy turns out to be more complex as regards joint morphology. This complexity in spinal morphology and architecture is the reason why it is more difficult to understand. Following the first concept of spinal stability by Nicoll (16) in 1949, various stability theories have been proposed. Decoulx and Rieunau (5) in 1958 pointed out that the "posterior vertebral body wall" was the mainstay of spine stability. Ramadier and Bombart (18) in 1963 emphasized the role of the facet joint in stability. Holdsworth (8) in 1963 described the "posterior ligamentous complex" required to maintain spinal stability; the posterior ligament complex includes supra- and interspinous ligaments, ligamenta flava, and posterior joint capsules. Roy-Camille (19) in 1979 reported that spine stability was maintained by the "middle segment" including the posterior wall of intervertebral disc and vertebral body, the pedicles, and facets. Kirkaldy-Willis and Farfan (9) in 1982 defined instability as "the abnormal increased joint deformation with stress." For them the increased motion may become a severe clinical problem by reduction of the lateral nerve root canal and by central spinal stenosis; the primary lesions are located on the annulus fibrosus as a result of torsional stress and extend finally to facet joints. In 1983, Denis (6) put forward a three-column spine concept: the anterior spinal column is formed by the anterior half of vertebral bodies and intervertebral discs, the middle spinal column includes the posterior half of vertebral bodies and discs and the posterior longitudinal ligament, and the posterior column corresponds to the facet joints and the posterior ligamentous complex. In this regard, Denis proposed a physiopathological classification of severe spinal injuries with a definition of unstable lesions.

In 1975, Louis et al. (12) described a three-column spine concept, different from that of Denis. This theory was proposed to explain comprehensively what the other theories appeared to do only in part.

Materials and Methods

Data from three separate disciplines support my concept of spinal stability: morphological studies on dry skeletons, biomechemical studies on cadaver spines taken early without chemical fixation, and clinical data from various spinal diseases collected for 20 years.

Morphological Studies

Morphological studies were based on the study of a large number of skeletons of Blacks and Caucasians made in the Department of Anatomy in Marseilles and Dakar (Senegal). Attention was given in particular to the architectural factors responsible in spinal stability.

Biomechanical Studies

Ten cadaver spines were studied, all removed within 24 hours after death and preserved in plastic bags at 4°C. Increasingly extensive cuts were made in the intervertebral ligaments, capsules, and discs to assess changes in segmental spinal mobility. Five cadaver spines were used to study ligament and disc resistance under shearing forces after cutting either the disc or the posterior ligamentous complex of three young and two elderly subjects. Dynamometers were used for measurements of forces applied to pairs of adjacent vertebrae.

Clinical Studies

Clinical studies were based on 20 years of spinal surgery, 5 in West Africa (Dakar, Senegal), which permitted the accumulation of a vast number of interesting pathological cases. During the period in Africa one also had the opportunity to perform autopsy examinations on advanced spinal diseases (severe paralysis due to Pott's disease or spinal injury). Studies were also carried out on diseases affecting the spine in 14 children (spinal malformation, scoliosis, Pott's disease) in order to evaluate the effects of lesions on the growing spine. Finally, these clinical and anatomopathological cases provided interesting data toward understanding unstable lesions and their consequences as related to neural structures and spinal growth.

Results: The Three-Column Spine Concept

It is necessary to consider spinal stability in both the vertical axis and transverse plane.

Vertical Axial Stability (Fig. 2.1)

In order to appreciate vertical axial stability, it is necessary to consider the morphology of the individual vertebrae and the structure of the spine as a single unit.

Vertebral Morphology

From the atlas to the sacrum it is possible to identify those structures in the complex morphology of the vertebrae that resist the forces of gravity. The atlas can be likened to two lateral masses joined by two arches. The axis can be reduced to three pillars, a vertical conical pillar lying medially and anteriorly (dens and body) and two lateral oblique pillars. These three pillars are fused above in the body of C2 and diverge below, with respect to stability. The axis does not have true pedicles and the structures referred to as such are actually isthmuses or partes interarticulares, since they are interarticular structures. The structural features of C3 to L4 are analogous to those of the axis, i.e., these vertebrae are composed of three pillars: the anterior pillar formed by the vertebral body and the two pillars formed by the articular processes lying posteriorly. The three pillars are reinforced by horizontal bars, namely the pedicles and laminae. A similar configuration is found at L5 except that the vertebra is wedge-shaped and the posterior pillars are angled at the isthmic zones. The sacrum provides three points of support for the three pillars, i.e., the sacral base and two sacral facets. The weight-bearing forces are then transferred from the sacrum to the pelvic girdle by the two sacroiliac joints.

Overall Architecture of the Spine

The juxtaposition of the various vertebral structures makes it possible to follow the lines of load-bearing forces from the cranium to the pelvis. The cranium transfers its weight to the spine through the two pillars of the atlas lying in the same coronal plane. The two pillars become three columns in the body of the axis, which is thus a veritable crossroad for the transmission of the forces. The forces are then transferred down the three columns, which are arranged in a triangle with an anterior apex. The larger anterior column takes on the aspect of a quadrangular pyramid formed by the alternating vertebral bodies and intervertebral discs down to the sacral base. The two posterior columns lying in a coronal plane are composed of the successive articular processes. At C2 and L5 these columns present an isthmic angulation. This may be one reason for the

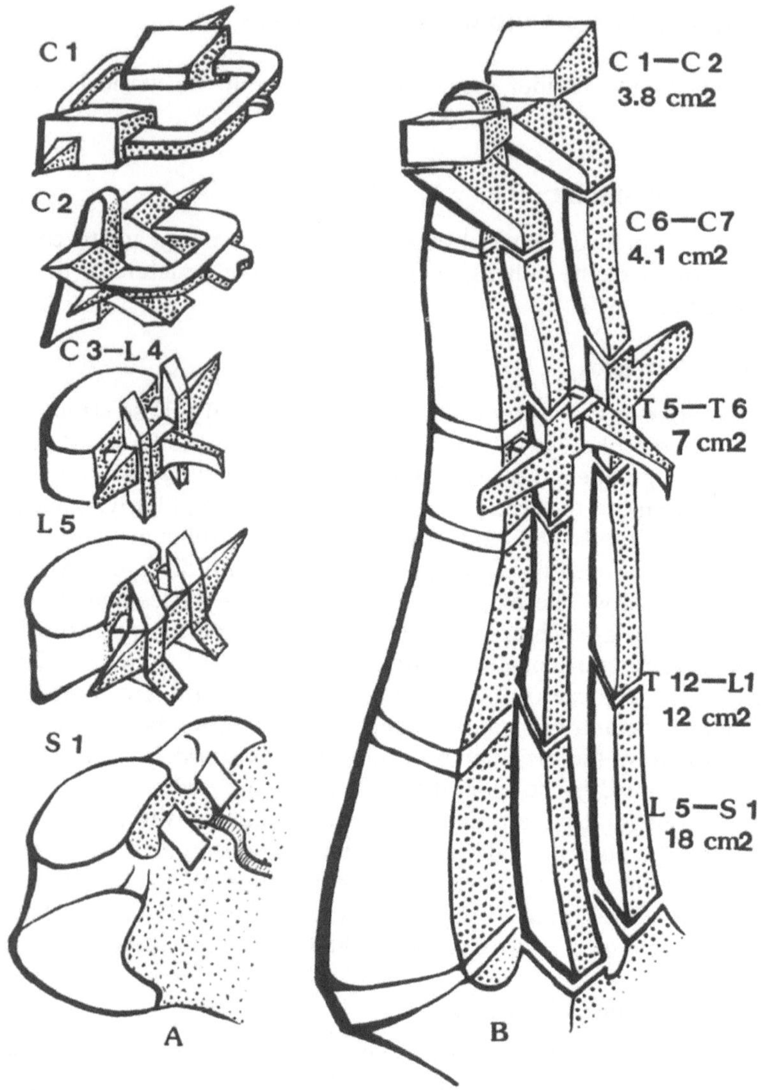

Figure 2.1. Illustrations of morphology of vertebrae (**A**), and overall architecture of the spine (**B**), showing the vertical columns, which are two columns at the Cl-C2 level and three columns from C2 to the sacrum. The total joint surface of a motion segment is increasing from the Cl-C2 level to the L5-S1 segment (*figures on the right*).

occurrence of spondylolysis in these regions. The sacrum also constitutes a crossroad of the descending forces, since it receives them at three points but transmits them to pelvis and lower limbs through two laterally placed sacroiliac joints. This vertical system of columns is reinforced by horizontal struts that at the level of each vertebra solidly join the columns to each other. The struts are the two arches of C1, the posterior arch of C2 and the pedicles and laminae of the vertebrae lying below C2. The spinous and transverse processes participate in the system of axial stability through muscular action. Under static and dynamic conditions the spinal curvatures modify the axis of the vertical columns but in no way change the principles of axial stability. This three-column structure of the spine, like a three-legged stool, provides the simplest and most efficient system of stability. This system also provides protection for the spinal cord and permits the exit of the segmental nerves at the intervertebral foramina.

Transverse Stability (Fig. 2.2)

When the spine is subjected to forces perpendicular to its axis, the points of weakness are located in the intervertebral motion segments. At any spinal level there are the same mechanisms to stabilize the spine: the coupling of bony stops and ligamentous brakes, or in other words the three-opposing-joint complex.

The Coupling of Bony Stops and Ligamentous Brakes

Any extreme intervertebral motion is stopped by the coupled action of bony stops and ligamentous brakes.

During flexion, the bony stops or buttresses are, in the C1-C2 motion unit, the dens against the anterior arch; between C2-C3 and L5-S1 motion units, the articular processes and the anterior edge of end plates against each other. The ligamentous brakes are, in the C1-C2 motion unit, the transverse ligament, the posterior atlantoaxial membrane, and the articular capsules of the lateral atlantoaxial joints; between C2-C3 and L5-S1 motion segments, the ligamentous brakes are all the ligaments located posterior to the nucleus pulposus, i.e. the posterior part of the annulus fibrosus, the posterior longitudinal ligament, the articular capsules, the ligamenta flava, and the inter- and supraspinous ligaments.

During extension, the bony stops lie at the three angles of a triangle, i.e., the most posterior parts of the articular and spinous processes coming into contact with each other and with laminae, and the posterior margin of the end plate. At the craniovertebral junction, the bony buttresses are the anterior arch contacting the dens, the posterior arches, and occipital bone. The ligamentous brakes brought into play are those situated anterior to the nucleus pulposus, i.e., the anterior longitudinal ligament and the anterior part of the annulus fibrosus.

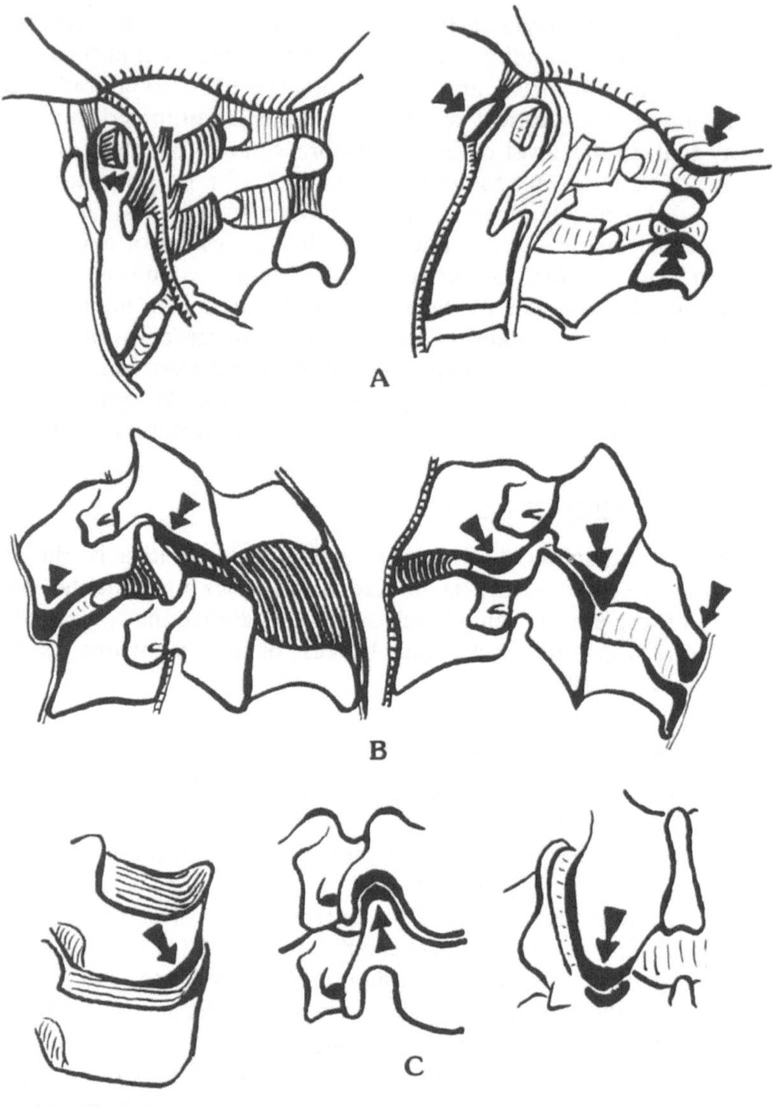

Figure 2.2. Illustrations of the transverse instability of the spine during flexion-extension at the Cl-C2 level (**A**), and the lower cervical region (**B**), and during inclination-rotation at the lower cervical region (**C** *left and middle*) and the lumbar area (**C** *right*). *Dark arrows* show the bony buttresses combined with ligamentous brakes for stabilizing vertebrae during excessive motions.

During inclination coupled with rotation, the bony stops are the articular processes, plus in the cervical spine the uncinate processes and the reciprocal pseudoarticulations between the lower surface of the cervical transverse processes and the upper articular processes (Fig. 2.2C). In the thoracic spine lateral inclination and rotation are considerably limited by the costovertebral joints, despite the facility of such movement afforded by the circular orientation of the articular facets in this region. In the lumbar region the sagittal aspect of the facets and the lateral margin of the end plates are acting as bony stops. The ligamentous brakes are the intervertebral ligaments of the side opposite the tilt.

The Three-Opposing-Joint Complex

Each mobile spinal segment is formed by a set of three joints located at each angle of a triangle and lying in nearly perpendicular planes. These three joints are the intervertebral disc and the two zygapophyseal joints. With the exception of the biarticular atlanto-occipital segment, all the mobile spinal segments are triarticular. At each level the posterior articulations lie in a plane that opposes that of the intervertebral disc; this is approximately 45° in the cervical area, 60° in the thoracic region, and 90° in the lumbar spine (Fig. 2.3). In addition, the unco-vertebral and costovertebral joint spaces oppose the disc and posterior joint spaces. This concept also applies to the Cl-C2 level where the median atlantoaxial joint is perpendicular to the lateral atlantoaxial joints. This configuration creates an orthogonal articular system whose mode of participation during effort differs according to the orientation of the axis of the spine relative to the forces acting upon it. In the vertical position the forces of gravity and weight bearing coupled with opposing muscular forces produce a compressive effect on the discs and a shearing effect on the posterior articulations. Conversely, when lifting a weight with the trunk in the horizontal position the different forces produce essentially compression of the posterior articulations and a shearing on the discs, although the required rigidity of the spine is nevertheless accompanied by an accessory effect of axial compression of muscular origin (1,15). Consequently, during the movements and efforts exerted by the spine, the posterior articulations share with the discs the bearing of the constraints applied to the vertebrae; thus there exists a modulated system of leverage involving these different structures. Accordingly, the total area of the discal and zygapophyseal articular surfaces in each motion segment increases in the craniocaudal direction to meet the increasing physical constraints. We calculated the mean total articular surface area at different spinal levels as follows: C1-C2 = 3.8 cm^2, C6-C7 = 4.1 cm^2, T5-T6 = 7 cm^2, T12-L1 = 12 cm^2, L5-S1 = 18 cm^2 (Fig. 2.1). Furthermore, the caliber of the flexor and extensor muscles of the trunk similarly increases caudally down to the gluteal muscles. Consequently the zygapophyseal joints should not be considered

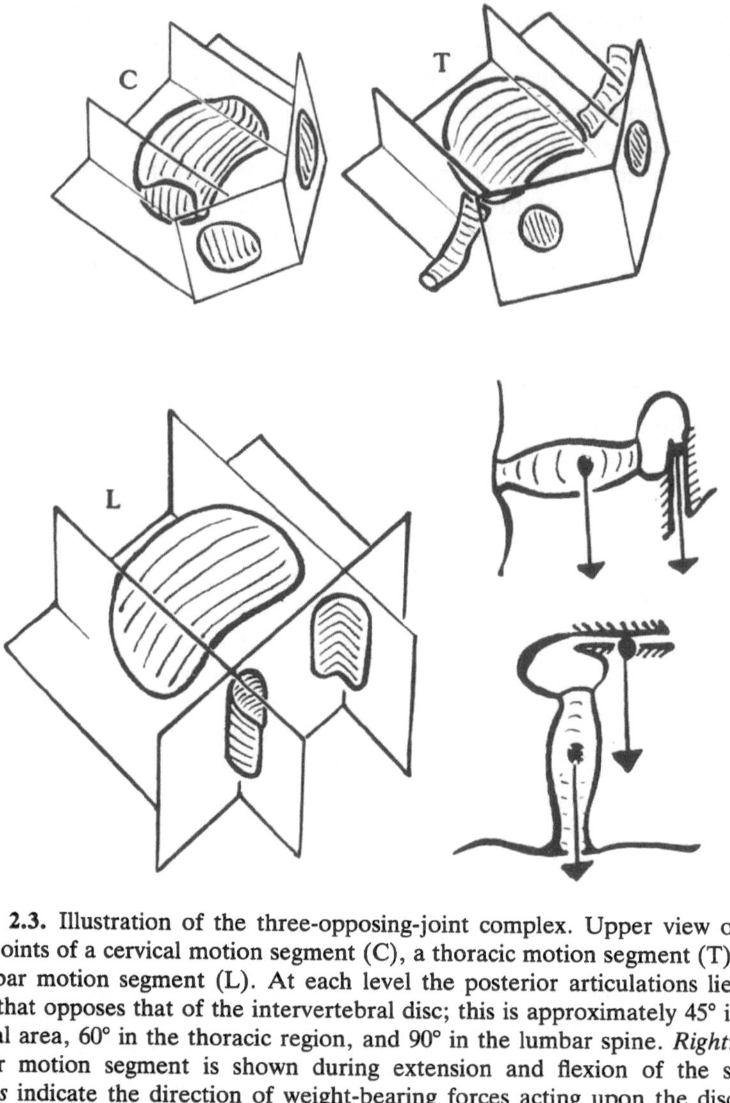

Figure 2.3. Illustration of the three-opposing-joint complex. Upper view of the three joints of a cervical motion segment (C), a thoracic motion segment (T), and a lumbar motion segment (L). At each level the posterior articulations lie in a plane that opposes that of the intervertebral disc; this is approximately 45° in the cervical area, 60° in the thoracic region, and 90° in the lumbar spine. *Right*: The lumbar motion segment is shown during extension and flexion of the spine. *Arrows* indicate the direction of weight-bearing forces acting upon the disc and the posterior joint. When the disc resists compression forces the posterior facets resist shearing forces and vice versa.

merely as being involved in the orientation of spinal movements, but also as weight-bearing structures subject to the pathological alterations of effort (sprain, spondylosis).

Discussion and Clinical Relevance

In this section, the various theories on spinal stability will be discussed and the clinical relevance will be considered in relation to spinal instability, development of the spine, and adaptations to wear.

Critical Review of Existing Concepts of Spinal Stability

The "posterior vertebral body wall theory" (5) easily explains wedge fractures and anterior damage of neural structures due to bone projection into the spinal canal. This theory, however, does not take into account the possible consequences of intervertebral ligament damage and subsequent bony displacement. By contrast, Holdsworth's (2,3,4,8,14) theory explains subluxation due to tearing of "the posterior ligamentous complex" but does not explain backward subluxation resulting from a rupture of the anterior longitudinal ligament and the anterior part of the annulus fibrosus. This classification also passes over the unstable Chance fracture characterized by the horizontal section of the spine in its bony structure.

The "middle segment" theory of Roy-Camille (19) emphasizes some important factors of spinal stability such as the posterior wall of discs and vertebral bodies, the pedicles, and facets. Despite the integrity of the middle segment, however, a coronal fracture of the vertebral body or a severe wedge fracture may unbalance the spine by progressive kyphosis. In addition, a posterior subluxation by tearing of the annulus anterior to the nucleus may be an unstable lesion. The Denis "three-column spine" concept affords a biomechanical explanation for many spinal injury lesions (6). However, this theory is not supported by anatomical data but by anatomopathological and radiological investigations. The division of vertebrae into three parts appears somewhat artificial, especially with respect to anterior and middle columns through the vertebral bodies. This theory does not explain why a normal spine is stable along its axis and how a motion segment maintains its stability during physiological movements.

Kirkaldy-Willis and Farfan (9) offer an excellent explanation for "instability in spondylosis." However, the instability associated with spondylosis is not the same as that associated with fracture-dislocation of the spine. This concept challenges the usual mechanisms put forward by chiropractors, osteopaths, and manipulators ("displaced vertebra," "subluxation," and "internal articular disorder") (20). Nevertheless the author accepts in the clinical instability concept both abnormal decrease and increase in the range of motion of a spinal joint. In my opinion the term "instability" must be kept only for abnormal increased motion, and to cover both abnormal decreased and increased motion I prefer the term "dysfunction."

Spinal Instability (Figs. 2.4 and 2.5)

My experiment on cadaver spines in 1976 (3) demonstrated that any instability with forward displacement requires at least a complete tear of ligaments and the annulus fibrosus posterior to the nucleus pulposus. A bilateral dislocation requires a complete division of all the intervertebral fibrous connections. The sectioning of one ligament, disc, or facet does not produce instability, i.e., an abnormal displacement of a vertebra beyond the physiological limits. On radiological grounds, the solution of continuity of a vertical column is easily recognized when located at the level of the bony parts of the column. Conversely, when the solution of continuity is situated through a motion segment, it might be difficult to be evidenced except in dislocation. Consequently flexion-extension x-rays are required for proving the instability through the following signs:

Flexion-extension motion superior to 11° for one vertebral unit.
Vertebral translation superior to 3.5 mm above C4 and to 2.5 mm below C4 through S1.
Loss of parallelism of facets.
Loss of contact of facets superior to 50%.
Interspinous widening.
Spinous process rotation superior to 8°.
Open posterior joint on the computed tomography (CT) scan (Fig. 2.5).

As a result of these biomechanical data and of anatomopathological observations, I proposed in 1975 (12) an instability theory with classification of lesions in order to determine therapeutic indications (Fig. 2.4). Each vertical column ruptured is given a score of 1, so the Chance fracture (slice fracture of the three columns in their bony structure) and the bilateral dislocation (horizontal shear through a motion segment) would score 3. The score for an incomplete lesion of the vertebral body and the fracture of pedicles or laminae is 0.5. The fracture of transverse or spinous processes is scored 0.25. The lack of substance in the anterior column is assessed as 2. This is the case with severe wedge compression fractures that have been reduced by a conservative method; so the vertebral body substance contains several gaps that yield a recurrence of the kyphotic deformity despite prolonged immobilization. Otherwise, a coronal fracture of the vertebral body sometimes produces a loss of substance under the anteroinferior edge of the vertebra above, inducing automatically a further kyphotic focus. Consequently an unstable lesion corresponds to a score equal or superior to 2. The loss of substance of one posterior

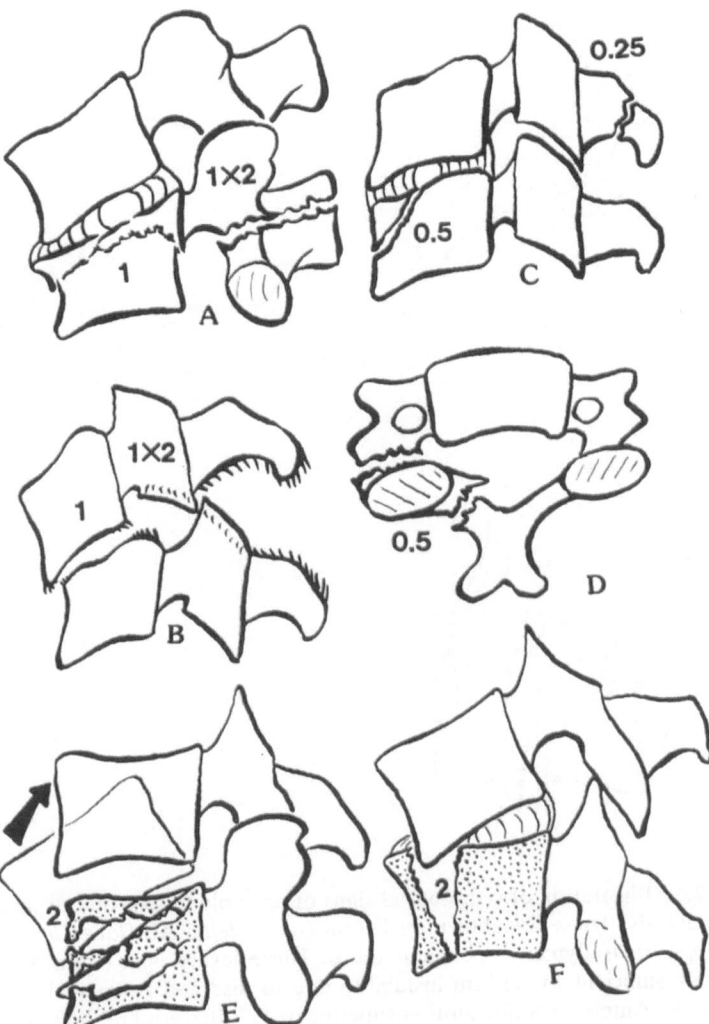

Figure 2.4. Classification and scoring of severe traumatic lesions of the spine. Each vertical column ruptured is given a score of 1 **(A,B)**. The score for an incomplete lesion of the vertebral body **(C)** and the fracture of pedicles or laminae is 0.5 **(D)**. The fracture of a transverse or spinous process is scored 0.25 **(C)**. The lack of substance of a vertical column **(E)** is assessed as coronal fracture of the vertebral body with tilt of the vertebra above **(F)**. A lesion is unstable when the sum score is equal to or greater than 2.

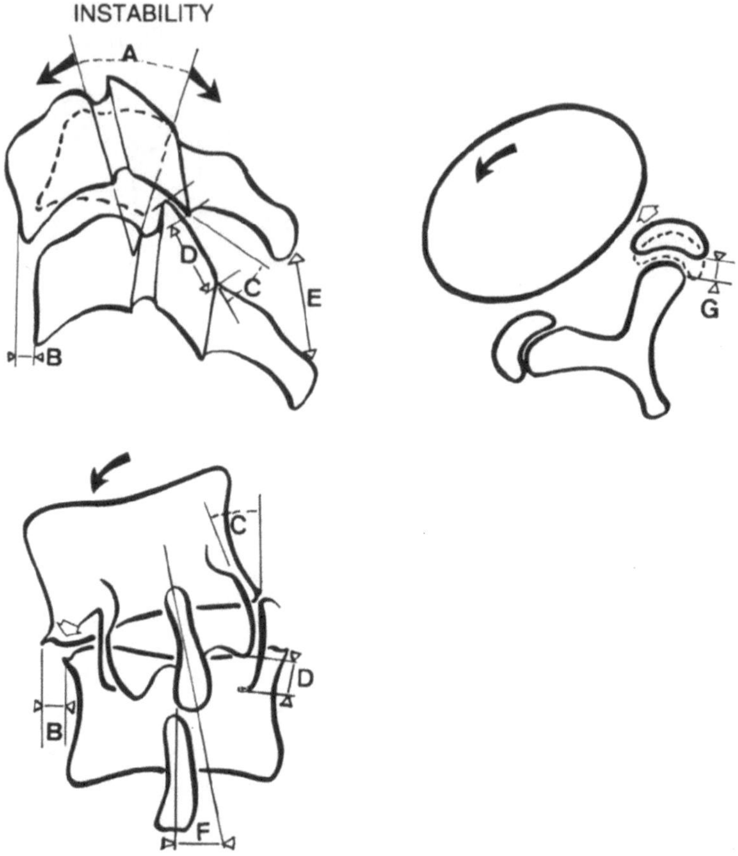

Figure 2.5. Illustration of radiological signs of unstable lesions due to subluxation or spondylosis. These are shown on lateral (*upper left*), AP (*lower left*), and CT scan (*upper right*) dynamic roentgenograms. These severe signs (from A to G) are separately sufficient to confirm instability due to disc and ligament loosening or rupture. A: Anteroposterior motion superior to 11°, B: vertebral body translation C1-C4 sup. to 3.5 mm, C4-S1 sup. to 2.5 mm; C: loss of parallelism; D: loss of facet contact sup. to 50%; E: interspinous widening; F: spinous rotation; G: open posterior joint. (Reprinted with permission from ref. 9.)

column is assessed as 1.5. Unstable lesions might be separated into three groups: first, a "temporary bony instability" such as a Chance fracture for instance, with bony lesions being likely to heal after reduction and immobilization without surgery; second, a "permanent ligamentous instability" such as a bilateral dislocation involving ligament and disc lesions, which is likely to yield weak scar so that surgical stabilization and fusion are advocated; thirdly, a "vertebral gap instability" such as a severe wedge fracture after reduction, a coronal fracture, an osteolytic lesion, or

Figure 2.6. Our construct after total vertebrectomy with reconstruction of the three pillars of the spine by autogenous bone grafting and screw-plate internal fixation.

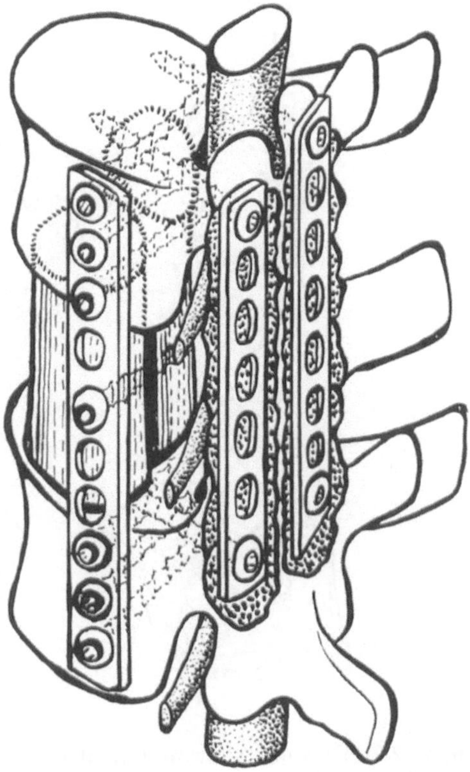

a surgical excision are liable to produce a progressive collapse with or without neurological compromise so that surgical repair is indicated (21).

Spinal surgery with removal of lesions might alter the spinal stability (3). The lack of substance after surgery is evaluated in the same way as spinal injuries: 2 for the damaged anterior column and 1.5 for one damaged posterior column by facetectomy. As a result, reconstruction of each column is mandatory with bone grafts and internal fixation, especially by screw-held plates in my practice. For severe spondylolisthesis or total vertebrectomy for malignant tumor, it is necessary to perform a reconstruction of the three columns by a combined approach (Fig. 2.6). We can define "partial instabilities" such as flexion instability, extension instability, rotation instability, and "total instability". Some partial instabilities can be combined.

Degenerative changes are likely to provoke instability but usually with moderate displacement (degenerative spondylolisthesis). I think that the symptoms of the spondylotic instability described by Kirkaldy-Willis and Farfan (9) are also common to "spinal sprains" and "subluxations" of the three-joint motion segments. These authors divide the spinal degenera-

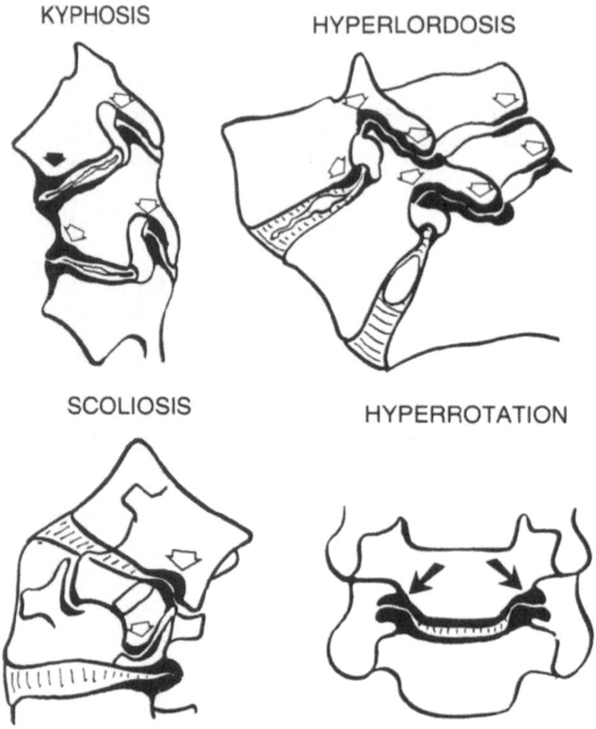

Figure 2.7. Drawings showing how the spine adapts to wear in different conditions: hyperflexion or kyphosis, hyperextension or hyperlordosis, and inclination-rotation such as scoliosis or uncarthrosis. Osteophytes, narrowing of the articular space, and bony condensation appear where constraints are excessive at bony stop zones. In addition, stretched ligamentous brakes result in spinal sprain, and then spondylotic instability. (Reprinted with permission from ref. 13.)

tive process into three stages: (a) temporary dysfunction, (b) unstable phase, and (c) stabilization.

The history of patients suffering from spinal pain demonstrates that pain is preceded by "spinal sprains" due to excessive or violent movements of some motion segments that can later lead to degenerative changes with fibrous and articular damage (Fig. 2.7). These lesions of the stabilizing factors (bony stops and ligamentous brakes) make the motion spinal segment work loose with progressive development of radiographic spondylotic signs. Dynamic radiograms using anteroposterior (AP) and lateral projections are necessary to confirm this fact clinically. Lately Kirkaldy-Willis and Farfan proposed the use of CT scans in the diagnosis of instability. When there is an "increased motion the cartilage space increases on rotation and the superior articular process on that side is dis-

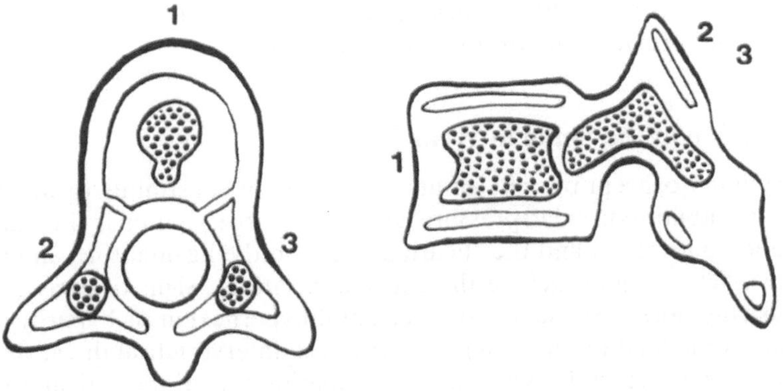

Figure 2.8. Ossification pattern of vertebra. There are three single primary ossification centers, one for each vertical column of the three-column spine concept.

placed forward to narrow the lateral canal" (9) (Fig. 2.5). This instability evidenced on flexion-extension radiograms can be called "macroscopic instability." Conversely some authors are extending the instability concept to changes in the instantaneous rotation center of a motion segment through computerized studies of spinal motion. Physiologically the instantaneous center of rotation of a motion segment is varying inside a small area, making it difficult to consider as pathological some limited variations. This "microscopic instability" does not seem liable to yield surgical considerations (10,11).

The Three-Column Spinal Concept and Spinal Growth (Fig. 2.8)

As a result of the three-column spinal concept we uphold that normal axial spine growth needs harmonious growth of each column. In fact, some congenital anomalies of the spine (hemivertebrae, incomplete spinal block, lateral spinal bar) or some surgical excisions with fusion limited to one column produce further increasing deformities due to the asymmetric nature of spinal growth. The pathological region of the spine limits the growth rate of a column while the two other columns maintain their growth rate. Consequently the disturbance of growth leads to scoliosis, kyphosis, or hyperlordosis.

The ossification pattern of vertebrae supports my concept. Each column originates from a single primary ossification center: the centrum for the anterior column and the two vertebral arch centers for the two posterior columns. As a consequence of this and to avoid deformity, it is important when operating on the growing spine of a child to perform a symmetrical fusion of all three columns for any limited disease requiring stabilization.

A posterior fusion of the thoracic spine for scoliosis may be an exception to this rule, provided the fusion is long and thick.

Adaptation of the Spine to Wear (Fig. 2.5)

My stability concept permits an understanding of constraints to which the spine is submitted: axial pressure along the three columns, pressure on the bony buttresses, and the shearing effect on the ligamentous and discal brakes. When a joint acts in the extreme positions, signs of early fatigue are usually noted. Subsequently, vertebral hyperflexion or hyperkyphosis increases the load on the anterior part of the intervertebral discs, the end plates of the vertebral bodies, and the superior part of the articular facets where osteophytes will be located. Hyperextension or hyperlordosis transfers forces toward the posterior arch and to the posterior part of the intervertebral disc. Thus it is not uncommon to observe signs of age-related arthrosis localized principally on the posterior articulations with zones of neocontact between normally distant structures, i.e., between the spinous processes, between the inferior part of the articular facets and the pedicular or isthmic regions. Lateral flexion with rotation or scoliosis increases the load on the lateral part of the discs, the intervertebral pseudoarticulation, and the homolateral posterior articulation, with neocontact between the cervical transverse processes and the tips of the superior articular facets. At an advanced age, the deformity of scoliosis shows signs of arthrosis with dislocation due to shearing of the most horizontally inclined disc and arthrosis of the posterior articulation. Cervical uncarthrosis reflects a wearing of the cervical vertebrae in lateral flexion and rotation.

Pal and Sherk (17) demonstrated through their experiments about vertebral stability of the cervical spine that 36% of the total load applied on the top of the cervical spine is transmitted through the anterior column and 32% each through the two posterior columns.

References

1. Bartelink DL. The role of abdominal pressure in relieving the pressure of the lumbar intervertebral discs. *J Bone Joint Surg*. 1957;39B:718.
2. Bedbrook GM. Stability of spinal fractures and fracture-dislocation. *Paraplegia*. 1971;9:23.
3. Catel HS, Clark GL. Cervical kyphosis and instability following multiples laminectomias in children. *J Bone Joint Surg*. 1967;49A:713.
4. Cheshire DJE. The stability of the cervical spine following the conservative treatment of fractures and fracture-dislocation. *Paraplegia*. 1969;7:193.
5. Decoulx R, Rieunau G. Rapport à la 23e réunion annuelle de la Societé Nationale Française de Chirurgie Orthopédique et Traumatologique. *Rev Chir Orthop*. 1958;44:244; 1959;45:237.

6. Denis F. The three-column spine and its significance in the classification of acute thoracolumbar spinal injuries. *Spine.* 1983;8:817.
7. Hausfeld JN. *A Biomechanical Analysis of Clinical Stability in the Thoracic and Thoracolumbar Spine.* Thesis, Yale University School of Medicine, New Haven, 1977.
8. Holdsworth FW. Fractures, dislocations and fracture-dislocations of the spine. *J Bone Joint Surg.* 1963;45B:6.
9. Kirkaldy-Willis WH, Farfan HF. Instability of the lumbar spine. *Clin Orthop.* 1982;165:110.
10. Louis R. Chirurgie du Rachis. (Surgery of the Spine.) Berlin, Heidelberg, New York, Tokyo: Springer Verlag; 1982.
11. Louis R. Spinal stability as defined by the three-column spine concept. *Ann Clin.* 1985;7:33–42.
12. Louis R, Bonsignour JP, Ouiminga R. Réduction orthopédique contrôlée des fractures du rachis. *Rev Chir Orthop.* 1975;61:323.
13. Louis R, Goutallier D. Fractures instables du rachis. *Rev Chir Orthop.* 1977;63:5–415.
14. Munro D. The factors that govern the stability of the spine. *Paraplegia.* 1965;3:219.
15. Nachemson A, Morris JM. In vivo measurements of intradiscal pressure. *J Bone Joint Surg.* 1964;46A:1077.
16. Nicoll EA. Fractures of the dorso-lumbar spine. *J Bone Joint Surg.* 1949;31B:376.
17. Pal G. Sherk H. The vertical stability of the cervical spine. *Spine.* 1988;13: S447–449.
18. Ramadier JO, Bombart M. Fractures et luxations du rachis cervical sans lésion médullaire. *Rev Chir Orthop.* 1963;49:741.
19. Roy-Camillie R. *Rachis Cervical Traumatique non Neurologique.* Paris, France: Masson; 1979.
20. Schafer RC *Clinical Biomechanics.* Baltimore: William Wilkins; 1983.
21. White A, Panjabi M. *Clinical biomechanics of the Spine.* Philadelphia: JB Lippincott; 1978.

Discussion

The Term "Spinal Instability"—Is There a Proper Definition at Present?

Dr. Kostuik opened the discussion by stating that he could understand the three-column concept of Louis in terms of trauma and tumor, but the problem remains as to how to interpret this concept in terms of degenerative diseases. Dr. Panjabi added that vertebral instability may be directional, namely, there may be instability in flexion, but not in extension. We have done work on the upper cervical spine studying Jefferson fractures and have shown that there may be instability in flexion and extension, but no instability in rotation. Dr. Panjabi felt it was important to talk about instability in terms of its direction and just using the word "instability" was imprecise.

He continued that instability is always conceived of as a large vertebral displacement of at least 3.5 mm in the cervical spine, but this displacement per se does not explain where the pain comes from. Perhaps it is associated with smaller motions. Instability must be related to magnitude and it is appropriate to consider the terms "major instability" and "micro-instability."

Dr. Kostuik continued that we seem to be coming closer and closer to a mechanical definition of instability. In the process of approaching this definition are we going to say that we all have unstable spines? All of us here, with a few exceptions, have experienced back pain problems on a chronic basis—a little bit of back pain every day. Does that mean we all have unstable spines because we have pain? The original definition by Augustus White and yourself involved loads that were beyond physiologic limits and resulted in some form of dysfunction. Pain was one of those elements.

Bjorn Rydevik added that there must be something more than just motion itself that may be physiologic within certain limits, which can be defined in degrees or millimeters. However, some individuals experience very significant pain, whereas others with the same x-ray appearance do not experience any significant pain at all. The painful component in his opinion is related to something more than actual motion, more than actual pressure—there must be some biochemical or inflammatory component. Some problems may be related to the overlap of innervation both craniocaudal and across the midline so that the injection of local anesthesia may not always help.

Dr. Kostuik added that there is considerable criticism by neurosurgeons in North America who do not do much surgery of those who do spinal fusions for so-called instability. The problem relates to the difficulty surgeons have in defining what instability is on a "micro" basis. We do not, as yet, have any way of documenting or actually defining what Dr. Panjabi has been referring to as microscopic instability. It's great if you have a nice flexion-extension film or other film that shows something very gross; everyone will accept those examples, but not necessarily cases where such documentation is not at hand. We should remember at this tine in this country 80,000 spinal fusions are performed every year for pain. That represents a large number of cases.

CHAPTER 3

Dysfunction of the Spinal Stability System and Its Restabilization

Manohar M. Panjabi

Low back pain is a significant problem of Western society, costing an estimated sum of $15 to $50 billion per year in the United States (2,8,11,21). There is a 50% to 70% chance of having low back pain during one's lifetime (3), with a prevalence of about 18% (13). Thus, more than 30 million people have low back pain at any time in the United States, of whom 10 million people have chronic symptoms (8). Specific causes for most of the low back pains are unknown. It is believed that a significant portion of the low back problem is of mechanical origin and that the underlying cause is spinal instability (12).

The spinal stabilizing system of the body may be thought of as a three-component system (Fig. 3.1): (a) passive subsystem—spinal column; (b) active subsystem—spinal muscles (surrounding the spinal column); and (c) neural control unit (controlling the spinal muscles) (15). We will first look at the normal function, and then look at the dysfunctions caused by injuries and degeneration of the various components of the spinal column. Next, we will examine the muscular system, followed by a brief analysis of the neural control of the spinal muscles.

Spinal Column and its Components

As a prelude to the discussion of the effect of injuries to the various spinal column components on the overall function of the spinal column, it is necessary to know the normal function. As for any structure that shows elastic behavior, one can apply a force and measure the deformation, or vice versa. The first method is called the flexibility method and the second is called the stiffness method. The slope of the curve (independent parameter on the x-axis and dependent on the y-axis) in the first method represents flexibility of the structure, whereas the same quantity in the second method represents stiffness. The flexibility method allows the spine to move in a physiological manner, and therefore is to be preferred. However, the spine is a three-dimensional structure, and therefore its

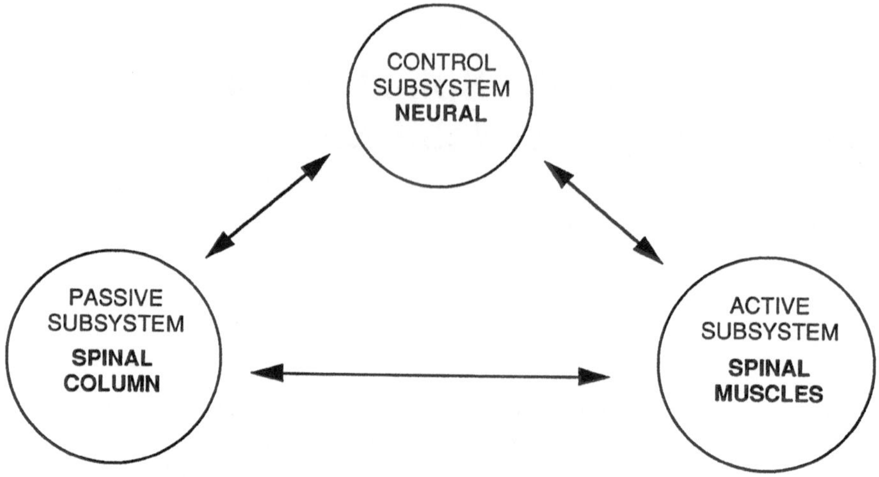

Figure 3.1. The spinal stability system consists of three subsystems: passive spinal column, active spinal muscles, and neural control unit. (Adapted from Ref. 15)

physical properties should be obtained in different directions. The way to do this is to set up a coordinate system that is three-dimensional and is oriented so as to represent the anatomic directions of the spine (23). This is shown in Fig. 3.2, where forces and moments applied to the spine specimen are shown by the large arrows, and the resulting six degrees of freedom motion of the vertebra are represented by thin arrows. The set of relationships between the motion response and the loads applied represent a complete description of the physical properties of the spine. If we consider only those motions that are produced in the same direction as the applied load, then these motions are called main motions. All other motions that result due to the application of the load are called coupled motions.

Neutral Zone

Physical properties represented by a load-displacement curve are often quantified in the form of ranges of motion (ROM). However, the ROM does not represent the nonlinear characteristics of the load-displacement curve. Several years ago, we introduced another parameter that does it (17). This is the neutral zone (NZ). It is a range of motion around the neutral position where the spine can be moved with very little resistance. Beyond the NZ, the spine offers resistance and this part of the range of motion is called the elastic zone (EZ). The sum of the neutral and elastic zones is the range of motion as it is traditionally called. The concepts of NZ, EZ, and ROM are depicted in Fig. 3.3.

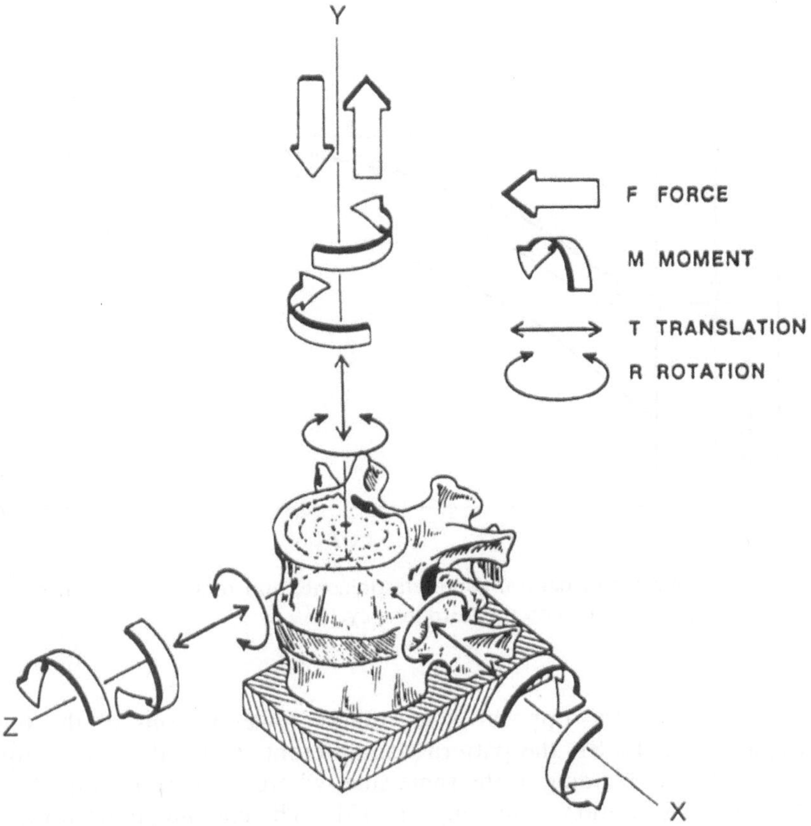

Figure 3.2. A functional spinal unit and a three-dimensional coordinate system placed at the center H of the upper vertebral body. Twelve load components and the resulting six components of motion are indicated. (Adapted from Ref. 23.)

Normal Physical Properties

Average values of the main motions of flexion-extension, bilateral axial rotations, and bilateral lateral bendings of the lumbar spine are shown in Fig. 3.4. Notice that the NZ and EZ shares of the ROM change in different physiological movements and for different spinal levels.

To a certain extent, the ranges of motion characterize the magnitude of the motion, whereas the coupling motions characterize the quality of motion. As there is large variability in the ranges of motion in the general population, the coupled motions have the potential of characterizing injury in a more precise manner. In a recent study of normal coupled motions in the lumbar spine, the following conclusions were reached (19): At the upper levels, e.g., L2-L3, axial torque resulted in lateral bending to the opposite side. When lateral bending was applied, it resulted in axial

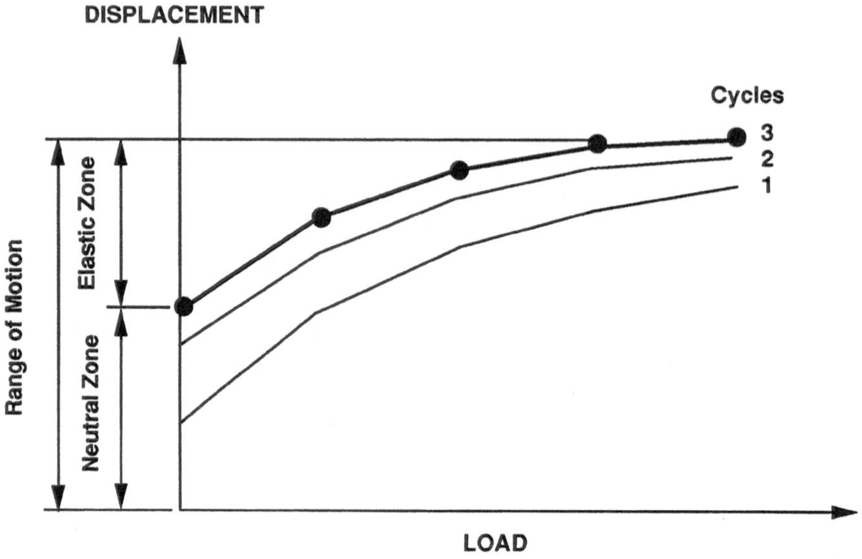

Figure 3.3. Concepts of neutral zone, elastic zone, and range of motion. Notice that the readings are taken on the third load cycle.

rotation, also to the opposite side. In the lower regions of the lumbar spine, e.g., L5-S1, the pattern was different. Here, the axial torque produced lateral bending to the same side, whereas lateral bending loads produced axial rotation to the opposite side. The coupling pattern is also affected by the posture of the spine. At the upper levels, flexion posture resulted in larger lateral bending motions irrespective of the applied load. However, at the lower levels this motion was unaffected by posture. This indicates a complex behavior of the lumbar spine that must be taken into account when interpreting measurements made in vivo.

The normal function of the spinal column is affected by injuries. Depending upon the severity of the injury, the spine can become unstable. The working definition of mechanical instability is that the spinal column after injury has significantly more motion than the intact motion. As the spine is a three-dimensional structure, the spine can be stable in one direction and unstable in another direction. Below is a description of some experimental findings concerning the injuries produced in discs, ligaments, and facet joints.

Disc Injuries

The disc is the main load-bearing component of the spinal column. An injury to the disc can affect the overall spinal mechanics. For example, it can lead to altered sharing of the load between the disc and the

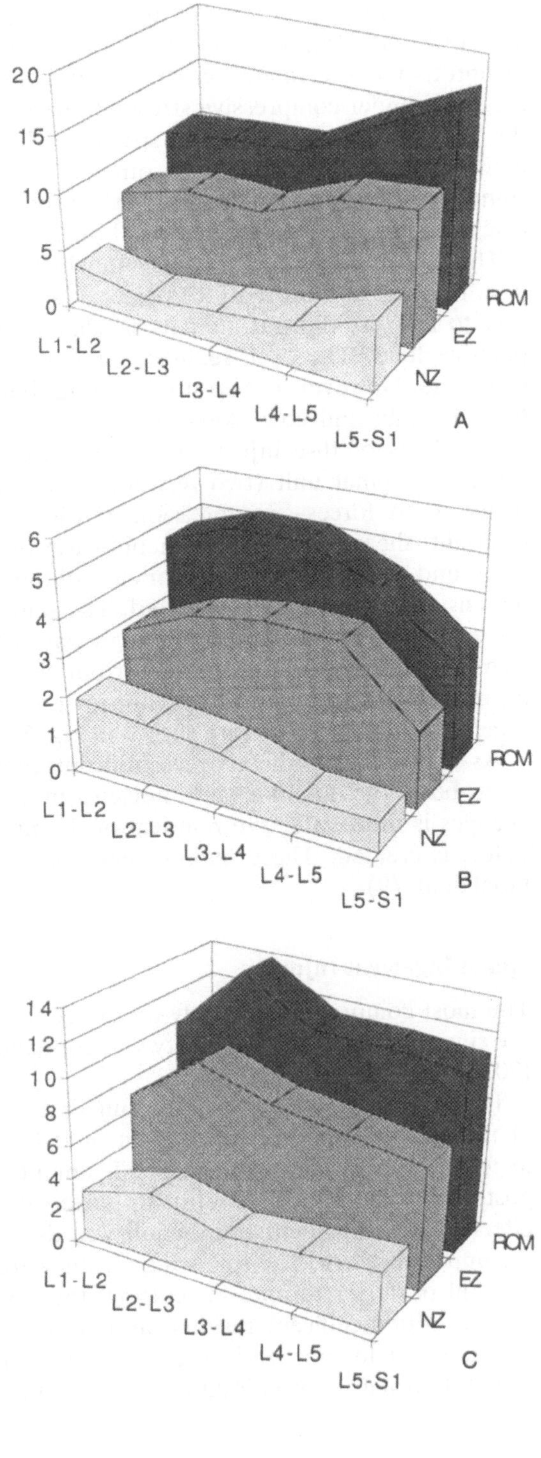

Figure 3.4 Main motions of whole lumbar spine. Neutral zone (NZ), elastic zone (EZ), and range of motion (ROM) are shown for **(A)** flexion-extension (about x axis), **(B)** left-right axial rotation (about y axis), and **(C)** left-right lateral bending (about z axis).

apophyseal joints. The two load-bearing components of the disc are the nucleus in the central region surrounded by the annulus fibrosis consisting of fibrous tissue arranged in concentric laminated bands. The nucleus is generally under compressive stress, whereas the annular layers, especially the outer layers, carry tensile stresses. The stresses in the two components of the disc balance each other as well as the load applied to the spine. A disturbance in the physical properties of any component of the disc will alter its over all mechanical behavior.

There have been several studies in which an injury was produced in the disc. Markolf and Morris (10) performed experiments to show that an injury to the disc did not alter its mechanical properties under axial compressive load. The "self-sealing" phenomena would be interesting if it were true. However, in two studies, it has been shown that the opposite is true. Panjabi and coworkers (18) did a comprehensive study of the in vitro effects of disc injury. They measured the response of the intact functional spinal unit (two-vertebra segment without the muscles) subjected to six forces—compression, tension, anterior/posterior shear, and left/right shear—and six moments—flexion, extension, left/right rotations, and left/right bendings. For each of these load types, complete three-dimensional motion was measured. The same testing was conducted after the specimen was injured by taking away (a) part of the annulus on the right inside, and (b) the nucleus from the window created by the first injury. Schematics of the two injuries and the resulting motions of the intact and injured spines are shown in Fig. 3.5.

As can be seen, there are significant changes in the spinal behavior after both the annular and nucleus injuries. The magnitude of the changes is more after the removal of the nucleus than when the annulus defect is created. These findings have been independently confirmed by Goel et al. (9).

Spinal Ligament Injuries

The most comprehensive study on the effects of ligament transections on the spinal flexibility or instability was conducted by Posner and coworkers (20).

The Posner experiment used 18 functional spinal units from three levels of the lumbar spine: L1-L2, L3-L4, and L5-S1. The specimen was subjected to flexion and loadings. The ligaments were transected either from posterior to anterior or anterior to posterior in a sequential manner. The effect to each ligament transection was documented from the motion of the upper vertebra. The following results were found: Under flexion loading and posterior to anterior cutting, there were incremental motion increases with significant residual motion after the facet joint transection. In extension loading and anterior to posterior cutting, a significant residual deformation was found after the anterior half of the disc was cut.

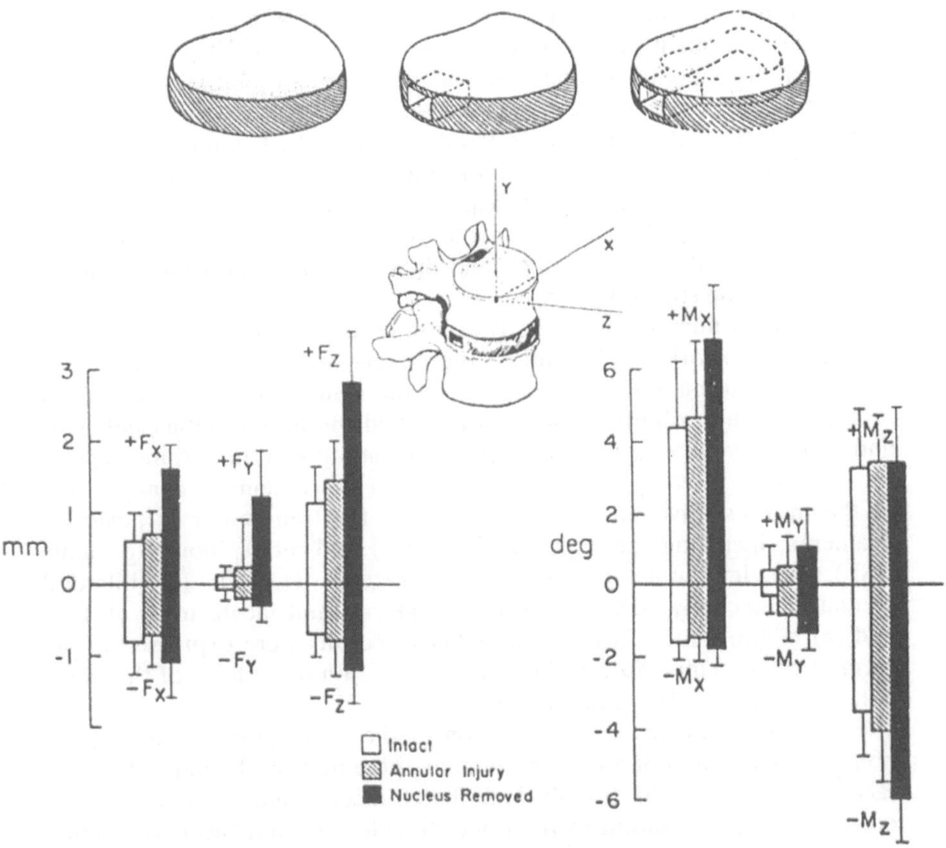

Figure 3.5. The *bars* represent main motions at maximum load values (150 N for forces and 7.5 Nm for moments) for all 12 loads as well as for the three states of the specimen: intact, with annulus injury, and after nucleus removal. Also shown with 1 SD. (Adapted from Ref. 17)

As residual deformation is equivalent to the neutral zone, the critical change in the physical properties took place at the facet joint transection in flexion and the anterior half of the disc in extension. Result of this study formed the basis for developing a checklist for the diagnosis of clinical instability in the lumbar spine (23).

Injury to the Facets

It is generally accepted in the clinical literature that facets are two of the three joints that transmit the load from one vertebra to the next. It has been estimated that they transmit from 18% to 36% of the load, depending upon the spinal posture (21). The other role of the facets that has also been well documented is that in axial rotation. As noted earlier, normal rotational movement in the lumbar spine is about 1° to 2° to either side. This small movement is the result of highly congruent joint surfaces of the inferior facets of the top vertebra and the superior facets of the bottom vertebra. It has been shown by several experiments, beginning with Farfan et al. (6), that transection of the facets significantly increases axial rotation. However, there are two aspects of facets that have not been studied as extensively. These are the role of injury to the facets in the coupled motions of the lumbar spine, and the effect of partial transections of the facets on the spinal motion.

Using fresh human cadaveric two-vertebrae lumbar spine specimens, Abumi and coworkers (1) studied the effects of sequentially increasing injury to the facets on the kinematics of the spine. Using the techniques of noninvasive flexibility testing, they studied the normal intact behavior and motion increases after each injury. The study was three-dimensional, thus providing a complete documentation of the kinematic changes due to the injuries. Five injuries were studied: (a) transection of posterior ligaments, including the supraspinous (SSL) and intraspinous ligaments (ISL); (b) left unilateral medial facetectomy (UMF); (c) bilateral medial facetectomy (BMF); (d) left unilateral total facetectomy (UTF); and (e) bilateral total facetectomy (BTF). Results were expressed in the form of relative increases in the ranges of motion over those of the intact behavior, and are shown in Fig. 3.6.

They concluded that the transection of the supraspinous and intraspinous ligaments did not affect any lumbar spine motion. Unilateral medial facetectomy increased the flexion. Total facetectomy of one side increased the axial rotation to the opposite side, i.e., left facet transection increased the right axial rotation. Total facetectomy increased the axial rotation to both sides. The extension and lateral bending movements were not increased by any of the injuries. Results of this study are helpful in making judgments concerning the facetectomies used in spinal stenosis surgery.

In a new study, Oxland et al. (14) looked at the motions of the lumbosacral joint, a frequent site of low back pain problems, as a function of the injury. The focus was not on the main motions, but instead on the coupled movements of the lumbar spine. Using fresh cadaveric human spine specimens, L1-S1, they studied the three-dimensional physiological movements of the lumbosacral joint of the intact spine and after each of the three injuries. The injuries were (a) transection of all ligaments posterior to the spinal canal, (b) a transverse tunnel (2 cm times the disc height) through the middle of the disc, and (c) bilateral removal of the inferior articulations of L5. The following conclusions were drawn: injury to the intervertebral disc increased the coupled lateral rotation, due to the application of axial torque; injury to the articular facets increased the coupled axial rotation under the application of lateral bending moment;

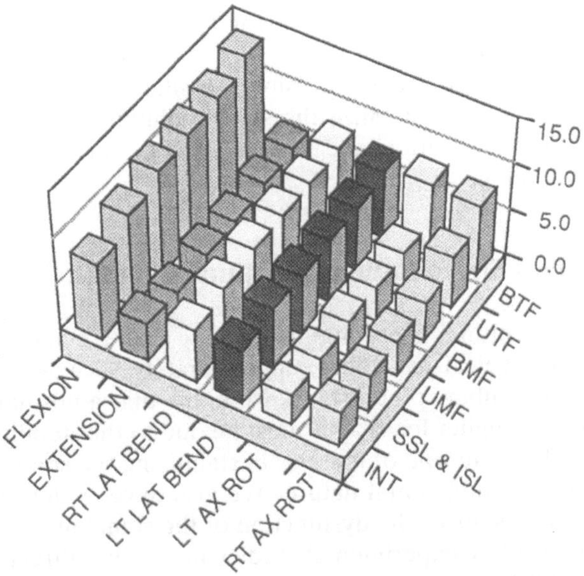

Figure 3.6. Relative increases in ranges of motion in multiple directions and due to sequential partial facetectomies. Five injuries were studied: (a) transection of posterior ligaments, including supraspinous (SSL) and intraspinous ligaments (ISL); (b) left unilateral medial facetectomy (UMF); (c) bilateral medial facetectomy (BMF); (d) left unilateral total facetectomy (UTF); and (e) bilateral total facetectomy (BTF). (Adapted from Ref. 1)

and injury to the articular facets changed the coupled flexion rotation under axial torque to extension rotation.

Thus, injuries to the various components of the spinal column alter its mechanics acutely, and may also produce adaptive changes in adjacent joints. There is some evidence to support the hypothesis that changes in the adjacent joints may be clinically significant (7).

In summary, the stabilizing role of the various spinal column components has been studied by creating experimental injuries and determining the effect on the stiffness and ranges of motion of the spinal specimen. The reason for the abundance of this experimental work is not necessarily due to the greater importance of the spinal column in low back pain problems, but more likely due to the difficulties of studying the other two components of the spinal stabilizing system.

Stability of the spinal column may also be compromised due to degeneration and microtrauma, and may manifest itself in additional micro-movements and/or macro-movements; the latter may be visualized on x-rays, whereas the former cannot be seen. Presently, it is not established what magnitude (micro or macro) or type (rotation, translation main or coupled) of movement is responsible for low back pain problems characterized as spinal instability.

Osteophyte formation and, possibly, ossification of ligaments are attempts by the body to stabilize the spinal column by stiffening its own components. Spinal fixation and fusion are the surgeon's attempts at doing the same thing.

Spinal Muscles Surrounding the Spinal Column

An intact spinal column is capable of carrying only a small load, without buckling or mechanical instability, approximately 90 newtons (about 20 pounds) for the lumbar spine (5). As we know that a normal person can carry significantly higher loads, this must be due to the stabilizing effect of the muscles. Thus, the role of muscles in stabilizing the spine is extremely important and of fundamental nature. We also have evidence, e.g., polio patients, for the results of the dysfunction of the spinal muscles.

There are very few experimental studies in which a direct relationship has been established between the muscle function and dysfunction and the effect on the stability of the spinal column. Electromyographic (EMG) studies are not very helpful in this respect as the EMG signal *does not* equate to the force generated by the muscle. An attempt was made in our laboratory to simulate the muscle force by a spring and applying it to the spine specimen in vitro. We have found that in a fresh cadaveric spine specimen after it is injured, the spinal stability can be restored to the normal value by applying simulated muscle forces (15). This aspect of muscle function was found to be even more significant if one considered the neutral zone (a displacement range around the neutral position within which the spine provides minimal resistance to external load), instead of the range of motion, as a measure of spinal instability.

There is clinical experience to support the compensating and enhancing effect of the muscles on an injured joint. The most common example of this is the injury to the knee joint. In an established case of increased laxity of the knee, the joint stability and function can be restored by training appropriate muscles surrounding the knee joint. Again, here the concept of neutral zone is relevant, as the laxity may be equated to the neutral zone.

Neural Control Unit of Spinal Muscles

This is the most important component of the stabilizing system. The neuromuscular control system monitors the requirements of spinal stability and provides these requirements with the help of the muscles at its command. The complexity and sensitivity of this task is to be realized. The stability requirements change with spinal posture, external load supported by the spine, and the inertial loads imposed due to the dynamic movements of the body parts. Once the stability requirements are computed for a certain instance of time, the precise force magnitude of each muscle attached to the spine must be computed, taking further into account such factors as maintaining the desired posture, not overloading any muscle, and using minimal energy to accomplish the stabilizing task.

Accomplishing this complex task is our daily experience. However, there seems to be no experimental study that has examined the function and dysfunction of this neuromuscular control. There is some evidence to suggest that there may be a disturbance in the control mechanism in low back pain patients. In a recent study, the low back pain patients had increased sway while standing, compared to the normal subjects (4). The compensating role of the neuromuscular control is exemplified by the case of an injured knee that an athlete voluntarily stabilizes in anticipation of increased stability requirements during a game.

Summary

The spinal stabilizing system consists of three subsystems: passive subsystem—the spinal column, active subsystem—spinal muscles, and neural subsystem—control of the spinal muscles. The elastic components holding the spinal column together and providing stability are the ligaments, disc, and the facet articulations. A significant injury to any of these components may lead to mechanical instability, both acutely and over time. Several biomechanical studies have documented the acute effects of the spinal column injuries. Muscles play a very important role in stabilizing the spinal column. Muscle spasm is the body's attempt at stabilizing a potentially unstable spine. Little biomechanical research has been done in this area. Neural control of the muscles is essential for providing optimal stabilization of the spinal column through activation of the spinal muscles. A dysfunction of the control system may result in unbalanced activation of the muscle groups, leading to increased loads on the muscles and the spinal column components. Practically no research has been done on this aspect of the stabilizing system.

References

1. Abumi K, Panjabi MM, Kramer KM, Duranceau J, Oxland T, Crisco JJ. Biomechanical evaluation of lumbar spinal stability after graded facetectomies. *Spine*. 1990;15(11):1142–1147.
2. Andersson GBJ, Pope MH, Frymoyer JW. Epidemiology. In: Pope MH, Frymoyer JW, Andersson G, eds. *Occupational Low Back Pain*. New York: Praeger; 1982:101–114.
3. Biering-Sorenson F. Low back trouble in a general population of 30-, 40-, 50-, and 60-year-old men and women: Study design, representativeness and basic results. *Dan Med Bull*. 1982;29:289–299.

4. Byl NN, Sinnott PL. Variations in balance and body sway in middle aged adults: Subjects with healthy backs compared with subjects with low-back dysfunction. *Spine*. 1991;16(3):325–330.
5. Crisco JJ. *The Biomechanical Stability of the Human Lumbar Spine: Experimental and Theoretical Investigations*. Doctoral dissertation, Yale University, New Haven, Connecticut, 1989.
6. Farfan HF, Cossette JW, Robertson GH, Wells RV, Kraus H. The effects of torsion on the lumbar intervertebral joints: The role of torsion in the production of disc degeneration. *J Bone Joint Surg*. 1970;52A:468.
7. Frymoyer J, Hanley E, Howe J, Kuhlmann D, Matteri R. A comparison of radiographic findings in fusion and nonfusion patients ten or more years following lumbar disc surgery. *Spine*. 1979;4(5):435–440.
8. Frymoyer JW, Pope MH, Clements JH, et al. Risk factors in low-back pain: An epidemiological study. *J Bone Joint Surg*. 1983;65A:213–218.
9. Goel VK, Goyal S, Clark C, Nishiyama K, Nye T. Kinematics of the whole lumbar spine. Effect of discectomy. *Spine*. 1985;10:543–554.
10. Markolf KL, Morris JM. The structural components of intervertebral disc. *J Bone Joint Surg*. 1974;56A:675–687.
11. Morris A. Identifying workers at risk to back injury is not guesswork. *Occup Health Saf*. 1985;55:16–20.
12. Nachemson AL. Advances in low-back pain. *Clin Orthop*. 1985;200:266–278.
13. Nagi SZ, Riley LE, Newby LG. A social epidemiology of back pain in a general population. *J Chronic Dis*. 1973;26:769–779.
14. Oxland TR, Crisco JJ, Panjabi MM, Yamamoto I. The effect of injury on rotational coupling at the lumbosacral joint: A biomechanical investigation. *Spine*. 1992;17(1):74–80.
15. Panjabi MM. The stabilizing system of the spine. Part I. Function, dysfunction, adaptation, and enhancement. *J Spinal Disorders*. 1992;5(4):383–389.
16. Panjabi MM, Abumi K, Duranceau J, Oxland T. Spinal stability and intersegmental muscle forces: A biomechanical model. *Spine*. 1989;14(2):194–200.
17. Panjabi MM, Goel VK, Takata K. 1981 Volvo Award in Biomechanics. Physiological strains in lumbar spinal ligaments, an in vitro biomechanical study. *Spine*. 1982:7(3):192–203.
18. Panjabi MM, Krag MH, Chung TQ. Effects of disc injury on mechanical behavior of the human spine. *Spine*. 1984;9(7):707–713.
19. Panjabi M, Yamamoto I, Oxland T, Crisco J. How does posture affect coupling in the lumbar spine? *Spine*. 1989;14(9):1002–1011.
20. Posner I, White AA, Edwards WT, Hayes WC. A biomechanical analysis of the clinical stability of the lumbar and lumbosacral spine. *Proceedings of the International Society on the Study of the Lumbar Spine*, 1980.
21. Prasad P, King AI, Ewing CL. The role of articular facets during +Gz acceleration. *J Appl Mech*. 1974;41:321.
22. Spengler DM, Bigos SJ, Martin NA, et al. Back injuries in industry: A retrospective study. I. Overview and cost analysis. *Spine*. 1986;11:241–245.
23. White AA, Panjabi M. *Clinical Biomechanics of the Spine*. 2nd ed. Philadelphia; JB Lippincott; 1990.

Discussion

The Load Sharing by the Facet Joints During Spinal Compression

Dr. O'Leary suggested that it is very hard conceptually to imagine that the facet joints carry 18% of a compression load during normal posture or in the course of any loading activity or position. It may look good on paper, but it has very little practical application. Dr. Panjabi responded that this is the work of Prasad et al. (1), showing that facet loads varied from 0% to 33% depending on the posture in the sagittal plane. When there is deviation from the sagittal plane in rotation or bending, the forces are shared differently, not only between the disc and the facets, but also between the right and left facets.

Dr. O'Leary continued: To even assume that there is only 33% in maximum extension, I would question that seriously. If you maximally hyperextend someone's spine you may completely unload the discs and I would expect the forces to be much higher if the patient remains in an upright posture with upright balancing mechanisms. The weight should be totally taken away from the discs. Dr. Panjabi responded that he did not think so. You may lie down on a bed and unload the spine, but not if you are standing. You may have changed the pattern, decreasing the load on the disc, but you will not eliminate it completely.

Dr. O'Leary continued: What happens if a gymnast walks across a pole and does a back somersault landing on her hands? Would you tell me that she had 30% of facet loading? Dr. Panjabi responded: No, somewhere it might be 0%, but this will not occur with you and me during walking or conducting normal activities. If you hang yourself upside down you may have 0% loading. That is not what I am talking about. I am refering to loading during normal activities. In the work by Prasad et al. (1) they had a cadaver sitting on a sled with a pressure transducer fitted into the disc. They looked at disc loading as a function of stretching. Dr. O'Leary interjected: In this setting the muscle forces are absent and I don't believe that it is applicable to our patients in the clinical setting.

The Mechanics of Intervertebral Disc Failure

Dr. O'Leary inquired if Dr. Panjabi felt that disc failure was primarily due to mechanical forces or were there other factors. From my standpoint injury has very little bearing on disc degeneration. I suspect that injury is just the final phase when a given event causes the already damaged disc to fail. Dr. Panjabi agreed, saying; That's true! Injury happens when the stress at a particular level exceeds the strength at that level or point. Obviously, the strength of a structure will decrease over time in association with degenerative changes within that structure. At that point smaller loads are capable of producing injury. Farfan et al. (2) have shown that strength and compressibility are not related to the degenerative changes. Nachemson (3) indicated that the physical properties of the spine do not change with age. This may be surprising, but he also has indicated that sex and age do not affect the physical properties of the spine.

The Validity of One-Segment versus Multiple-Segment Studies

Dr. Farcy pointed out that most of this work has been based upon studies of one spinal unit. For an orthopedic surgeon the most important view is an overall view of the spine related to its alignment. The alignment phenomenon is not taken into account in single-segment specimens. My goal is to restore the alignment of the spine and my concept of a spine with four curves differs from your experimental mode, which shows the spine as a straight beam. Dr. Kostuik interjected that we tried such experiments for years in the laboratory and they are hard to do in vitro. That is where mathematical models based upon unit motion segment data can perhaps help. Dr. Farcy continued: That is still creating an uncertain mathematical model that does not totally account for reality and leaves us puzzled. Dr. Panjabi continued: I think what you are saying is very true and I attempted to conduct my experiments in vivo and in vitro states. However, reality is much more complex and involves the remote as well as the direct observations. Remote observations are more difficult to assess, but may be quite accurate. In my recent work I have begun to use the entire lumbar spine from Ll to the sacrum. This is much more compatible with reality than a two vertebral segment model. Yet, many of the two vertebral segment studies produced useful information because they have readily reproducible information, not as easily obtained from whole lumbar spine segments.

Further Comments on the Definition of Instability

Dr. Kostuik suggested along with Dr. Rydevik that there may be a need for multiple definitions of instability vis-à-vis different pathological conditions including trauma, infectious processes, and degenerative states. Dr. Rydevik included the statement that pain is a significant parameter in the definition and the checklist compiled by Dr. Augustus White and Dr. Manohar Panjabi should be subjected to continuing attempts at validation.

Stabilization Training

Dr. Arthur White began: As you know, Dr. Panjabi, your work goes along very well with our theories of spine training. We do a lot of rehabilitation in San Francisco and utilize your concepts. What we do is to identify the neutral zone by doing a clinical workup with scans evaluating any underlying pathology such as spinal stenosis. Then we put the patients through a trial and error period to see what they can tolerate, and we identify their neutral zone. We try to activate their neural control unit by changing movement patterns and teaching them that they do have control of the position and posture of their spines. Then we concentrate on building up the musculature to bring the spine back into the neutral zone with strength and using the control unit. This is what we call stabilization training and what we offer patients to avoid surgery.

The comparative costs are much less than surgery and in many cases surgery is not just postponed, but avoided in our present follow-up. The study in Massachusetts where patients on the operating schedule for spine surgery were given stabilization training rather than surgery demonstrated a 92% avoidance of surgery and return to full normal working activities.

Dr. Kostuik emphasized that that sort of study must be repeated in various demographic surveys to assess its reproducibility.

The Natural History of Spinal Stability

Dr. Holtzman raised the question of considering the natural development of spinal stability. The more lax spine of the pediatric age group becomes a more rigidly flexible structure in adulthood and less elastic in the aged. Are we seeing a natural tendency for the adult spine to develop its neutral zones to accommodate a variety of loads that are added to it by increasing body weight and increasing activity in certain types of stress-related situations? Are we seeing ligamentous injury with protruding intervertebral discs and changing ligamentous length with aging? Dr. Kostuik suggested that changes in the ligaments with aging might be related to collagen cross-linkages. It was concluded that the evolution of spinal stability remains to be studied.

References

1. Prasad P, King AI, Ewing CL. The role of articular facets during $+G_3$ acceleration. *J Appl Mech*. 1974;41:321.
2. Farfan HF, Cossette JW, Robertson GH, Wells RV, Kraus H. The effects of torsion on the lumbar intervertebral joints: The role of torsion in the production of disc degeneration. *J Bone Joint Surg*. 1970;52A:468.
3. Nachemson AL. Advances in low-back pain. *Clin Orthop*. 1985;200:266–278.

CHAPTER 4

Pathophysiology of the Nerve Roots in the Lumbar Spine

Björn L. Rydevik and Kjell Olmarker

Spinal nerve roots are often mechanically deformed in connection with degenerative conditions of the spine, such as disc herniation and spinal stenosis, including segmental instability, and in association with spine trauma. Limited information is available regarding the reaction of spinal nerve roots to mechanical trauma, which is different from peripheral nerves for which the trauma effects have been explored in more detail. However, data from experiments on peripheral nerve compression cannot always be directly transferred to spinal nerve root compression because of certain anatomical and physiological differences between peripheral nerves and spinal nerve roots.

Anatomy and Physiology of Spinal Nerve Roots

The spinal nerve roots constitute the anatomical connection between the central nervous system and the peripheral nervous system. The nerve roots have a complex anatomy, comprising sensory nerve root with dorsal root ganglion and motor nerve root. The anatomical arrangements are different in the central spinal canal, i.e., in the cauda equina, and laterally in the intervertebral foramina. In the cauda equina, the nerve roots lack epineurium and perineurium, but the roots are surrounded by the cerebrospinal fluid. The dorsal root ganglion is critically located at each level in or near the intervertebral foramen. The nerve roots have a blood supply that is less well developed than for peripheral nerves. However, the nerve roots seem to derive some of their nutrition via diffusion from the cerebrospinal fluid. Such a nutritional mechanism might be considered to be an analogy with nutrition of the cartilage in the synovial joints via diffusion from the synovial fluid.

Effects of Compression on Nerve Roots

Previous data on experimental nerve root compression indicate that nerve roots may be more susceptible to eompression than peripheral nerves. Recently, a model has been developed for graded nerve root compression in vivo in the pig lumbosacral spine. Using this model, the effects of graded compression of nerve roots have been analyzed regarding intraneural microcirculation (vital nticroscopy), edema formation in the nerve roots (fluorescence microscopy), nutritional supply to the nerve roots (isotope tracing methodology), and impulse propagation (neurophysiological techniques). Data obtained indicate that the nutritional supply to the nerve roots in the cauda equina, in terms of reduced solute transport to the roots and impaired intraneural blood flow, can be acutely affected at pressure levels of 10 to 20 mm Hg or greater. Long-standing eompression of nerve roots at these pressure levels might, therefore, lead to a reduction of the nutritional supply to the nerve fibers and accumulation of waste products within the nerve root tissue. Intraneural edema, as seen with fluorescence microscopy by extravasation of serum albumin labeled with Evans blue, was induced after compression at 50 mm Hg for only 2 minutes. Experimental compression during 2 hours in the pig model revealed an acute pressure threshold between 50 and 75 mm Hg for impairment of nerve root impulse conduction.

The dorsal root ganglion has attracted certain interest as a possible mediator of pain in the lumbar spine. The dorsal root ganglion seems to be mechanosensitive, and mechanical deformations of the ganglion can lead to increased pressure in the ganglion and may give rise to pain-production. Experimental whole body vibration may induce significant changes in neuropeptide synthesis in the dorsal root ganglion. Other investigations have indicated a probable role of whole body vibration as a risk factor for low back pain.

Pain Mechanisms of Spinal Nerve Roots

Acute compression of a normal peripheral nerve or nerve root does not always cause pain, but rather numbness, paresthesia, motor weakness, and related signs and symptoms. However, if a nerve root has become irritated because of, for example, a herniated disc, even minimal mechanical deformation can result in severe radiating pain. Thus, it seems, that nerve root irritation is a significant factor that has to be present before mechanical root deformation gives rise to pain. Mechanical factors, such as compression and/or traction of the nerve roots, can induce a sequence of tissue reactions in the nerve roots that may lead to intraneural inflammation. The exact nature of this inflammation is not known, but there is evidence that the tissue reactions may be characterized by edema, inflammatory cell reaction, and local demyelination.

It has also been suggested that chemical mechanisms might be involved in the production of nerve root inflammation. Breakdown products from degenerating nucleus pulposus might leak from the disc and induce a "chemical radiculitis" in the nearby root. Intraoperative measurements of pH in the nucleus pulposus has demonstrated low pH values particularly in patients with extensive adhesion formation around the nerve root. Autoimmune mechanisms might be involved in this context and/or direct irritating effects of proteoglycans from the disc on the nerve root.

The functional changes induced by mechanical and/or chemical mechanisms in nerve root syndromes may be of two different modalities: (a) *loss of nerve function* (seen as sensory deficit and/or muscle weakness), and/or (b) *hyperexcitability of the nerve tissue.* The latter phenomenon means that a nerve root can easily be further stimulated by even minor mechanical deformations, i.e., being the site of ectopic impulse generation, which is likely to be related to pain production. The loss of nerve function can be demonstrated clinically with electrophysiologic measurements such as nerve conduction velocity determination and electromyogram (EMG) analyses. It is likely that the two types of functional changes can be present at the same time in nerve roots.

Experimental-Clinical Correlations

Experimental postmortem dural constriction and pressure measurements among the nerve roots in the cauda equina have indicated that reduction of the cross-sectional area of the dural sac to about 65 mm^2 (37% of the normal area) can induce pressure levels of about 50 mm Hg. The pressure among the nerve roots started to build up at the cross-sectional area of the dural sac of about 75 mm^2, a value that corresponds well to values reported for patients with central spinal stenosis. The animal experimental data indicate significant physiological change at corresponding pressure levels. For disc herniation there is less information regarding pressure levels acting on the nerve roots, but the disc height seems to be a critical factor in this regard. The effects of repeated mechanical nerve root deformation such as in segmental instability are incompletely understood, but are likely to include various acute and chronic changes in nerve root physiology.

Conclusion

The nerve roots in the lumbar spine have a complex anatomy and physiology. Current knowledge regarding pathophysiology and pathoanatomy of nerve root compression as based on experimental data and clinical observations indicates that impairment of the nutritional supply including the microcirculation of the nerve roots may occur even at low pressure level compression. Prolonged low pressure compression is likely to lead to functional changes. Thus, a correlation between mechanical nerve root deformation, physiological changes, and clinical symptoms may be defined.

Bibliography

Bobechko WP, Hirsch C. Autoimmune response to nucleus pulposus In the rabbit. *J Bone Joint Surg*. 1965;47B:574–580.

Fowler RJ, Danta G, Gilliatt RW. Recovery of nerve conduction after a pneumatic tourniquet: Observations on the hind-limb of a baboon. *J Neurol Neurosurg Psychiatry*. 1972;35:638.

Gelfan S, Tarlov IM. Physiology of spinal cord, nerve root and peripheral nerve compression. *Am J Physiol*. 1956;185:217–229.

Gertzbein SD. Degenerative disc disease of the lumbar spine. *Clin Orthop*. 1977;12:68–71.

Jackson RP, Montesano PX, Jacobs RR. *Facet joint injections in mechanical low back pain patients*. Abstract, International Society for the Study of the Lumbar Spine, Dallas, Texas, 1986.

Lindahl O. Experimental skin pain—induced by water soluble substances in humans. *Acta Physiol Scand*. 1961;51(Suppl):179.

Lundborg G. Structure and function of the intraneural microvessels as related to trauma, edema formation, and nerve function. *J Bone Joint Surg*. 1975;57A:938–948.

Lundborg G. *Nerve Injury and Repair*. Edinburgh: Churchill-Livingstone; 1988.

Lundborg G, Myers R, Powell H. Nerve compression injury and increased endoneurial fluid pressure: a "miniature compartment syndrome." *J Neurol Neurosurg Psychiatry*. 1983;46:1119–1124.

Marshall LL, Trethewie ER. Chemical irritation of nerve root in disc prolapse. *Lancet*. 1973;2:320.

Nachemson A. Intradiscal measurements of pH in patients with lumbar rhizopathies. *Acta Orthop Scand*. 1969;40:23–42.

Ochoa J, Fowler TJ, Gilliat RW. Anatormical changes in peripheral nerves compressed by a pneumatic tourniquet. *J Anat*. 1972;113:433.

Olmarker K. *Spinal Nerve Root Compression. Experimental Studies on Effects of Acute, Graded Compression on Nerve Root Nutrition and Function, with an In Vivo Compression Model of the Porcine Cauda Equina*. Thesis, Göteborg, Sweden, 1990.

Olmarker K, Holm S, Rosenqvist A-L, Rydevik B. Experimental nerve root compression. Presentation of a model for acute, graded compression of the porcine cauda equina, with analyses of neural and vascular anatomy. *Spine*. 1991;16:61–69.

Olmarker K, Holm S, Rydevik B. Importance of compression onset rate for the degree of impairment of impulse propagation in experimental compression injury of the porcine cauda equina. *Spine*. 1990;15:416–419.

Olmarker K, Rydevik B, Hansson T, Holm S. Compression-induced changes of the nutritional supply to the porcine cauda equina. *J Spinal Dis*. 1990;3:25–29.

Olmarker K, Rydevik B, Holm S. Edema formation in spinal nerve roots induced by experimental, graded compression. An experimental study on the pig cauda equina with special reference to differences in effects between rapid and slow onset of compression. *Spine*. 1989;14:579–563.

Olmarker K, Rydevik B, Holm S, Bagge U. Effects of experimental graded compression on blood flow in spinal nerve roots. A vital microscopic study on the porcine cauda equina. *J Orthop Res*. 1989;7:817–823.

Parke WW, Watanabe R. The intrinsic vasculature of the lumbosacral spinal nerve roots. *Spine*. 1985;10:508–515.

Rydevik B, Brown MD, Lundborg G. Pathoanatomy and pathophysiology of nerve root compression. *Spine*. 1984;9:7–15.

Rydevik B, Holm S, Brown MD, Lundborg G. Diffusion from the cerebrospinal fluid as a nutritional pathway for spinal nerve roots. *Acta Physiol Scand*. 1990;138:247–248.

Rydevik B, Lundborg G. Permeability of intraneural microvessels and perineurium following acute, graded nerve compression. *Scand J Plast Reconstr Surg*. 1977;11:179–187.

Rydevik B, Lundborg G, Bagge U. Effects of graded compression on intraneural blood flow. *J Hand Surg*. 1981;6:3–12.

Rydevik B, Lundborg G, Skalak R. Biomechanics of peripheral nerves. In: Nordin M, VH Frankel, eds. *Basic Biomechanics of the Musculoskeletal System*. Lea and Febiger; Philadelphia: 1989:75–87.

Rydevik B, McLean WG, Sjöstrand J, Lundborg G. Blockage of axonal transport induced by acute, graded compression of the rabbit vagus nerve. *J Neurol Neurosurg Psychiatry*. 1980;43:690–698.

Rydevik B, Myers RR, Powell HC. Pressure increase in the dorsal root ganglion following mechanical compression. Closed compartment syndrome in nerve roots. *Spine*. 1989;14:574–576.

Rydevik B, Nordborg C. Changes in nerve function and nerve fiber structure induced by acute, graded compression. *J Neurol Neurosurg Psychiatry*. 1980;43:1070–1082.

Rydevik BL, Pedowitz RA, Hargens AR, Swenson MR, Myers RR, Garfin SR. Effects of acute graded compression on spinal nerve root function and structure: An experimental study on the pig cauda equina. *Spine*. 1991;16:487–493.

Sharpless SK. Susceptibility of spinal nerve roots to compression block. The research status of spinal manipulative therapy. NIH workshop, February 2–4, 1975. In: Goldstein M, ed. *NINCDS Monography*, no. 15. NIH; Bethesda, Maryland: 1975:155–161.

Sunderland S. *Nerves and Nerve Injuries*. 2nd ed. Edinburg: Churchill Livingstone; 1978.

Weinstein JN, Pope M, Schmidt R, Serroussi R. Effects of low frequency vibration on the dorsal root ganglion. *Neuroorthopaedics*. 1987;4:24–30.

Discussion

Some Considerations Regarding Radicular Pain

Dr. Bennett M. Stein noted that the present manner of treating the most frequent pain syndromes such as neuralgia is to either cut the sensory root or to further damage the dorsal root ganglion. I can appreciate that compression will reduce nerve conduction, but I do not fully understand how that generates pain. I wonder if you could add to the physiological studies some intraspinal cord studies to try to determine if there is some sort of release mechanism in the Rexed laminae that gives rise to the spinothalamic fibers. It might be possible to determine if there is hyperexcitability of Rexed's third and fourth lamina or even to perform thalamic recordings.

My other thought concerns whether anyone has studied pain receptors in the dural sleeves about the roots and the dorsal root ganglia or for that matter in the annulus or the joint capsules.

Dr. Rydevik responded that the first part of the question was beyond what we have done so far, but it is an area—the area of deafferentation pain—that should definitely be explored. The second question relates to dural sensitivity. It is a subject to which we have given considerable thought, but which remains theoretical at this time. We have reason to speculate that mechanical factors may in some way relate to myelin breakdown and the release of biochemical factors. These may in some way produce a dural irritation or an intradural nerve root inflammation that is accompanied by reflex muscle spasms and pain. Nociceptors in the ligaments and annulus may similarly be implicated.

Spinal Instability and Pain

Dr. Arthur White asked Dr. Rydevik if vertebral instability need be painful in and of itself. Dr. Rydevik responded that you must think of the time factor here. An initial event may take off in various directions. There may be healing with recovery to normal, partial healing, or nonhealing. Cases that are characterized by partial healing or nonhealing may be characterized by chronic inflammation and chronic root irritation. The fibrosis that ensues causes impaired sliding of the neural structures in the vertebral canal. We know that nerve roots may normally slide 6 to 8 mm with motions of the spine and if that capacity is impaired due to adhesions or fibrosis in the region of the nerves then entrapment and or tethering may yield painful symptomatology.

Pain and the Facet Joint

Dr. Hughes mentioned that Dr. Edward Schlesinger, the former Chief of Neurosurgery at the New York Neurological Institute, used to make an effort to denervate the facet joints by removing their synovial linings and claimed that this was important for the relief of pain. Similarly some patients will improve dramatically after bilateral-lateral fusions. Can anyone put this in perspective in terms of the validity of back pain arising from the facet joint?

Dr. Rydevik responded that this is a very controversial issue. The popularity of the facet joint has swayed up and down over the past 20 years. Clinical studies by Jackson et al. on the clinical results of facet joint injections have not been conclusive. Mechanical stretching of the facet joint capsule may result in a very strong neurophysiologic response in the small sensory nerves that innervate that joint in animals. However, clinically this is difficult to assess because of the two- to three-level overlap in innervation and the overlap across the midline.

Dr. Kostuik agreed that "facet pain" was due to something else. Dr. Rydevik added that painful instability, as Dr. Panjabi mentioned, may not always be associated with a large degree of vertebral displacement. There may also be micro-instability associated with exquisite pain, but a paucity of radiographic findings.

Observations on the Threshold for Applied Pressure

Dr. Panjabi stated that he wished to ask a question that was more technical. The starting point in all this relates to the mechanical factors and you are trying to find a threshold. The threshold that you had was for slowly applied pressures. Then you showed that if you applied the same pressure at a higher rate, the threshold is much lower. In addition you have compression and stretching. I suggest three factors: compression, stretching, and the rate of loading; all three of them coming together gives the threshold ratio.

In most of your work the loading rate, that is, the pressure increase per unit time, is not well defined. Do you plan in the future to delineate the mechanical factor definitions with greater precision? Similarly, what actually happened to the nerves?

These observations on the significance of the rate of deformation came about by chance. One of our collaborators just happened to initiate the pressure in a different manner one day and we thought there was something wrong with the experimental setup. Later, when we reviewed the protocol it became apparent that the pressure was increased slowly rather than abruptly and that is how that observation was made.

I must admit that I am not aware of any good model in the literature or anywhere else to study the reaction of the neural elements in experimental instability in animals. Therefore at this time we have to rely on related studies and draw conclusions regarding static compression.

CHAPTER 5

Biocompatibility of Metallic Spinal Implants

Gregory J. Bennett

Lumbar stabilization surgery has increasingly utilized metallic implants in various forms. The intended effect of most implants is to provide sufficient stiffness to the spine to facilitate a bone fusion across motion segments. Spinal implants may have many other effects including local and systemic chemical and immunological effects, and biomechanically induced changes in surrounding bone, such as pressure necrosis, remodeling, and osteopenia (8,13). Because of the biomechanical variations in spinal instability syndromes and possibly also the biological capability for bone formation and incorporation, the implant design and surgical construct remain diverse and their relative merits are poorly understood. However, in general, the implants are considered temporary "splints" for support and load sharing with the spine in anticipation of an eventual bone fusion. Once the fusion has occurred, their contribution to spine stability and patient comfort and activities becomes less apparent. Nevertheless, most implants are left in place after the fusion matures. This raises the possibility of deriving additional long-term benefits from the presence of the implant or, alternatively, the possibility of accumulative biologic toxicity or undesirable biomechanical consequences.

Osteointegration has been defined by Branemark et al. (7) as "direct structural and functional connection between ordered, living bone and the surface of a load-carrying implant." The concept of osteointegration was derived from observations by Albrektsson et al. (1,2) using titanium devices to permit studies of bone circulation and repair mechanisms. In the course of this research, the unanticipated observation that the titanium bone "windows" became densely attached to the bone itself led to further work on the unique bone-metal interface associated with titanium. Freshly machined titanium is covered by a thin oxide coating within seconds upon exposure to air (Fig. 5.1). This has the amorphous crystalline structure of a ceramic and creates a composite material. The predominant molecular form is TiO_2, which is corrosion resistant, catalytically active, and has strong van der Waals forces due to its high dielectric constant (Fig. 5.2). The interaction between oxide coating and

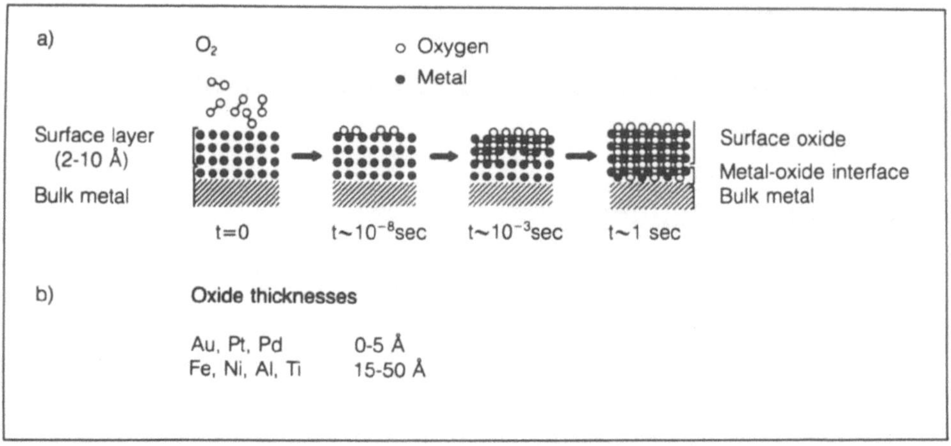

Figure 5.1. Aspects of metal oxidation. (Reproduced with permission from ref. 7.)

biologic macromolecules is a dynamic process associated with gradual thickening of the oxide layer up to approximately 100 Å and the gradual incorporation of Ti-Ca-P complexes into bone tissue (Fig. 5.3). If this process is not altered by trauma or chemical interference, such as occurs with fluorine contamination, then eventually a steady state is reached that is associated with a stable mechanical relationship and little further change in the oxide coating (Fig. 5.4). This permits load sharing with skeletal structures on a permanent basis. Thus, osteointegration completely reverses our thinking about the role of spinal implants as temporary load-sharing structures (6,9,15,18).

Metals may be pure, consisting of a high percentage of one element, or alloyed with other metals to combine the relative merits of the individual constituents into a material with more favorable properties. A coated material consists of a bulk material, which largely determines properties such as stiffness and machinability, and a surface layer. The surface properties, such as corrosion, wear, fatigue, and compatibility are determined by as little as the outer 15 to 30 atoms (Fig. 5.5). Surfaces commonly used on metals for alteration of these properties include carbide, oxide, and nitride coatings. The molecular interactions of osteointegration are, therefore, highly dependent upon this very small layer of atoms.

The surface topography, including such features as porosity, can greatly alter the tissue interactions with bone and appears to affect the biomechanical interaction as well (11). Irregularities on the 0.1 mm scale (10^6 Å) can enhance the mechanical linkage between bone and the implant with or without molecular osteointegration. Surface variations of 10 to 100 microns (10^4 to 10^5 Å) influence the organization of interface macro-

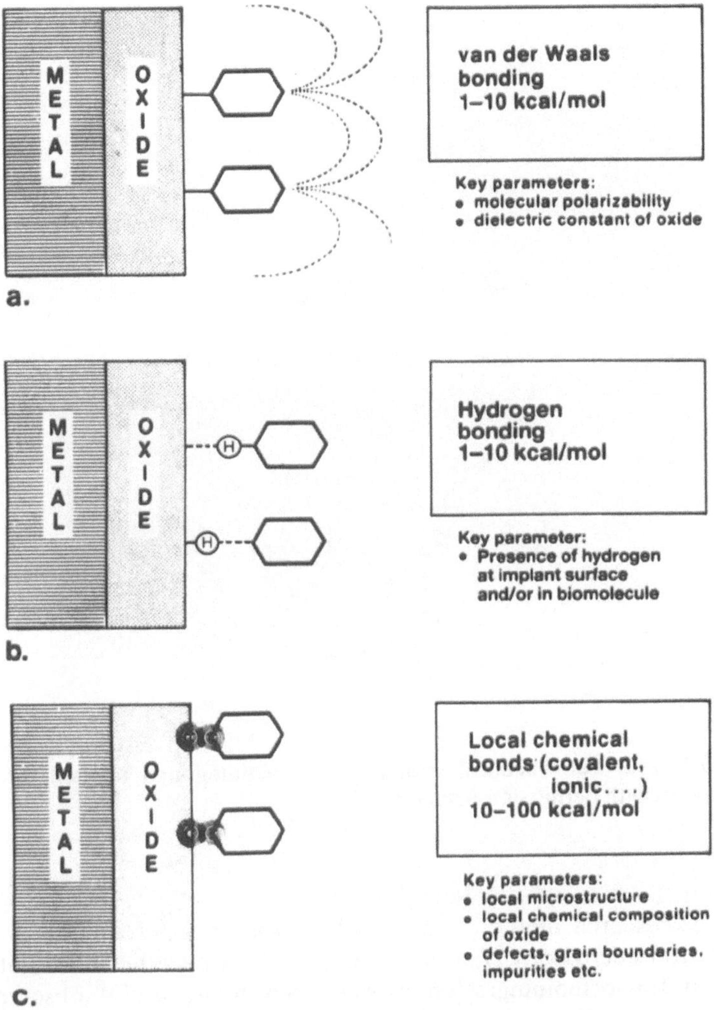

Figure 5.2. Bonding between biomolecule and an implant surface. (Reproduced with permission from ref. 7.)

molecules. At the 1 nm range (10 Å), chemical bonding energies and local electromagnetic fields can be altered. For practical purposes, metals cannot be machined or polished to surface specifications of less than 10 nm. The optimal surface configuration for macroscopic roughness (greater than 0.1 mm) and chemical interaction (0.01 to 0.1 mm) remains unknown and will likely vary with the biomechanical environment and other local material and host factors.

The chemical bond between titanium and bone can be described with

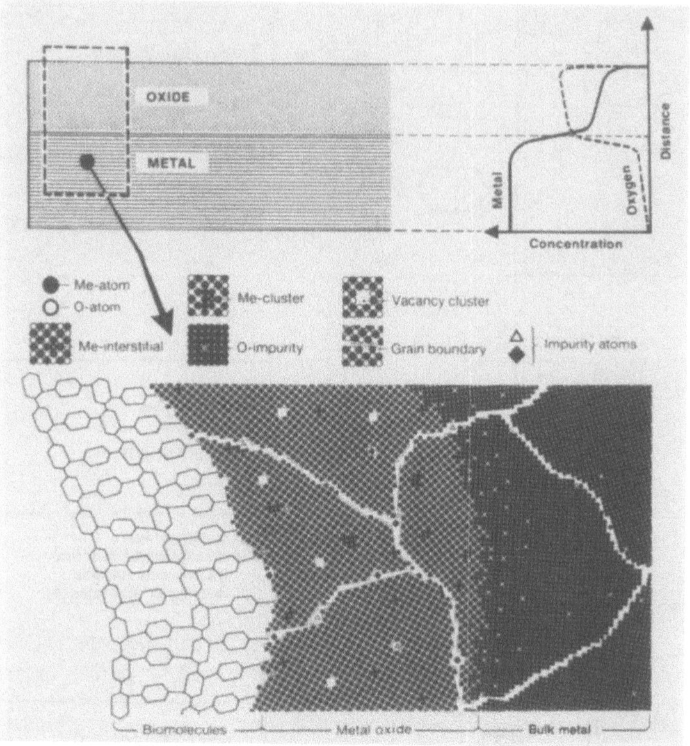

Figure 5.3. Proposed chemical structure of osteointegrated implant interface. (Reproduced with permission from ref. 7.)

numerous research methods, including various spectroscopic techniques and electron microscopy (Fig. 5.6). Surface science studies have not fully explained the osteointegration process, but many useful observations have been made. The oxide layer has been found to contain carbon, nitrogen, chloride, and calcium, with the calcium widely dispersed throughout. The calcium is found in complexes that include phosphate and titanium (Figs. 5.7 and 5.8). Energy dispersive x-ray (EDX) spectroscopy mapping of TiO_2 and adjacent cells has confirmed this by demonstrating the superimposition of these atoms as shown in Fig. 5.9. These complexes can be traced from the oxide layer in gradually diminishing quantities into the adjacent cellular structures. The chemical bonds between the oxide coat have not been directly demonstrated by EDX, but the dynamic exchange of Ti-Ca-P is highly suggestive of the presence of such direct chemical bonding.

The successful surgical use of titanium implants for osteointegration is highly dependent upon atraumatic technique for preparation of the sur-

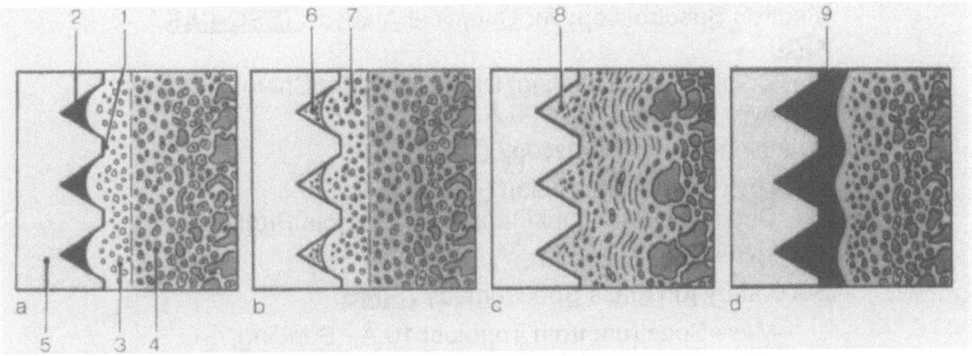

Figure 5.4. A diagrammatic representation of the biology of osteointegration. Note the initial traumatic phase including blood and damaged bone at the apex of the bone threads in (a); (b) and (c) show progressive maturation of the bone implant interface to a stable organized osteointegrated relationship; (d) illustrates loss of osteointegration with proliferation of nonmineralized connective tissue. (Reproduced with permission from ref. 7.)

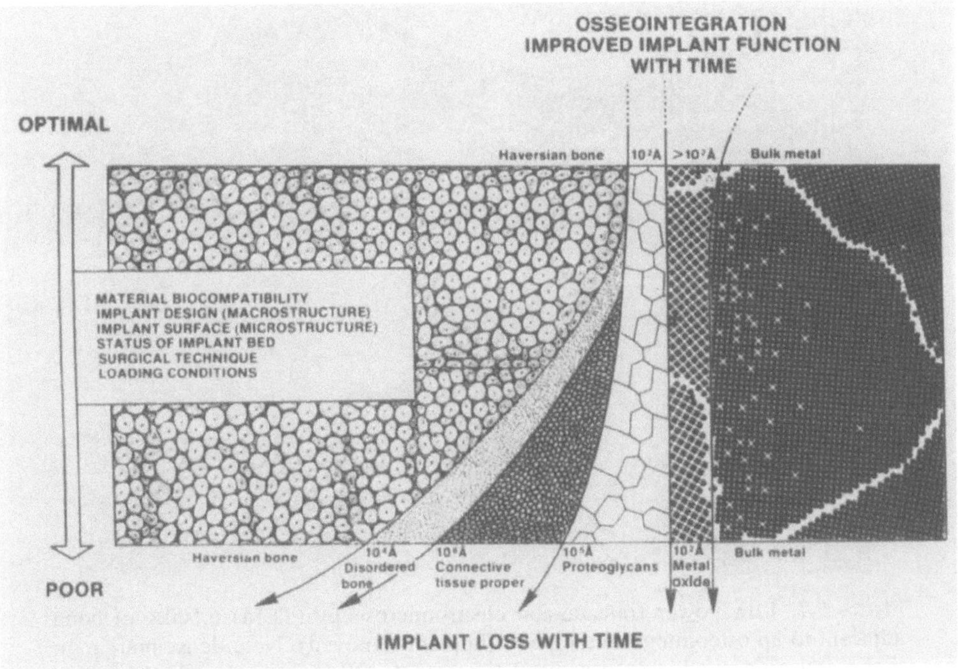

Figure 5.5. Factors influencing osteointegration. (Reproduced with permission from ref. 6.)

Electron Spectroscopy for Chemical Analysis (ESCA AKA XPS)

Composition, Bonding, Depth Profiling, Chemical States over Topmost 10 - 200 Å

Scanning Auger Microscopy (SAM)

High Spatial Resolution (~250 Å) with Chemical/Elemental Mapping and Depth Profiling, Composition, Image

Secondary Ion Mass Spectrometry (SIMS)

Mass Spectrum from Topmost 10 Å - Bonding, Structure, Reactivity and/or Ion Microscopy Imaging and Depth Profiling with ppb Elemental Sensitivity

Low Energy Ion Scattering Spectrometry (LEISS)

High Surface Sensitivity (3-5 Å), Structural and Compositional Information

Figure 5.6. Selected surface spectroscopy techniques useful in biocompatibility studies. (Courtesy of Michael A. Meenaghan, D.D.S., Ph.D., SUNY at Buffalo Dental School and Surface Science Center.)

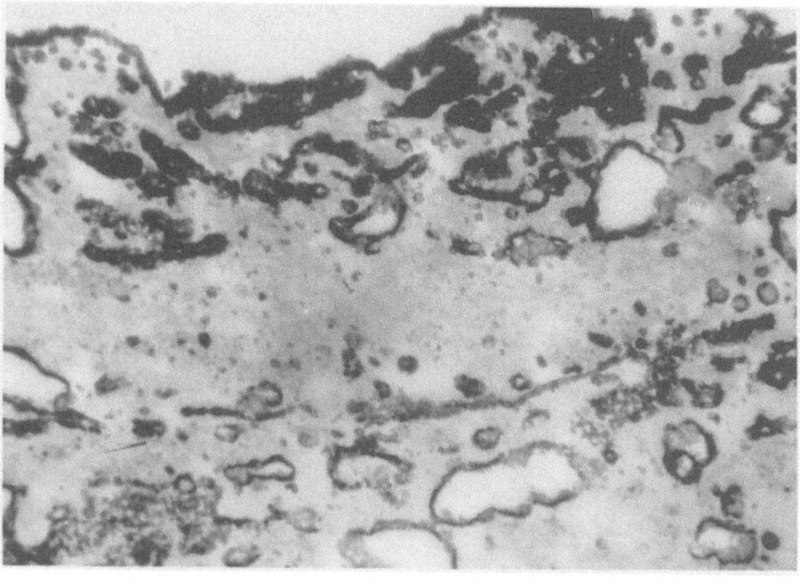

Figure 5.7. Low power transmission electromicroscopy (TEM) 6,500× of bone adjacent to an osteointegrated implant (implant removed). Note dense margin on tissue and adjacent highly organized tissue (osteoid). (Courtesy of Michael A. Meenaghan, D.D.S., Ph.D., SUNY at Buffalo Dental School and Surface Science Center.)

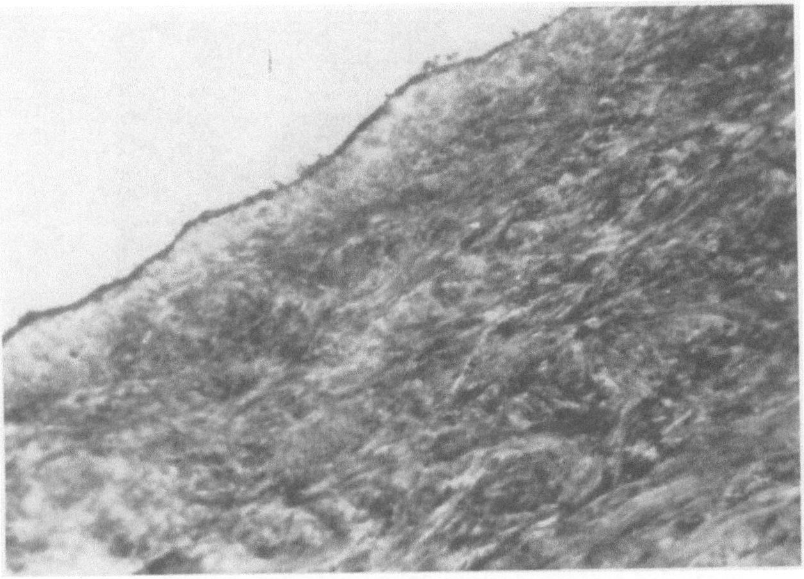

Figure 5.8. Unstained high power (100,000×) transmission electromicroscopy (TEM) demonstrating electron-dense titanium incorporated into bone tissue and adjacent to cytoplasmic organelles. (Courtesy of Michael A. Meenaghan, D.D.S., Ph.D., SUNY at Buffalo Dental School and Surface Science Center.)

rounding bone, and the surface preparation and sterilization procedures to remove organic residues from the implant (10,16). Branemark has recommended slow RPM drilling of the bone bed (15 RPMs), and a wide variety of surface cleaning techniques have been proposed including ultraviolet light and radiofrequency glow discharge, both of which have been found to be superior to conventional steam autoclave (3,4).

The surface energy of the implant (dynes/cm) is a useful screening test for implant appropriateness for osteointegration or other applications. Low surface energy (20 to 30 dynes/cm) is desirable for intravascular implants, such as heart valves, where biological nonadherence is required (5,12). In bone, however, a low surface energy implant becomes coated with glycoproteins, followed by poorly organized fibrous tissue with chronic inflammatory changes, and it eventually loosens. Implants with a high surface energy (greater than 40 dynes/cm) have extensive binding sites on the glycoprotein film for acid-base and polar molecular interactions, cell spreading along the implant surface, mitoses, and a dense connective tissue matrix that eventually adheres to the implant resulting in tissue integration (Figs. 5.10 to 5.11).

In addition to the local biochemical interactions important for osteointegration, more complex responses to metallic implants can occur includ-

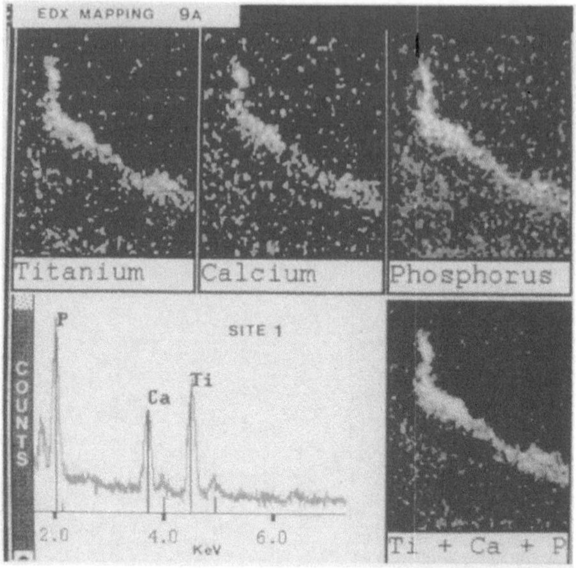

Figure 5.9. Energy dispersive x-ray (EDX) spectroscopy mapping of the electron-dense material in Figs. 5.6. and 5.7. Note the presence of distinct peaks of phosphorus, calcium, and titanium, which are identical when superimposed, suggesting that they are present in complexes. (Courtesy of Michael A. Meenaghan, D.D.S., Ph.D., SUNY at Buffalo Dental School and Surface Science Center.)

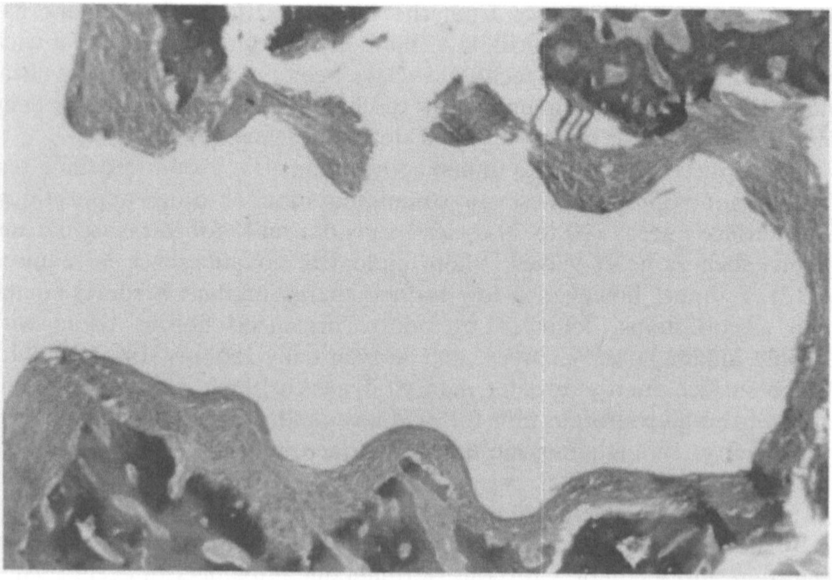

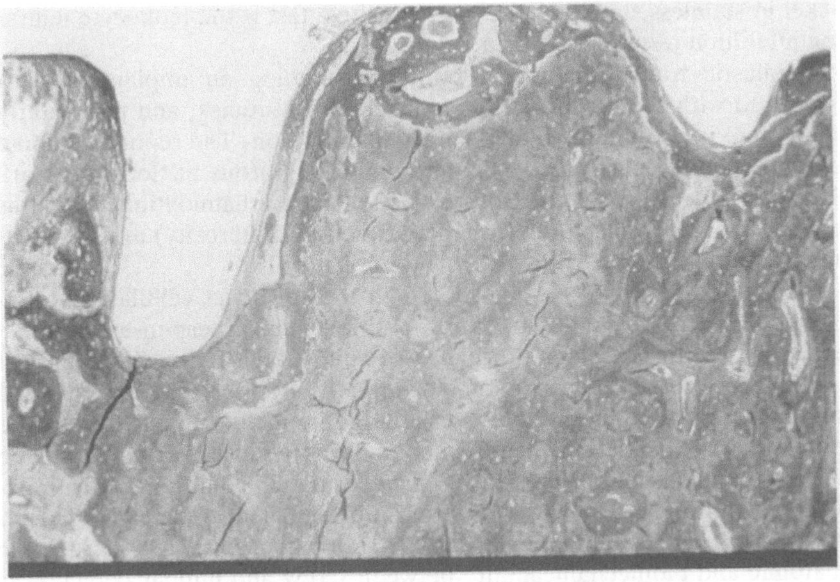

Figure 5.11. Bone adjacent to an osteointegrated implant. Note minimum of fibrous tissue and extensive new bone formation (osteoid). (Courtesy of Michael A. Meenaghan, D.D.S., Ph.D., SUNY at Buffalo Dental School and Surface Science Center.)

ing antibody and cell-mediated immune responses and, perhaps, neoplasia. For implants that do not become tissue integrated, there is an immediate inflammatory response consisting of foreign body giant cells and the formation of a type 1 collagen layer of approximately 20 to 200 microns in thickness. Subsequent implant loosening is associated with formation of synovial-like tissue and local fluid production with surface wear on the implant. Regional lymphadenopathy may be seen, particularly in the inguinal region with hip replacement. Occasionally, metal fragments can be transported systemically to the pulmonary circulation and be identified in the lungs. Cellular immunity is most frequently seen in women and is associated with previous exposure to nickel-containing jewelry. In men, previous occupational exposure to chromium can result in delayed hypersensitivity reactions to chromium-containing alloys. Skin testing is helpful in predicting these responses, such as the presence of

Figure 5.10. Bone surrounding a failed osteointegrated implant (implant removed). Note extensive fibrous tissue. (Courtesy of Michael A. Meenaghan, D.D.S., Ph.D., SUNY at Buffalo Dental School and Surface Science Center.)

nickel in stainless steel, but the most sensitive test is the leukocyte migration inhibition test (14).

Neoplastic transformation in bone surrounding an implant is most associated with the presence of cobalt in animal studies, and particularly when there is also infection or chronic inflammation. The reported human tumors including osteosarcomas and malignant fibrous histiocytomas are also correlated with cobalt alloys, infection, and inflammation as well as increased metal surface area (usually a function of porosity) and, in occasional reports, the use of stainless steel implants (17).

Biocompatibility can be considered to include local cellular and biochemical effects, regional, structural, and mechanical responses, and systemic effects. Improved performance of spine stabilization implants will probably utilize some aspects of biocompatibility to reduce the surgical trauma necessitated by the insertion of large implants and extensive bone grafting. Spine stabilization implants, such as pedicle screws, could be made as composite structures with a surface coating combining biocompatibility with fatigue resistance to permit more efficient transfer of loads to the implant and simultaneously reduce implant size. The macroscopic anatomic and biomechanical "fit" between screw and lumbar pedicles, as well as the optimal implant stiffness, and the local and systemic consequences of such an implant should be considered in its development.

Summary

Lumbar instability disorders have presented clinicians with difficulties in diagnosis and treatment. Pedicle fixation has permitted rigid segmental fixation in patients with defective or absent posterior elements. Since most pedicle screws are left in place after maturation of the bone fusion, the possibility of deriving long-term benefits from the stabilizing effects of the implant was proposed using the concept of osteointegration. The local and systemic consequences of prolonged metal exposure and the chemistry of biocompatibility and osteointegration was reviewed.

References

1. Albrektsson T, Branemark PI, Hansson HA, et al. The interface zone of inorganic implants in vivo: Titanium implants in bone. *Ann Biomed Eng.* 1983;11:1–27.
2. Albrektsson T, Branemark PI, Hansson HA, Lindstrom J. Osseointegrated titanium implants. Requirements for ensuring a long-lasting, direct bone-to-implant anchorage in man. *Acta Orthop Scand.* 1981;52:155–170.
3. Baier RE, Meyer AE. Aspects of bioadhesion. In: Lee L-H, ed. *Fundamentals of Adhesion.* New York: Plenum; 1991:407–425.
4. Baier RE, Meyer AE, Akers CK, Natiella JR, Meenaghan M, Carter JM.

Degradative effects of conventional steam sterilization on biomaterial surfaces. *Biomaterials.* 1982;3:241–245.
5. Baier RE, Meyer AE, Natiella JR, Natiella RR, Carter JM. Surface properties determine bioadhesive outcomes: Methods and results. *J Biomed Mater Res.* 1984;18:337–355.
6. Branemark PI, Hansson BO, Breine U, Lindstrom J, Hallen O. Osseointegrated implants in the treatment of edentulous jaw. Experience from a 10 year period. *Scand J Plast Reconstr Surg.* 1977;16(suppl):1–32.
7. Branemark PI, Zarb G, Albrektsson T. *Tissue Integrated Prosthesis: Osseointegration in Clinical Dentistry.* Chicago; Quintessence; 1985.
8. Goel VK, Lim TH, Gwon J, et al. Effects of rigidity of an internal fixation device: A comprehensive biomechanical investigation. *Spine.* 1991; 16(suppl):S155–S161.
9. Hansson HA, Albrektsson T, Branemark PE. Structural aspects of the interface between tissue and titanium implants. *J Prosthet Dent.* 1983;50:108–113.
10. Hartman LC, Meehaghan A, Schaaf NG, Hawker PB. Effects of pretreatment sterilization and cleaning methods on materials properties and osseoinductivity of a threaded implant. *Int J Oral Maxillofac Implants.* 1989;4:11–19.
11. Hayashi K, Matsuguchi N, Uenoyama K, Kanemaru T, Sugioka Y. Evaluation of metal implants coated with several types of ceramics as biomaterials. *J Biomed Mater Res.* 1989;23:1247–1259.
12. Kasemo B. Biocompatibility of titanium implants: Surface science aspects. *J Prosthet Dent.* 1983;49:832–837.
13. McAfee PC, Farey ID, Fracs BS, et al. Device-related osteoporosis with spinal instrumentation. *Spine.* 1989;14:919–926.
14. Merritt K, Brown SA. Hypersensitivity to metallic biomaterials. In: Williams DF, ed. *Systemic Aspects of Biocompatibility.* Boca Raton: CRC Press; 1981:33–48.
15. Parel SM, Holt GR, Branemark PI, Tjellstrom A. Osseointegration and facial prosthetics. *Int J Oral Maxillofac Implants.* 1989;1:27–29.
16. Singh S, Schaaf NG. Dynamic sterilization of titanium implants with ultraviolet light. *Int J Oral Maxillofac Implants.* 1989;4:139–146.
17. Sunderman FW. Recent advances in metal carcinogenesis. *Ann Clin Lab Sci.* 1984;14:93–122.
18. Tjellstrom A, Rosenhall U, Lindstrom J, Hallen O, Albrektsson T, Branemark PI. Five-year experience with skin-penetrating bone-anchored implants in the temporal bone. *Acta Otolaryngol.* 1983;95:568–575.

Discussion

Allergic Reactions to Implants

Dr. O'Leary inquired about the possible allergic reactions to implants and their treatment. Dr. Bennett responded that it depends on the type of allergic response one is seeing. If you are confronting anaphylaxis then treatment obviously consists of epinephrine and other medications. It is well known that patients with skin test positivity and it is even better known that those who have positive migration inhibiting factor (MIF) testing for sensitivity or increased risk of systemic symptoms usually will have minor skin symptoms from nickel-containing implants. Therefore, in patients where one is considering a nickel-bearing implant, particularly in women, it is wise to consider a test for sensitization. There is also a group of patients who are skin test negative and undergo placement of an implant, and a significant percentage become skin test positive without symptoms.

It is thought that cumulative exposure can eventually lead to an anaphylactic response and there is such a sensitization in dentists who have repeated exposure to metal implants.

Dr. Kostuik mentioned that some of the postoperative pain may be related to metal sensitivity. Dr. Bennett felt that there were so many other factors that might be implicated in spine pain that metal sensitivity would be less likely a cause. Dr. Kostuik added that there was the occasional case where it was felt that a mechanical problem was related to the implant and the implant was surgically removed, and the patients experienced a lasting improvement, not just from the effect of surgery.

Temporary versus Permanent Implants

Dr. Neuwirth stated that most of the research on the implant interface comes from prosthetic designing, either dental or orthopedic. Prostheses function quite differently from any of our spinal inplants. None of our spinal implants is meant to be a permanent or semipermanent replacement. At least not yet. With regard to the use of biologic fixation in spinal implants—since most of our implants really need work only a relatively short period of time—do you foresee a wide application with all its attendent problems such as toxicity or retrieval/removal, or do you think that biologic fixation will be devoted toward a more closely defined group of patients in which traditional fixation has had particularly difficult problems? The examples I would offer include sacral fixation and long fusions extending down to the sacrum. Dr. Bennett replied that it is difficult to conceptualize, but it has been shown that given appropriate loads in an optimum environment implants are capable of permanent load transfer characteristics. There is no question that this occurs. The problem is how to match the loading characteristics of the implant with the loading environment of the spine, which is complex. I would still imagine that a fusion would be part of the structure.

The Size of an Implant and its Potential Viability Without Bony Fusion

Dr. Bennett mentioned that if one wishes to downsize an implant, a smaller implant by virtue of enhanced load transfer might still get the job done and provide adequate stabilization. Also a more long-lasting implant might provide sufficient fixation to permit a stable surgical construct with less extensive soft tissue dissection and preparation and less native bone incorporation. I can make a massive fusion by stuffing an intervertebral disc space with large amounts of native bone; if one could design a smaller fusion construct and rely on the permanent stabilizing properties of an osteointegrating implant of small scale it might be possible to lessen the morbidity of a fusion such as the lumbar fusion.

Dr. Neuwirth commented: If you just use the example that you showed of the L5-S1 spondylolisthesis, if you do not perform a fusion, but just coat your screws and have a biologic integration at that level where you get rigid fixation of the screws, then your screw will fail or your plates or rods will fail. I think unless we conceptually change the way we treat these problems we are still going to have to achieve bony stability and not rely on the integration of the surface of the metallic implant.

Dr. Bennett added: I think the tissue healing response to surgery is very important, both in relation to the implant and in relation to the motion segments. I don't think one can take a position that all implants will predictably fail. Dr. Neuwirth said, I disagree.

Dr. Rydevik mentioned that osteointegration can achieve a permanent state of fixation to bone tissue, which is different from that seen with prosthetic fixation systems. However, with spine stabilization one would prefer to have temporary stabilization until healing has taken place. This is more like treating a fracture. I believe that though there may be some initial failures, once an integration has been achieved it will last for many years without deterioration. The interface is not only a matter of metal it is a matter of the bone, which is also the interacter.

Adverse Sequelae with Implants

Dr. Kostuik indicated that one of the big problems with metallic implants is postoperative imaging in situations such as the failed back syndrome. This is a very substantial problem nowadays, considering the pseudarthrosis rate. Conventional tomography and flexion-extension films are not useful in this situation. We must rely on computed tomography (CT) scanning to demonstrate failed fusions, and when there is metallic interference, even with the new techniques available at an institution such as Johns Hopkins, it is a difficult process.

Dr. Neuwirth added: At the Orthopedic Institute there has been some work of a preliminary nature, in the pediatric population, with bioabsorbable implants, and unfortunately they have not been strong enough even to withstand the smaller forces that they are subjected to in children. For example, the screw had to be quite a bit larger than the metallic screw to allow reasonable strength and then the screw holes became stress risers and they fractured. If one could devise an implant that was resorbable with time and could be associated with a biologic fixation, that would approximate our present aim.

Dr. Kostuik added: All the current materials including the sulfones are necessary in such large quantities in a procedure such as lumbar fusion that toxicity may become a very significant factor. It is not quite the same as putting in a plate and then if necessary, removing it.

II. CLINICAL ASPECTS OF INSTABILITY

A. BASIC CONCEPTS

CHAPTER 6

Spinal Stabilization: Is Fusion the Right Way?

Michael G. Neuwirth and Joseph Y. Margulies

This chapter discusses current concepts of spinal stabilization from the anatomic, biologic, and biomechanical point of view. Stability must be defined, understood, and referenced to the functional spinal unit. The functional spinal unit is defined as two adjacent vertebra with intervening soft tissues, disc, and articular structures that connect them (30). This functional unit must remain intact as it has forces applied to it creating various stresses and strains on its component. In order to maintain stability, its components move relative to each other. Each element in the construct has individual biomechanical and viscoelastic properties, but the unit as a whole has separate properties distinct from its component parts. Stability, therefore, may be defined as the ability of the functional spinal unit in which, under physiologic load, no abnormal strain or excessive motion occurs and the neural elements are protected. The proper word in this context should be equilibrium. Normal physiologic motion is part of the definition. When forces are excessive, the range of motion exceeds normal tolerance and instability results. Instability may be acute, such as in fractures or dislocations from a motor vehicle accident or chronic, such as the segmental lumbar instability that results with progressive degenerative disc and facet articular disease. It may produce pain, and it may result in neurologic injury. Scoliosis and kyphosis represent a specific type of instability with impairment of normal coronal and sagittal balance.

Appropriate treatment for spinal instability depends on a thorough understanding of the biologic, biomechanical, and anatomic elements that create stability. Orthopedists think of fusion as a solution to instability. This, however, implies either a less than complete understanding of what true stability is or an inability to repair it. True stability implies normal motion. Currently we can restore neither the ability of the functional spinal unit nor the spine in its entirety to function in its normal way. Fusion eliminates motion and therefore does not restore stability in the true sense of the word. Fusion protects the patient by eliminating motion, and by eliminating motion it may reduce pain and increase function.

Fusion is the common tool by which patients suffering from a variety of spinal problem are treated. Techniques of fusion have changed rapidly in the last 10 years with dramatic improvement in surgical and anesthetic techniques and material technology. For example, 12 to 15 years ago standard treatment of patients with idiopathic scoliosis involved a preoperative traction cast followed by internal fixation with one Harrington rod connected to the spine with two hooks. Postoperatively, these patients were maintained in plaster casts and/or braces for 6 to 9 months. Currently surgical treatment for idiopathic scoliosis use internal fixation with multiple rod systems that are fixed to multiple points on the spine with hooks, screws, or wires. Longitudinal rods are cross-linked for greater stability and the end result is that the patient is up and about within 2 to 3 days after surgery, requiring no external fixation as a rule (1,6).

Clearly, technology is much improved; however, conceptually there has been no change at all in treating spinal instability. In fact, the goal of treatment remains the same. Technically, we have made great strides that allow the patient a more efficient, less time-consuming treatment and an earlier return to function. But motion is sacrificed for stability.

Galen in ancient Rome proposed that one should not hang a patient with a cervical fracture upside down and shake him, which was a common treatment at the time, but rather recommended immobilization to secure healing. This, in fact, is no different conceptually from fusing a cervical spine fracture today.

A variety of conditions may be treated with fusion and these include fractures, tumors, deformities, and degenerative disc disease. The specific approach depends on the anatomy of the particular problem. If the bony elements are contiguous and intact, then posterior stabilization and fusion will suffice. In patients with a short life expectancy, stabilization alone without fusion is adequate (27,29). If there are large gaps of continuity such as those that may occur with tumors or burst fractures, then stable spacers are required. These spacers may be made from bone graft, cement, or metal. Complex problems often require circumferential fusion in order to achieve adequate stabilization.

Until recently, surgeons have dealt only with the bony elements in restoring spinal stability (10,25). Recent work in France on the repair of soft tissue disruptions and in this country and in Europe on disc replacement (14,32) may in the future come closer to the idea of restoring true spinal stability rather than just obtaining fusion.

Anatomically, the goal of fusion must be to preserve and if necessary restore normal coronal and sagittal alignment. Past failure to achieve this is evident in the common problem of iatrogenic and flat back (11,18). Clinically, with modern techniques of fixation we are better able to achieve the goal of proper spinal alignment (3). Biomechanically, there are several points of particular interest with regard to fusion.

First is the long-term effect of the fusion mass on adjacent unfused segments. Clearly the work of Cochran et al. (4) illustrates the deleterious effects of the long fusion in scoliosis down to L4. The effect of short fusion masses on the unfused spine and the role of an isolated or floating fusion in degenerative conditions of the back must be evaluated (24). The effect of combined anterior/posterior fusion on adjacent motion segments also needs to be evaluated since that seems to be a more common current solution to instability problems. Will longer fusions be better tolerated if proper spinal alignment is maintained?

A second, biomechanical question is the effect of rotation on spinal stability and the health of the adjacent unfused segments. Emphasis today is placed on derotational maneuvers in treating spinal deformity. The importance of this is unclear (8).

A third biomechanical question is the appropriate rigidity of a construct. We know from research in the application of rigid plates to long bones that these rigid plates result in stress shielding, which may result in impaired healing and excessive weakening of bone. This, of course, explains the current popularity of intramedullary fixation, which is a load-sharing device, as compared with plate fixation, which is load-sparing. The bone must share the load in order to remain healthy. Recent developments in spinal implant systems emphasize rigidity (16).

Is there an optimal stiffness for stabilization constructs and if so does it differ from patient to patient or from region to region in the spine? Stiffer is not necessarily better; recent works (28) address this question, but only in a preliminary fashion.

McAfee et al. (20), for example, have concluded that more rigid internal fixation constructs resulted in better fusion healing and did not result in significant stress shielding of the intervening vertebra.

Biodegradable fixation in spinal stabilization is another issue that requires specific attention. Biodegradable fixation is an important aspect of prosthesis design but its role in spinal stabilization, if any, is unclear. Spinal implants need work only until the fusion heals. This differs from a prosthesis, which must work indefinitely through the life of the patient. It is unclear whether biodegradable fixation will enhance our ability to stabilize the spine, and if so, what applications it may have. Removal of biodegradable fixed constructs may also be a problem.

The major biological question under active investigation at the present time is the problem of pseudarthrosis and what means are available to augment fusion. Efforts to augment bone healing are done through various approaches. There is some evidence to suggest that electrical and electromagnetic stimulation may improve the rate of bone healing in long bone fractures. There is also work that suggests that electrical and magnetic stimulation may increase the rate of the healing of spinal fusions (19,21).

Clearly, improving nutrition will help improve the healing rate for fusions. We note that patients who smoke (12) double the rate of failure of fusion and this probably relates to the tissue oxygen tension. Positive nitrogen balance allows soft tissues to heal and bony tissue must react the same way.

There is much current interest in the effect of bone graft on fusion healing. The gold standard of course is the iliac crest autograft. Allograft, however, can be obtained in a variety of forms; it may be in small pieces or solid. It may need only to provide material to increase fusion and it also may need to play a mechanical role in supporting the spine. There are also multiple types of allograft. These include fresh allograft, fresh frozen allograft, freeze-dried allograft, and chemically and gas sterilized and irradiated allograft (7,9,17,31). Clearly, using allograft introduces the risk to the patient of infection such as AIDS and this must be discussed preoperatively with all patients in whom allograft is a choice. The effectiveness of allograft in achieving fusion is variable.

There are differences in the type of allograft, as well as the specific problem to which it is being applied. These differences will affect success. Fresh allograft comes the closest to autograft in bone conduction and bone induction and this would appear to be the best (15,23). However, all forms of allograft induce a limited rejection response in the host. Antigenic manipulation that is necessary with tissue grafting such as kidney tranplants does not appear to be necessary for bone grafting.

Methods to increase the viability of allograft involve adding fresh autologous bone marrow to the allograft to increase its biologic potential (5). Autograft, although biologically the best bone graft, carries with it the liability of graft site morbidity, which may run as high as 7% in experienced hands (2). Current research also continues on the use of graft substitutes such as hydroxyapatite (13,22,26), which if successful, may eliminate the need for any biologic graft.

Summary

This chapter has addressed some of the biologic, anatomic, and biomechanical issues that relate to all fusions performed to treat spinal instability.

The goal of future research must be the restoration of normal function and not just eliminating motion to protect the spine. However, until that goal is achieved the current goal must be to increase the rate of fusion and to more reliably restore normal bony and neurologic anatomy through fusing as a short segment of the spine as possible.

References

1. Asher M, Carson W, Heinig C, Strippgen W, Arendt M, Lark R, Hartley M. A modular spinal rod linkage system to provide rotational stability. *Spine.* 1988;13:272–277.

2. Banwart J, Asher M. Is iliac crest donor site mobidity overstated? *6th Annual Meeting, North American Spine Society Proceedings*, 1991:228.
3. Bridwell KH, Betz R, Capell AM, Huss G, Harvey C. Sagittal plane analysis in idiopathic scoliosis patients treated with Cotrel-Dubousset instrumentation. *Spine.* 1990;15:644–659.
4. Cochran T, Irstam L, Nachemson A. Long-term anatomic and functional changes in patients with adolescent idiopathic acoliosis treated by Harrington rod fusion. *Spine.* 1983;8:576–584.
5. Connolly J, Guse R, Lipiello L, Dehne R. Development of an osteogenic bone marrow preparation. *J Bone Joint Surg.* 1989;71(A):684–691.
6. Cotrel Y, Dubousset J, Guillaumat M. New universal instrumentation in spinal surgery. *Clin Orthop.* 1988;227:12–23.
7. Dodd CA, Fergusson CM, Freedman L, Houghton GR, Thomas D. Allograft versus autograft bone in scoliosis surgery. *J Bone Joint Surg.* 1988;70B: 431–434.
8. Ecker AN, Betz RR, Trent PS, Trent AC. Computer tomography evaluation of Cotrel-Dubousset instrumentation in idiopathic scoliosis. *Spine.* 1988; 13:1141–1144.
9. Etaizeau JP, Czorny A, Miahle C, Kuhnast M, Prievot J. Use of vascularized bone grafts in surgery of the spine. Apropos of 6 cases. *Rev Chir Orthop.* 1989;75:166–171.
10. Graf H."Safir" commercial publication—personal communication.
11. Grobler LJ, MoE JH, Winter RB, Bradford DS, Lonstein LE. Loss of lumbar lordosis following surgical correction of thoracolumbar deformities. *Orthop Trans.* 1978;2:239.
12. Hanley EN, Levy JA. Surgical treatment of isthmic lumbosacral spondylolisthesis. *Spine.* 1989;14:45–50.
13. Heise U, Osborn JF, Duwe F. Hydroxyapatite ceramic as a bone substitute. *Int Orthop.* 1990;14:329–338.
14. Hellier WG, Hedman TP, Kostwik JP. Wear studies for a dynamic intervertebral disc prosthesis. *6th Annual Meeting, North American Spine Society Proceedings*, 1991:351.
15. Herron LD, Newman MN. The failure of ethylene oxide gas—sterlized freeze-dried bone graft for thoracic and lumbar spinal fusion. *Spine.* 1989;15:446–500.
16. Johnston CE, Ashman RB, Baird AM, Allard RN. Effects of spinal constructs stiffness on early fusion mass incorporated. *Spine.* 1990;15:408–912.
17. Knapp DR Jr, Jones ET. Use of cortical cancellous allograft for posterior spinal fusion. *Clin Orthop Rel Res.* 1988;229:99–106.
18. Kostuik JP, Maurais GR, Richardson WJ, Okajima Y. Combined single stage anterior and posterior osteotomy for corrections of iatrogenic lumbar kyphosis. *Spine.* 1988;13:257–266.
19. Lane WJ. Direct current electrical bone growth stimulations for spinal fusion. *Spine.* 1988;13:363–365.
20. McAfee PC, Farey ID, Sutterlin CE, Gurr KR, Warden KE, Cunningham BW. Device related osteoporosis with spinal instrumentation. *Spine.* 1989; 14:909–918.
21. Mooney V. A randomized double blind prospective study of the efficacy of

pulsed electromagnetic field for interbody lumbar fusion. *Spine*. 1990;15:708–717.
22. Nasca RJ, Lemons JE, Deinlein DA. Synthetic biomaterials for spinal fusion. *Orthopedics*. 1989;12:543–548.
23. Nasca RD, Whelchel JD. Use of cryopreserved bone in spinal surgery. *Spine*. 1987;12:222–227.
24. Brodsky AE, Hendricks RL, Khlil MA, Darden BV, Brotzman TT. Segmental ("floating") lumbar spine fusion. *Spine*. 1989;14:447–450.
25. Senegas J. Canal lombaire etroit. S.O.F.C.O.T. July 1989. *Rev Chir Orthop*. 1990;76(Suppl 10):59–67.
26. Senter HJ, Kortyna R, Kemp WR. Anterior cervical discectomy with hydroxyapatite fusion. *Neurosurgery*. 1989;25:39–42, 42–43.
27. Siegel T, Siegal T. Current consideration in the management of neoplastic spinal cord compression. *Spine*. 1989;17:223–228.
28. Smith KR, Hunty TR, Sher MA, Anderson HC, Robinson RG. A study of bone stress shielding in the canine lumbar spine *Orthop Trans*. 1990;14:17.
29. Thalgott JS, Gardner V, White J, Lowery G. Management of metastatic lesions of the spinal column with plate stabilization. *6th Annual Meeting, North American Spine Society Proceedings*, 1991:256.
30. White AA, Panjabi MM. *Clinical Biomechanics of the Spine*. 2nd ed. New York: JB Lippincott; 1990:6.
31. Wittenberg RH, Moeller J, Shea M, White AA 3d, Hayes WC. Compressive strength of autologous and allogenous bone grafts for thoracolumbar and cervical spine fusion. *Spine*. 1990;15:1073-B.
32. Zippel H, Schellnack, K Buttner K. Exchanging intervertebral disks. The concept and clinical experience using a cement-free intervertebral disk endoprosthesis of the "Charitie Modular SB." *Chir Narzadow Ruchu Ortop Pol*. 1986;51:245–248.

Discussion

The Concept of Restoring Proper Spinal Stability

This is a reiteration of what has been stated in the text, namely, that the restoration of true stability requires the repair of all damaged elements in a spinal segment—the ligaments, the damaged disc, and the damaged facet joints—such that normal motion and the capability of that joint segment to withstand normal stresses is assured. The term *internal fixation* implies ankylosis and is used to restore normal coronal and sagittal alignment. *Fusion* implies the creation of a bony union, but it does not restore stability in the full and true sense of the word. It protects the patient by eliminating motion and by eliminating motion it may reduce pain and increase function. However, it does not restore the stability of the intact spine.

Dr. Kostuik added that there are a few centers in France working on the problem of restoring stability through ligamentous replacements in the spine. This is controversial, but we should keep an open mind because that it may restore stability for a sufficient period of time to allow a patient to overcome that phase of healing during which there is significant pain.

Some Long-Term Data on Fusions

Dr. Kostuik noted that before the advent of rigid internal fixation the best study that was available on long-term effects came from the University of Iowa (Weinstein et al. Lumbar disc herniation, a comparison of the results of chemonucleolysis and open discectomy after 10 years, *J.B.J.S.* (PM). 1986;68(1):43–54) in which 30 years later 35% of people demonstrated radiological instability, 50% were taking some form of analgesic medication, and 15% carried the diagnosis of spinal stenosis. On the other hand, 85% of the patients were happy with their result. Of course this does not take into account random demographics.

Those procedures were simple posterior fusions. We now know that posterior fusions biomechanically had more motion, specifically *micromotion*, than intertransverse fusions, which was why intertransverse fusions were developed in the first place. Anterior fusions had the least motion of all. These are my contentions and when I lecture on the subject I mention that in a primary case one should not perform a 360° fusion. Dr. Bennett interjected: By a 360° fusion do you mean a combination of interbody and intertransverse or do you also include the posterior elements? Dr. Kostuik responded: No, posterior fusion plus anterior fusion. It does not matter what type of posterior fusion. Dr. Bennett continued: My experience with patients who have axial instability and high axial loads, typically big active males, is that they do much better acutely with a combination of interbody and intertransverse fusions accompanied by pedicle fixation and compression lock-in grafts.

Dr. Kostuik responded: Yes, I think you may well be right, except I don't think you are looking at the long-term problems. Dr. Bennett continued: I have one more question. Are most of your 360° fusions more than one level? Dr. Kostuik replied that most of them are two-level fusions.

Internal Fixation in Lumbar Fusions

Dr. McCormick asked if Dr. Neuwirth was using internal fixation in all of the lumbar fusions. Dr. Neuwirth responded: Yes, I use internal fixation in most cases except the occasional isolated lumbosacral fusion in a young healthy adult who can tolerate external fixation with a thoralolumbosacral orthoses (TLSO). I do not use internal fixation in children for spondylolisthesis. Overall, I would say that 90% of my cases involve internal fixation.

Dr. McCormick continued: Do you have any sense of changing your fusion rates now that you have gone to internal fixation as compared to when you were not using it as frequently? Dr. Neuwirth responded: It is hard to evaluate on the basis of my personal series since I believe that the cases I tend to see now are different than they were 5 years ago.

CHAPTER 7

The Diagnosis and Treatment of Instability in Collapsing Degenerative Lumbar Scoliosis

Arthur H. White, James B. Reynolds, and Joseph Grant

When there is gross instability that is measurable on x-rays and that creates obvious neurological damage and pain at a single level, the diagnosis and treatment are quite simple and clear. These are cases usually of spondylolisthesis, degenerative instability, or iatrogenic postoperative instability. Stabilizing one such unstable level with any type of fusion will readily give relief in the vast majority of cases.

Grades III and IV spondylolisthesis offer no diagnostic difficulty, but present the spine surgeon with a surgical challenge that usually requires anterior and posterior surgery in order to achieve success.

In our opinion the greatest challenge in spine surgery today is collapsing degenerative scoliosis. Although vertebral alignment is clearly disruptive in this condition, the purest definition of instability is not met. That is, there is not usually measurable hypermobility of any one segment. Why is there then any instability problem? The answer is that there is progressive malalignment, which causes deformity, nerve damage, and pain.

Of even greater interest to the student of instability is the challenge of surgical treatment. The surgeon who is unaware of instability in this condition will focus upon the obvious stenosis and proceed with a decompressive laminectomy and foraminotomy. Only then does the unsuspecting spine surgeon recognize the dangerous instability problem that this condition presents as he observes the open passage ways that he produced rapidly restenosing because of instability.

With our aging population and our improved tools to diagnosis and treat more simple low back problems, we are seeing an ever-growing number of patients with instability caused by collapsing degenerative scoliosis. There is very little in the literature on this subject. The following is our current experience with the condition and our current mode of treatment. Through this chapter, we would like to stimulate interest, research, and the development of multicenter studies on this complex instability problem.

Degenerative scoliosis occurs in the older age group and although it can start under the age of 60, it usually does not become symptomatic until beyond the age of 60. It can occur from a symmetric collapse of the disc space or it may be the progression of a standard type of curve.

Initially, there is usually not a great deal of reaction, but rotation rapidly becomes an important component of this scoliosis. Frequently, the L3-4 level is the level that is most involved.

A relative kyphosis also develops. There is frequently a great deal of disc space collapse and, for this reason, the loss of height in the anterior portion of the spine causes a relative kyphosis in the lumbar spine with a loss of the normal lordotic curve. Frequently, there will also be an element of anterior olisthesis of one vertebra or the other that is a degenerative spondylolisthesis. The pars, in this condition, remains intact. The signs of both degenerative scoliosis and degenerative spondylolisthesis are signs that this particular spine is quite unstable.

Central and foraminal stenoses are a common component of degenerative scoliosis. The asymmetric loading of the facets cause facet hypertrophy. The degeneration of the disc itself contributes to the narrowing of the spinal canal and there is a frequent occurrence of degenerative spondylolisthesis, all of which add to foraminal and central canal narrowing. The majority of these patients are female, so there is always a component of osteoporosis involved with these patients. The osteoporosis, at times, can be very severe.

The symptoms, as with all back problems, range from back pain to sciatica to pseudoclaudication. The initial care of these patients is much like other back problems. Backache and fatigue are common complaints. The patient may be comfortable at rest, but progressively have more pain and fatigue in the back as the length of time increases that the patient has been up. These patients can be improved by nonoperative care, e.g., physical therapy such as traction, ice, massage, and mobilization.

For those people who do not improve with physical therapy, a corset may be of some value and seems to be of more value in this condition than in most other back problems. Rarely, a Boston brace can be required.

People over the age of 60 do not like to wear Boston braces because they are cumbersome, difficult to apply, and very restrictive, but if they do give sufficient relief, they can be worn part-time or even full-time. The standard Boston brace is a rear-entry brace. It opens in the back and has straps that hook in the back. For these patients at this age, it is very difficult for them to utilize this type of brace. Boston braces are made that are front-opening and this is the type that should be ordered for this population. Epidurals and selective nerve root blocks are of great value in these patients. Because they are not particularly active, they will frequently get long-term relief from these epidurals. As with all epidurals, corticosteroids should be limited in their use. We would not advise a series of three epidurals. In this population, we would us them once every 3 to 4 months. Initially, two could be used, but on a long-term basis, every 3 to 4 months should be the maximum amount these patients are allowed because of the amount of corticosteroids.

Stabilization Training

Collapsing degenerative lumbar scoliosis is a progressive disease and a dynamic disorder. There are, therefore, personal and environmental factors that can aggravate the condition and those that can prevent or slow the development of the condition and symptoms. Factors that aggravate or hasten the development of the dynamic stenosis are obesity, weakness, spinal trauma (micro or macro), postural neglect, and disease processes such as arthritis affecting other joints like the knees and hips, which have a protective function for the spine.

Factors that prevent or slow down collapsing degenerative scoliosis are strength, lower extremity flexibility, and postural and body mechanics training.

Theoretically, if instability is the cause of symptoms, then the opposite of instability, stability, should prevent or decrease symptoms. We have, therefore, developed over the years a training program that promotes spinal stability, which we have termed stabilization training. Stabilization training works extremely well for younger individuals with spinal instability. Most patients with collapsing degenerative scoliosis are elderly and more difficult to train. We currently have patients with this condition who are as young as 53 and in extremely good physical condition. Every patient deserves an attempt at aggressive conservative care that includes education and exercise even when surgery is successful in relieving current signs and symptoms of instability. The natural history of collapsing degenerative scoliosis is progressive deformity and instability. There are almost always vertebral levels more proximal in the spine that demonstrate a precarious level of degenerative change. These levels need protection. Stabilization training is a superb tool for such protection.

Definition

After working with thousands of patients and many therapists of various backgrounds and training, we would define stabilization training as follows: A patient is trained to move his or her spine is such a way as to find the least painful position. The spine is then held in that "neutral" position while performing ever-increasing tasks. A simpler definition might be that stabilization means bracing, holding, or fusing a diseased and painful spinal segment in a pain-free, balanced, or neutral position through the sole use of voluntary musculature.

The simplest form of stabilization is abdominal bracing. The voluntary tightening of the abdominal muscles and the additional bracing of the diaphragm to increase intra-abdominal pressure has been known for decades to give support to the spine. This is a technique used in preventing spinal fracture in ski jumping and in pulling out of rapid dives in jet planes. We have all used such abdominal bracing when receiving blows during contact sports. With such abdominal bracing, the spine is not necessarily placed in any predetermined position. It is simply supported in whatever position it happens to be in at the time of the muscular diaphragmatic contraction.

Stabilization includes the practice of abdominal bracing. Before bracing, align the spine in a neutral position. This known or preconceived position can be determined strictly on the basis of pathological diagnosis. At other times the position is found and learned through the experience of pain. Since so many painful spinal conditions do not create pain at the time of change of position, it can sometimes take many hours, days, and even weeks to determine where the position of neutral balance is for a diseased segment. This may require doing a specific exercise program with the spine held in one position of flexion or extension, and then following the patient for 24 hours clinically to see whether or not that particular exercise program has had any ill effects on the patient. Of course, all other aspects of the patient's life and activity have to be controlled during such evaluation.

Technique

There is no one perfect technique for teaching individuals how to stabilize. The technique may depend upon the specific diagnosis, the coordination of the patient, the past experience of a patient with regard to athletic endeavors, and many other factors. For example, patients who have been highly trained in the martial arts will find that the concepts taught in stabilization come quite easily. Other individuals who have primitive or detrimental movement patterns may never be able to accomplish satisfactory levels of stabilization training. A short period of testing of an individual can determine which level of stabilization training a patient should enter, which could be anywhere from lying down to running.

An average patient with a disc problem but no significant neurological loss would begin stabilization training lying supine. Tightening the abdominal musculature is first practiced with the use of partial sit-up exercises, setting the diaphragm and learning to breathe while doing so. Various forms of pelvic tilt are practiced until a comfortable position of spinal pelvic alignment is obtained. A maximum level of pelvic tilt flattens the lumbar spine firmly against the surface on which the patient is lying. A hand can be placed behind the lumbar lordosis to ensure maximum forceful flattening. Some patients will need maximum lordosis for comfort. Once the optimum position is achieved, the abdominal musculature is contracted and the diaphragm is braced. Motion of the extremities can then begin, first by lifting one extremity at a time slowly as the therapist verifies the patient's ability to maintain the stabilized neutral position while doing so. The extremities are then raised faster and alternately until the patient is doing a bicycling motion with the legs at the same time as a waving motion of the arms from side to side and overhead. This is called a dying bug exercise because it looks like a bug expiring on its back with its legs waving. It is again necessary to stress that there should be no pain, and the patient should show no evidence of spinal motion. This can be accentuated by balancing a stick horizontally across the patient's abdomen or chest, or by placing a hand behind the patient's back with a finger in each interspinous space to feel for any motion that is occuring.

Stabilization training can also be done with the patient lying prone. This is slightly more difficult than lying supine for most patients. While lying prone the patient is asked to alternately raise one extremity, and then the other, and then two simultaneously. It is easier to observe the patient's spine for motion in this position.

The next logical progression from the prone position is that of kneeling. A patient kneels, finds the neutral, balanced, pain-free position with a cat-like rounding of the back and then relaxing into lordosis (the hump-sag exercises). Once the neutral, balanced, pain-free position is found in this kneeling position, the patient then practices raising one extremity, then another, and eventually two extremities without having pain or having any motion of the spine. Again, a good test to determine if pelvic stability is being maintained is to have the patient balance a stick horizontally across his or her back while watching in the mirror to see if the stick wavers or falls off.

There are numerous varieties of floor exercises with gym balls, large air-filled rubber balls that can be used for balancing the legs upon as the patient lies supine in a hip- and knee-flexed position (90/90°). The ball creates less stability than the floor and requires greater strength and stabilization control to avoid spinal motion. Stabilization can next be carried into the standing position. In standing stabilization, mirrors are extremely valuable for permitting patients to watch themselves as they find their neutral position. They may use a wall to back up against when they first attempt to find their neutral stabilized position. They then move away from the wall and begin moving one extremity after another, leading eventually to standing on one foot, perhaps even with a weight in one hand.

Increasing degrees of force to attempt to offset the patient's stability are then introduced. This includes such things as jousting between patient partners. Two patients face each other and grasp a stick or baton that is mutually held between them. They then try to force each other off center. This is somewhat akin to Little John fighting Robin Hood on the bridge with his staff. Instead of striking, however, the opponents simply slowly exert displacing forces, under the direction and supervision of a therapist. The therapist assesses each individual's stabilizing capabilities as the patients joust.

As a patient's physical demands increase in activities of heavy labor and contact sports, the stabilization training needs to be increasingly aggressive. Until this point in the training, the stabilization has been relatively impractical. The things that they have been doing are rarely applicable to daily activities. At this point in training, patients need to move about more freely and actively as they do in their daily lives. This can include such activities as walking rapidly with weights in their hands while maintaining stabilization. It can be done on a treadmill at first so that the therapist can easily test and verify good stabilization techniques.

Once verified, patients are allowed to take long walks on their own, remaining pain-free and testing their endurance for up to hours of walking stabilization. Low-impact aerobics and dancing programs can be done utilizing stabilization techniques under more enjoyable and aerobic circumstances. Jogging can be practiced on a treadmill with stabilization, and them practiced daily by the patient. This is a whole new way to jog. It is difficult to breath while tightening the abdominal musculature. The impact of the foot hitting the ground produces vibration through the leg and pelvis into the spine. This vibration is cushioned by stabilization of the spine, not only with the abdominal musculature, but also with the use of greater amounts of knee flexion and more use of the quadriceps and hamstring muscles to cushion part of the vibration on the spine.

Contact sports require patients to receive blows from other individuals. This frequently entails unexpected trauma or very short warning to allow preparation to receive a blow. Through practice, therefore, the patient must learn to stabilize rapidly and then receive blows of increasing intensity. We have developed training for professional athletes in competitive sports by having them train in martial arts. Martial artists, of course, have dealt with blow, trauma, an human interaction for centuries. Very specific techniques in different schools have been developed and honed to a very fine training program.

There is no activity simulation program better than the required activity itself. If a patient is a baseball player at second base, there is no better place to train than at second base. All of the required positions and motions are analyzed for efficiency, stabilization, and energy conservation. The required changes are taught and practiced until they virtually become a natural reflex for the patient. They may require jumping, falling, rolling, throwing, catching, or kicking.

It is amazing to us, and probably the crux of all low back pain problems, that many athletes and physically highly accomplished individuals are seemingly untrainable, with habit patterns of movement that lead to injury after injury. Perfect body mechanics are not a requirement for superb athletic performance. We have known for years that teaching patterns of movement and posture can greatly improve athletic and artistic prowess. Similarly, the martial arts can advance individuals from a brown belt to a black belt, for example, by demonstrating more and more perfect movement, posture, and body mechanics. There is no end to the training that we can do in posture, strength, body mechanics, and, now, stabilization.

Mental Stabilization

Simply to use stabilization exercises and expect a patient to become pain-free and normally active is not to take advantage of one of the biggest tools that we have in health care: the human brain. We can program the brain to help us accomplish any task in a more rapid fashion. It has been widely demonstrated that mental imaging and mental programming allow athletes to accomplish much greater feats of strength and coordination.

Some spinal practitioners have stated for years that the only training that is necessary to prevent and control back pain is an awareness of the back. They simply tell their patients, "think back" before they take on any task that may lead even remotely to back pain. This simple type of awareness conceivably puts an individual in a better position of preparedness for doing a physical activity. Even getting out of bed can be traumatic to a degenerative spine. An individual who is aware of the back problem before getting out bed is more likely to more slightly differently, to tighten the abdominal muscles and "reflexly" protect the spine without conscious attention and without having to take an extensive training program in stabilization.

Stabilization Education

Patients undergoing stabilization training generally have had basic back school. They are in stabilization training in order to accomplish higher levels of activity than they have been able to do previously, given their underlying pathological conditions. They want to be able to move more freely, more rapidly, and in a way that they might consider "normal." Their education, therefore, needs to constitute considerably more than helpful hints and first aid. They should have already been doing abdominal, gluteal, and quadriceps exercises for months. They should have made changes in their environment by altering their seats, workstations, and home environment.

Education for stabilization training, therefore, begins with motivation and theory. Patients already understand at their level of capability the underlying disease process that is creating their pain. It is explained that this underlying diseased spinal segment or other process can ensure voluntary efforts in a position of comfort and noninjury. Patients already know that there are times when they can be pain-free and can find positions of comfort. It is easy from there for the patients to understand that if they can maintain the diseased spine in the position of comfort (neutral position) they can increase physical activities if they are strong enough and coordinated enough to maintain that neutral position. When patients see some of the physical and coordinated feats that human beings are able to accomplish in athletics and acrobatics, it quickly becomes clear to them that it is simply a matter of practice, time, and strengthening to maintain spinal positioning and alignment.

Exaggeration is sometimes helpful in demonstration and motivation. For example, a clinician can demonstrate to a patient in the examining room that he or she can bend laterally to fully 45° and still run around in circles maintaining the neutral position. Similarly, patients can see that if they have a rock in their shoe under the heel that they could, if necessary, walk for miles on their toes without putting pressure on the rock. When these types of examples are extrapolated to spinal positioning and maintenance of stabilization, the patient can at least understand the theory. Additional motivation is accomplished by getting patients to express what they are willing to do to regain normalcy in life activities. Patients frequently make statements such as, "I would do anything to be able to golf again," or "Surgery is such a frightening thing to me that if there is anything also known to medical science, I will do it." The clinician can quickly capitalize on these statements by countering with, "There is something you can do, but it won't be easy," or "How hard are you willing to work?" or "There is no limit to how strong you can get, how coordinated you can get, and how well you can balance your diseased spine."

If the patient still does not understand the condition, the principles to be used, and the theory of stabilization, then demonstrations are in order. It may take a few sessions to get a patient to feel that he is accomplishing what has been described.

Some therapists prefer to simply train patients and let them gain the understanding and feeling for stabilization in the process. The process can go much more quickly with informed and highly motivated patients. Simply doing the stabilization training for an hour a day and spending the other 23 hours in nontraining will take much longer, cost more money, and be much less successful than working with a knowledgeable, well-motivated patient who will attempt to use the basic principles 24 hours per day. Occasional sessions with a therapist to problem-solve and learn new techniques will permit advancement rapidly to higher levels of stabilization.

A quick demonstration by the clinician of one of the stabilization, t'ai chi, or yoga positions, which are somewhat difficult to achieve for the average person, can serve as a good example to the patient of what can be achieved and will challenge some patients to perform. The patient can then be asked to achieve the same position, such as a one-legged, straight back stance. Most patients will not be able to achieve this position. If they can, they have high stabilization potential. After just a few tries, they find they are able to do it better and better, and begin already to understand the principles, theory, and challenge.

Surgery

The operative treatment of stenosis patients with degenerative scoliosis is far less successful as compared to similar patients without degenerative scoliosis. Decompression and stability both must be carefully considered. Because of the asymmetric pressures that occur at the facet levels, facet arthrosis and hypertrophy occur. This, in combination with other factors, will lead to both central and foraminal stenosis. When considering surgery on these patients, it is very important to isolate the source of the pain. Degenerative discs, arthritic facets, and stenosis, be it central or foraminal, can all be a source of pain. Various diagnostic blocks including discograms, selective nerve root blocks, and facet injections all can help in selecting those areas that are the most symptomatic and where surgery is most likely to relieve the patient's symptoms.

Any symptoms should have at least an 80% relief from either facet injections or selective nerve root blocks or epidurals to be considered as a good prognostic sign for surgery. Electrodiagnostic testing can be helpful. Electromyograms (EMGs) are helpful in the lower lumbar spine with L4, L5, and S1. EMGs are particularly sensitive for L5 and S1 lesions. They frequently will detect L4 lesions. Somatosensory evoked potentials (SSEPs) are helpful for the upper lumbar regions including L4. They also can be used for the upper lumbar regions including L4. They also can be used for L5 and S1. Computed tomography (CT) with sagittal reformations usually are much more helpful in this condition than magnetic resonance imaging (MRI). The sagittal reformations will yield bony details, and this is usually stenosis that arises from either osteophytes originating from the vertebral end plates or from the facets themselves. MRI is not nearly as accurate in detecting the exact dimensions of the foramen. Much of the surgical planning should be based on CT. The CT must have multiplanar reformations in order to be accurate and helpful in planning the surgical procedures.

Plain films are extremely valuable. These must be taken with the patient in the upright position. Most radiologists prefer to take their films with the patient lying down, but for an orthopedist particularly planning a surgical procedure involving scoliosis, the upright position is absolutely necessary.

In reviewing the plain films, there are several points that are of interest. Osteophytes are important as a stabilizing factor in this condition.

Those patients who have osteophytes are much more likely to do well than those patients without osteophytes, but simply narrowed and degenerative discs.

Translation, or rotatory translation, is of critical importance. L3-4 will frequently have a lateral translation into the convex side of the curve. This usually forebodes instability. In addition, an anterior olisthesis is a very poor prognostic sign.

Bending films, both flexion, extension, and side-bending, are important. When looking at bending films, it is important to see if the motion is present throughout the curve or if there is one isolated level that has the most motion occurring. It is important to look for the amount of lateral translation, the amount of forward translation, and the amount of wedging, both in the anteroposterior (AP) and lateral, that occur at each disc space. If the curve is very stable and there is very little motion present, this is a good prognostic sign. If there is motion present of more than a few degrees, then fusion must be considered. If fusion is considered, then the levels to be fused and whether instrumentation is used are all important decisions that will need to be made. The amount of stability found at the time of surgery can also help in deciding the levels to fuse.

At times, in order to decompress the foramen adequately, it is necessary to remove the facet or to remove the entire pedicle. If a pedicle is removed, you are destabilizing not only the level where the foraminotomy is being performed, but also the level above it.

The other factor that must be considered when you are considering fusion and instrumentation is the degree of osteoporosis. A severe degree of osteoporosis precludes considering any instrumentation. Moderate osteoporosis will make your fixation less rigid. It may be necessary to place your pedicle screws through the anterior portion of the vertebral body for better purchase. There is some risk to vascular structures when penetrating the anterior cortex of the vertebral body.

Instrumentation in these older patients has a very high incidence of infection. It is very difficult to do Steffee instrumentation on these patients because of the curve. Wiltse instrumentation is very adaptable to this situation and can easily be made to conform to these curves. The Luque system of plate fixation is much like the Steffee system, but not as rigid. It is just as difficult to use in this situation. The Cotrel-Dubousset (CD) can be used, but it is difficult to implant in the lumbar spine and has loosening problems that occur because of the small contact point between the lock nut and rod.

Summary

Collapsing degenerative spondylolisthesis is an instability problem that must be recognized and not treated as routine spinal stenosis. One should not try to surgically correct all areas of visible pathology, i.e., scoliosis, stenosis, bulging discs, and displaced vertebrae. Thorough diagnostic testing can lead to an accurate determination of the pain generator.

Surgery on elderly individuals with this condition is fraught with complications. Exhaust all conservative measures before considering surgery and accept a reasonable amount of disability.

If surgery is going to be performed, accurately localize the pain generator and try to determine the current and potential degree of instability. Make your final assessment regarding fusion at the time of surgery after decompression has been accomplished and stability has been manually tested.

Limit the type and extent of fusion to fit the condition. Do not try to choose all scoliotic curvatures or all displaced vertebrae. These patients are usually elderly with osteoporosis and do not fuse well or maintain internal fixation well.

Decompression to adequately relieve stenosis in these patients frequently requires total facetectomy and significant destabilization. This may leave inadequate area to accomplish a posterior lateral fusion. In such cases, an interbody fusion may be necessary to prevent recurrent symptoms from instability.

We have not found any single criterion that helps us consistently predict a successful outcome of surgery. There is a slight but not statistically significant reason to consider fusion when there is hypermobility on bending films, a vacuum phenomenon, and major degrees of lateral translation. The only statistically significant finding that has been found to correlate with surgical failure is a lower compensatory curve of L5 greater than 10°.

At first thought, one would consider a fusion even with internal fixation when there was a high risk of failure due to several of the above criteria. Fusions, however, especially with internal fixation carry a high degree of complication especially in these elderly, osteoporotic debilitated individuals. Infection rates as high as 8% and internal fixation failures as high as 20% have been reported in the literature. Such morbidity should give the surgeon pause in his decision as to whether to do a fusion with internal fixation.

Another interesting and as yet unstudied alternative may be extensive decompression without fusion. This frequently requires total facetectomy and even total excision of the pedicle on the concave side of the L5 compensatory curve. Superficial biomechanics would lead one to believe that such extensive decompression would so greatly destabilize the L5 segment that further curvature and lateral translation would be inevitable. This is not always the case. These segments when tested at surgery or with bending films are not generally hypermobile and frequently are quite stiff. We have successfully decompressed these cases extensively without fusion and experienced no further instability or slip. Aside from the compensatory curve being greater than 10°, we do not have good predictors for this possibility. We have also, surprisingly, not experienced "breakdown" at the level above a fusion. Because of the great morbidity in this group, we do not recommend trying to fuse the entire primary curvature, which frequently extends through the entire lumbar spine. It is usually only the lower one or two levels (L4-5, L5-S1) that are the primary cause of pain and disability. Occasionally, the L3 level will also be involved.

Bibliography

Benner B, Ehni G. Degenerative lumbar scoliosis. *Spine*. 1979;4:548–552.

Briad JL, Jegon D, Cauchoix J. Adult lumbar scoliosis. *Spine*. 1979;4:526–532.

Epstein JA, Epstein BS, Jones MD. Symptomatic lumbar scoliosis with degenerative changes in the elderly. *Spine*. 1979;4:542–547.

Grubb SA, Lipscomb HJ, Coonrad RW. Degenerative adult onset scoliosis. *Spine*. 1988;13(3):241–245.

Sano S, Yokokura S, Nagata Y, et al. Unstable lumbar spine without hypermobility in postlaminectomy cases: Mechanism of symptoms and effect of spinal fusion with and without spinal instrumentation. *Spine*. 1990;15(11):1190–1197.

Discussion

Collapsing Degenerative Scoliosis: Its Nature and Whether it Should be Surgically Corrected

Dr. Neuwirth began with a question about degenerative scoliosis. It seems that the series presented by Dr. White had fairly small spinal curves, not average. One case presented had a curve larger than the series suggested. I do not routinely take erect films on all these patients to make a diagnosis of scoliosis. My first question is, Are your x-ray films supine or erect? And my second question relates to whether a patient with a 12° degenerative scoliosis with back and leg pain and elements of central and foraminal stenosis and degenerative disc disease is really any different from the patient with a smaller degree of deformity?

Dr. Kostuik interjected and asked if he might answer that question. The answer is absolutely no. Measurement errors are 7°. I do not think that degenerative scoliosis is any different from a degenerative spine that appears straight in an x-ray. I believe that the business of degenerative scoliosis is overtalked about and overrated. It is not scoliosis you are treating. Dr. White pointed that out because he did not do long extensive fusions in those people. He dealt with the local problem.

Dr. White said: It is an instability problem. Dr. Kostuik continued: Sure it is an instability problem. Sure, they collapse on one side more than the other. One of the last things I am going to do in my career is to get rid of the terminology "degenerative scoliosis."

Dr. Neuwirth inquired: At what point does the curve become important? Dr. Kostuik responded: I don't think the curve ever becomes important in adult life because you can have curves of 100° and the patients may not have any pain. The main question becomes if in adulthood a patient has a deformity you will deal with the patients symptoms primarily, not the deformity. If patients wish to have an extra benefit because they don't like the imbalance of a 50° imbalanced lumbar curve, the surgeon can offer to correct that imbalance, but certainly not for a 20° curve.

Dr. Neuwirth agreed: No, not a curve of 20°, but if you isolate some cases of adult degenerative disc disease, you may clearly find some types of pain that are related to the size of the curve, its degree of rotation, and so forth. If their functional complaint is pain I think it does become necessary to correct the curve, although not absolutely in the cases we have seen here.

Dr. Kostuik said: I don't agree with having to correct degenerative curves, but various orthopedists are doing just that particularly in North Carolina and Cleveland, Ohio.

Dr. Neuwirth continued: What about the case of a woman who has a 50° lumbar curve and functions perfectly well? Dr. Kostuik responded: That is not degenerative scoliosis. Dr. Neuwirth agreed that it is not a degenerative scoliosis, but she and others present in adulthood with a scoliotic curve that has progressed and is painful. I believe that a portion of the painful symptomatology in some of those patients may be related to the curve itself. Dr. Kostuik concurred, saying: Sure, because the curve has progressed. The best way to assess that is to ask the patients what their height was when they were about 20. If they have lost two inches the curve has progressed. Dr. O'Leary commented that you cannot discount the fact that degenerative scoliosis is a reality. Dr. Kostuik said: Certainly it is a realilty, but you are looking at an x-ray. Dr. O'Leary added that if there is a progression of the curve from 20° to 45° over a 1- to 2-year period, then what is your terminology? Dr. Kostuik replied: That is not a degenerative scoliosis. That is an idiopathic curve that developed degenerative changes on top. Dr. O'Leary continued: Suppose you see a 50-year-old patient with a scoliotic curve measuring 15° to 20° and he returns after 5 years with a 45° curve, what is occurring? Dr. Kostuik said: I suspect that that patient always had a thoracolumbar or lumbar curve since adolescence. On the other hand, if you see a patient whose spine is straight at the age of 60 and at 65 he has a curve of 45°, I don't specifically have a term for that; is that degenerative? I don't know. My definition of *degenerative scoliosis* is an unstable spine due to asymmetric changes or asymmetric loading or a failure of the elements on one side to a greater extent than the other. We don't really know the cause of real scoliosis. In terms of pain the patients will have problems more commonly on the concave side or in the compensatory curve, but they can also get root problems on the convexity, particularly if they have a prefixed root coming very tightly around the pedicle as opposed to the more common emergence of the root from the dura at a 50° angle.

CHAPTER 8

Vertebral Injury and Instability

Sanford J. Larson

A number of classifications have been proposed for vertebral injury. Some have been based on the radiographic appearance, using terms such as burst, wedge, teardrop, and fracture dislocation. Eponyms have been used, as for example Jefferson or Chance, and others have been based on the mechanism of injury. Reliable communication of information is a major reason for a classification system. Terms such as burst, which mean different things to different people, or fracture dislocation, which can cover a wide variety of injury, or eponyms, which may not be universally recognized, have obvious disadvantages. Classification employing accepted anatomical terms and based on the mechanism of injury (3,9,10,12) has definite advantages in this regard.

The mechanism of injury also has a considerable influence on the stability of the injured vertebral column. Different methods have been developed to define stability, some of which include neurological deficit as a factor. Although neurological deficit may be an indication for surgical treatment, it does not affect the mechanical properties of the vertebral column and therefore is irrelevant to a definition of stability. A stable vertebral injury can be defined as one in which progression of deformity should not occur unless a load is applied greater than that which produced the original injury. Conversely, in an unstable injury progression of deformity can be anticipated under physiological loads. Holdsworth (4) emphasized the importance of the posterior ligamentous complex and related bony structures in the maintenance of stability, and his views have been supported by the observations of others (5,7–9). This view has been criticized (2) on the basis of laboratory experiments, which have demonstrated that division of the posterior ligamentous complex is not followed by instability. This criticism, however, equates cutting with tearing. If the posterior ligamentous complex is cut, the posterior longitudinal ligament, the intervertebral disc, and the anterior longitudinal ligament remain intact. However, if the supraspinous and intraspinous ligaments are torn sufficiently to allow significant separation of the spinous processes, then the joint capsules, the posterior longitudinal ligament, and at least a portion of the disc or vertebral body must necessarily be involved in the same process, and progressive deformity can be anticipated. Disruption of the posterior ligamentous complex by flexion cannot occur without concomitant injury to the vertebral body or intervertebral disc, nor can disruption of the disc by extension occur without injury to the posterior elements. On the other hand, the vertebral body can be extensively injured while the posterior elements remain intact, and progression of deformity should not occur under ordinary circumstances (4–9,13,14).

In vertebral injury, the most common deforming forces can be categorized as axial compression, axial distraction, flexion, flexion compression, flexion distraction, extension, rotation, and shear. These may also occur in combination, as for example, rotation and shear, or extension and shear.

Axial Compression

In axial compression, the load falls principally upon the vertebral body. The exception is C1, where it falls on the medially directed wedge-shaped articular pillar, producing fracture of the atlas. The resulting lateral displacement may injure the C1-C2 joint capsule and avulse the transverse atlantal ligament (Fig. 8.1) with consequent decrease in resistance to

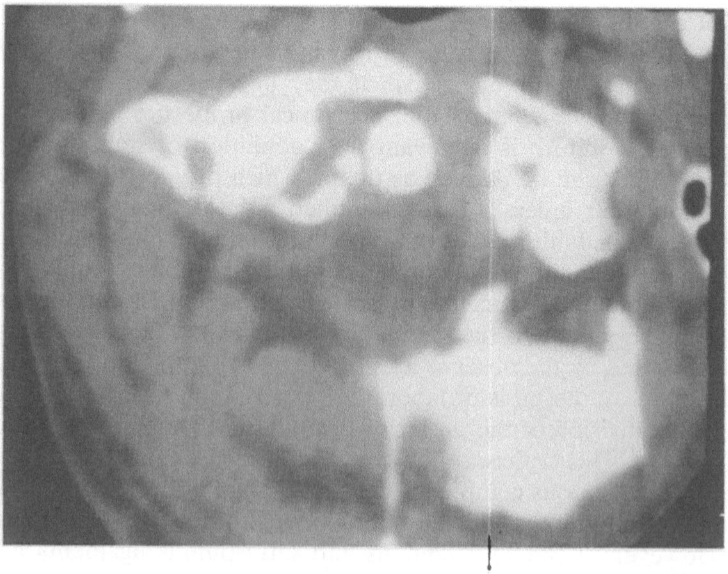

Figure 8.1. Axial compression fracture of C2. The tubercles for attachment of the transverse ligament have been avulsed from the lateral mass.

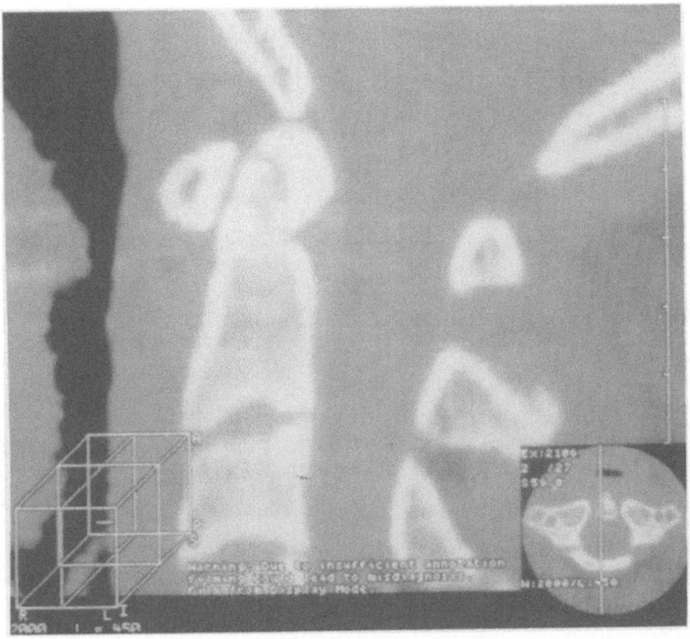

Figure 8.2. Odontoid fracture produced by contact with the rim of the foramen magnum.

translational movement. Therefore, this should be considered an unstable fracture. Rarely, the anterior rim of the foramen magnum may impinge on the odontoid process, producing a somewhat vertical fracture (Fig. 8.2). Since the joint capsules and transverse ligament are preserved, stability should not be impaired.

If the cervical and lumbar vertebral bodies are subjected to an axial load, they are shortened vertically, but widened circumferentially. This injury can be considered stable if the posterior elements are intact (Fig. 8.3) because flexion will be resisted by the posterior ligamentous complex, and axial translation by the preserved apophyseal joints. However, this is not the case if the posterior elements are disrupted (Fig. 8.4A). This patient was operated upon because of significant neurological deficit. The lateral approach (6) was used for reconstruction of the spinal canal, interbody fusion, and application of Cotrel-Dubousset rods. Although neurological recovery was excellent, mild flexion deformity developed (Fig. 8.4B,C), which was not associated with pain or other symptoms. However, when the posterior elements remain intact, flexion deformity should not develop despite resection of part of the vertebral body (Fig. 8.5).

Axial loads to the thoracic vertebral column tend to produce a tele-

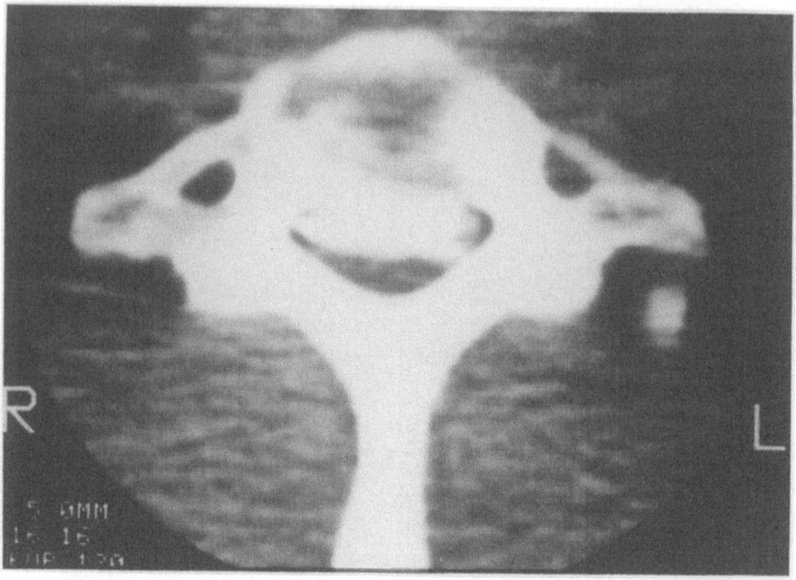

A

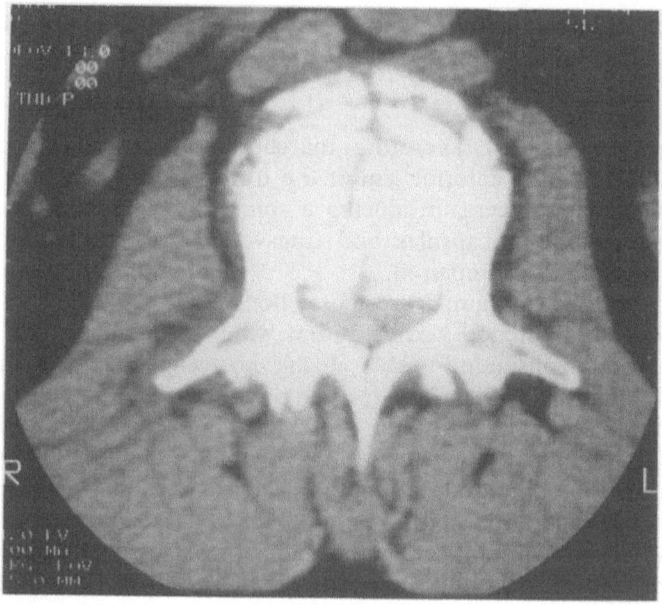

B

Figure 8.3. **A:** Fracture of C6 with bone displaced into the spinal canal. The neural arch waa not injured. **B:** Axial load fracture of L3. Although the vertebral body has expanded circumferentially with consequent greenstick fracture of the lamina, the posterior elements have not been disrupted. **C:** Axial load fracture of

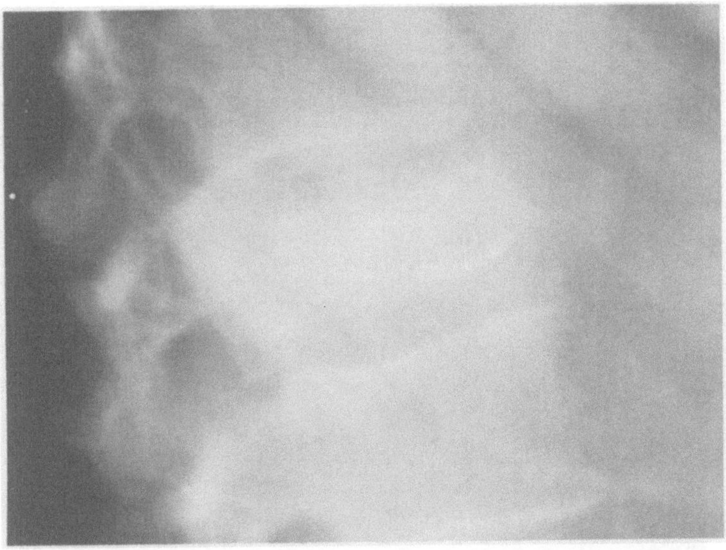

C

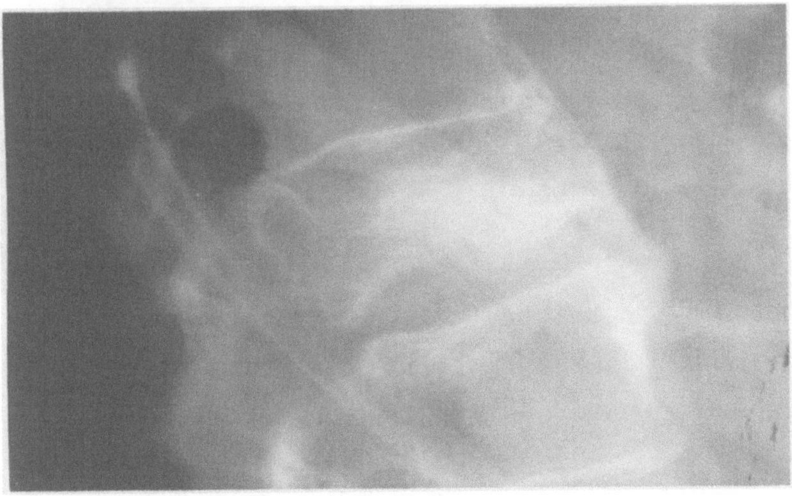

D

L3. Bone is displaced into the spinal canal, but neurological deficit was mild and transient. Treatment was nonsurgical. (By permission.) **D:** Same patient as in C2 years later. Bony union developed from L2-L4 without change in alignment. (Reproduced with permission from ref. 6.)

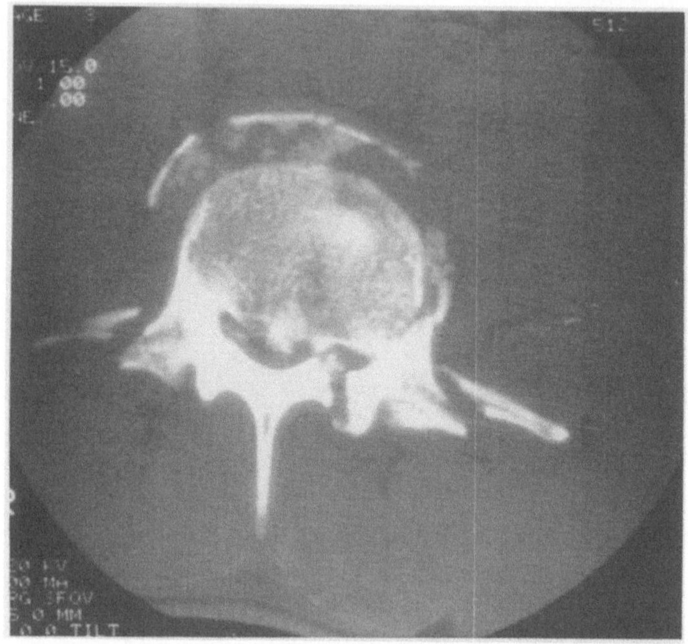

B

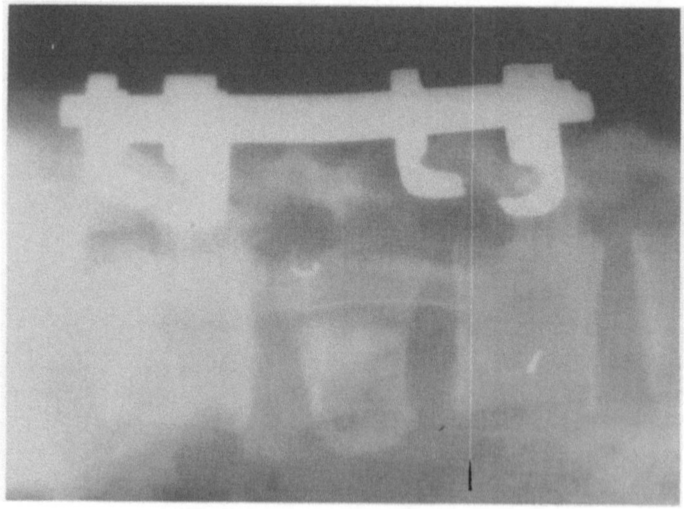

Figure 8.4. **A:** Axial load fracture of L3. Both pedicles are fractured. Although the fracture line on the right is not clearly visible, it can be inferred from the position of the vertebral body relative to the pedicle. **B:** Film made shortly after operation. **C:** Film taken 1 year later. The flexion deformity of 15° developed during the first 3 postoperative months.

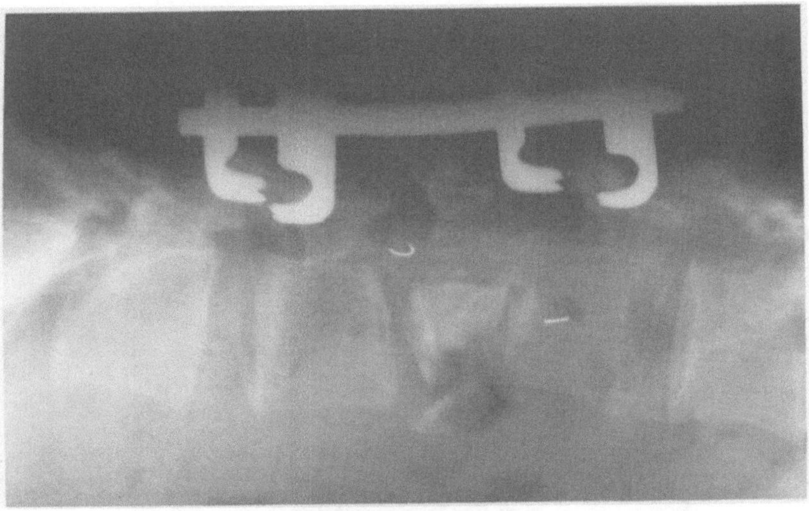

C

Figure 8.4. (*cont.*)

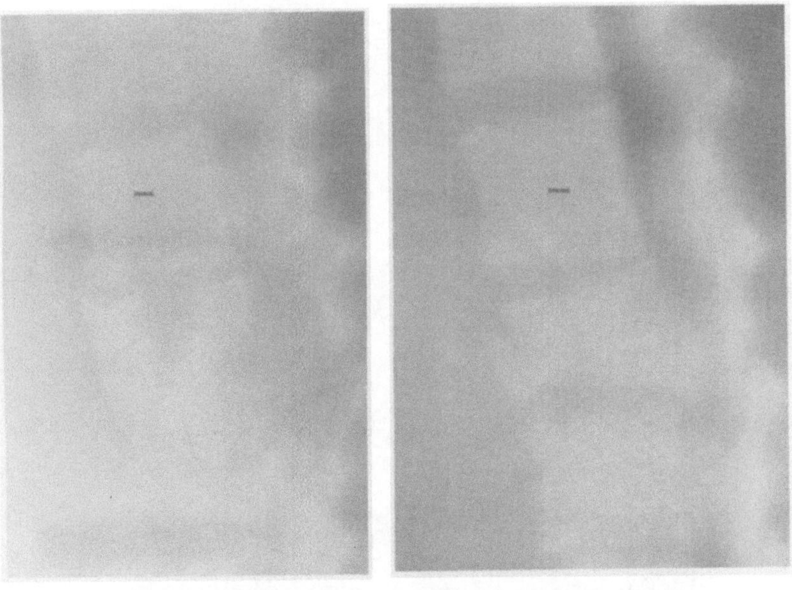

Figure 8.5. Preoperative film (*left*) in patient with paraparesis. The posterior elements were intact. Lateral approach for reconstruction of the spinal canal and interbody fusion was done. The patient had full functional recovery. Vertebral alignment was unchanged 1 year following surgery (*right*).

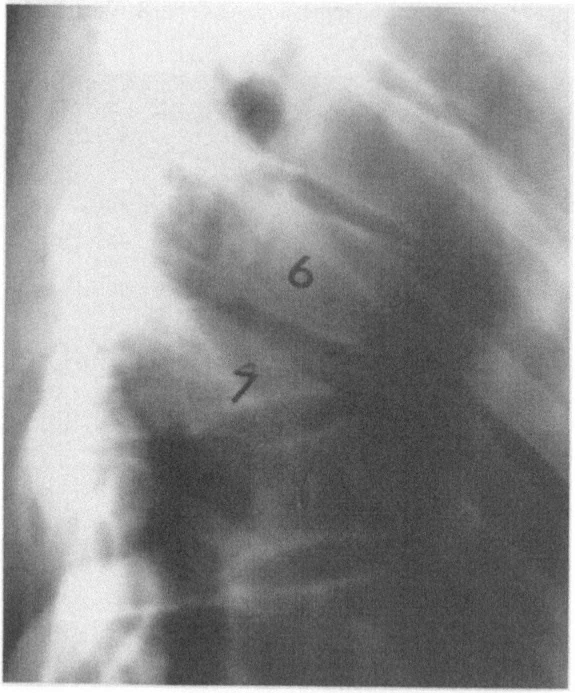

A

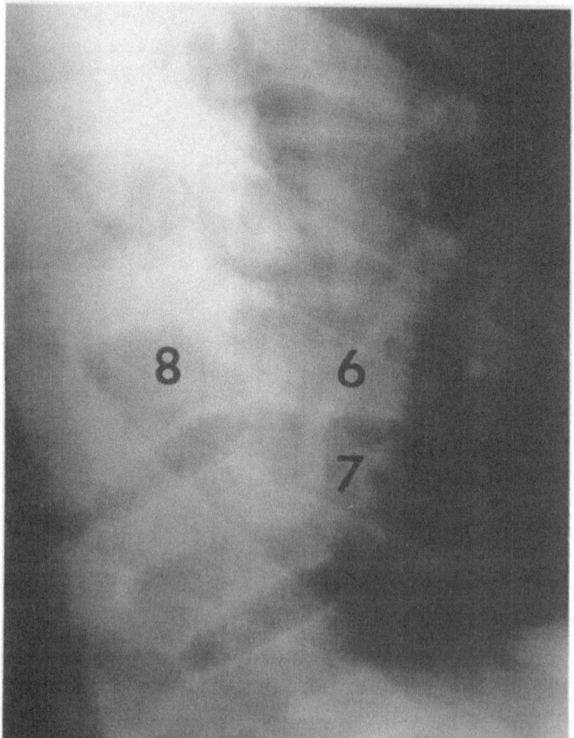

B

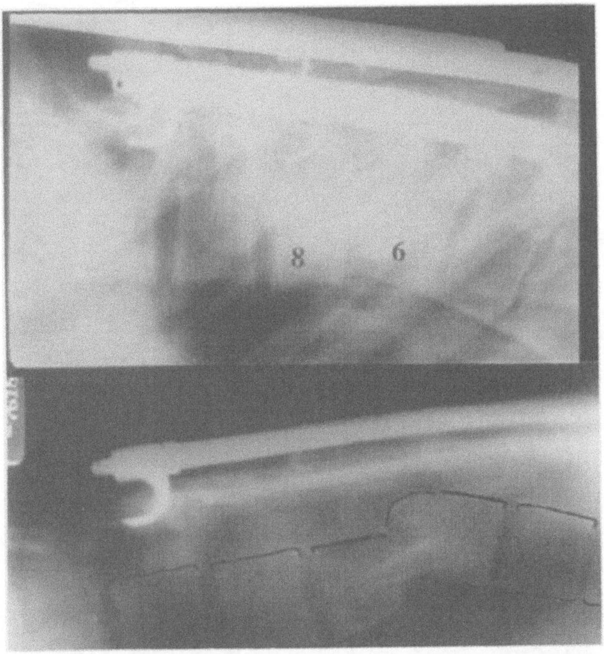

C

Figure 8.6. **A:** The patient had fallen 40 ft and sustained multiple injuries including this fracture of T7 and a complete myelopathy. **B:** Film taken 6 weeks later after transfer for treatment of the vertebral injury. Part of T7 remains attached to T6 and part to T8. Attempts at reduction with halo-femoral traction were unsuccessful. **C:** A bilateral lateral approach was used for reduction, interbody fusion, and application of Harrington rods. The upper film was taken shortly after surgery and the lower, 1 year later.

scoping injury, probably related to the thoracic kyphosis. Because the neural arch and vertebral body are injured, these are unstable fractures, and deformity may progress substantially (Fig. 8.6).

In the low lumbar area, axial loads may, in addition to the characteristic fracture of the vertebral body, produce a fracture of the pars interarticularis, presumably related to the lumbosacral angle (Fig. 8.7). Since translational movement may not be effectively opposed, this can be considered an unstable lesion.

Axial Distraction

Axial distraction injuries are limited to the upper cervical vertebrae. They usually occur in pedestrian vehicular accidents where the body accelerates relative to the head and neck. Those who have survived usually have

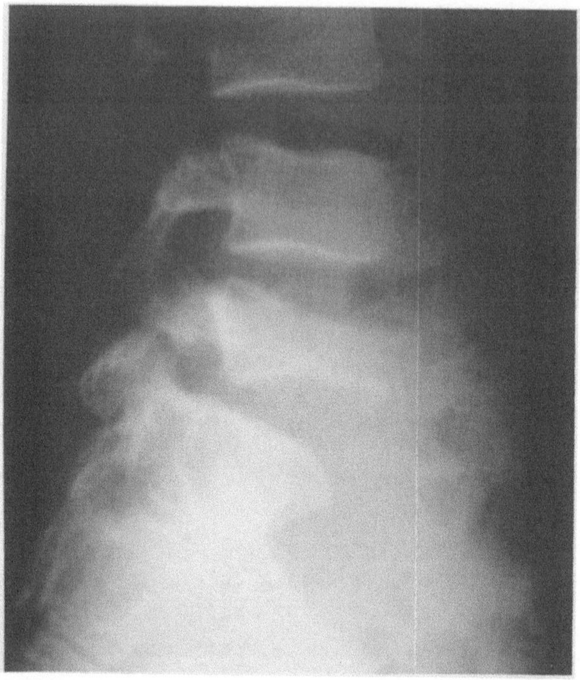

A

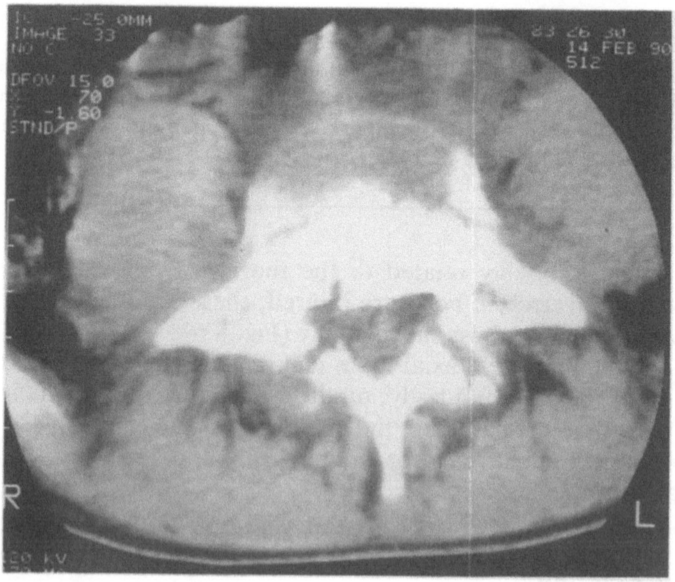

B

Figure 8.7. A: This patient had fallen 30 ft, sustaining bilateral os calcis fractures in addition to fractures of the body and pars interarticularis of L5. **B:** CT scan in the same patient.

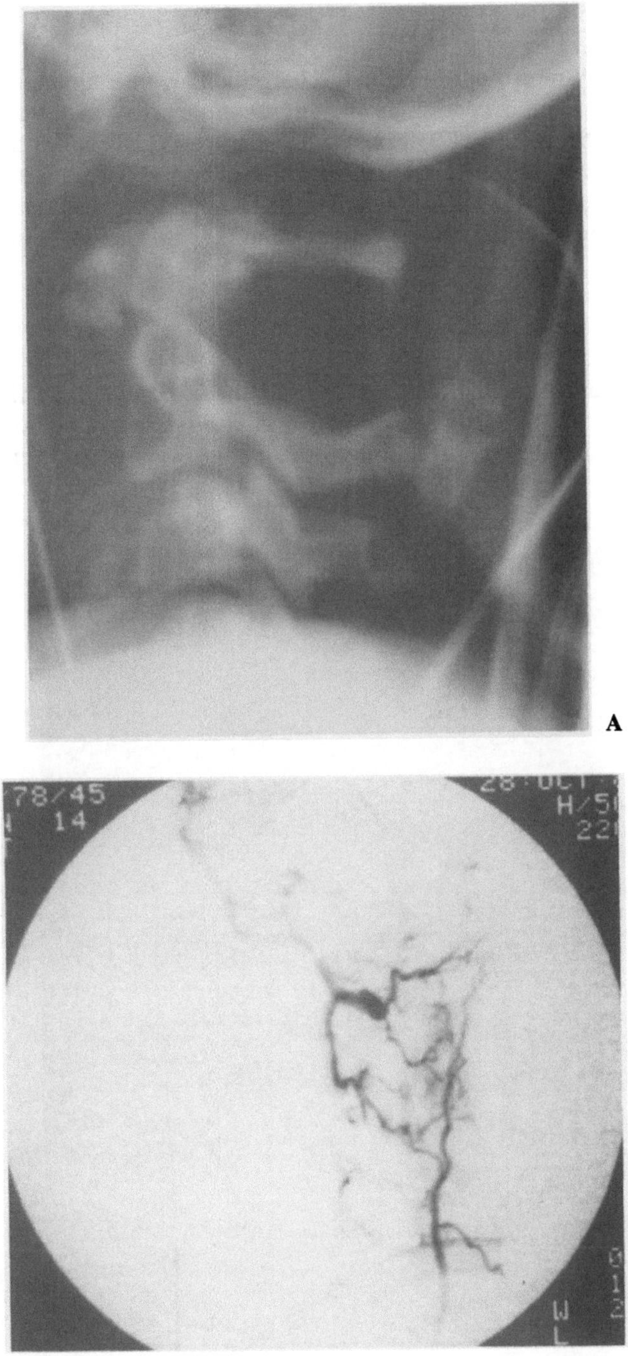

A

B

Figure 8.8. A: Atlantoaxial separation in a pedestrian who had been struck by an automobile. The anterior portion of C1 has also been fractured transversely. **B:** The spinal angiogram done 3 days after injury demonstrated interruption of flow in both vertebral arteries with distal filling by collateral vessels.

minimal if any neurological deficit. The patient whose films are shown in Fig. 8.8 had a mild cerebellar deficit secondary to what was probably avulsion of the vertebral arteries and which resolved within a few days. The patient was placed in an orthosis, and after reduction by muscle contraction an occiput-C2 fusion was done. The loss of resistance to motion in all directions except axial compression makes this an unstable injury.

Flexion

Flexion produces a ligamentous injury and is confined to the cervical spine. Films taken shortly after injury may show minimal or no abnormality because of reflex contraction of the extensor muscles. Separation of

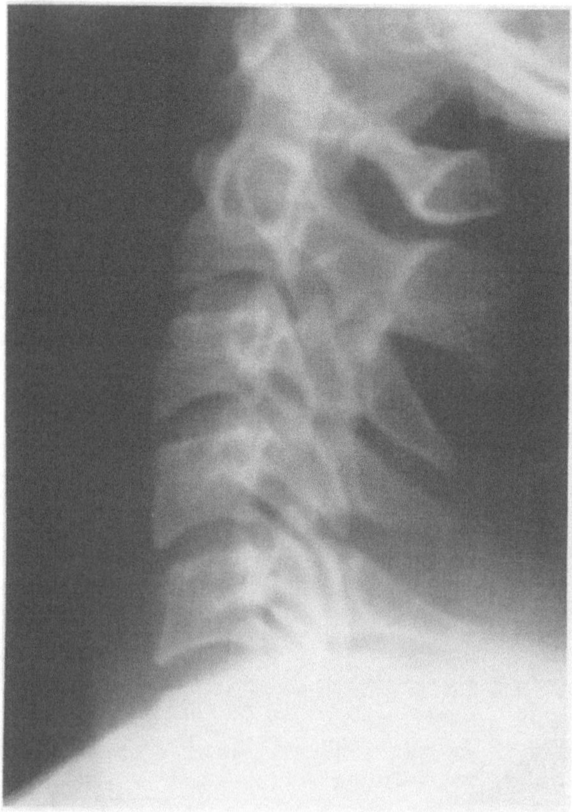

A

Figure 8.9. A: This film taken shortly after injury had been interpreted as normal although the spinous processes of C4-C5 are asymmetrically separated. **B:** Film taken 2 weeks later. A mild myelopathy had developed.

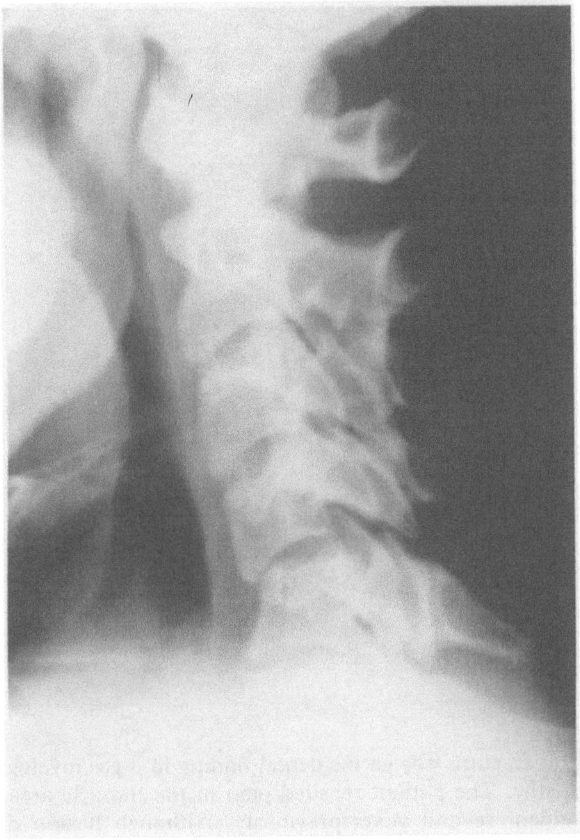

B

Figure 8.9. (*cont.*)

the spinous processes beyond physiological limits implies pathological stretch of the supraspinous and intraspinous ligaments with concomitant injury to the joint capsules, posterior longitudinal ligament, and intervertebral disc (Fig. 8.9). The loss of retraint to additional deformity makes this an unstable injury (7).

Flexion Compression

If compression is added to flexion, a wedge-shaped vertebral fracture may be produced and the possibility of posterior element injury also exists. Despite extensive injury to the vertebral body, the fracture may be considered stable if the posterior elements are preserved (Fig. 8.10). However, if disruption of the posterior elements is added to vertebral body injury, then progression can be expected under physiological loads (Fig. 8.11).

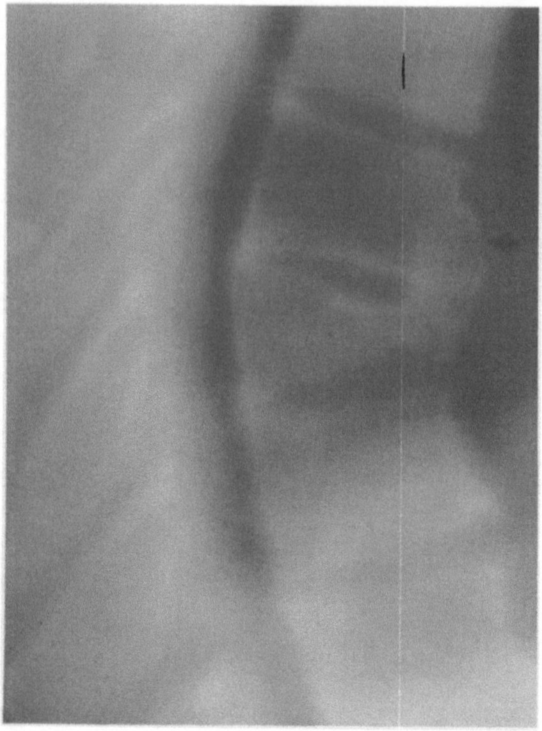

Figure 8.10. This fracture was an incidental finding in a gas myelogram done for cervical myelopathy. The patient recalled pain in the thoracic area following an automobile accident several years previously. Although flexion deformity was greater than 30°, and loss of height anteriorly more than 70%, the posterior elements were intact, and bony union had taken place (*arrow*).

The appearance of both the stable and unstable flexion compression injury is much the same in the cervical, thoracic, and lumbar portions of the vertebral column.

Flexion Distraction

Because of the configuration of the articular processes, flexion and distraction in the cervical portion of the vertebral column produces bilaterally locked facets (Fig. 8.12A). Attempts at reduction by skeletal traction may result in overdistraction (Fig. 8.12B). This patient, although quadriplegic, had preserved diaphragmatic function. Subsequent to application of skeletal traction, he became apneic, and required assisted ventilation. After transfer to the VA Spinal Cord Injury Center in Milwaukee, open

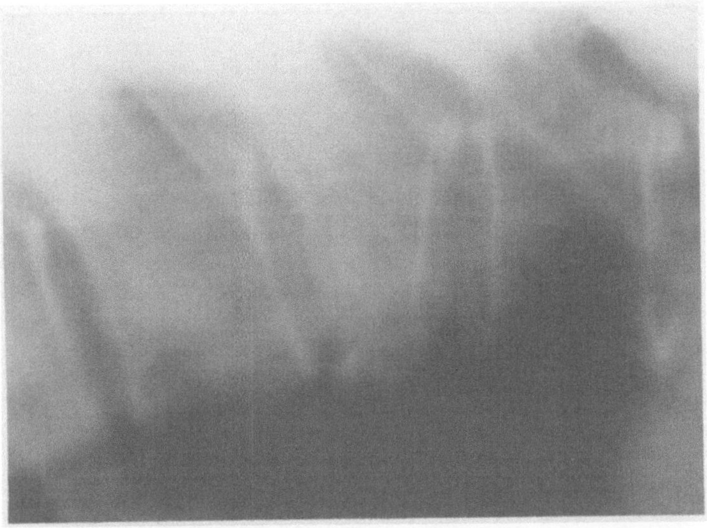

A

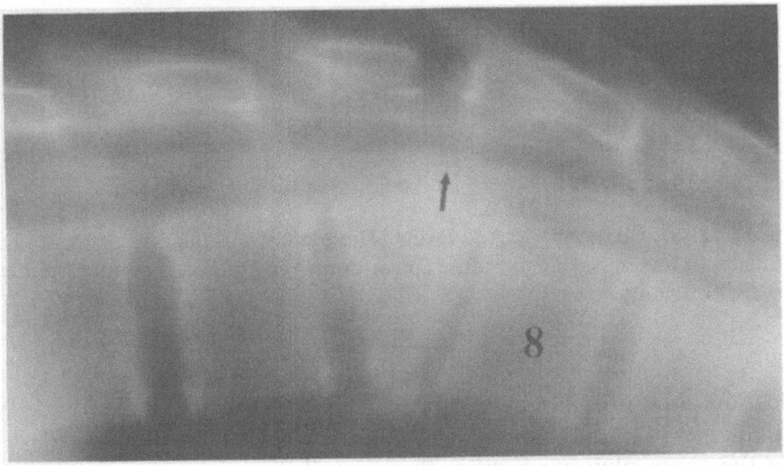

B

tion in vertical dimension anteriorly. **B:** The patient was allowed up and significant myelopathy developed within 2 days. The flexion deformity had increased, stretching the spinal cord over the gibbus (*arrow*). A lateral approach was used for reconstruction of the spinal canal and application of Harrington rods. The patient had full recovery of neurological function. (Reproduced with permission from S. Larson, et al., Lateral Extracavitary Approach to Traumatic Lesions of the Thoracic and Lumbar Spine. J Neurosurg, 1976;45:628–637.)

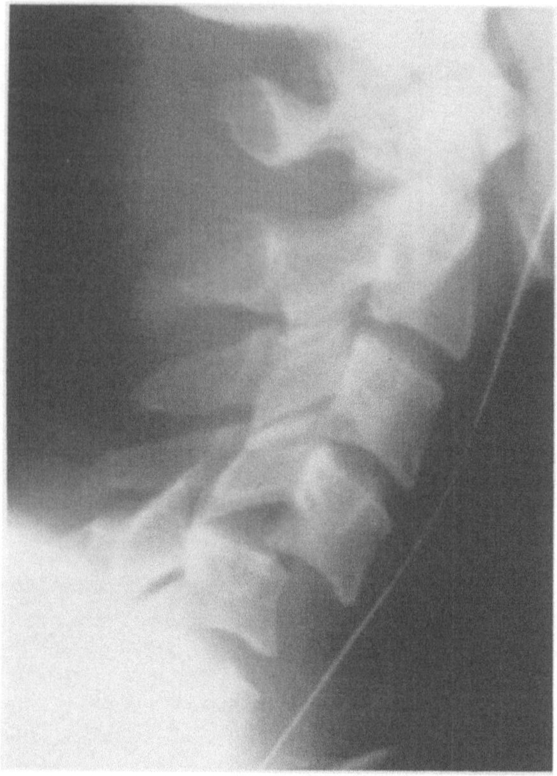

A

Figure 8.12. A: Bilaterally locked facets. The patient was quadriplegic but had diaphragmatic function. **B:** Film after apnea developed during attempted reduction by skeletal traction.

reduction and fusion was performed, but ventilator dependence was permanent.

In the thoracolumbar region, flexion and distraction produces separation beginning posteriorly in the spinous process or interspinous ligament, and moving anteriorly into the vertebral body or disc. Since posterior and anterior elements are disrupted, resistance to further deformity is diminished. Immobilization is necessary, although this need not require surgical fixation. The patient whose films are shown in Fig. 8.13 was placed in a body cast and the fracture healed satisfactorily.

Extension

In the upper portion of the vertebral column, extension can produce fracture of the C1 lamina or the pars interarticularis of C2. If the anterior lon-

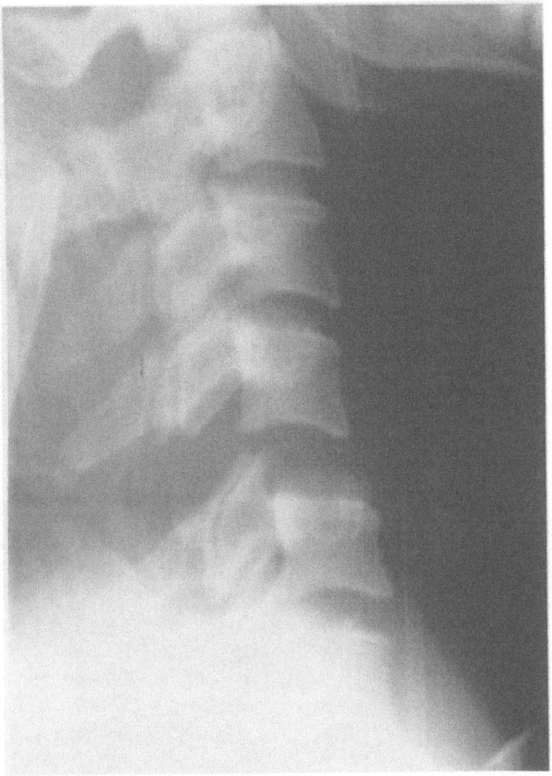

B

Figure 8.12. (*cont.*)

gitudinal ligament and intervertebral disc are also disrupted, resistance to translational movement is decreased and the fracture should be considered unstable (Fig. 8.14). In the lower cervical vertebrae, extension injuries are of two types. In one, the anterior longitudinal ligament and the disc are disrupted as are the joint capsules. The spinous processes may also be fractured (Fig. 8.15). Although stable in flexion because the posterior ligamentus complex is intact, this injury is unstable in extension, and if the cervical spine is not adequately immobilized, significant spinal cord injury may develop (1,11). In the other type, the intervertebral disc and associated ligaments fail and pedicle or articular pillar fracture occurs. The vertebral body is then displaced anteriorly (Fig. 8.16). Because both anterior and posterior elements are disrupted, this is an unstable injury. Shear added to extension results in anterior displacement of the vertebral body and severe posterior comminution (Fig. 8.17). Because distruption is circumferential, this is a very unstable lesion.

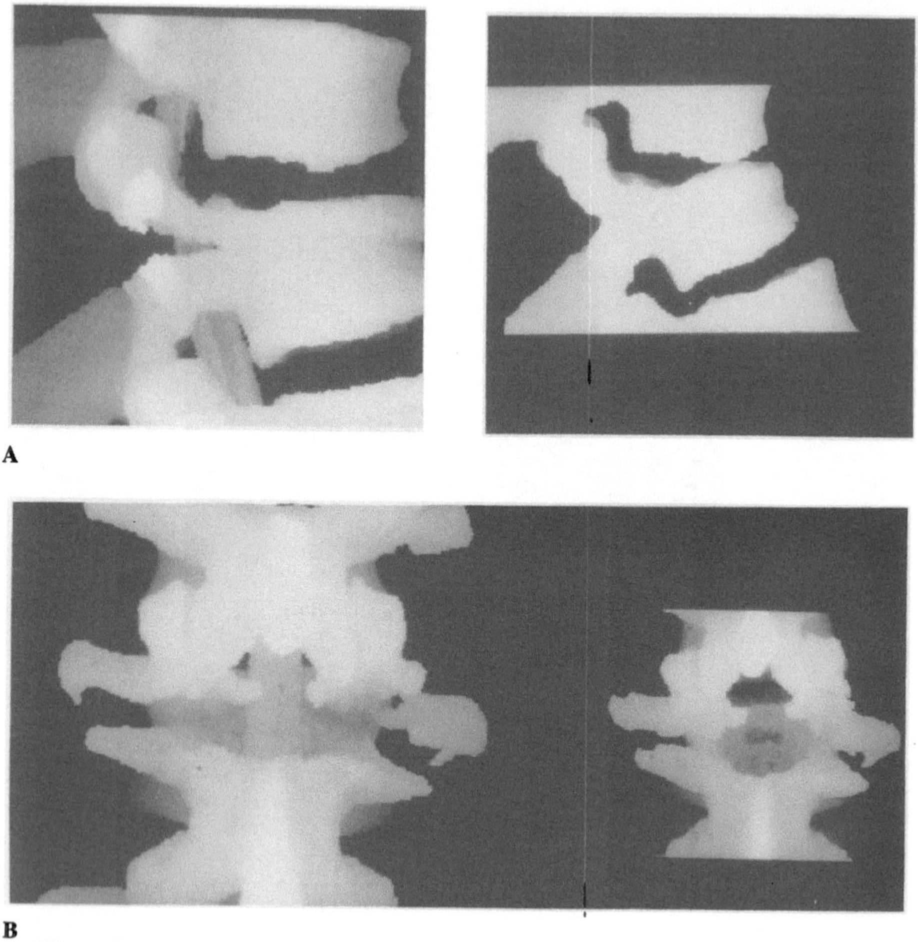

Figure 8.13. **A:** Post myelogram 3D-CT in a patient with a lap belt injury (*left*). Neurological function was normal and film 3 months later demonstrated bony union (*right*). **B:** Same patient immediately postinjury (*left*) and 3 months later (*right*).

Extension injuries may also occur in the thoracolumbar area, but are less common (Fig. 8.18). Like the corresponding cervical injury (Fig. 8.15), it is unstable in extension.

Rotation

In the cervical spine, rotation produces the unilaterally locked facet, and is an unstable injury because the disc and related ligaments are also in-

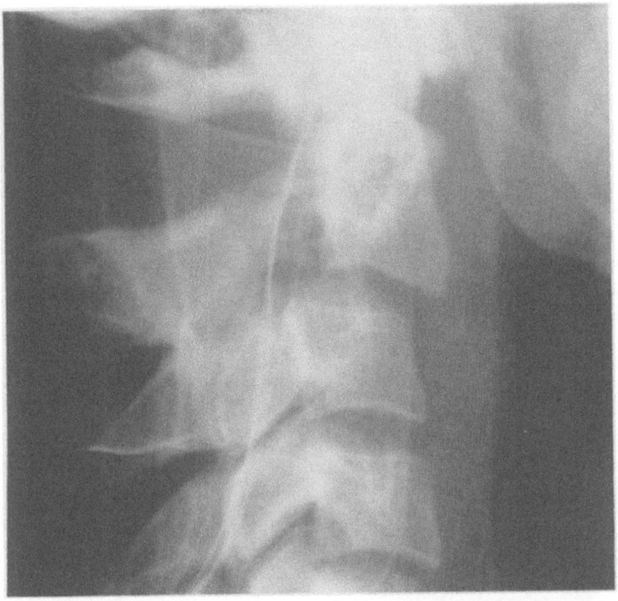

A

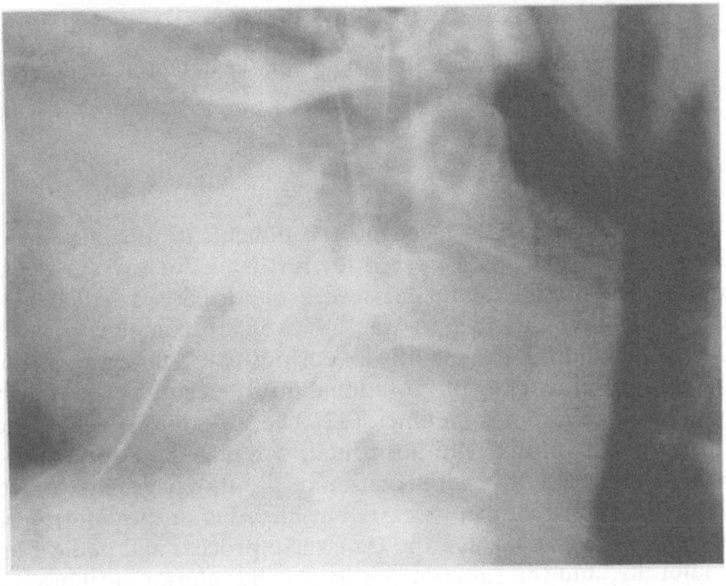

B

Figure 8.14. A: Fracture of the pars interarticularis of C2. **B:** Progressive displacement has occurred despite immobilization in a halo vest.

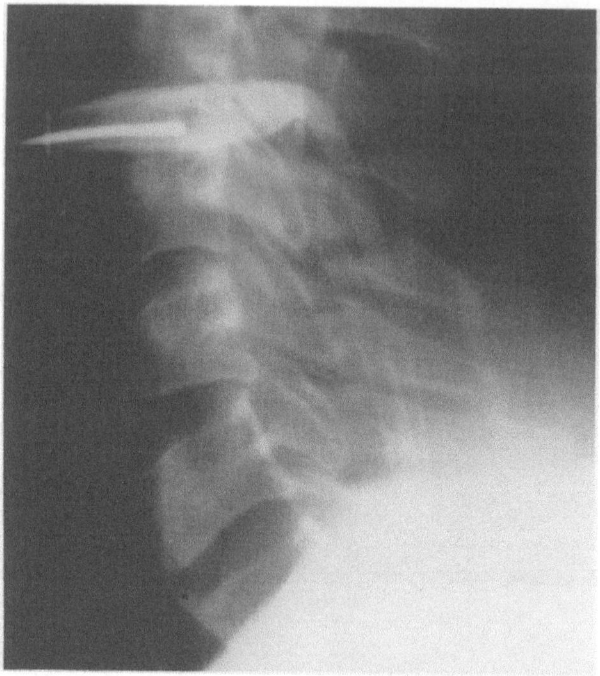

Figure 8.15. Lateral view demonstrates anterior separation at C5-C6 and fractured spinous processes of C3-C4.

jured. A unilaterally locked facet may be difficult to recognize at C1-C2 (Fig. 8.19). This patient was treated for torticollis for several weeks. By the time the diagnosis was made, severe quadriparesis had developed. Reduction and skeletal traction was followed by complete recovery of neurological function. Subsequently an occiput-to-C2 fusion was done.

In the thoracolumbar region, rotational injury occurs at the transitional vertebra, usually T11 but sometimes T12. The superior articular processes of the transitional vertebra are horizontal, whereas the inferior processes are vertical. Consequently, with rotation of the thoracic spine, movement is permitted at the superior processes but impeded at the inferior processes. When the fracture occurs, the transverse process and pedicle are displaced laterally, and the superior portion of the inferior vertebra remains attached to the rotating vertebra (Fig. 8.20). Because of the complete circumferential disruption, this is a most unstable lesion and change in alignment may occur even if the patient is kept recumbent (Fig. 8.21). Distraction instrumentation should be avoided, not only because overdistraction may increase the neurological deficit (Fig. 8.22), but because the absence

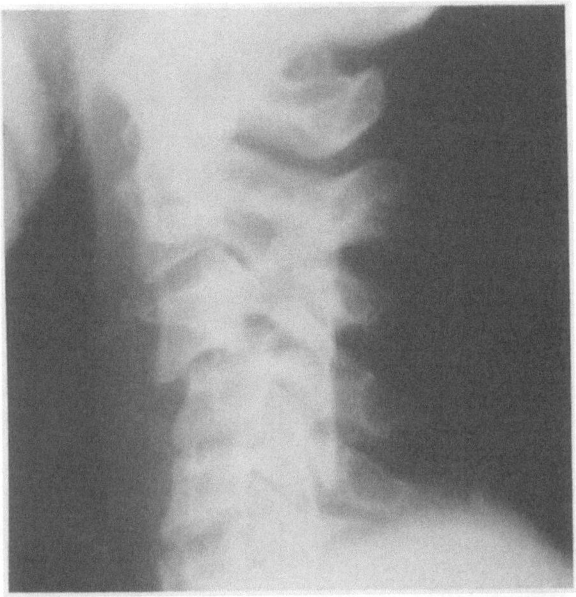

A

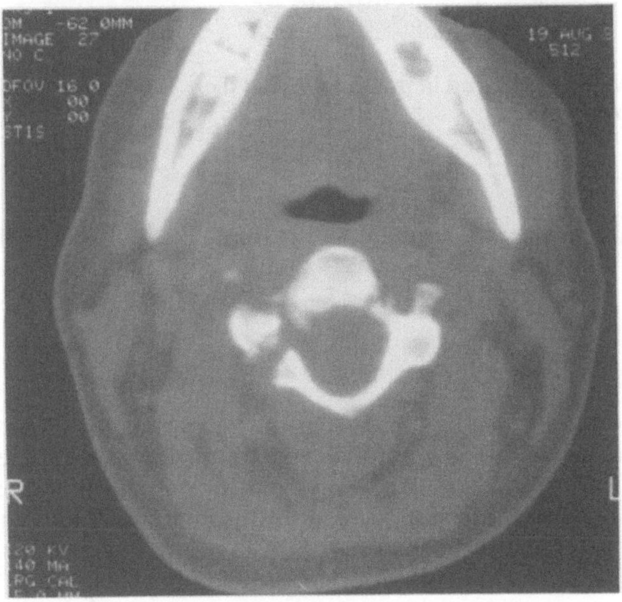

B

Figure 8.16. A: C4 is displaced anteriorly on C5. **B:** The posterior elements are fractured bilaterally.

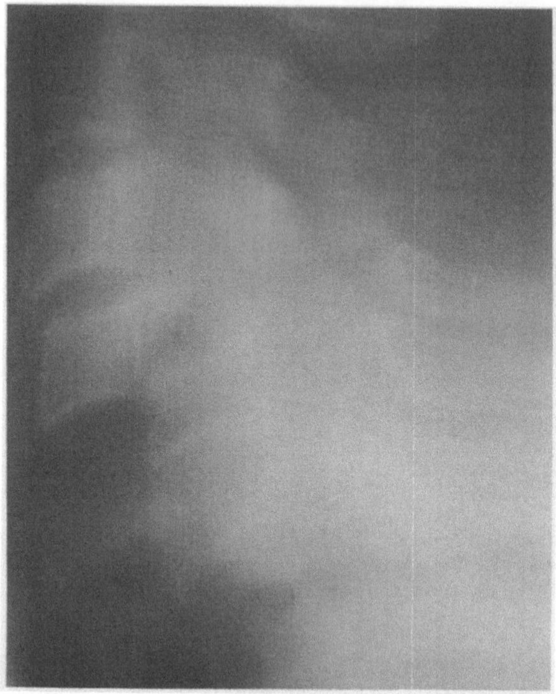

Figure 8.17. C6 is displaced in front of C7, and there is extensive comminution of the posterior elements.

of resistance to distraction may permit dislocation of the hooks if Harrington rods are used.

Shear

Shear produces translational movement, disrupting both anterior and posterior elements. Because resistance to further displacement is decreased, these injuries are unstable. Type II odontoid fractures can also be considered shear injuries. At other levels of the vertebral column, the disruption is largely through soft tissues (Figs. 8.23 and 8.24) and adequate healing may therefore not occur without internal fixation.

Figure 8.18. A: Lateral view demonstrates anterior disruption at L1-L2. **B:** Both pedicles are fractured.

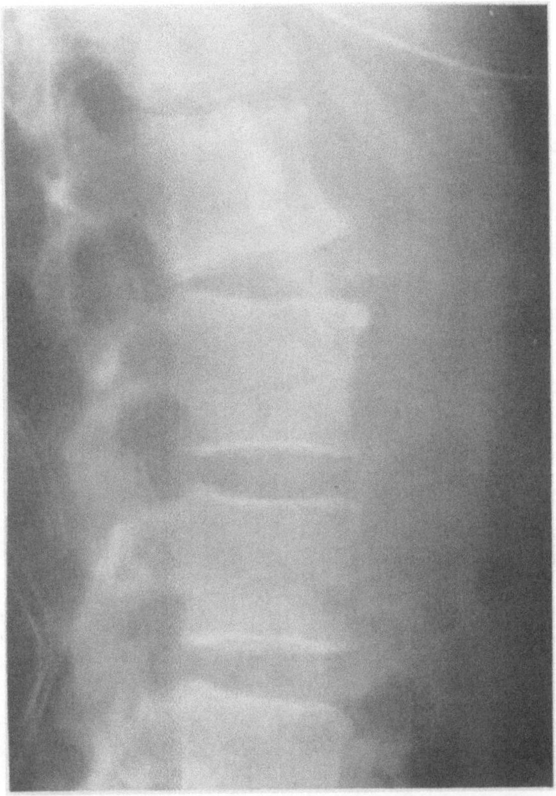

A

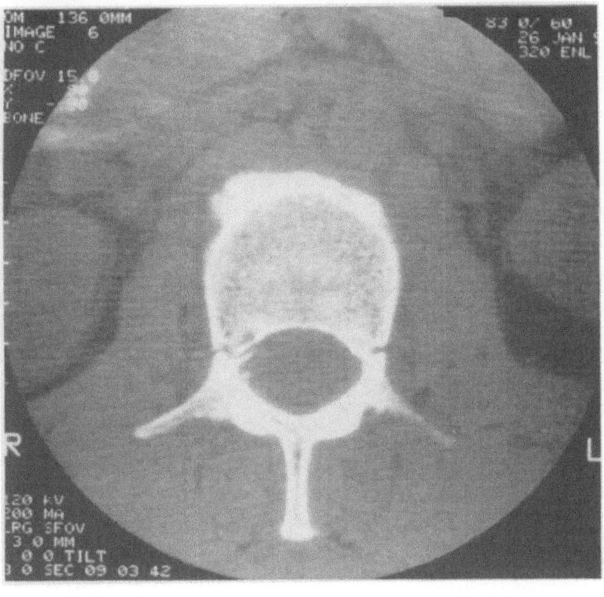
136 0MM
IMAGE 6
NO C
26 JAN
320 ENL
R
L
120 kV
200 MA
LRG SFOV
3 0 MM
0 0 TILT
SEC 09 03 42

B

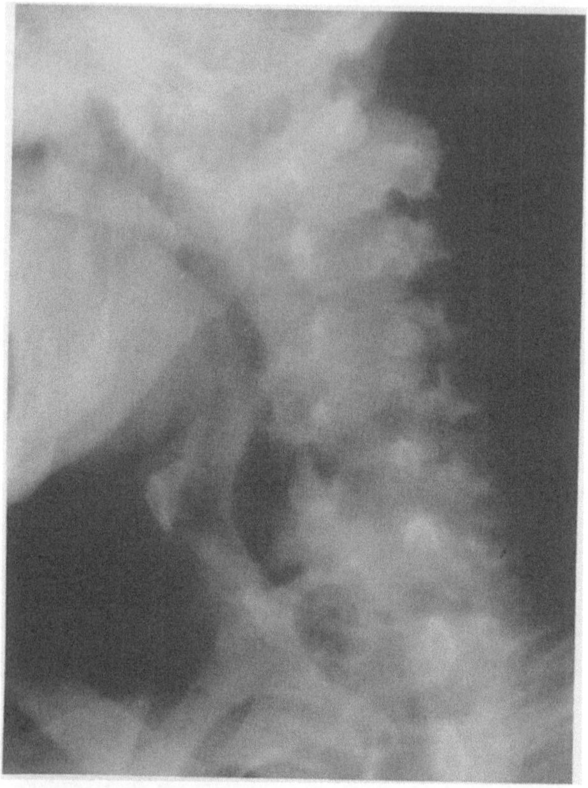

A

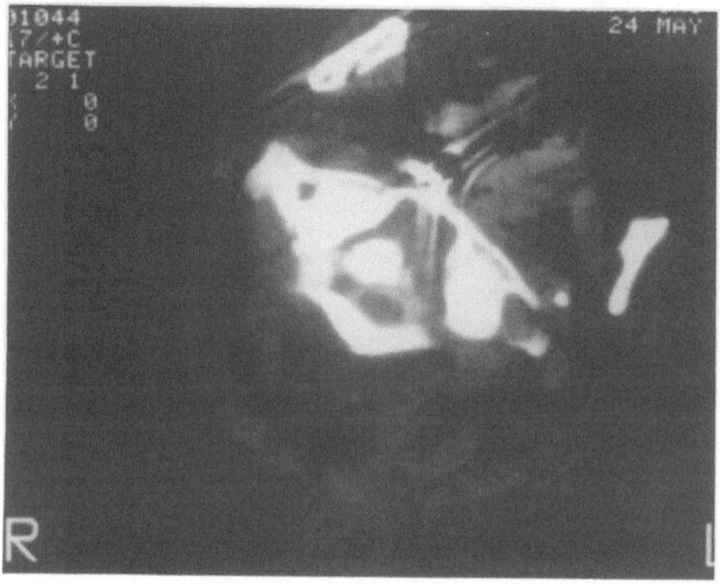

B

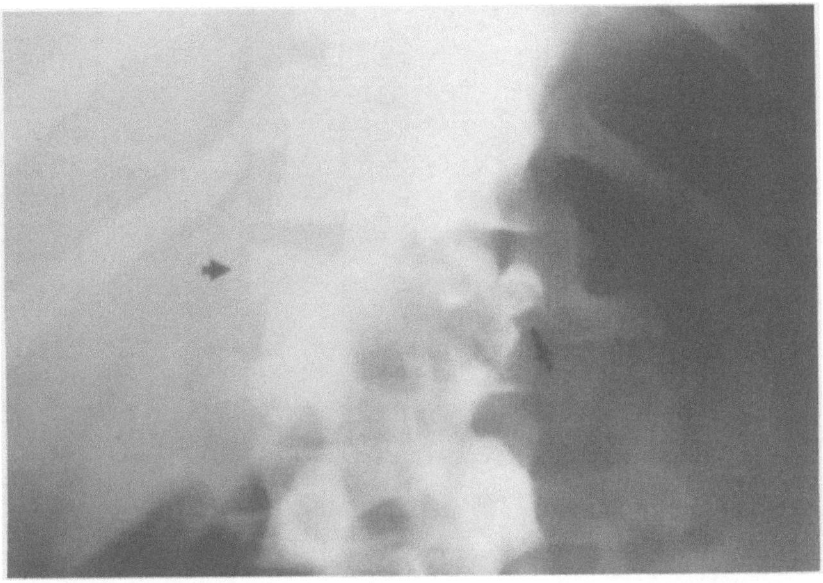

Figure 8.20. The pedicle and transverse processes are displaced laterally (*long arrow*). The superior portion of L1 remains attached to T12 (*short arrow*).

Combined

In some instances, the injury may be produced by a combination of forces as for example, flexion, compression, and shear (Fig. 8.25). This patient had a severe neurological deficit and obvious instability. The lateral approach was used for reconstruction of the spinal canal, realignment of the vertebral column, and interbody fusion with posterior instrumentation. Recovery of neurological function was complete.

Summary

Identification of the force or forces producing vertebral injury can help determine whether or not the vertebral column is stable. Stable injuries are those restricted to the anterior column and occur in conjunction with axial compression and flexion compression. These forces may also disrupt the posterior elements with consequent instability. Injuries caused by

Figure 8.19. A: Lateral film in a patient with unilateral dislocation of C1-C2. **B:** CT scan in the same patient.

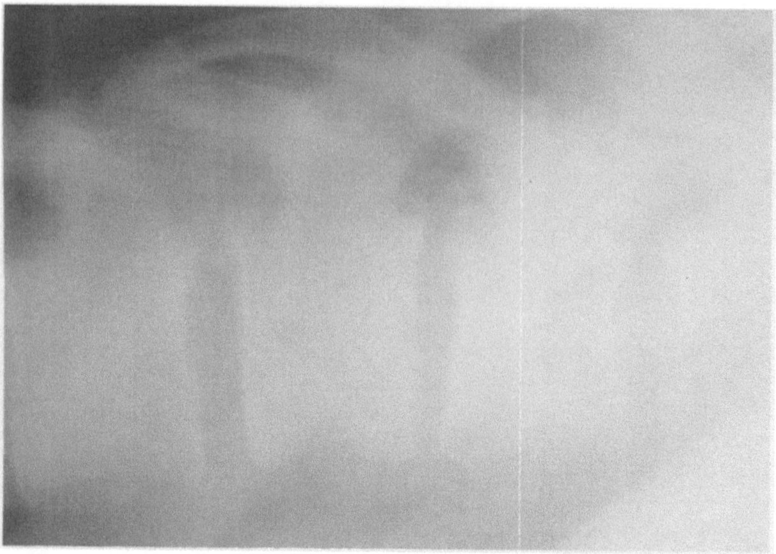

A

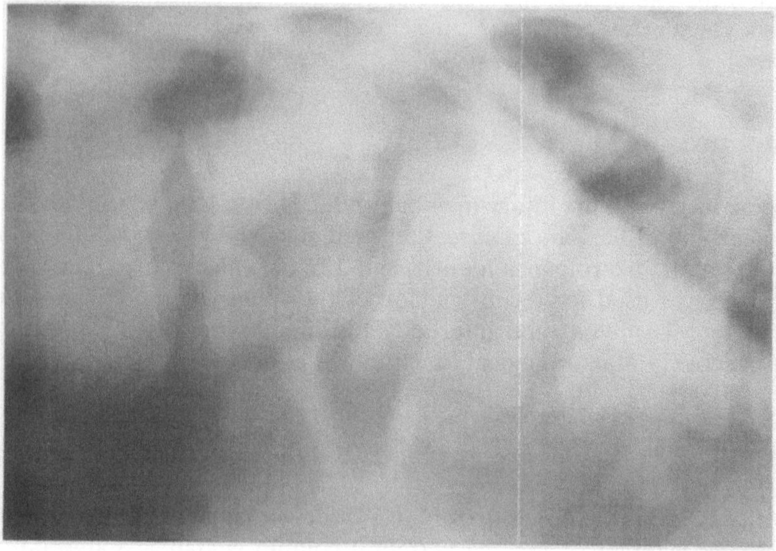

B

Figure 8.21. **A:** Film taken shortly after a rotational injury at T12-L1. Alignment is nearly normal. **B:** Film made 2 days later. The patient had been kept recumbent and had been log rolled. **C:** Same patient after lateral approach for reduction, interbody fusion, and Cotrel-Dubousset instrumentation.

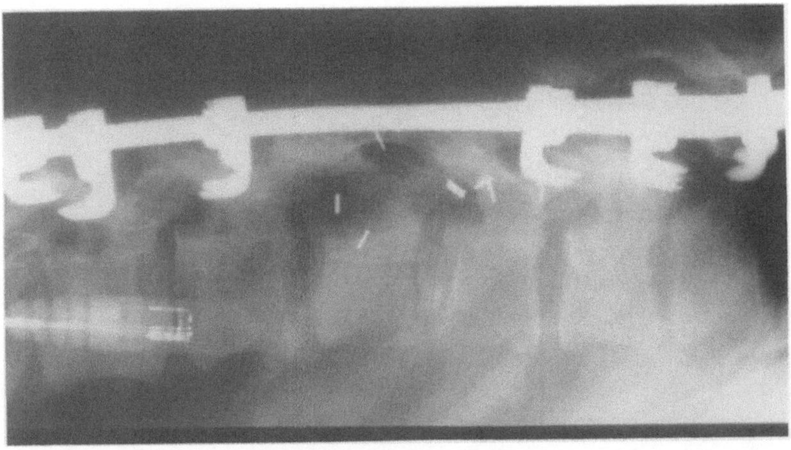

C

Figure 8.21. (*cont.*)

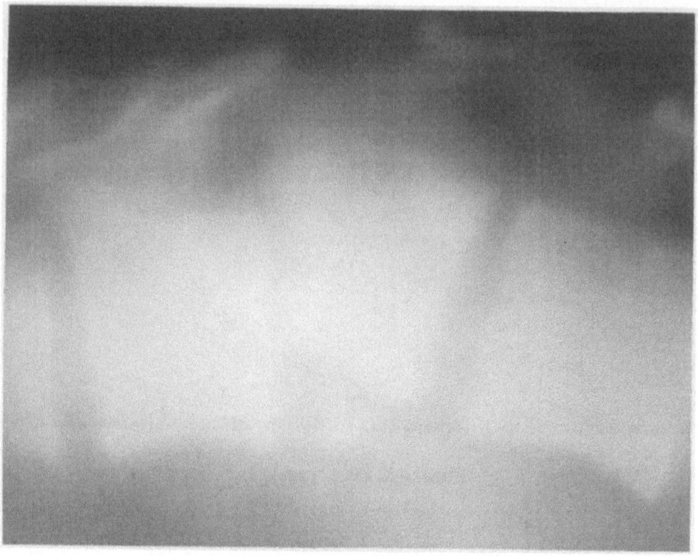

A

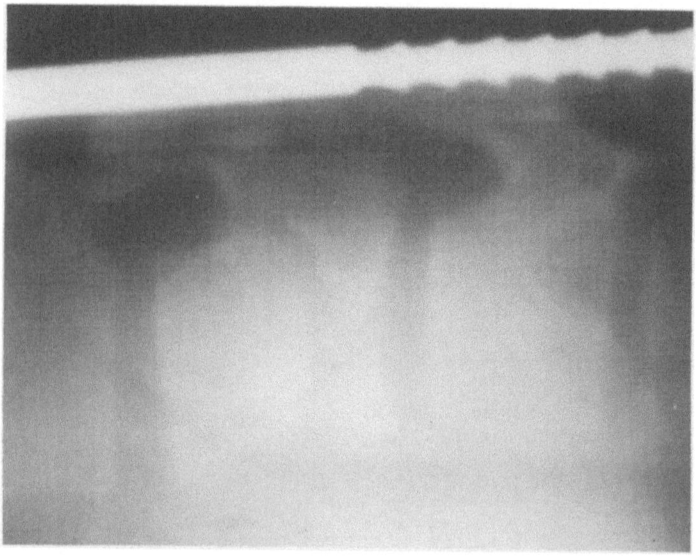

B

Figure 8.22. **A:** Film taken shortly after a rotational injury. **B:** Lateral film after application of Harrington rods, which had produced significant overdistraction.

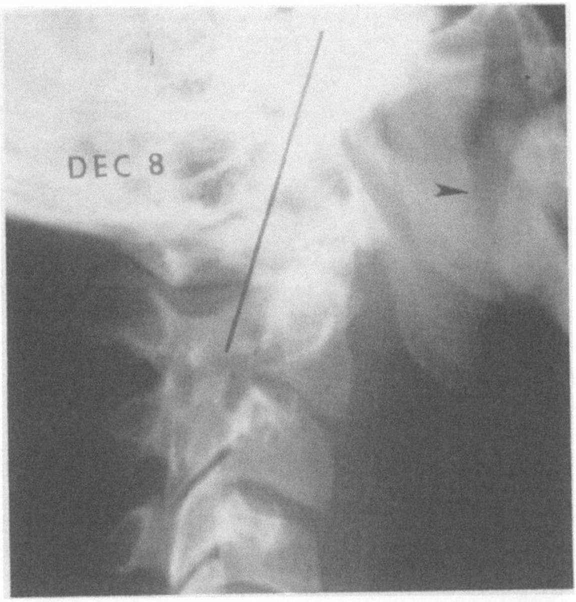

A

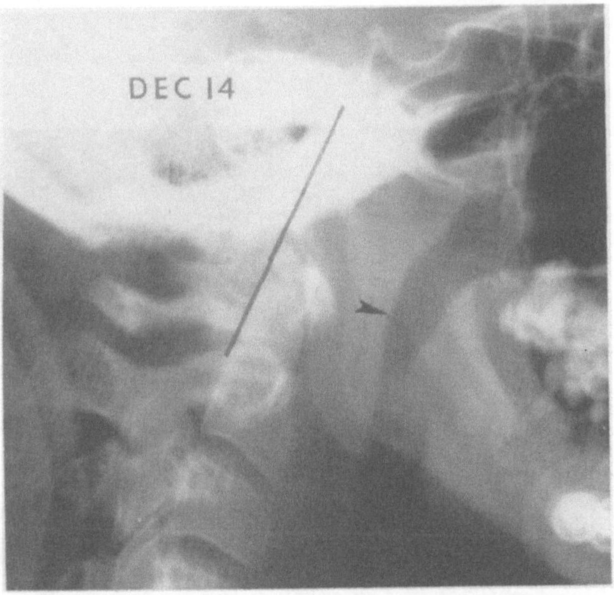

B

Figure 8.23. A: Posterior occipital atlantal dislocation. The prevertebral space is substantially enlarged (*arrow*). The line follows the basilar process of the occipital bone and passes well behind the odontoid process. **B:** Postural reduction was achieved. The prevertebral space has contracted (*arrow*).

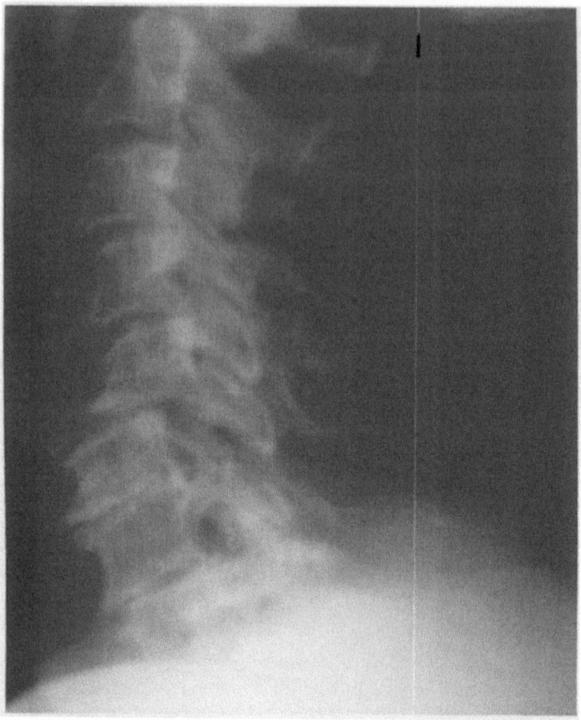

A

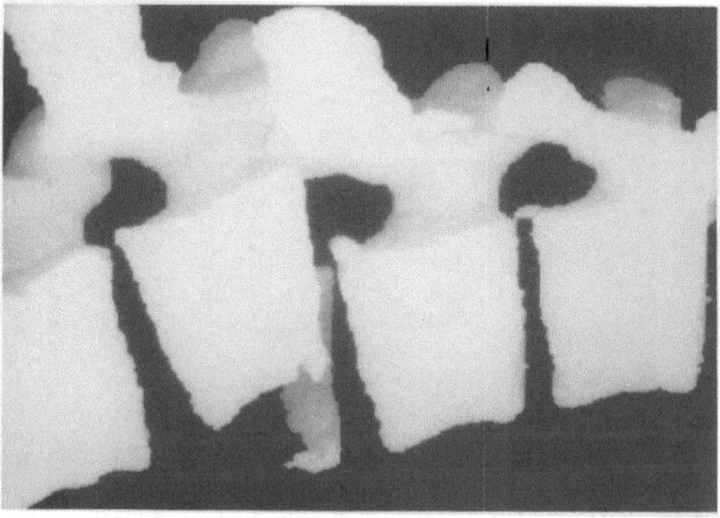

B

Figure 8.24. **A:** Posterior displacement of C5 on C6. **B:** Anterior displacement of T12 on L1. **C:** AP view demonstrates dislocation of the apophyseal joints at T12-L1 in the same patient.

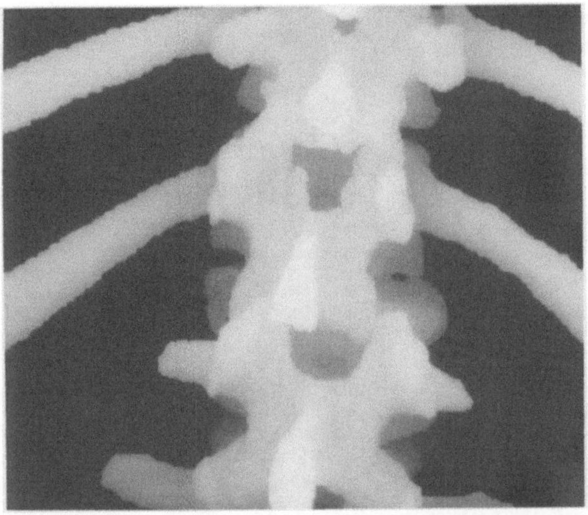

C

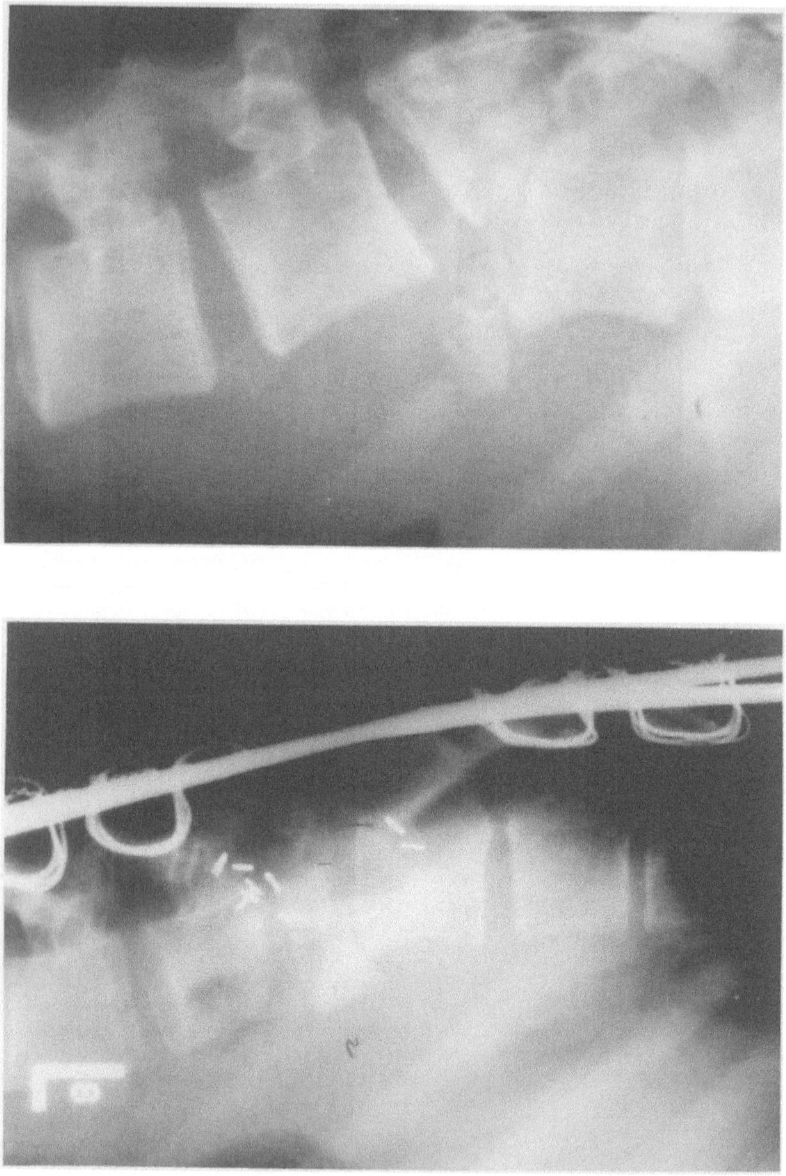

A

B

Figure 8.25. **A:** Fracture dislocation at L1-L2 produced by flexion, compression, and shear. **B:** Same patient after lateral approach for reconstruction of the spinal canal, interbody fusion, and reduction with Luque segmental instrumentation.

flexion, extension, rotation, and shear should always be considered unstable since the posterior elements are necessarily involved. Although instability is not an absolute indication for surgical treatment, it does mandate adequate immobilization. Identification of the forces producing an unstable injury is also important for the selection of the most appropriate method of stabilization. The major value of any classification system is as a guide, but never a substitute for thought, and as a means for communication of information. Although no system is perfect, a mechanistic classification has distinct advantages over the other types that have been proposed.

References

1. Cintron E, Gilula LA, Murphy WA, Gehweiler JA. The widened disc space: A sign of cervical hyperextension injury. *Radiology*. 1981;141:639–644.
2. Denis F. The three column spine and its significance in the classification of acute thoracolumbar spinal injuries. *Spine*. 1983;8:817–831.
3. Gehweiler JA Jr, Osborne RL Jr, Becker RF. *The Radiology of Vertebral Trauma*. Philadelphia: WB Saundera; 1980.
4. Holdsworth FW. Fractures, dislocations, and fracture dislocations of the spine. *J Bone Joint Surg*. 1963;45B:6–20.
5. Kelly RP, Whitesides TE Jr. Treatment of lumbar fracture dislocation. *Ann Surg*. 1968;167:705–717.
6. Larson SJ. The thoracolumbar junction. In: Dunsker SB, Kahn A, Schmidek H, Frymoyer J, eds. *The Unstable Spine*. Philadelphia: W.B. Saunders Co. 1986:127–152.
7. Larson SJ. Post traumatic spinal instability. In: Pitts LH, Wagner FC Jr, eds. *Craniospinal Trauma*. Thieme Medical Publishers; New York: 1990:159–170.
8. McAfee PC, Yuan HA, Frederickson BE, Lubicky JP. The value of computed tomography in thoracolumbar fractures. *J Bone Joint Surg*. 1983; 65A:461–473.
9. McAfee PC, Yuan HA, Lasda NA. The unstable burst fracture. *Spine*. 1982;7:365–373.
10. Roaf R. International classification of spinal injuries. *Paraplegia*. 1972; 10:78–84.
11. Scher AT. Hyperextension trauma in the elderly. An easily overlooked spinal injury. *J Trauma*. 1983;23:1066–1068.
12. Whitely JE, Forsyth HF. The classification of cervical spine injuries. *Am J Roentgenol*. 1960;83:633–644.
13. Whitesides TE Jr. Traumatic kyphosis of the thoracolumbar spine. *Clin Orthop*. 1977;128:78–92.
14. Whitesides TE Jr, Ali Shah SG. On the management of unstable fractures of the thoracolumbar spine. *Spine*. 1976;1:99–107.

Discussion

Classification Systems: Their Attributes and Shortcomings

Dr. Kostuik began the discussion by saying, I think the purpose of any classification is to allow us to be able to treat people and to provide a treatment protocol. There are tremendous problems with any classification. In the last 10 years we have seen a number of different systems proposed around the world and I would refer those of you who are interested to our chapter in *Trauma in the Adult Spine*. I feel that there is no good classification system that covers all situations. The best attempts that I have seen in recent years include the systems of Marlboro, Harms from Germany, Gertzbein from Toronto, and Pavy from Switzerland, all of whom worked very hard to put together a comprehensive classification. Unfortunately, it is a bit unwieldy unless you are someone who does trauma on a daily basis.

I think the problem with the Holdsworth classification is that it really does not tell us which ones we need to operate on and which ones we do not. Obviously, in your case, Dr. Larson it is easy because you have 30 years or more of experience, like many people around here, and we know what to do; it becomes intuitive, but it does not allow us to teach younger people properly. That is my criticism of all the older classifications including the Holdsworth classification, which was a tremendous advance because prior to that time there was no classification system.

Prof. René Louis, speaking to Dr. Larson, noted: You are saying that instability depends on the integrity of the posterior complex, but if you add neck extension with only the anterior part of the ligament ruptured, the anterior longitudinal ligament and the anterior part of the annulus with the posterior complex intact so there is extension injury—your role is reversed.

Dr. Larson responded: No, because in the extension injuries that I showed with opening of the fish mouth, the spinous processes were fractured, the articular pillar is fractured and there is anterior disruption. The anterior pillar is fractured for that to occur. I think the posterior longitudinal ligament and the annulus posteriorly also has to be fractured, otherwise that will not separate. So I think it is implied. You cannot see it, obviously. Our radiologists now say they can see posterior and anterior longitudinal ligament injuries on the MRI. I am not convinced from what they have shown me, but they say they can see it. I think it is inferred that the articular pillar is fractured for the separation to occur. I also think that the posterior longitudinal ligament must also have had to separate or to at least have been stretched.

Prof. René Louis continued: I have some autopsy specimens. They are not ruptured. The posterior facets sometimes are ruptured. The posterior ligaments are loosened, but not ruptured. Not always, because it is difficult to say "always" or "never." Dr. Larson said: They may be stretched rather than actually torn; they may be more lax than they had been. Prof. Louis added that the margin must be crushed and really completely open for the ligament to be torn.

Dr. Kostuik interjected: One of the big problems I have is with the flexion-distraction injuries. We have been shown a number of examples of those cases being treated with Harrington distraction rods. This is difficult conceptually because you are applying a distractive force to something that has already been distracted and in some cases, as was shown, there was the development of paraparesis. This is something I have recognized and tried to avoid. I would like to emphasize that a classification system has to allow us to treat the patient with appropriate measures. If there are fractures one must provide the reverse force to correct them whether it is an axial fracture in the lower extremity or a fracture in the spine. That is why I am critical of the classification systems that currently exist.

Dr. Larson noted that the classification he is using is by no means the original. It was initiated in 1925 with elaborations added over the years. The advantage of it is that, as was mentioned, it is based on the direction of the deforming force. If you have a distraction force you do not distract farther. If you have a flexion deformity, one tends to go toward extension and vice versa. Obviously, there is no classification that is perfect, but this one at least gives a direction as to how treatment should be carried out. As to what absolutely should be done, I do not believe any classification will do that. One may classify brain tumors, but that does not tell one whether the tumor should be removed. That depends on what is happening to the patient.

Dr. Kostuik noted that some of the newer classifications come pretty close. In the current AO manual the work of Magro comes pretty close. Dr. Neuwirth added that in terms of classification the point is for classifications to be useful in teaching they have to be fairly simple, which is not the case with most of these very complicated classification systems. Therefore I do not know if we will ever achieve the goal of having a classification system that is precise enough to instruct everyone in how fractures occur and what is the best approach to deal with them and at the same time simple enough to be taught widely. There was a study by the Scoliosis Research Society quite a few years ago looking at who operated upon fractures of the spine. Were they spine surgeons? Were they orthopedists in the community? Were they neurosurgeons? Many were being done by people not particularly trained in spine. Dr. Kostuik said: That is absolutely correct. Dr. Neuwirth continued: So if this is the goal of the individual you are trying to reach with a classification system that is useful, if it is too complex no one is going to use it. The thought I have and I am not sure if its applicable to the spine relates to the classification of ankle fractures—the Langenhousen classification. It is a very accurate classification because it looks not only at the mechanism of injury, but also the position of the body within, prior to the application of force. I think that probably has something to do with the way fractures in the spine develop and I wonder if you think about the application of forces to the spine; for example, it may help to explain what must be done after the event. In view of the complex presentation of severely traumatized individuals, I wonder if indeed this is possible and whether there is any validity to incorporating such an idea in the classification system.

Dr. Kostuik responded: I think the best example of that is the seatbelt injury. I mean the old lapbelt injury. Dr. Bennett added that that is continuing to happen today since some individuals are removing the strap to avoid wrinkling their clothes.

Dr. Hal Dick inquired if there are any classifications that include an overview of the functional deficit that goes along with the mechanism of injury that also provides a view as to the type of treatment that should be initiated. Dr. Kostuik asked: You mean the functional deficit in terms of neurological function? Yes. Dr. Kostuik continued: I think that would be almost impossible. I'd like to hear Dr. Larson's opinion because there is such tremendous variation in the neurological presentation related to various fracture patterns. In the cauda equina, for example, one can see an almost completely occluded canal without any neurological deficit and in a separate instance with a 30% occluded canal have a major neurological deficit.

Dr. Larson responded: I think two things happen at the time of impact in a fracture. First, there is energy absorption by the spinal cord or neural elements, which takes place at impact. There is nothing that one can do about that. If the energy absorption is sufficient to totally knock out the neural elements, then that's that. The second thing is persisting deformity. It is always easier to predict from the patient's symptoms and findings what the x-rays are going to show than to predict a patient's neurological symptoms from an x-ray.

Dr. Kostuik noted that there appears to be a consensus that if the neurological deficit in the cauda equina is due to bony intrusion, that everyone would operate on the patient.

Dr. Bennett noted that the Dennis classification is probably the most uniformly used in determining the presence of instability and the type of treatment. It is relatively simple. Dr. Farcy also agreed that the Dennis classification was a very useful guideline. Dr. Larson added that the only basic practical difference between the Dennis system and the Holdsworth system is in the axial load fracture.

The Need for Acute Care in Spinal Cord Centers

Dr. White added: The level of spine training at which treatment in the emergency room setting is usually conducted is by generalists without specific training. They are not going to grasp a classification in the middle of the night. It is our responsibility to teach them, to talk to them about the mechanisms of injury, to teach them the neurological examination, and then to get x-rays and CT scans and have them become proficient in reading those studies including motion studies of the spine; afterward to attempt a trial of treatment without giving up, but watching the patient closely to avert paralysis. With that kind of a system classification, better care might be rendered on a general basis.

In essence, Dr. Kostuik continued, that is an idealization of the present imperfect world in which we live. Under these circumstances I would have to say that I do not think spinal injuries should ever be treated by generalist. I believe they should be treated in special centers and on this continent there are enough such centers to provide this care.

Dr. Larson said: I agree with you entirely. The problem is that people are at a distance and I do not think we are at a point yet where the medical community at large is accepting of that concept. Dr. Kostuik said emphatically that the medical profession has got to accept that notion of spinal injury care because too many problems are occurring.

The Early Surgical Treatment of Unstable Spine Injuries

Dr. Kostuik noted that there is more and more evidence that the morbidity from respiratory disease and other complications including duration of stay in the ICU was significantly decreased if the unstable spine was operated upon in the first 24 hours, and that has been our practice now for some time. It makes nursing care easier as well. Dr. Sonntag agreed that early intervention, either conservative or operative, stabilizes the patient and decompresses the neural structures, if necessary, and then gets him mobilized as soon as possible. Dr. Larson disagreed with the need for early operation, specifically for the patients with bilateral locked facets. I do not try to reduce them because I am going to fuse them anyway; therefore, I may as well do an open reduction and fuse at the same time. Dr. Sonntag stipulated that there are many ways to reduce bilateral locked facets and certainly we do not take films every 30 minutes. We take films every 5 minutes and have a resident at the bedside until the reduction is completed. If after 6 to 8 hours there is no reduction, we then take them to surgery.

CHAPTER 9

Nonoperative Stabilization of the Adult Cervical Spine

Robert N.N. Holtzman

External stabilization of the adult cervical spine is provided by a number of devices. The soft collar and Philadelphia collar serve well for the management of minor cervical injuries without evidence of instability or "subtle" instability of 1 mm or less motion between adjacent vertebrae. However, when gross instability exists, manifested by motion between adjacent vertebrae on flexion-extension radiographs greater than 1 mm in the young adult and perhaps up to 2 mm in the elderly adult, by pain, or neurological deficits following a traumatic event, the current trend among spinal neurosurgeons and orthopedic spine surgeons is to proceed with internal fixation and fusion. Alternatively, rigid external stabilization in the form of the Halo-Vest system as the primary and/or sole therapeutic modality is considered an option in selected cases. This becomes particularly relevant when the patient's age or medical condition militates against surgical intervention. A significant corollary to Halo-Vest application is delayed surgical intervention for those patients who fail to achieve a fusion despite an adequate period of rigid immobilization or whose occupation or activities involve extremes of physical exertion and endurance.

External stabilization is best provided at present by the Halo-Vest apparatus. Periods of stabilization usually range from 2 months to 6 months but may extend up to 1 year in selected instances to insure satisfactory fusion of the unstable elements.

This chapter describes 27 instances of cervical spine instability managed primarily with external stabilization, or with a combination of external stabilization and internal fixation and fusion. It serves to emphasize that external stabilization is an appropriate and often necessary adjunct, either preceding or following internal stabilization. It also attempts to clarify those instances where external nonoperative stabilization alone is sufficient in providing lasting stability, thereby justifying its position as a substantive element in the armamentarium of the spine surgeon.

Indications for External Stabilization

For each of the 27 cases decribed below a specific rationale was employed for the initial institution of Halo-Vest stabilization. They include the following:

1. Application of the Halo ring or Universal for the purpose of instituting traction to achieve reduction and realignment of a subluxation or fracture dislocation with immediate or delayed vest immobilization. This was particularly pertinent when the amount of weight required for reduction exceeded the stress and grasping tolerances of Gardner-Wells, Vincke, and Crutchfield tongs.
2. External stabilization in preparation for surgical internal stabilization.
3. Patients with a medical contraindication to surgery.
4. Patients whose age was over 80 years and whose general condition placed them at significant risk for general anesthesia and surgery.
5. Situations in outlying hospitals where surgical equipment was not available to achieve optimum internal fixation.
6. Patients with moderate to severe osteoporosis.
7. Patients who unequivocally refused surgical intervention despite an unbiased presentation of the therapeutic options of surgery versus external stabilization.
8. Medical-legal inplications.
9. Selected instances where internal fixation has failed.

Medical Contraindications to Surgical Intervention

1. Myocardial infarction of recent or undetermined age.
2. Pulmonary embolus or severe pulmonary insufficiency.
3. Coagulopathy.
4. Respiratory arrest and coma.
5. Renal failure.

Complications of the Use of the Halo Stabilization Device

1. Pressure ulceration from the jacket in patients with:
   a. extreme thoracic kyphosis
   b. impaired nutrition and poor skin turgor
   c. moderate to severe obesity.
2. Pin site infection:
   a. bacterial
   b. fungal.
3. Insecure pin fixation and loosening with Halo ring disruption.

4. Pain from the jacket or pin sites.
5. Failure of fusion despite an adequate period of immobilization.
6. Settling of the Halo-Vest in the erect posture with repeated resubluxation.
7. Confinement psychosis.
8. Residual scars at the site of pin placement.
9. Improper pin placement with resultant pain on chewing and/or inability to close the eyelids.
10. Dysphagia for either solids or liquids.
11. Pin penetration of the dura.

Cases Exemplifying the Application of External Stabilization Devices

C1-C2 Level

Case 1

This 93-year-old former nurse sustained a fall with blunt head trauma. A left Babinski sign was noted along with lethargy attributed to sedation ordered in the emergency room. Lateral x-ray (Fig. 9.1A) and computed tomography (CT) demonstrated a type III odontoid fracture with subluxation of C1 anteriorly on C2 (Fig. 9.1B). The patient was reduced with 10 lbs of traction after Halo placement. Because of her extreme age surgery was felt to be a less of an option and vest fixation was achieved. After 6 months, fusion had occurred and was documented on flexion-extension views (Fig. 9.1C,D) along with a persisting 5-mm subluxation. An interval hospitalization for pin placement revision for pin site infection took place at 3 months. Otherwise, she was independently ambulatory at home and wore a Philadephia collar for several months. She succumbed 1 year later to gastric carcinoma.

Case 2

This 66-year-old woman was evaluated for chronic neck pain and found to have a subluxation of C1-C2 (Fig. 9.2A) without neurological deficit. Reduction was achieved with the Halo (Fig. 9.2B) and stable fixation with the vest. She was discharged home fully ambulatory and struck her head a number of times against the walls of her house ultimately dislodging the pins and disrupting the reduction. Reinstitution of the Halo fixation was attempted on two occasions with subsequent repeated pin dislodgment. She underwent C1, C2, and C3 wiring without bony fusion. Disruption of the internal fixation was noted 12 years later (Fig. 9.2C,D). She complained of neck pain, but remained fully ambulatory.

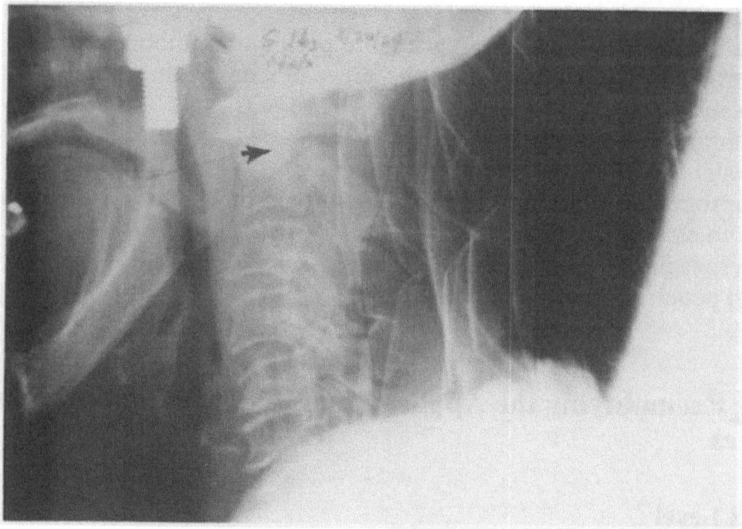

A

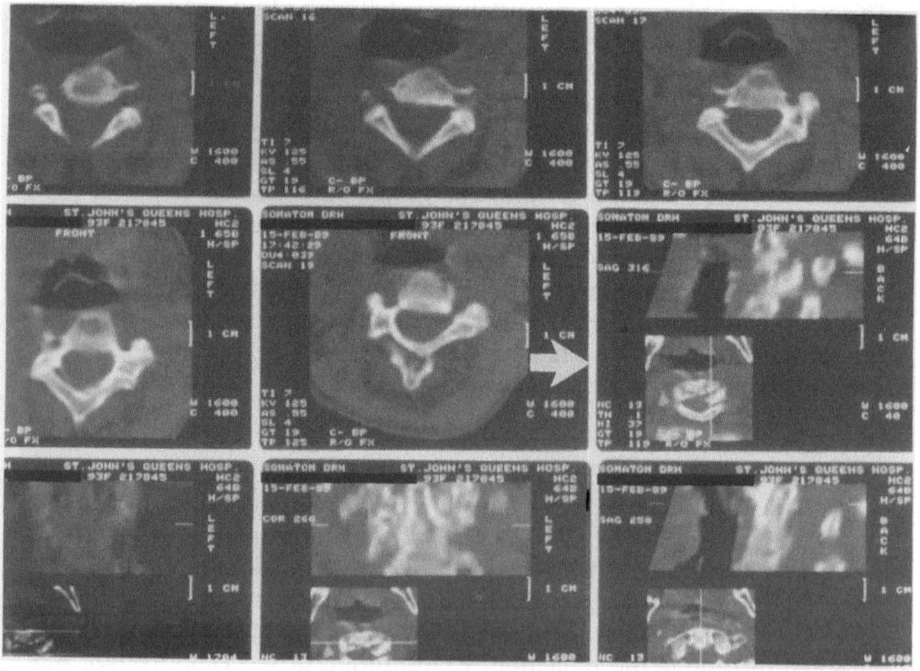

B

Figure 9.1. A: Lateral radiograph demonstrates the Cl-C2 subluxation (*black arrow*). **B:** CT scan demonstrates the odontoid type III fracture (*white arrow*). **C,D:** Flexion-extension views at 6 months with the Halo removed document stability with a persisting 5-mm subluxation (*small black arrows*).

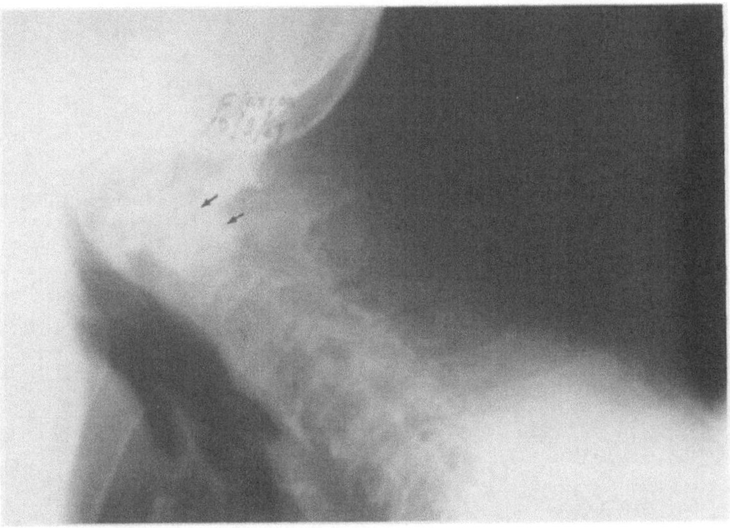

C

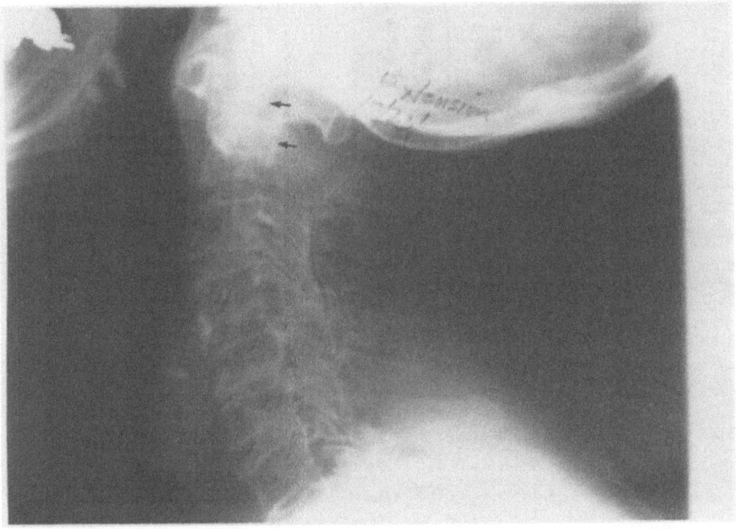

D

Figure 9.1. (*cont.*)

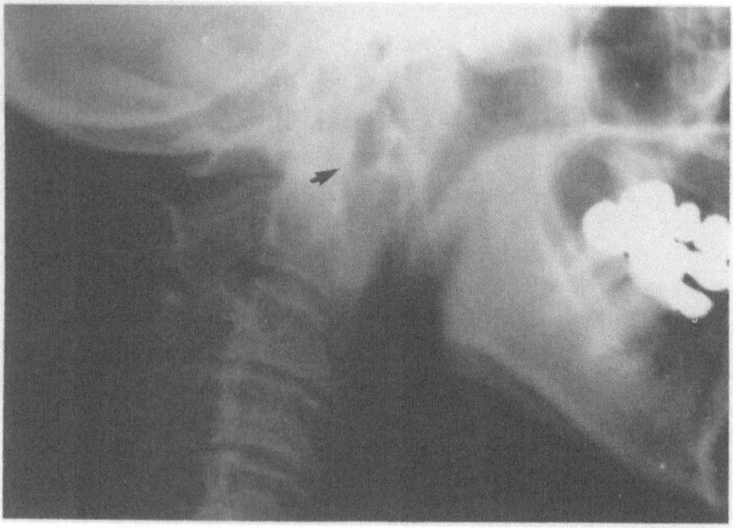

A

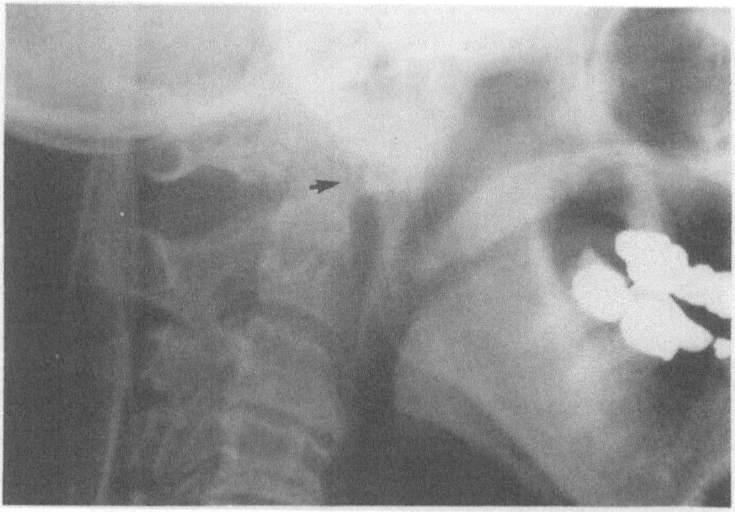

B

Figure 9.2. **A:** Subluxation C1-C2 without fracture (*black arrow*). **B:** Reduction and maintained in the Halo-Vest (*black arrow*). **C,D:** Disruption of the wire fixation.

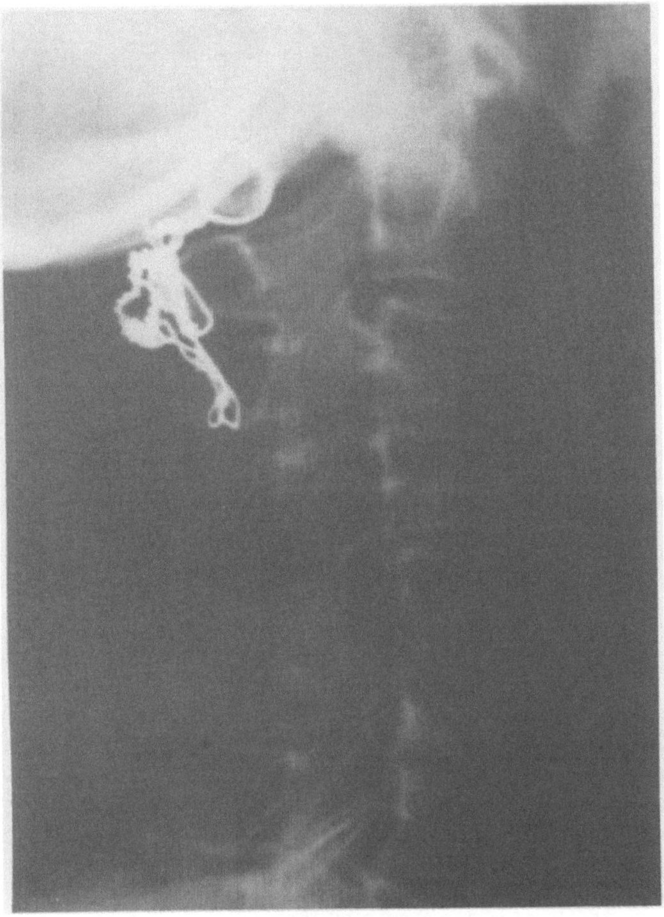

C

Figure 9.2. (*cont.*)

Case 3

This 81-year-old man suffered a fall from a second story balcony landing on the vertex of his skull. He arrived in the emergency room apneic, was intubed, resuscitated, and subsequently regained full consciousness, but suffered a moderate central cord syndrome with paraparesis. His examination and laboratory data were consistent with the diagnosis of rheumatoid arthritis. Plain radiographs of the neck demonstrated a type II odontoid fracture, C1-C2 subluxation, and a Jefferson fracture (Fig. 9.3A). Halo reduction and vest fixation were provided (Fig. 9.3B). Because of the patient's girth the vest was not well tolerated. Ultimately, he

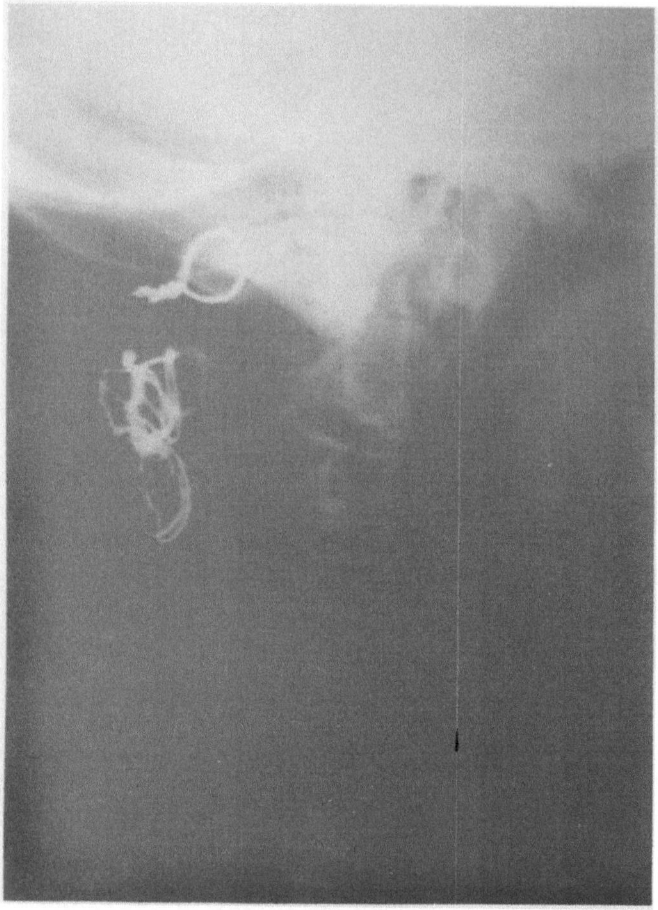

D

Figure 9.2. (*cont.*)

was able to sit erect, feed himself, and begin to stand when he succumbed to intractable congestive heart failure 3 months later and expired.

Case 4

An 89-year-old man with agitated senile dementia and loud abusive verbalizations presented with neck pain. Examination disclosed Babinski signs without overt paresis. Plain radiographs in flexion and extension demonstrated C1-C2 subluxation with a type II odontoid fracture (Fig. 9.4). In view of the patient's state of agitation it was clear that he would not tolerate Halo-Vest fixation. A Philadelphia collar was applied and the patient scheduled for internal fixation when he developed *Staphylococcus*

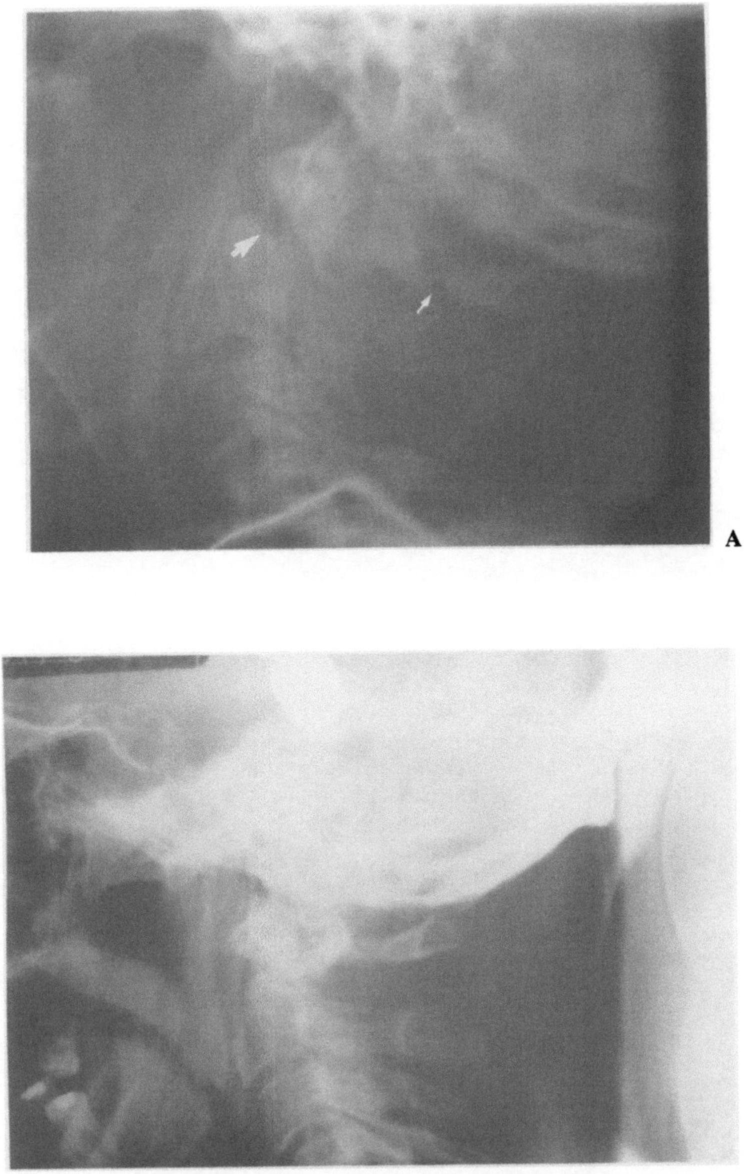

A

B

Figure 9.3. **A:** C1-C2 subluxation; type II odontoid fracture (*large white arrow*); Jefferson fracture (*small white arrow*). **B:** Reduction in Gardner-Wells tongs before Halo stabilization.

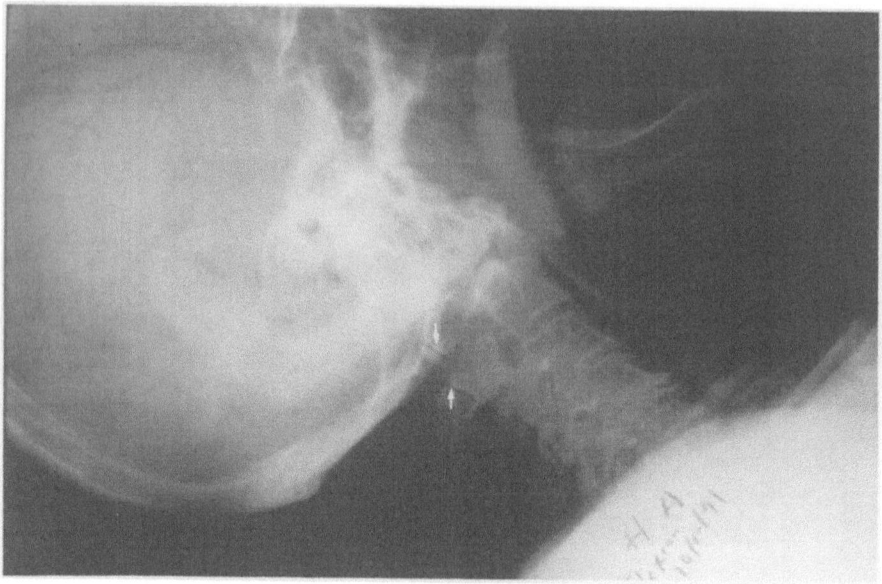

A

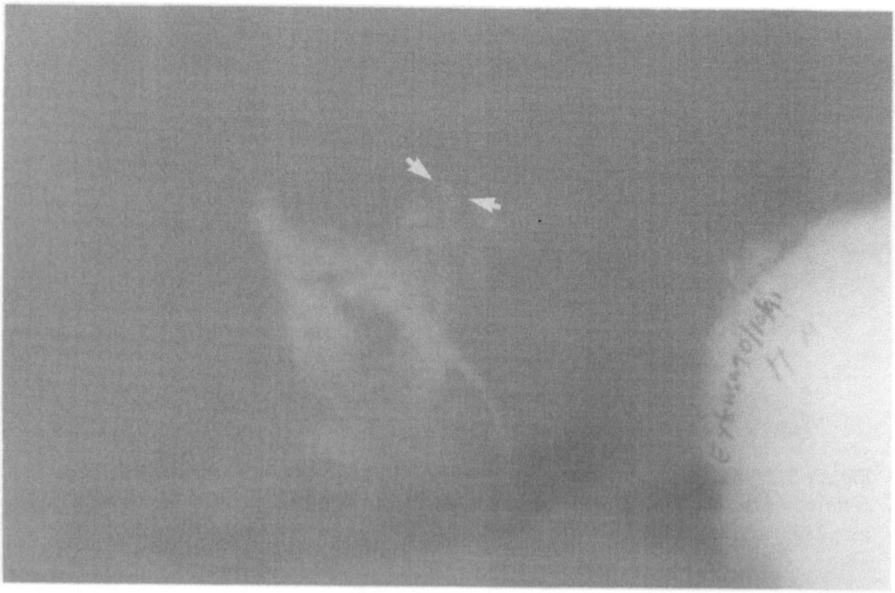

B

Figure 9.4. **A:** C1-C2 subluxation; flexion film (*small white arrows*). **B:** Extension film showing reduction and type II odontoid fracture (*large white arrows*).

aureus sepsis including meningitis, GI bleeding, and cardiorespiratory arrest.

Case 5

A 49-year-old man sustained a gunshot wound to the cervical spine with the bullet lodged in the lateral aspect of the arch of C1 (Fig. 9.5A,B). A Jefferson fracture was documented on CT scanning (Fig. 9.5C). The neurological examination disclosed no deficits. The patient was felt to have a stable cervical mechanism and was treated successfully with a Philadelphia collar.

Case 6

This 67-year-old man with documented rheumatoid arthritis had a history of progressively worsening neck pain after arising one morning from bed. The patient was of small stature and appeared quite frail. The neurologi-

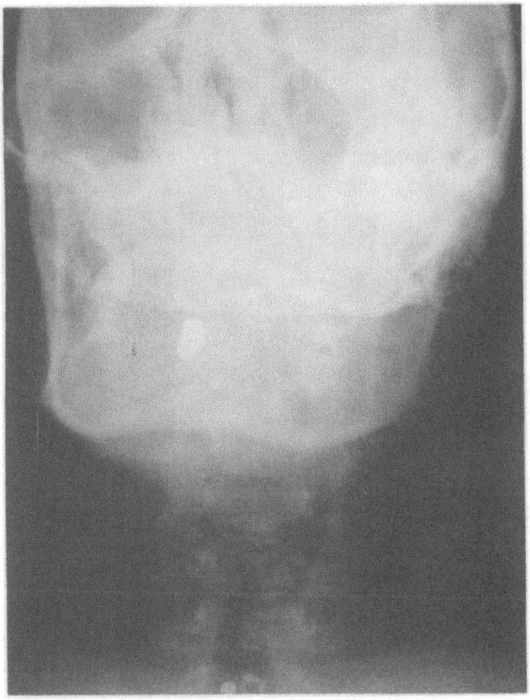

A

Figure 9.5. A: AP view of the cervical spine with bullet lodged in the left lateral mass of C1. **B:** Lateral view of the same. **C:** Axial CT of C1 showing the bullet and the unilateral Jefferson fracture (*small white arrows*).

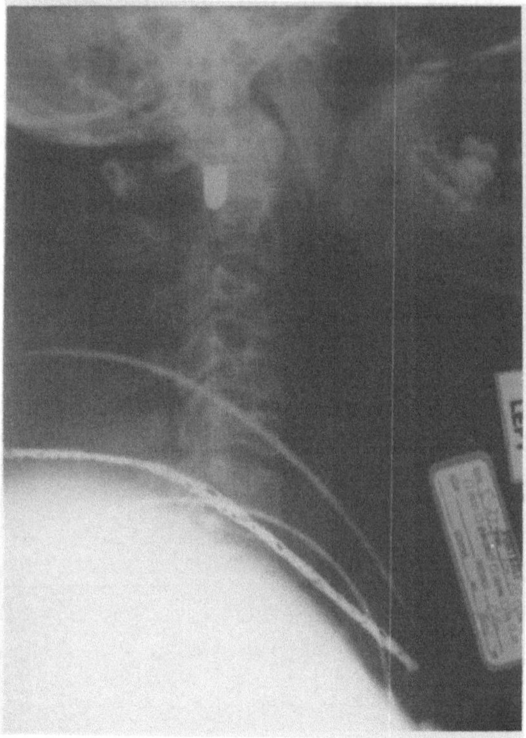

B

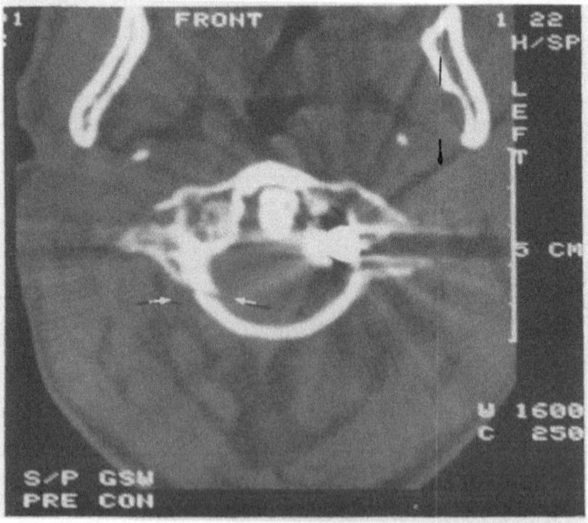

C

Figure 9.5. (*cont.*)

cal examination was normal. Plain radiographs disclosed the C1-C2 subluxation (Fig. 9.6A,B). Halo application and reduction was performed with only 5 lbs to avoid overdistraction, and vest fixation was instituted. One week later he underwent C1-C2 sublaminar wiring and iliac graft fusion (Fig. 9.6C). Assimilation of the arch of C1 to the occiput necessitated a partial suboccipital craniectomy for the wire placement and a spina bifida of the arch of C1 suggested a tenuousness to that structure that mandated the iliac graft fusion. Postoperative myelogram CT scan demonstrated the rotational subluxation and partial block (Fig. 9.6D). The patient remained stable and independently ambulatory after discharge, but complained of right occipital neuralgia. The Halo was removed after 2 months (Fig. 9.6E) and the patient was maintained in a Philadelphia collar. The rotational subluxation could not be corrected leaving the patient with a mild left head tilt. He died $1\frac{1}{2}$ years later of gastrointestinal bleeding and pneumonia.

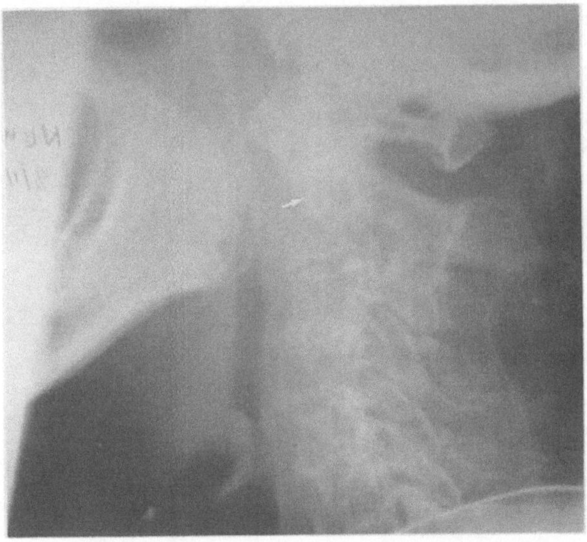

A

Figure 9.6. A: Plain radiograph in neutral position showing severe osteoporosis; and questionable subluxation C1-C2. (*white arrow*). **B:** Flexion film documenting the subluxation (*small black arrows*). **C:** Postoperative film of the sublaminar wiring and iliac bone graft fusion; odontoid type II fracture is seen (*large white arrow*). **D:** Postmyelogram CT scan showing rotational subluxation and incomplete filling of the C1 subarachnoid space with dye. **E:** Post-Halo removal with persisting subluxation (*white arrows*).

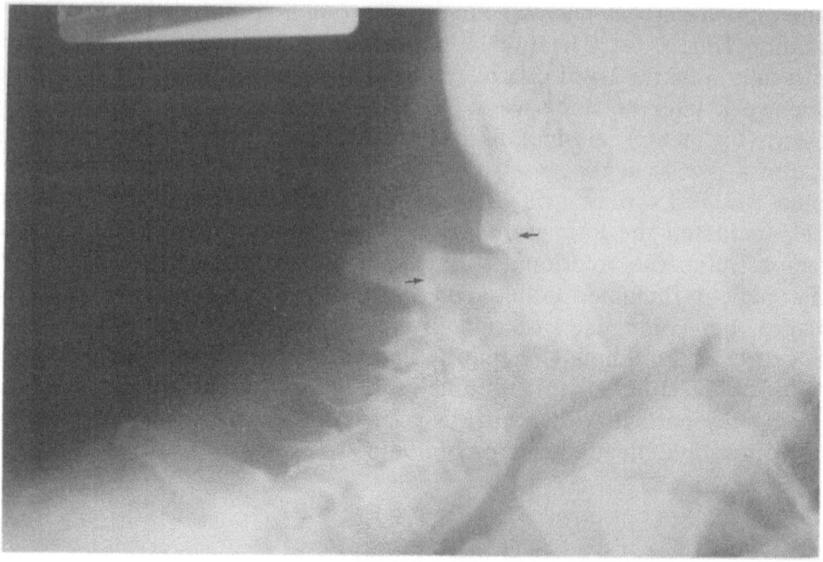

B

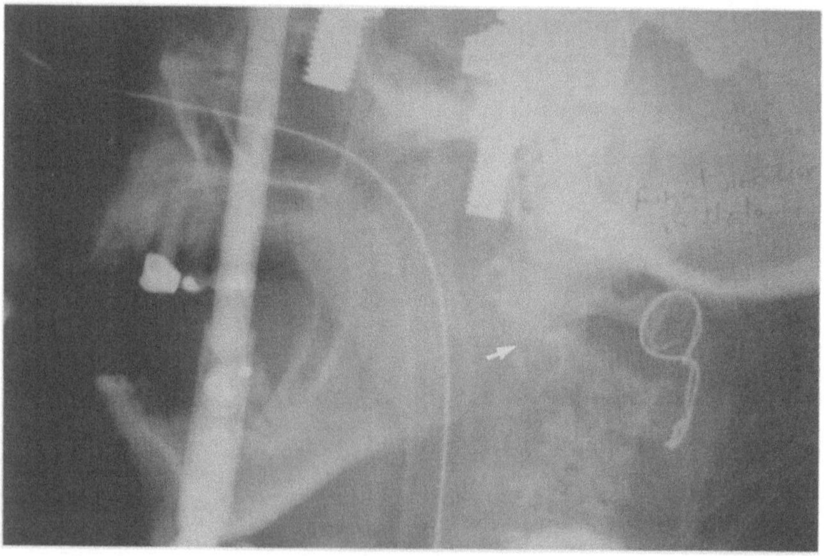

C

Figure 9.6. (*cont.*)

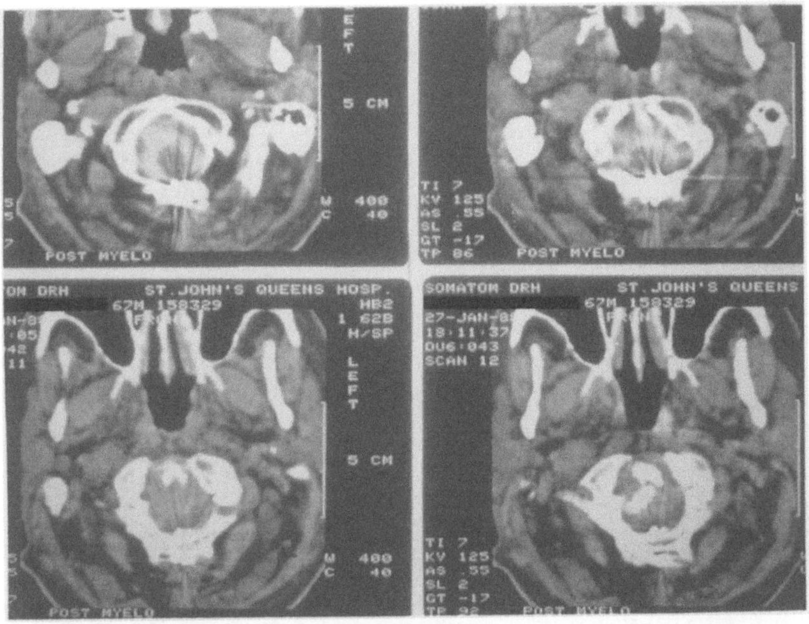

D

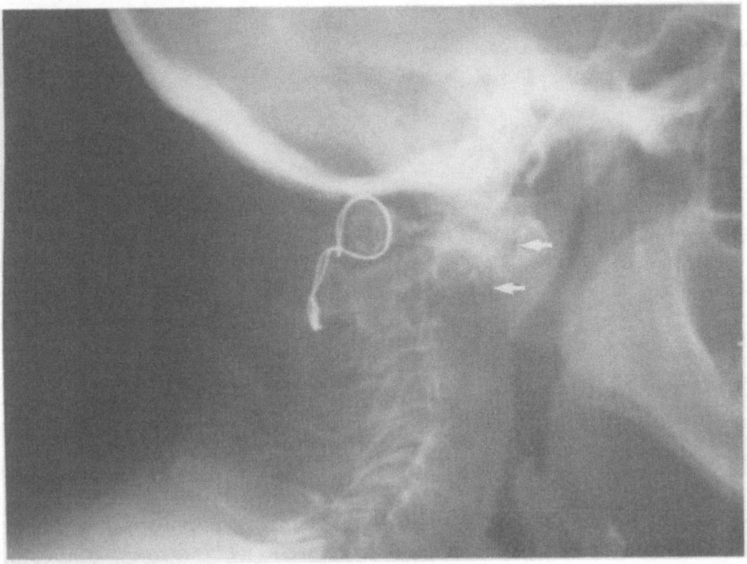

E

Figure 9.6. (*cont.*)

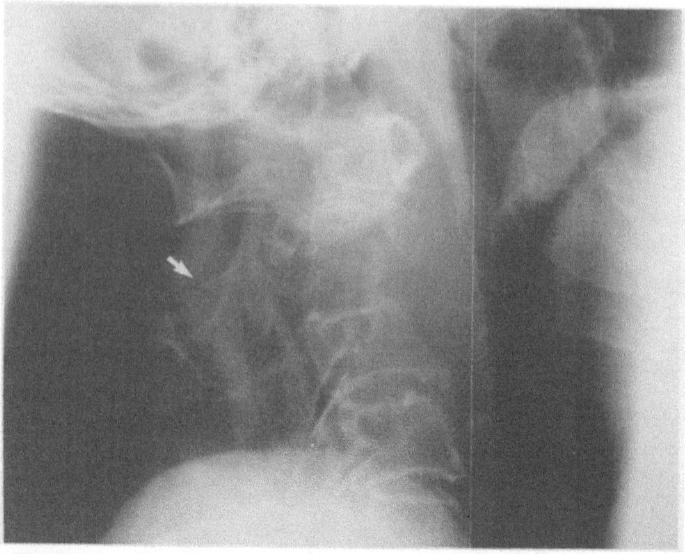

A

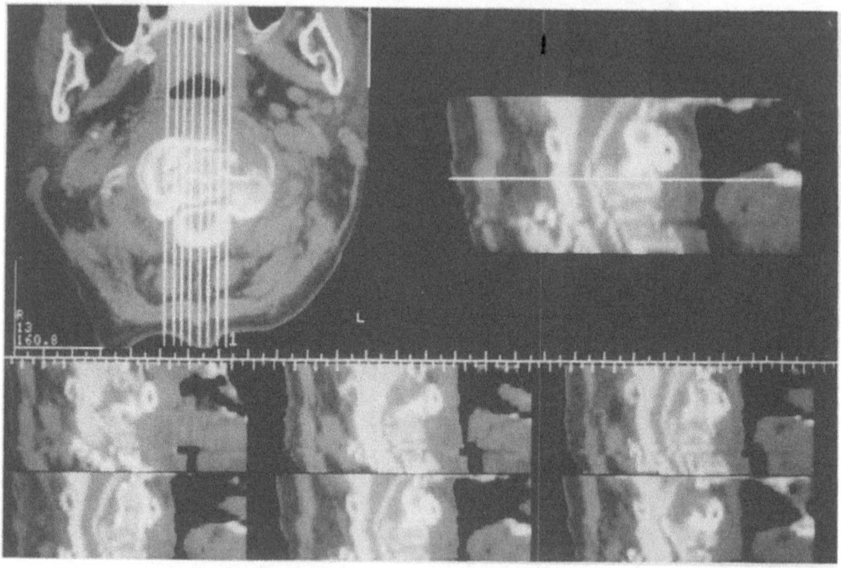

B

Figure 9.7. **A:** Lateral radiograph showing severe osteoporosis and hangman's fracture with caudal displacement of the C2 arch (*white arrow*). **B:** Postmyelogram CT scan demonstrating the C1-C2 subluxation, type III odontoid fracture without impingement upon the spinal cord. **C:** "Settling" with progressive anterior slippage of C1 on C2 (*small white arrow*). **D:** Flexion-extension and attempted distraction with 30 lbs demonstrated complete fusion of the odontoid to its base (*large black arrow*). **E:** Pressure ulceration from the vest over the T2-T3 spinous processes.

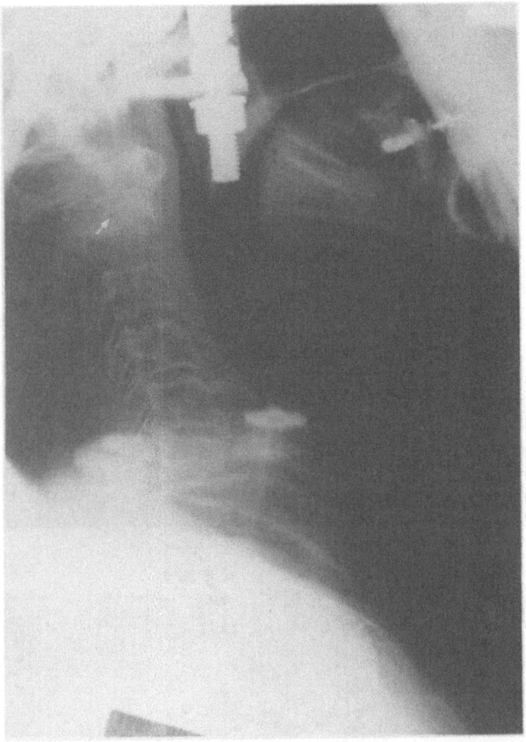
C

Figure 9.7. (*cont.*)

Case 7

This 69-year-old woman, a known ethanol abuser, fell and presented in the emergency room with neck pain, limitation of neck movements, and a left Babinski sign. Her plain radiographs showed severe osteoporosis and a hangman's fracture with caudal displacement of the C2 arch (Fig. 9.7A). Postmyelogram CT scan demonstrated the C1-C2 subluxation, type III odontoid fracture without impingement upon the spinal cord (Fig. 9.7B). She was maintained in the Halo-Vest for 3 months and progressive anterior slippage was noted (Fig. 9.7C). Flexion-extension and distraction films with 30 lbs of weight demonstrated complete fusion of the odontoid to its base and stability of the C1-C2 level (Fig. 9.7D). A pressure ulceration from the vest developed over the T2-T3 spinous processes due to her kyphosis, which was successfully managed with conservative measures (Fig. 9.7E). She was discharged and has remained well. It is acknowledged that a laminectomy of the arch of C1 may be required in the future.

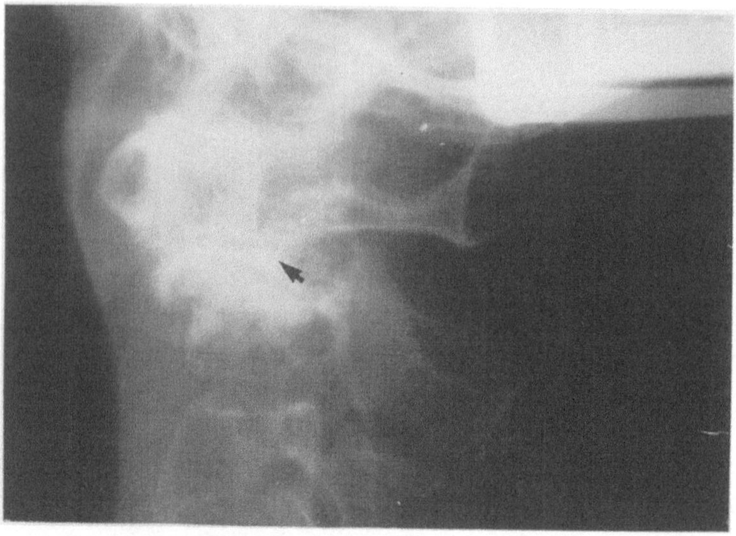

D

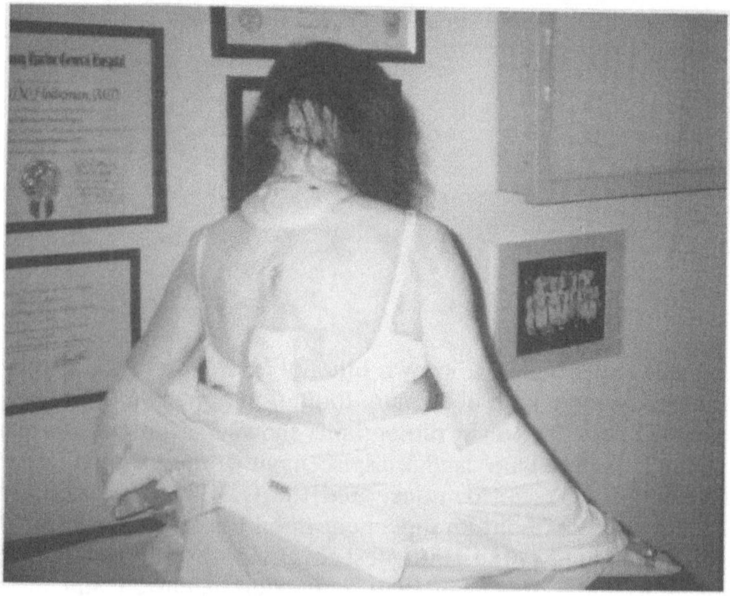

E

Figure 9.7. (*cont.*)

C2 Level

Case 8

This 38-year-old man dived into an empty swimming pool while inebriated. He presented with neck pain without any neurological deficits. Plain radiographs demonstrated a typical hangman's fracture of the arch of C2 (Fig. 9.8A). Halo-Vest fixation was instituted and maintained for 3 months. Progressive healing was documented radiographically with complete bony union seen at 7 months (Fig. 9.8B).

C3-C4 Level

Case 9

This 82-year-old man was involved in a motor vehicle accident with loss of consciousness. Past history included right rotator cuff injury with loss of throwing motion, transient ischemic attacks (TIAs) with syncope, labyrinthitis, and a cardiac arrythmia consisting of premature ventricular contractions. His neurological examination was normal. EKG showed deep Q waves in V1-V6. A myocardial infarction (MI) could not be excluded. Plain radiographs disclosed a C3-C4 subluxation (Fig. 9.9A) with a subtle, but definite change in position when compared to the scout film of the CT scan. Gardner-Wells tongs were inserted and the patient was maintained at bed rest. Halo-Vest stabilization was instituted 10 days later when the pain from the right clavicular fracture had subsided and demonstrated "reduction" (Fig. 9.9B). The Halo-Vest was removed 9 weeks later. Pressure ulcerations were managed conservatively during the last 3 weeks and after vest removal with complete healing. Stability at the C3-C4 level was seen on subsequent radiographs at 3 and 4 months (Fig. 9.9C,D,E). Consideration was given to the fact that the subluxation was not acute, but perhaps represented a spondolytic subluxation of the aged due to ligamentous weakening.

Case 10

This 72-year-old woman presented with neck pain, paresthesias, numbness and weakness of her hands, and episodes of falling. Her examination disclosed a spastic cervical myeloradiculopathy and a severe hearing disturbance. The EKG could not exclude a myocardial infarction. Magnetic resonance imaging (MRI) demonstrated C3-C4 subluxation and cervical spinal cord compression at that level by the subluxation and ventral soft tissue (Fig. 9.10A). Halo traction was instituted and reduction achieved with 141bs (Fig. 9.10B), whereupon vest stabilization was added. An erect film showed no motion (Fig. 9.10C). Initially there was a mild improvement in her myeloradiculopathy. She developed lower extremity phlebitis, as she was largely bed- and chair-ridden, which was managed

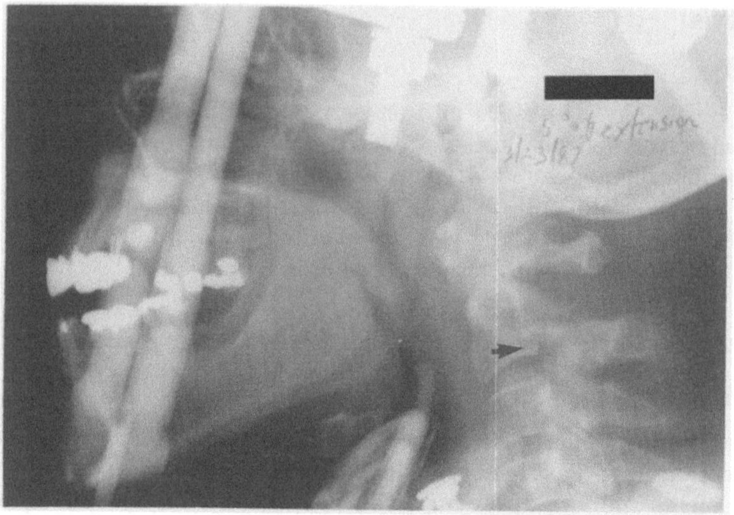

A

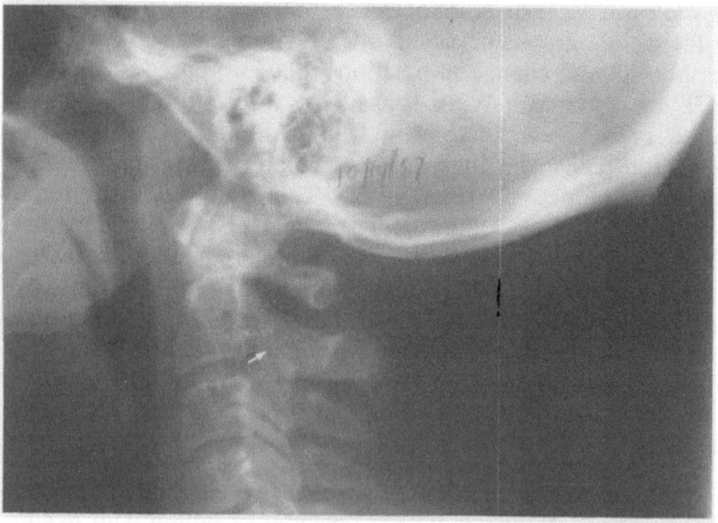

B

Figure 9.8. A: Typical hangman's fracture (*large black arrow*). **B:** Complete bony union at 7 months (*small white arrow*).

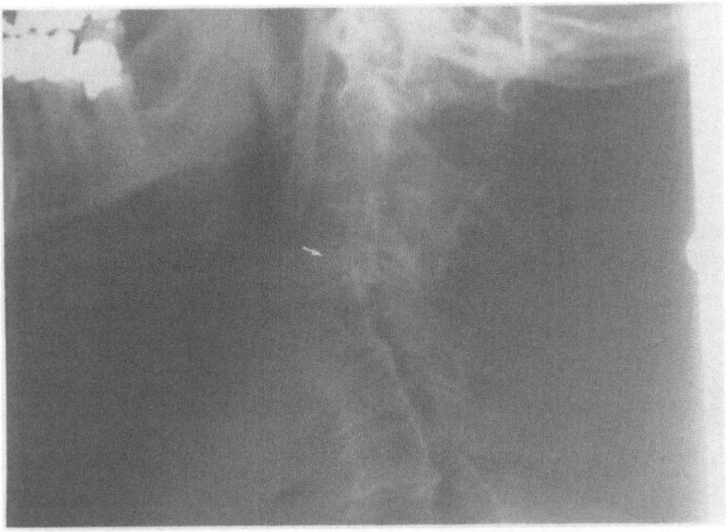

A

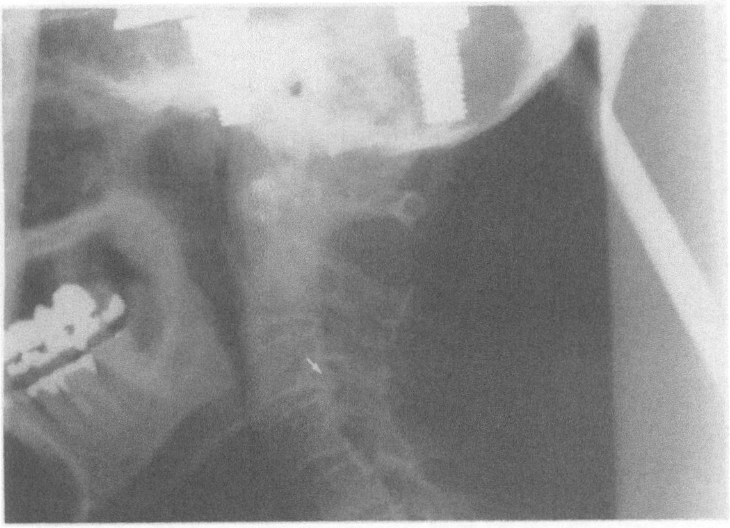

B

Figure 9.9. **A:** Subluxation at C3-C4 with definite motion when compared to the scout film of the CT scan (*small white arrow*). **B:** Reduction and fixation in the Halo-Vest (*small white arrow*). **C,D,E:** Stability documented on motion films at 3 and 4 months.

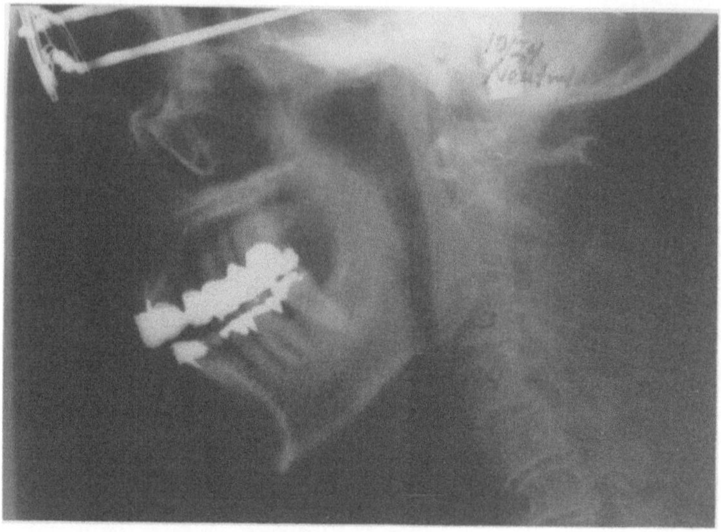

C

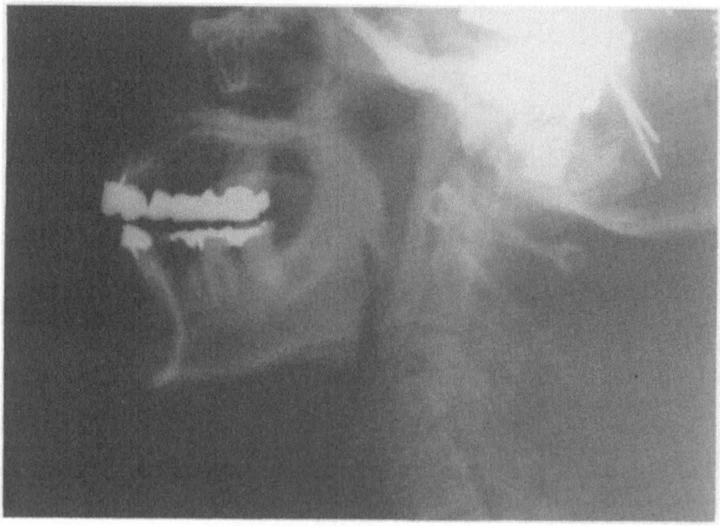

D

Figure 9.9. (*cont.*)

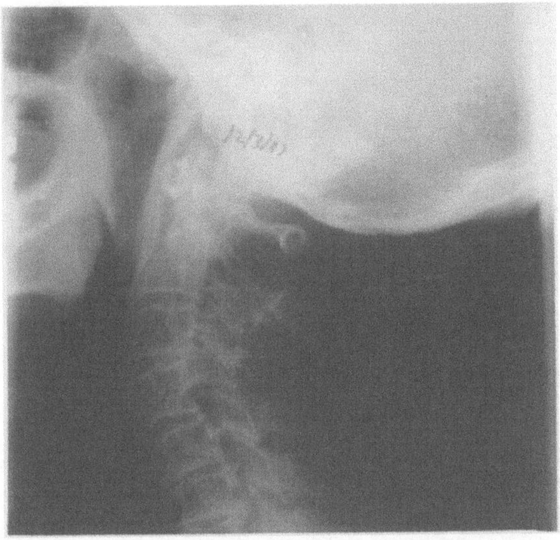

E

Figure 9.9. (*cont.*)

successfully with anticoagulation. The Halo-Vest was removed at 3 months. Plain radiographs demonstrated 4 mm of subluxation, almost certainly a consequence of "settling," and stability on flexion-extension views (Fig. 9.10D,E). MRI showed the subluxation and some resolution of the epidural soft tissue mass (Fig. 9.10F). Her neurological profile improved, characterized by independent ambulation and the ability to dress and feed herself. A mild residual myeloradiculopathy persisted.

Case 11

This 69-year-old man was involved in a motor vehicle accident. He complained of neck pain. The neurological examination was normal. Plain films demonstrated a C3-C4 subluxation without fracture (Fig. 9.11A,B). The option of internal fixation was offered and the patient refused. Halo application and retroflexion effected a reduction. Vest fixation was added. The patient was fully ambulatory and discharged home. One month later a 3-mm resubluxation was seen presumably related to "settling" of the Halo. Realignment was achieved (Fig. 9.11C). One more month of external stabilization demonstrated an incomplete fusion with a 4-mm step-off posteriorly and a 3 to 4-mm persisting subluxation on flexion-extension films (Fig. 9.11D,E). Philadelphia collar support was provided in the interim with the anticipation of fusion taking place or proceeding with internal fixation and fusion.

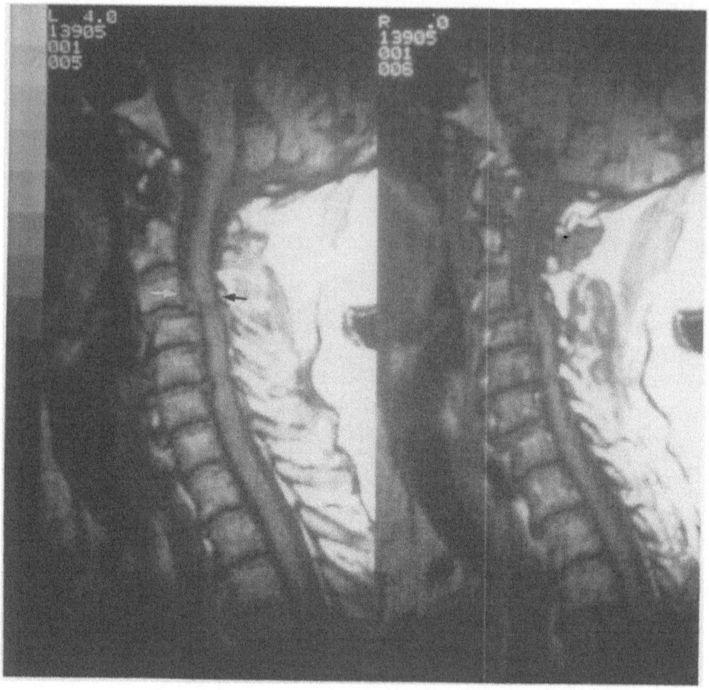

A

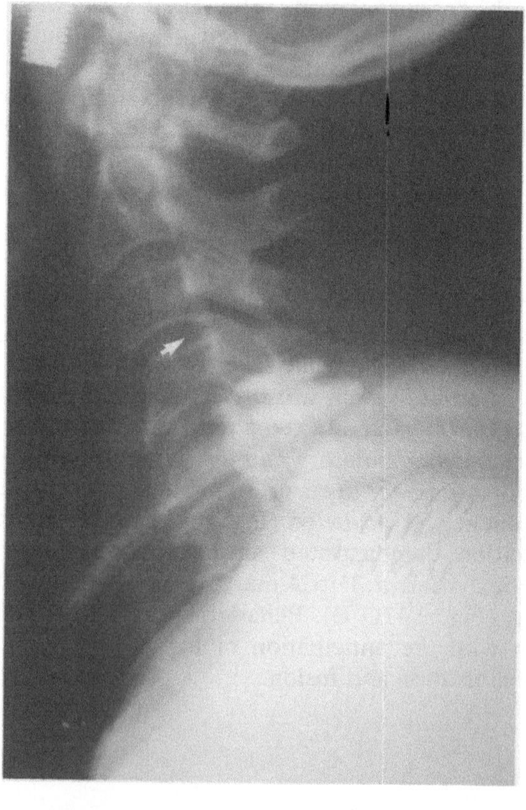

B

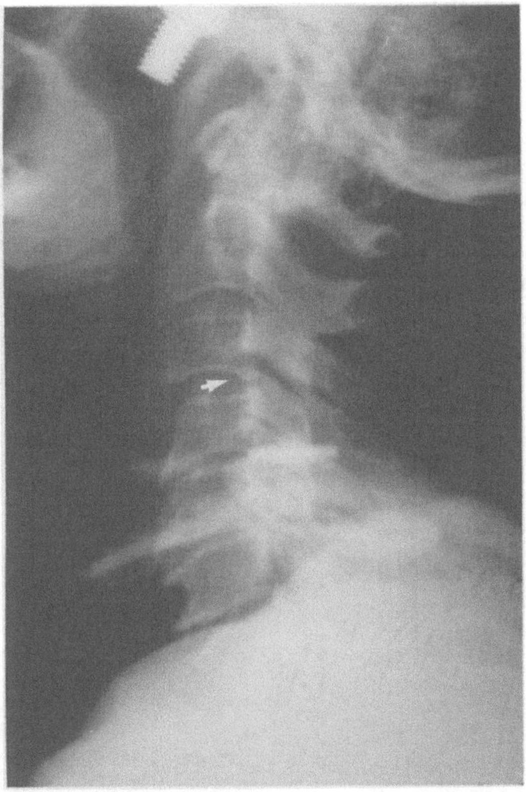
C

C4-C5 Level

Case 12

This 76-year-old woman presented with neck pain after a fall. There was a long history of ethanol abuse. Her complex medical history included myocardial infarction ×2; pulmonary emboli with ligation of the vena cava; chronic atrial fibrillation; TIAs; diabetes mellitus and mitral insufficiency. Plain cervical spine films, normal 5 years ago (Fig. 9.12A), now showed a subluxation at C4-C5 (Fig. 9.12B,C). Left C5 and C6 radiculopathies were noted. Halo application and 25 lbs of traction produced a satisfactory reduction that was maintained with the attachment of the vest

---

Figure 9.10. **A:** C3-C4 subluxation with ventral extradural soft tissue mass (*small white and black arrows*). **B:** Plain radiograph showing perfect reduction with 14 lbs (*large white arrow*). **C:** Upright film in Halo—no slippage (*large white arrow*). **D,E:** Flexion-extension films after 3 months show "settling" with 4-mm stable subluxation. **F:** MRI with T1-weighted imaging shows persisting subluxation with smaller ventral extradural mass (*small white arrow*).

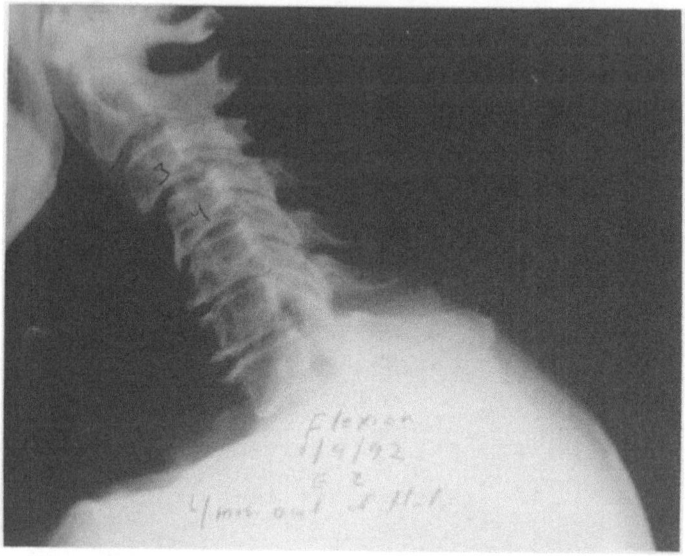

D

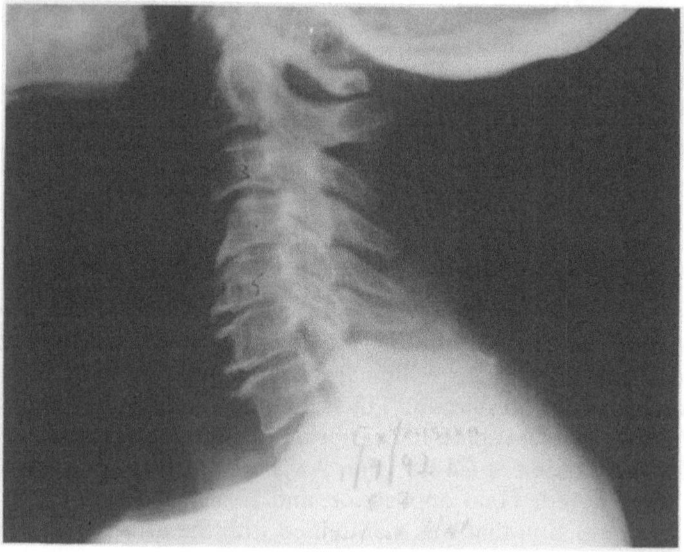

E

Figure 9.10. (*cont.*)

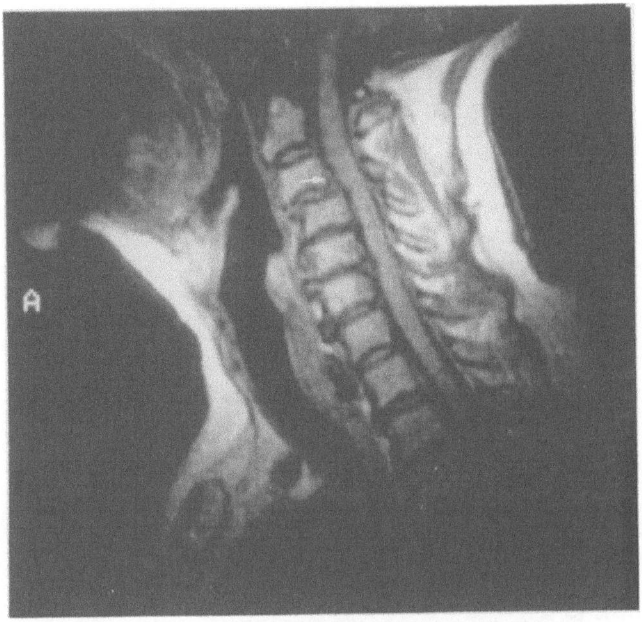

F

Figure 9.10. (*cont.*)

(Fig. 9.12D). One week later the patient loosened the Halo with the tools left at her bedside and re-reduction was required. A 1-mm subluxation persisted. With settling of the Halo-Vest in the erect posture a resubluxation became apparent, necessitating a third reduction. At this sitting, in an attempt to achieve perfect alignment in the erect posture, additional subluxation, to a lesser extent, at C3-C4 was evident (Fig. 9.12E). This instability was ascribed to multilevel spondolytic ligamentous weakening. Pin site infections became evident with a cellulitis surrounding the frontal pins not responsive to bacitracin. *Candida albicans* was cultured along with *Staphylococcus aureus* and there was a partial response to Mycostatin and changing the pin positions. In view of the incomplete response and the inability to maintain long-term external stabilization inplantation of a Luque rectangle over the C2-C6 spinous processes, wiring of C3 bilaterally, and subsequent wiring of C5 and C6 as a second unit, was performed 11 weeks after admission. This was followed by iliac grafting (Fig. 9.12F). The patient tolerated the procedure well and began to ambulate independently. Her radiculopathies substantially resolved and she was discharged.

A

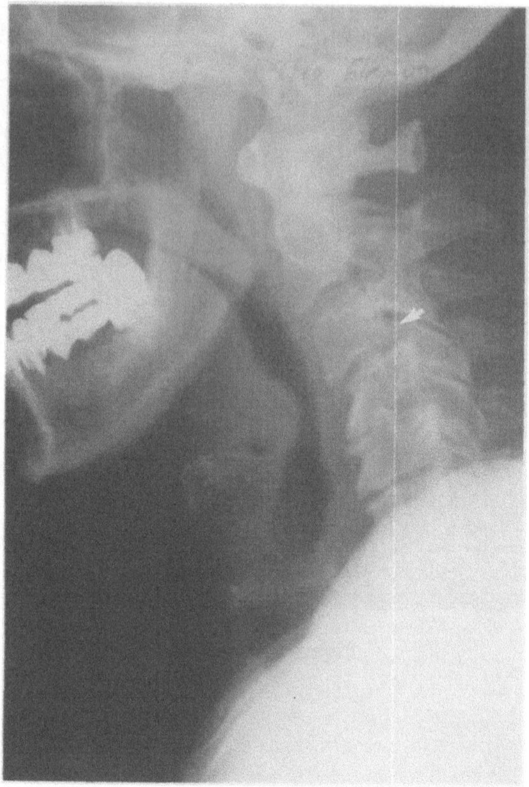

Figure 9.11. A: Plain radiograph demonstrating C3-C4 subluxation in flexion (*large white arrow*). **B:** Film in extreme extension demonstrating reduction (*large white arrow*). **C:** Two months later 3-mm resubluxation compatible with "settling." **E:** At 3 months with Halo removed 3 to 4-mm of persisting subluxation is seen on flexion-extension films (*large white arrows*).

Case 13

This 82-year-old woman was involved in a motor vehicle accident and suffered blunt forehead trauma with lacerations. Neurological examination disclosed a left Babinski sign. Plain radiographs demonstrated a 3-mm subluxation at C4-C5 (Fig. 9.13A). A flexion film confirmed instability (Fig. 9.13B). Halo reduction was achieved and the vest attached (Fig. 9.13C). The patient was discharged home after 1 month, but complained of increasing neck pain. CT myelography did not disclose spinal cord compression, but facet fracture with sclerosis was noted (Fig. 9.13D). She developed a confinement psychosis that was managed medi-

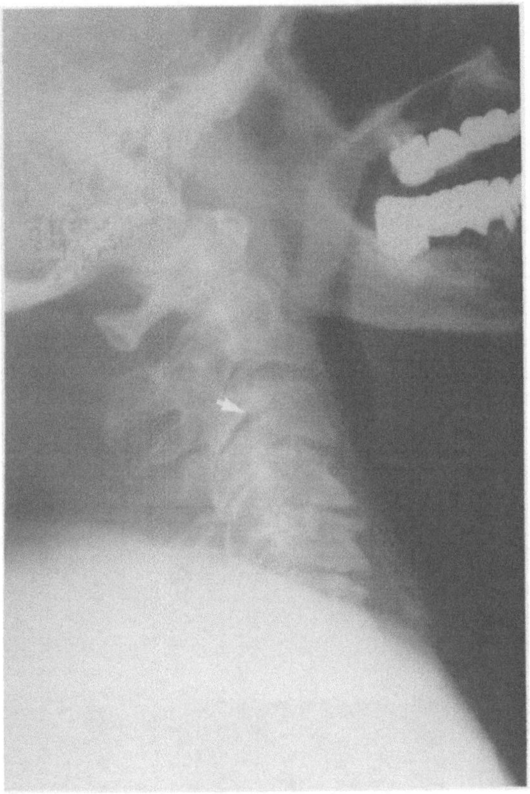

B

Figure 9.11. (*cont.*)

cally. She recovered and had the Halo removed at 3 months with satisfactory stabilization achieved.

Case 14

This 25-year-old man suffered blunt trauma and was found to have a C4-C5 subluxation on plain radiographs (Fig. 9.14A). Halo traction reduced the subluxation and vest fixation was added (Fig. 9.14B). After 2 months the Halo was removed with satisfactory stabilization.

Case 15

This 32-year-old man was involved in a motor vehicle accident in Florida, with loss of consciousness. He returned to New York and was admitted to the hospital 16 days later because of severe neck pain, left shoulder pain, and left arm weakness. His examination demonstrated a left C5 radiculo-

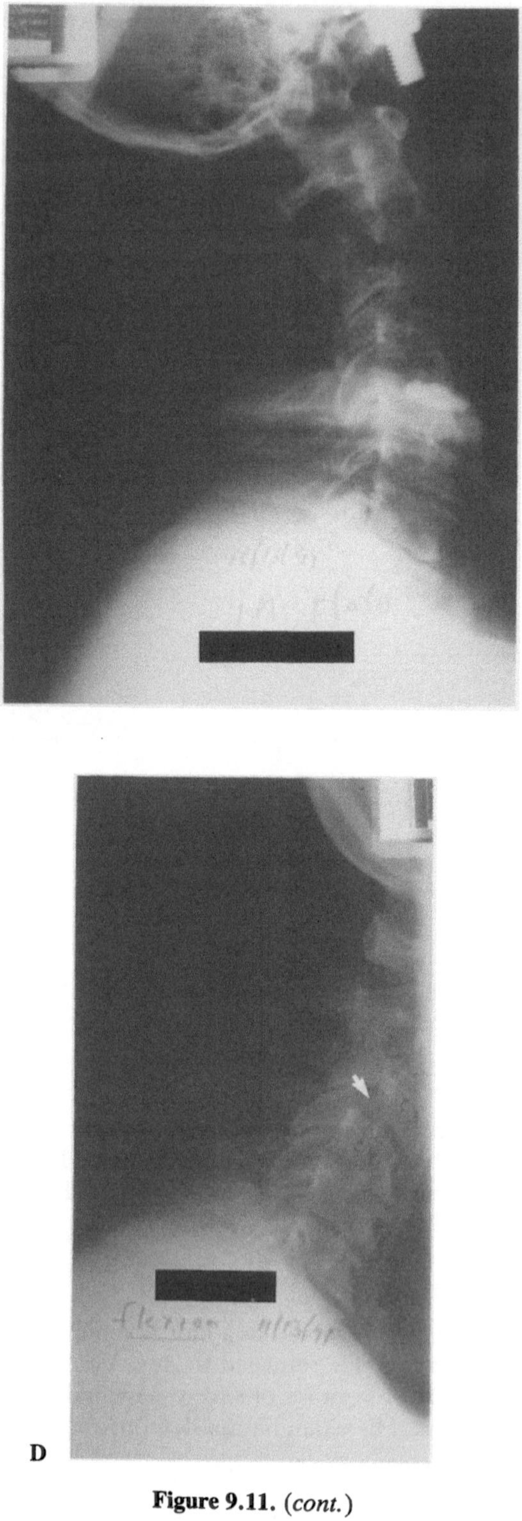

C

D

Figure 9.11. (*cont.*)

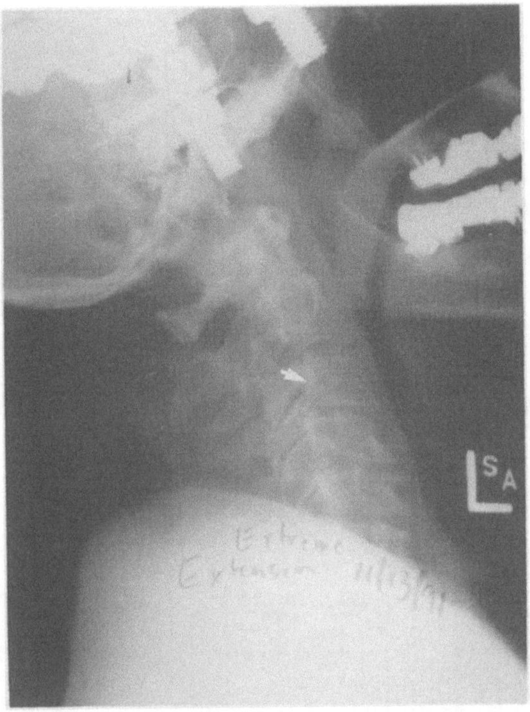

E

Figure 9.11. (*cont.*)

pathy, bilateral C6 radiculopathies and a myelopathy characterized as a partial Brown-Séquard syndrome. Plain radiographs demonstrated subluxation at C4-C5 (Fig. 9.15A) with a fracture of the left uncinate process (Fig. 9.15B). Halo traction with 15 lbs effected a reduction (Fig. 9.15C) and jacket fixation was added. There was a dramatic neurological improvement. He was discharged home, where he fell and dislodged the Halo pins. Neck and left arm pain recurred. He was readmitted and, because of his unreliability, was placed in Gardner-Wells tongs and traction for 6 weeks with stabilization documented at the C4-C5 level, but a persisting 2-mm subluxation (Fig. 9.15D). Neurologically he was asymptomatic with resolution of his deficits.

Case 16

A 69-year-old man with syncope struck his occiput. He complained of neck pain without other symptoms. His neurological examination was normal. Plain x-rays demonstrated a subluxation at C4-C5 with abnormal motion on flexion and extension (Fig. 9.16A,B). He was completely re-

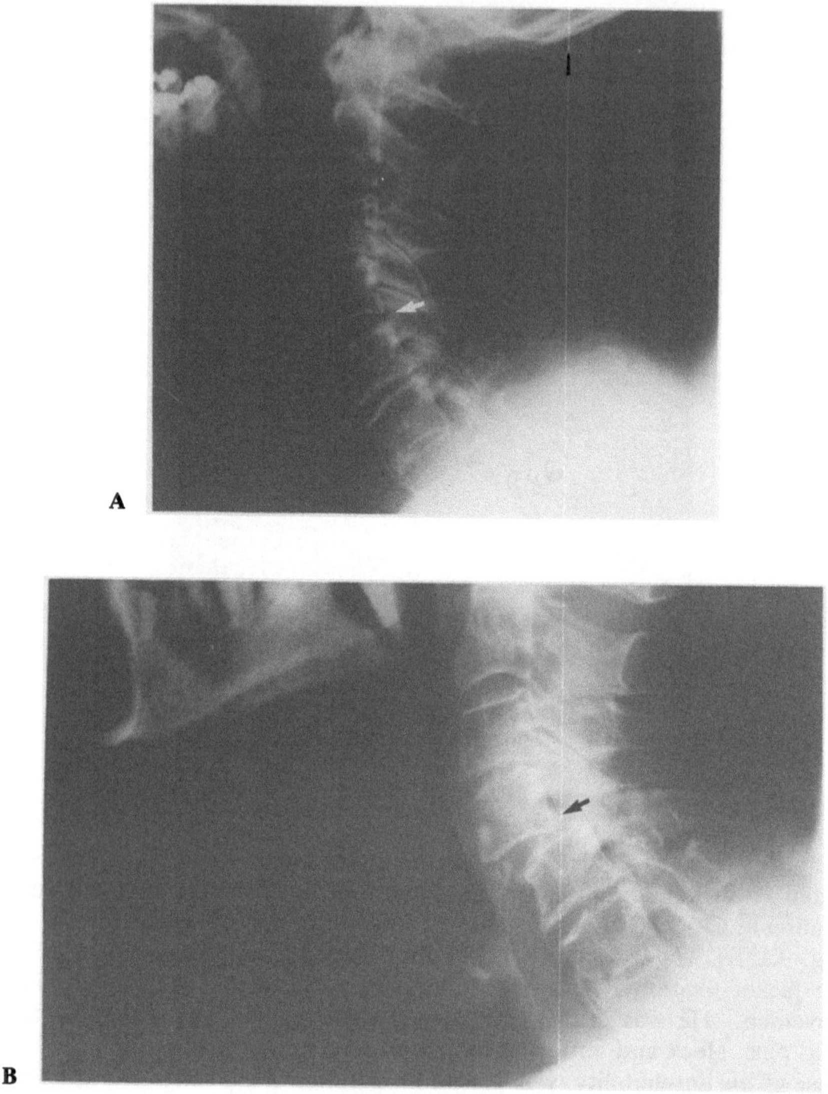

Figure 9.12. A: Plain radiograph 5 years ago demonstrates normal alignment of the cervical spine. B: Film demonstrating C4-C5 subluxation (*large black arrow*). C: CT scan and reconstruction demonstrate the subluxation. D: Film demonstrating Halo-Vest reduction and fixation (*large white arrow*). E: Film demonstrating "settling" with resubluxation C4-C5 (*lower large white arrow*) and some subluxation C3-C4 (*upper large white arrow*). F: Implantation of Luque rectangle C2-C6 with sublaminar wiring and iliac bone graft fusion.

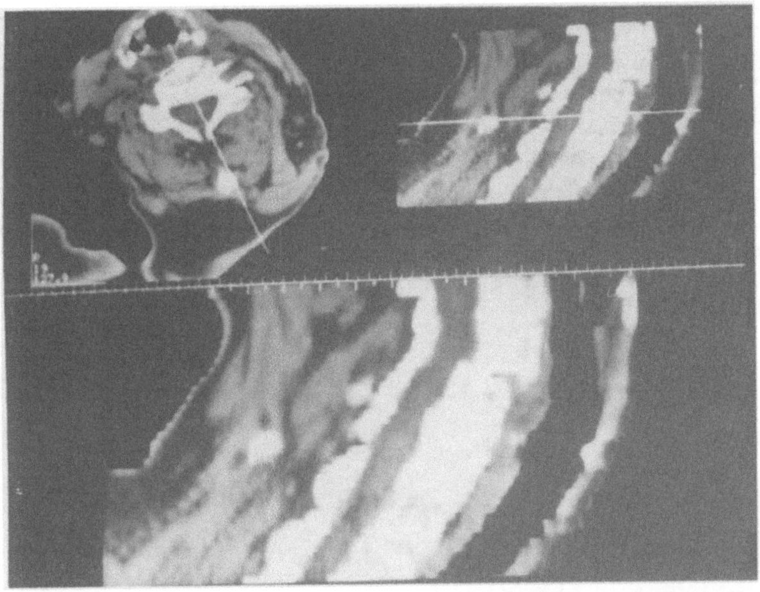

C

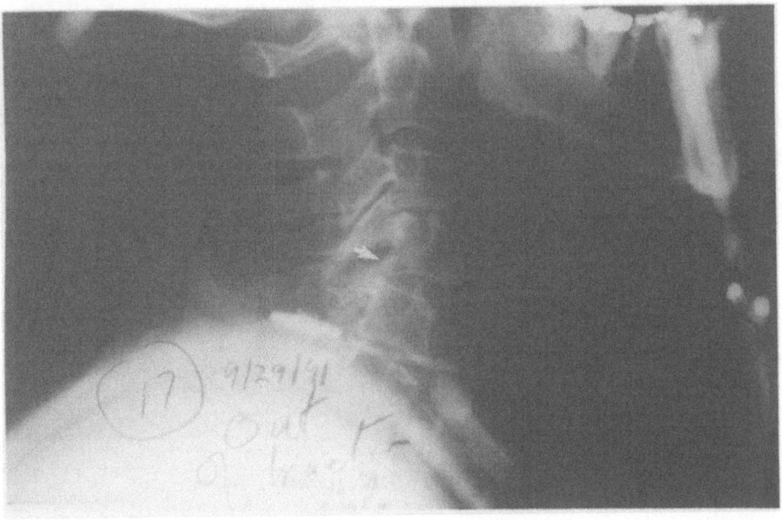

D

Figure 9.12. (*cont.*)

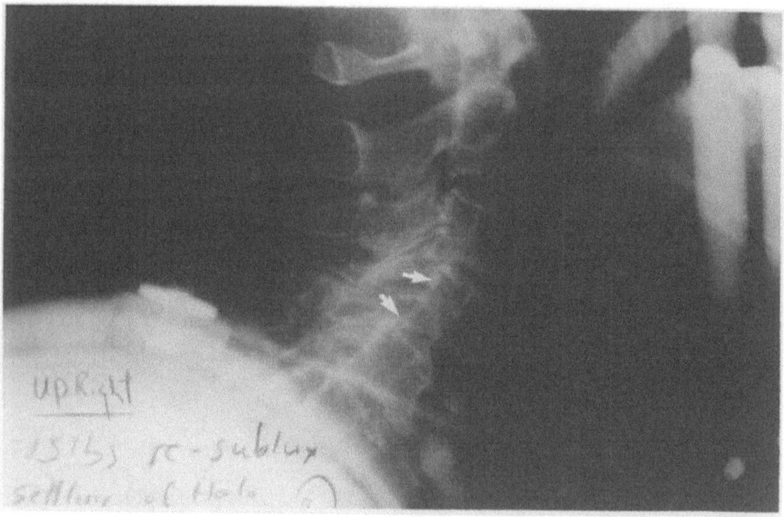

E

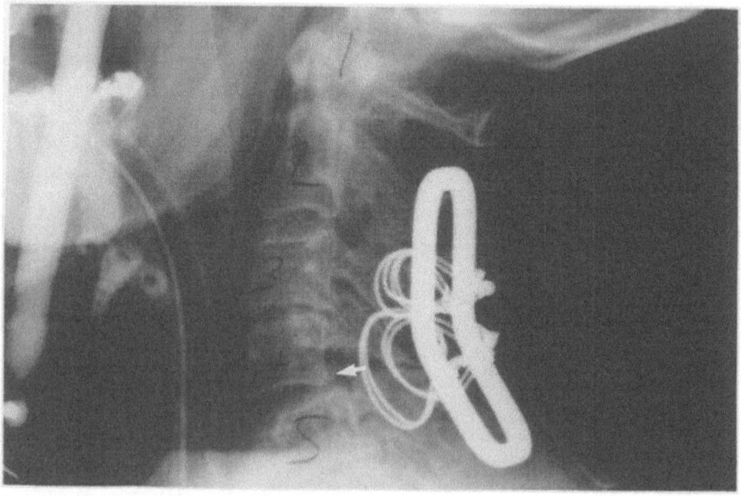

F

Figure 9.12. (*cont.*)

duced in extension. CT scan demonstrated a left C4-C5 pedicle and facet fracture (Fig. 9.16C). A posterior approach was carried out under general anesthesia, the laminae exposed, and Haid/Camille plates were screwed down across C4-C5 on the right and C5-C3 on the left (Fig. 9.16D). Postoperatively the left plate became dislodged and resubluxation occurred (Fig. 9.16E). Reoperation was performed for removal of the disrupted

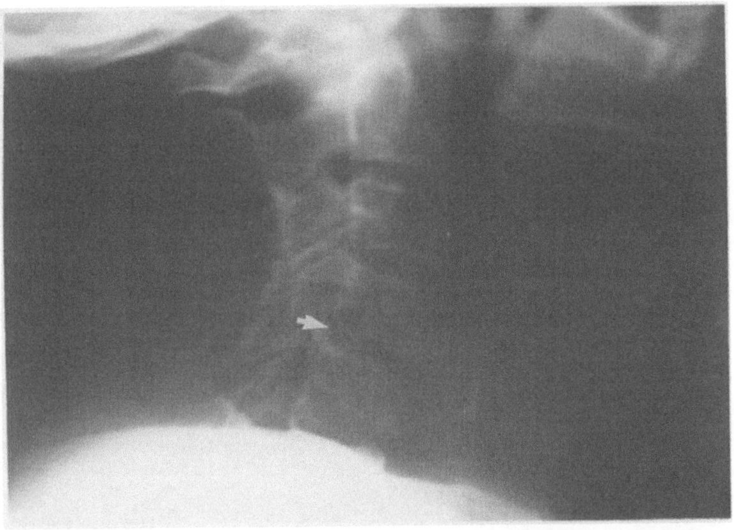

A

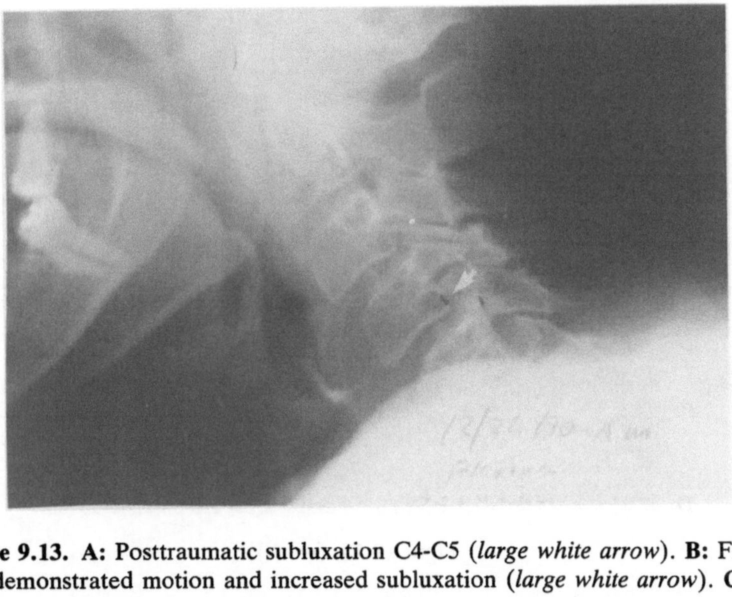

B

Figure 9.13. **A:** Posttraumatic subluxation C4-C5 (*large white arrow*). **B:** Flexion film demonstrated motion and increased subluxation (*large white arrow*). **C:** Reduction and fixation in the Halo is seen (*large white arrow*). **D:** Postmyelogram CT scan demonstrated a facet compression fracture with sclerosis (*large white arrow*) without evidence of spinal cord compression.

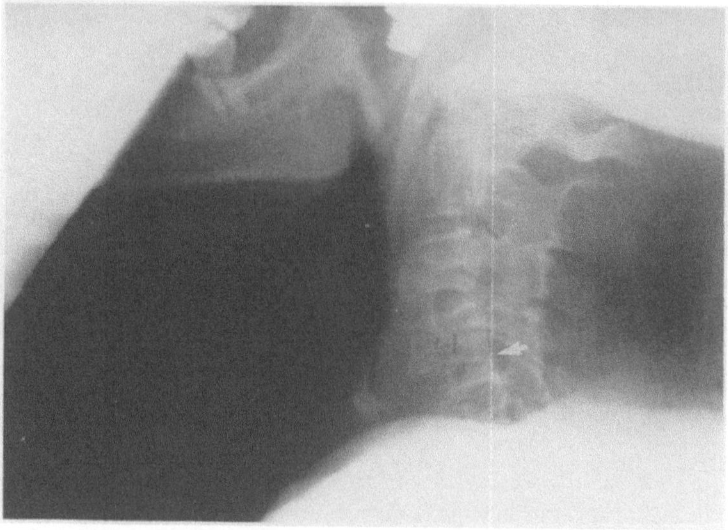

C

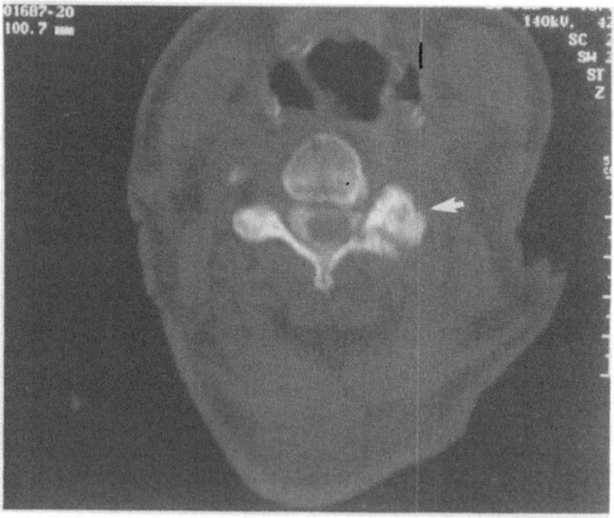

D

Figure 9.13. (*cont.*)

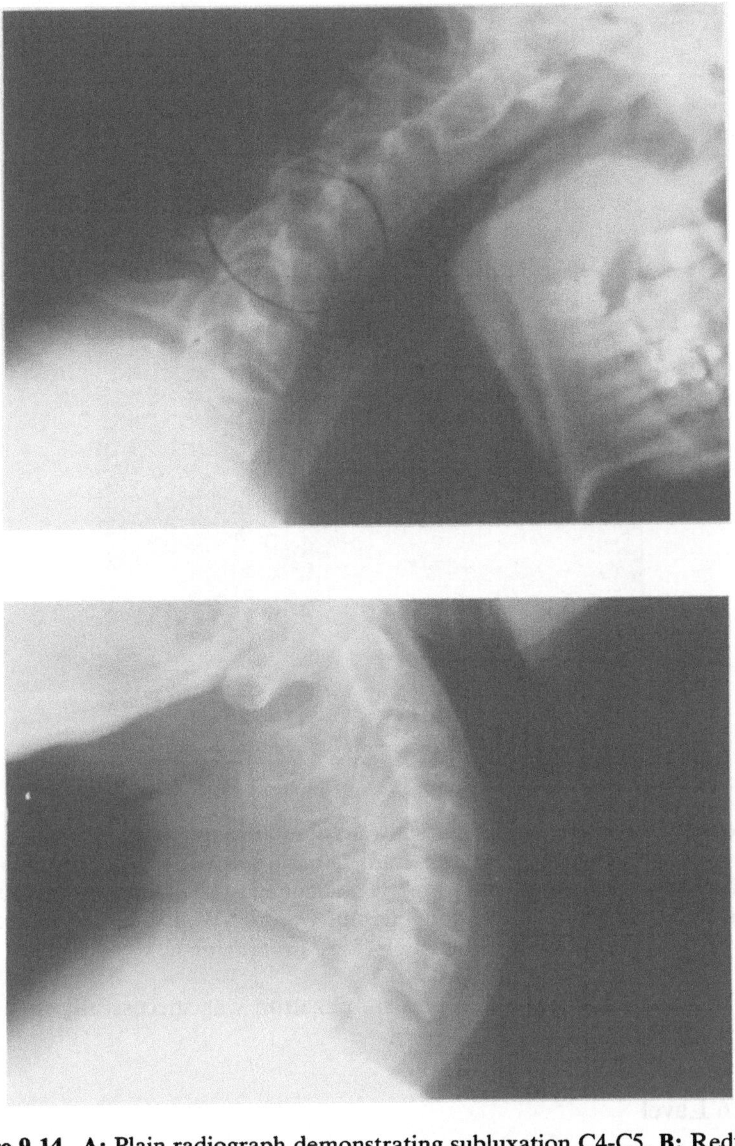

A

B

Figure 9.14. **A:** Plain radiograph demonstrating subluxation C4-C5. **B:** Reduction of the subluxation in extension.

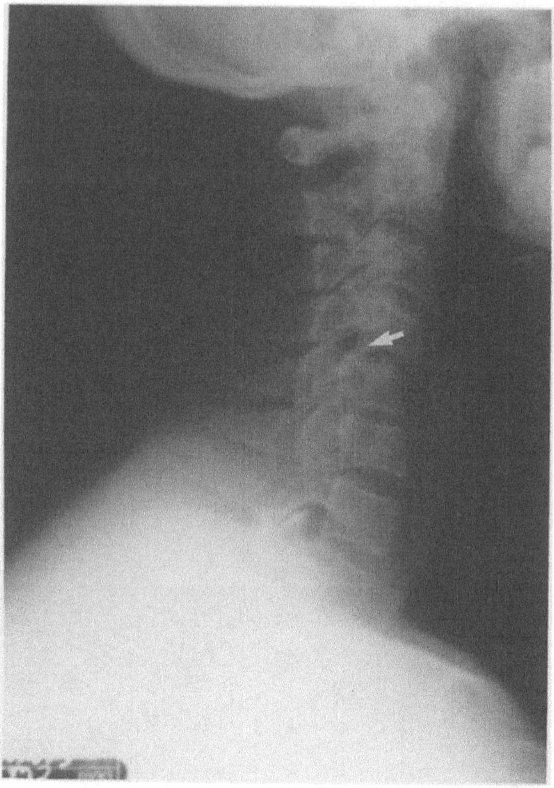

A

Figure 9.15. **A:** Plain radiograph showing a subluxation at C4-C5 (*large white arrow*) **B:** Left uncinate process fracture (*large white arrow*). **C:** Reduction and stabilization in the Halo-Vest with perfect alignment (*large white arrow*). **D:** Following Halo removal and discontinuation of Gardner-Wells traction stability was seen with a persisting 2-mm subluxation (*large white arrow*).

left plate and Halo reduction and stabilization was successfully instituted (Fig. 9.16F).

C5-C6 Level

Case 17

This 83-year-old woman with congenitally dislocated hips fell and was thereafter unable to walk. Her neck was in a position of extreme flexion. Examination was consistent with severe myeloradiculopathy. Plain radiographs showed a fracture dislocation at C5-C6 (Fig. 9.17A). Initial traction was instituted using Gardner-Wells tongs with 10 lbs of weight (Fig. 9.17B). A Halo ring replaced the Gardner-Wells 4 days later. Fifty lbs was used to achieve reduction (Fig. 9.17C), and it produced a signif-

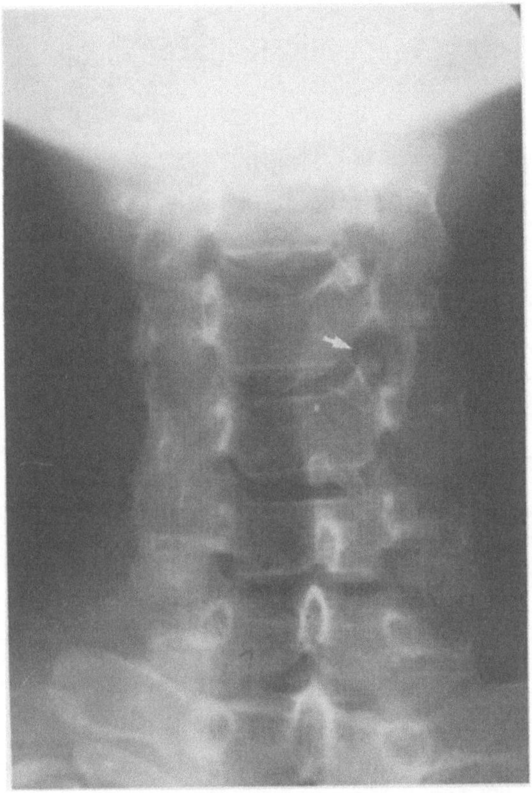

B

Figure 9.15. (*cont.*)

icant vertebral distraction. With reduction of weight to 20 lbs the patient became quadriplegic and had difficulty breathing (Fig. 9.17D). Weight was immediately restored to 40 lbs (Fig. 9.17E) with reversal of the quadriparesis and resumption of her ability to talk. A C1-C2 myelogram was performed demonstrating a block at C5-C6 (Fig. 9.17F). On the following day a laminectomy was performed from C3-C7 inclusively relieving the constriction at C5-C6 caused in part by the encroaching lateral masses and in part by redundant posterior longitudinal ligament. Postoperatively she remained very weak with a persisting myeloradiculopathy simulating the central cord syndrome. After 2 months the Halo-Vest was removed and the patient could sit erect, but could not walk and had difficulty with fine motor functions in both hands. She developed a urinary tract infection, refused all attempts at treatment, and died from sepsis 5 months after the initial injury. Postmortem studies of the spine show the area of fracture and healing (Fig. 9.17G,H).

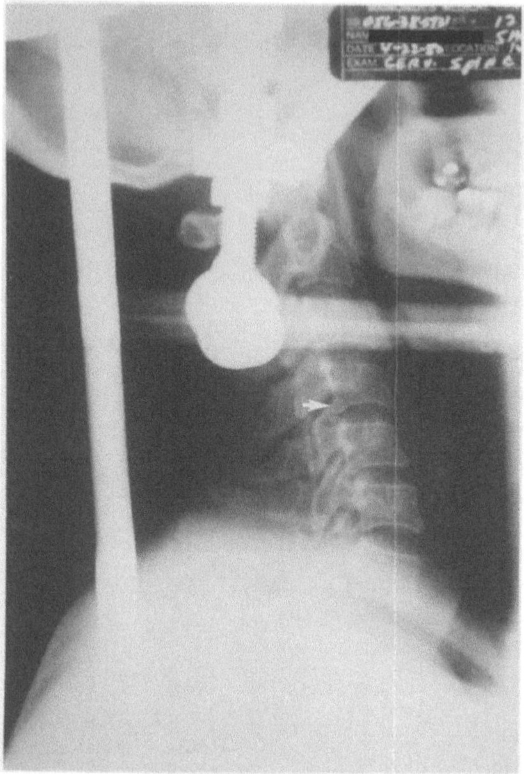

C

Figure 9.15. (*cont.*)

Case 18

This 28-year-old man was involved in a high-speed motor vehicle accident. There was no loss of consciousness and he complained of severe neck pain. Examination disclosed an incomplete quadriparesis. Initial cervical spine films missed the lesion (Fig. 9.18A), but a swimmer's view detected a dislocation at the C5-C6 level (Fig. 9.18B). A CT scan demonstrated unilateral facet, pedicle and laminar fractures (Fig. 9.18C,D). Halo Universal was applied and reduction achieved with morphine, Valium, and the slow application of weight over a 6-hour period. Halo-Vest fixation was established (Fig. 9.18E). The patient was transferred to another hospital for spinal rehabilitation and it was elected there to perform surgery and internal fixation. Six months later he was ambulatory, having returned to work, with a mild to moderate myeloradiculopathy involving primarily the left upper extremity.

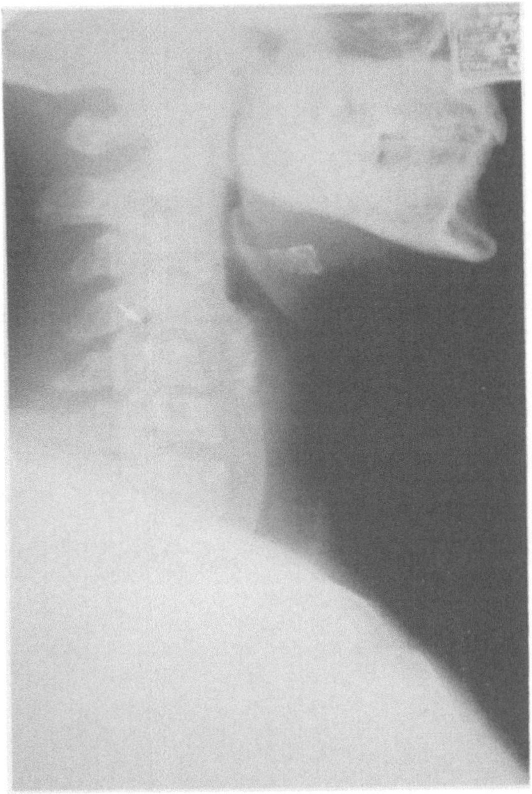

D

Figure 9.15. (*cont.*)

Case 19

This 47-year-old man with a history of drug abuse presented with severe neck pain and rapidly progressive weakness in all extremities. His examination disclosed a moderate quadriparesis with more pronounced distal weakness in his upper extremities. Plain radiographs demonstrated a collapse at the C5-C6 disc space with bony changes indicative of osteomyelitis with a retrolithesis of C5 on C6 (Fig. 9.19A). A myelogram was performed demonstrating a high-grade incomplete block (Fig. 9.19B). An anterior cervical approach for decompression and debridement was performed with dramatic improvement in the neurological profile. Halo-Vest fixation was employed to ensure the rapid mobilization of the patient (Fig. 9.19C). The patient was difficult to manage. He loosened the Halo-Vest on a number of occasions. Because of this a progressive subluxation was demonstrated as healing and fusion took place (Fig. 9.19D).

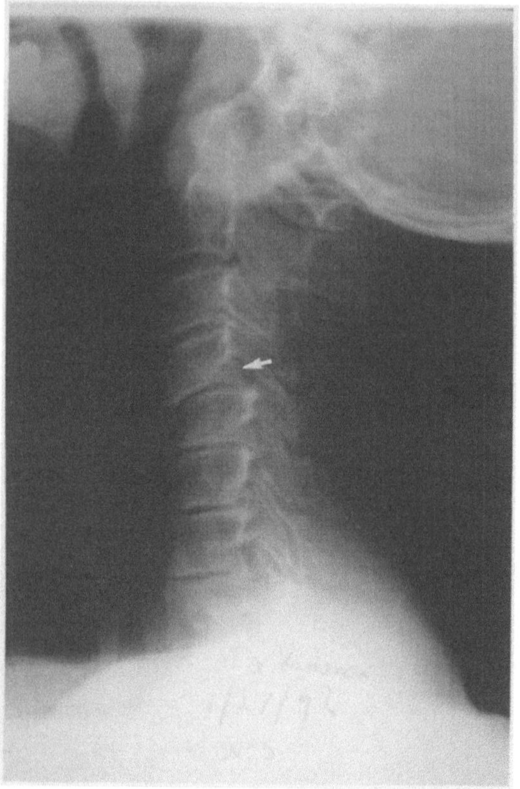

A

Figure 9.16. **A:** Plain radiograph in extension showing a subluxation at C4-C5 (*large white arrow*). **B:** Film in flexion showing increase in the C4-C5 subluxation (*large white arrow*). **C:** CT scan axial view showing the left facet and pedicle fractures (*large white arrows*). **D:** Internal fixation with Haid/Camille plates. **E:** Spontaneous dislodging of the left screws and plate with resubluxation (*large white arrow*). **F:** Reoperation, removal of the left plate and screws. Institution of traction with Gardner-Wells tongs and conversion to a Halo-Vest with restoration of alignment (*large white arrow*).

The patient became neurologically normal and fully independent. He was discharged from the hospital still wearing the Halo-Vest. He removed it himself and was lost to follow-up.

Case 20

This 67-year-old insulin-dependent diabetic man was initially admitted for cellulitis involving the right olecranon bursa. Blood cultures were positive for group B streptococcus and therapy was initiated with penicillin G and

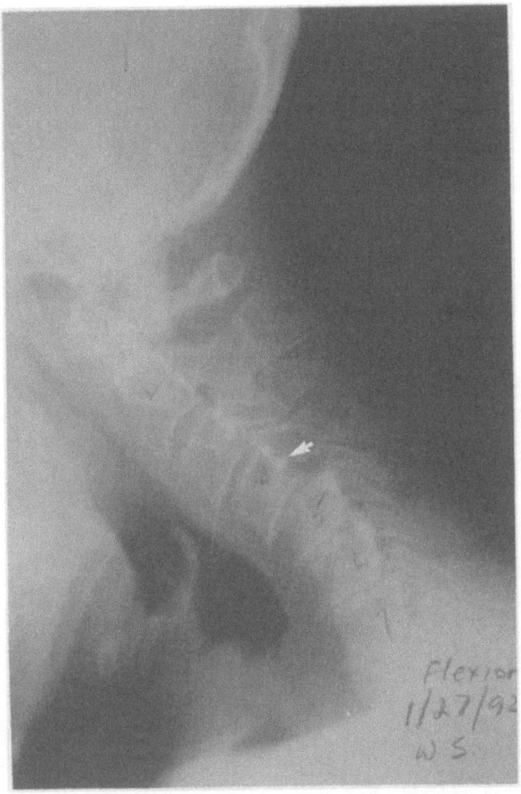

B

Figure 9.16. (*cont.*)

oxacillin. Surgical drainage was performed. Pathology showed acute inflammation. Incidental cervical spine films were negative (Fig. 9.20A). One and one-half months later an osteomyelitic process was documented involving the C5-C6 intervertebral space (Fig. 9.20B,C). Needle aspiration was not diagnostic (Fig. 9.20D). The patient had severe bilateral C5, C6, and C7 radiculopathies without long tract signs. These were confirmed on nerve conduction studies and were felt to be superimposed on a diabetic polyneuropathy. MRI documented moderately severe spinal cord compression at that level (Fig. 9.20E). Surgical intervention for definitive bacteriologic diagnosis, debridement, and fusion was offered to the patient and he refused. Halo ring and vest fixation were accepted by the patient. Pin loosening occurred, requiring replacement. Antibiotics were continued, but the neurological profile did not improve. One month later, after exhaustive discussions, the patient consented to surgery and underwent anterior approach, debridement, C5 and C6 resection, and C4-C7

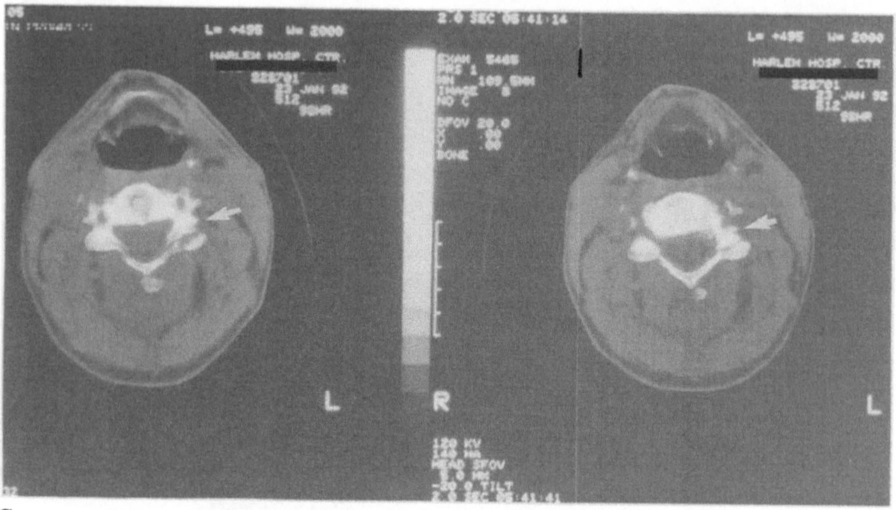

C

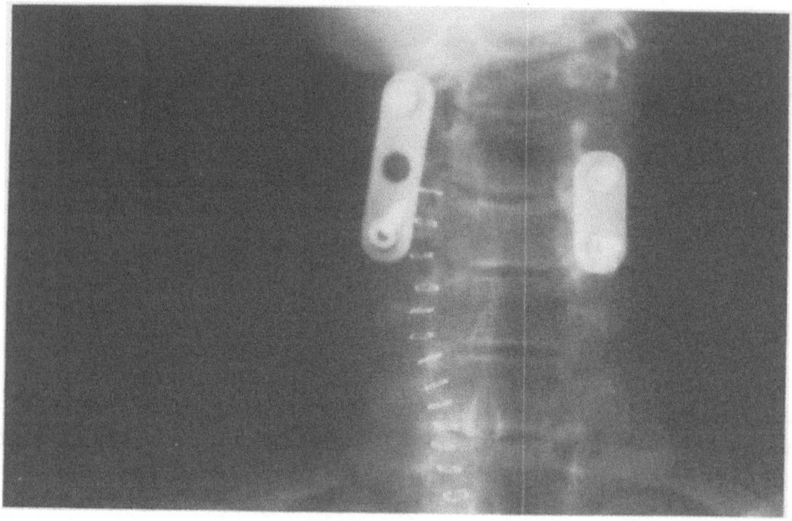

D

Figure 9.16. (*cont.*)

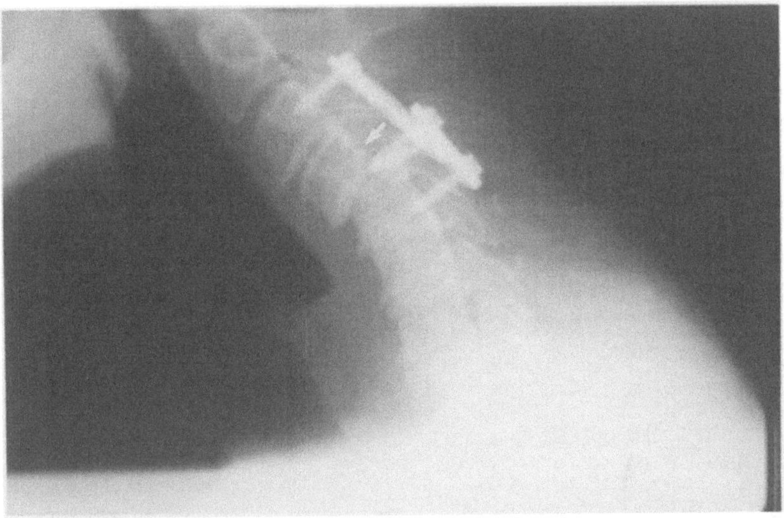

E

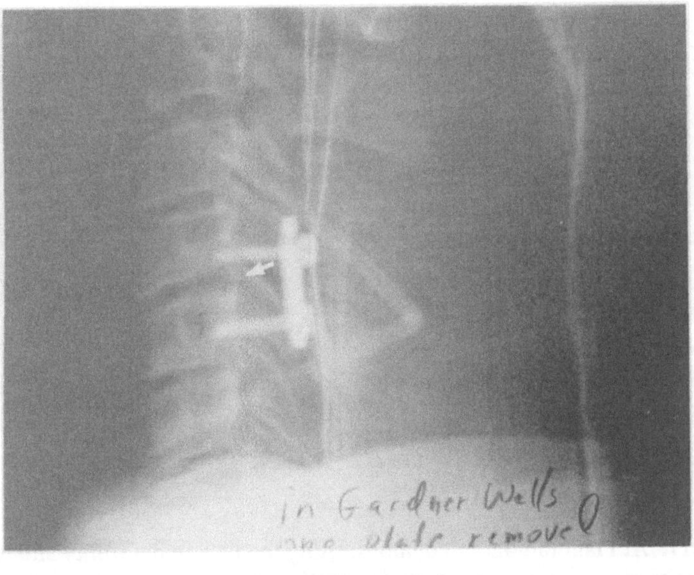

F

Figure 9.16. (*cont.*)

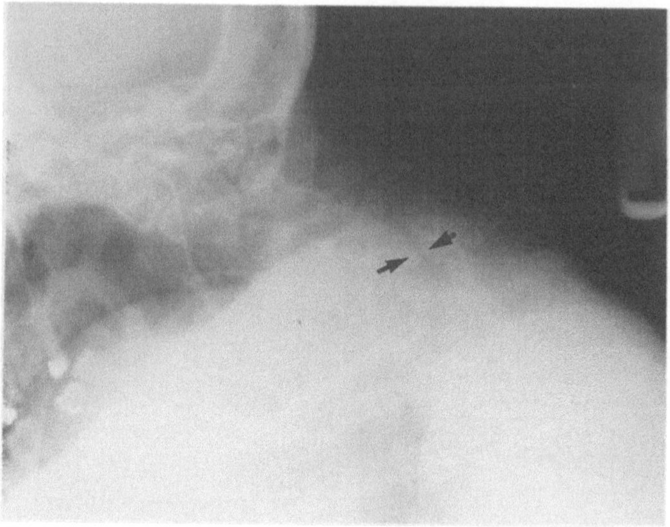

A

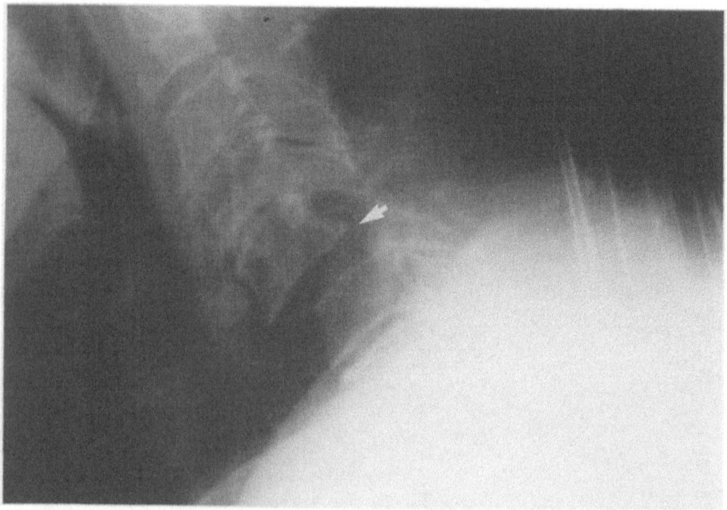

B

Figure 9.17. A: Plain radiograph demonstrating the flexion deformity and fracture C5-C6 (*large black arrows*). **B:** Partial reduction of the flexion deformity with 10 lbs of traction (*large white arrow*). **C:** Overdistraction and reduction of the subluxation with 50 lbs (*large white arrows*). **D:** Reduction of traction weight to 20 lbs to relieve the overdistraction with resultant loss of speech and quadriparesis (*large white arrow*). **E:** Restoration of traction weight to 40 lbs with recovery (*large white arrow*). **F:** Myelogram via C1-C2 puncture demonstrating a block at C5-C6 (*large white arrow*). **G,H:** Postmortem photographs of the cervical spine demonstrating the area of fracture and healing and the spondolytic ridges (*large white and black arrows*).

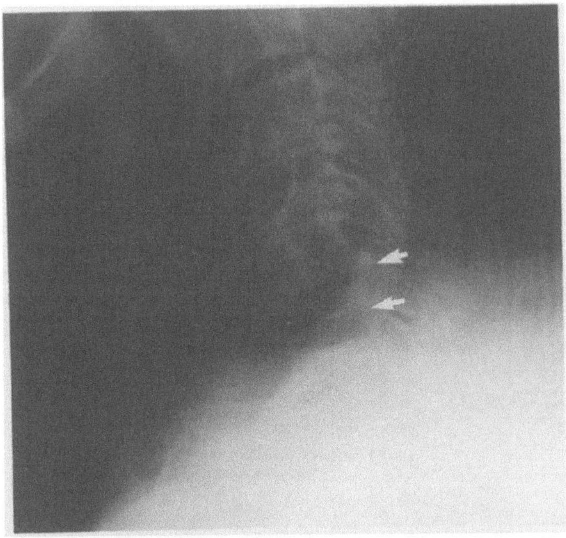

C

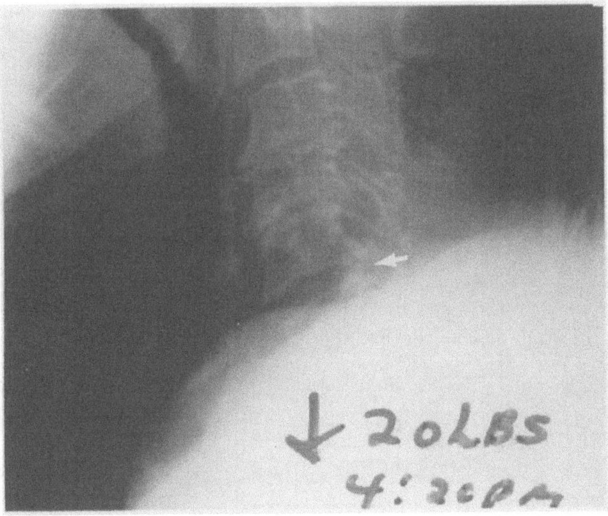

D

Figure 9.17. (*cont.*)

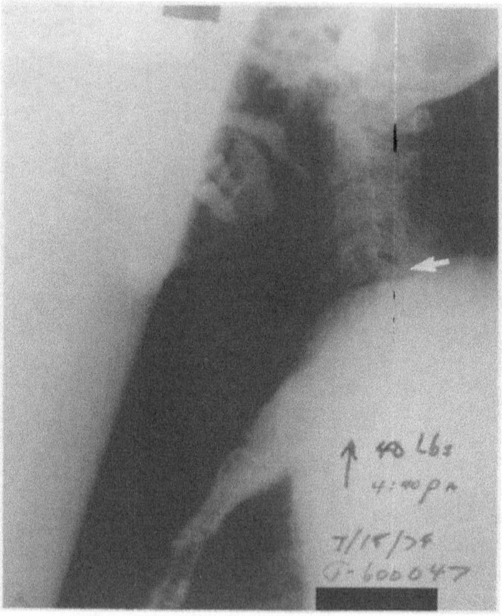

E

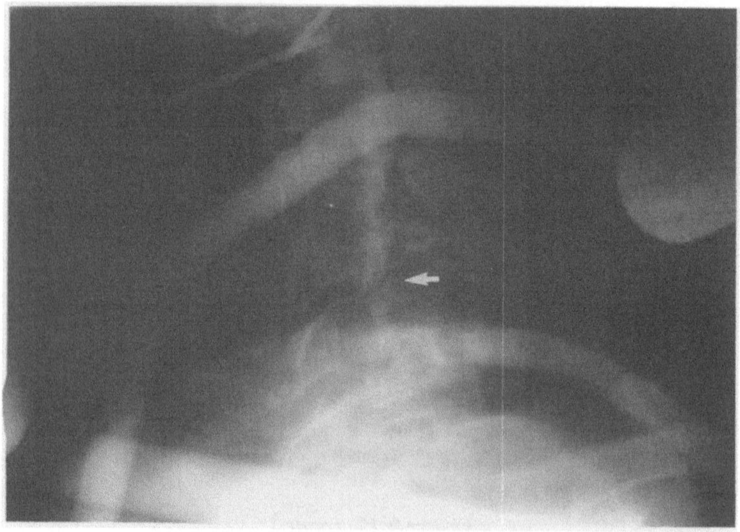

F

Figure 9.17. (*cont.*)

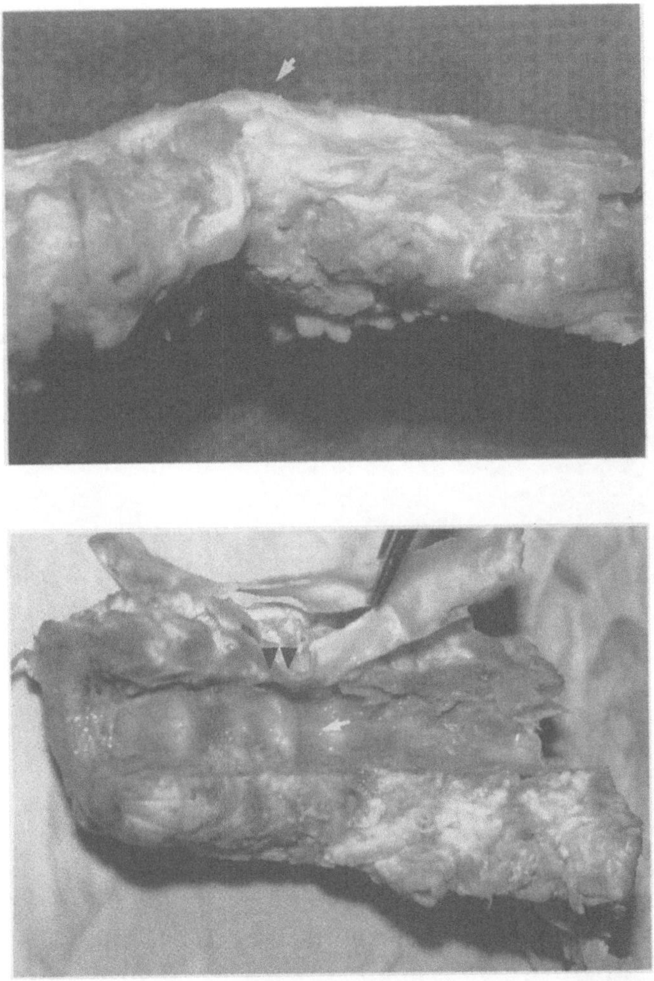

G

H

Figure 9.17. (*cont.*)

autogenous iliac bone graft fusion. Reoperation was required for spontaneous anterior migration of the superior portion of the strut graft (Fig. 9.20F). The postoperative MRI showed peridural fibrosis. The patient slowly improved over the ensuing 5 months.

C6-C7 Level

Case 21

This 42-year-old man was involved in a motor vehicle accident and sustained a questionable loss of consciousness. Neurological examination dis-

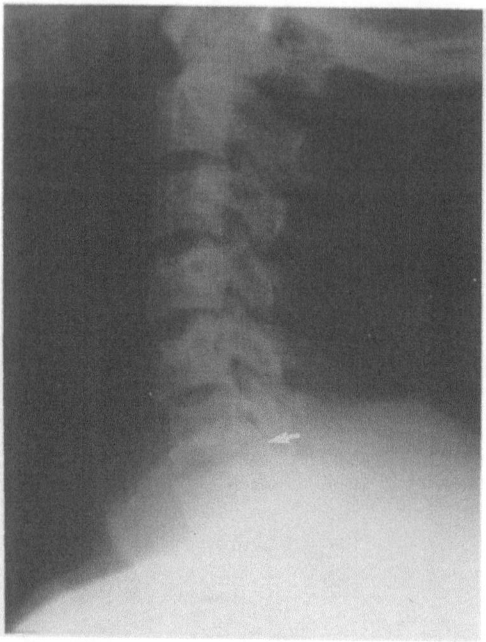

A

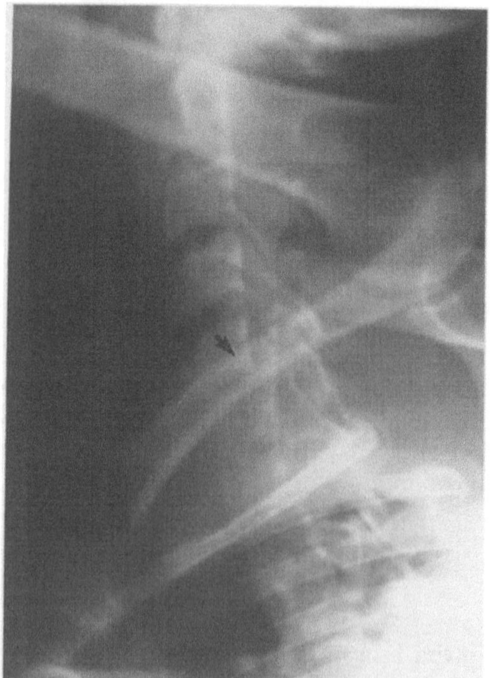

B

Figure 9.18. A: Initial plain radiographs of the cervical spine missed the lesion (*large white arrow*). **B:** Swimmer's view documented the C5-C6 subluxation (*large black arrow*). **C,D:** CT scan axial views showed the unilateral pedicle, facet, and laminar fractures (*large white arrows*). **E:** Halo fixation achieved reduction and stabilization (*large black arrow*).

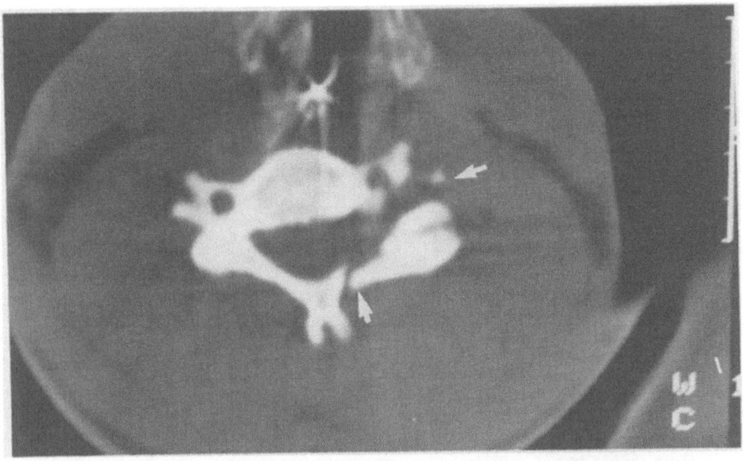

C

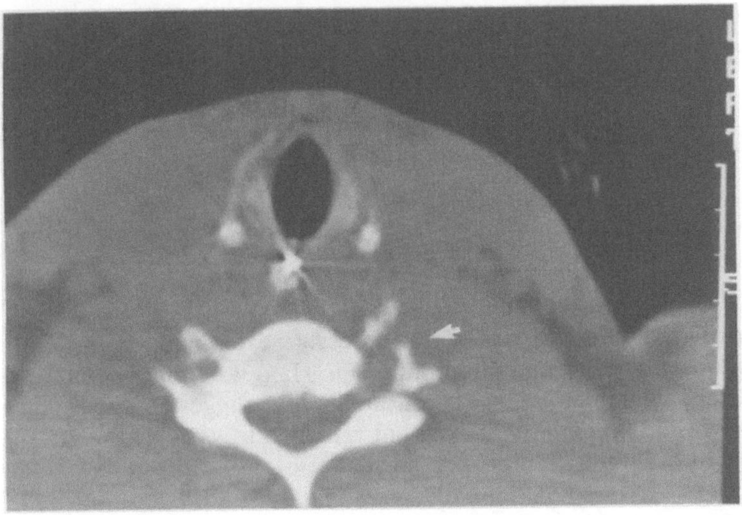

D

Figure 9.18. (*cont.*)

closed no deficits. Plain radiographs demonstrated a 65% subluxation of C6 posteriorly on C7 with locked facets (Fig. 9.21A). Gardner-Wells tongs were applied with 60 lbs added in increments of 5 to 10 lbs with sedation and ultimately unlocking of one facet (Fig. 9.21B). Due to deformation of the tongs a Halo ring was substituted for the Gardner-Wells and with the steady incremental addition of weight in 5- to 10-lb units the other facet was unlocked with the manual addition of flexion and rotation to the 70 lbs (Fig. 9.21C). Halo-Vest fixation in 20 lbs of traction was maintained. A single loose pin required replacement at 1 month. Some

E
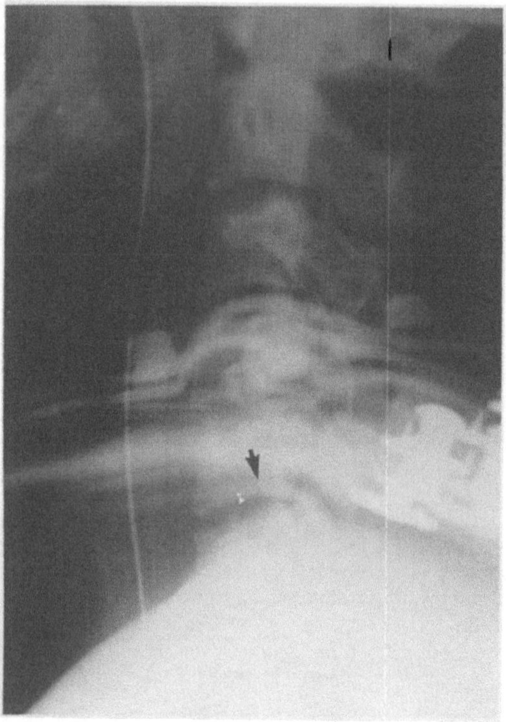

Figure 9.18. (*cont.*)

left-sided weakness was noted on successive examinations, which began to improve at the 3rd and 4th month. The Halo was removed at 3 months and a Philadelphia collar was substituted. MRI suggested a herniated disc at C5-C6 (Fig. 9.21D,E). The patient returned to work in the 7th month. MRI at 1 year was interpreted as normal.

Case 22

This 35-year-old woman sustained a fall and suffered a subluxation at C6-C7 (Fig. 9.22A) without neurological deficits. Neck pain was her predominant complaint. Halo reduction and vest fixation were performed with normal alignment achieved (Fig. 9.22B). The Halo was removed at 2 months with no adverse sequelae. Good alignment was maintained out of the Halo (Fig. 9.22C).

Case 23

This 21-year-old woman was involved in a motor vehicle accident without loss of consciousness. She experienced immediate pain in her neck, both

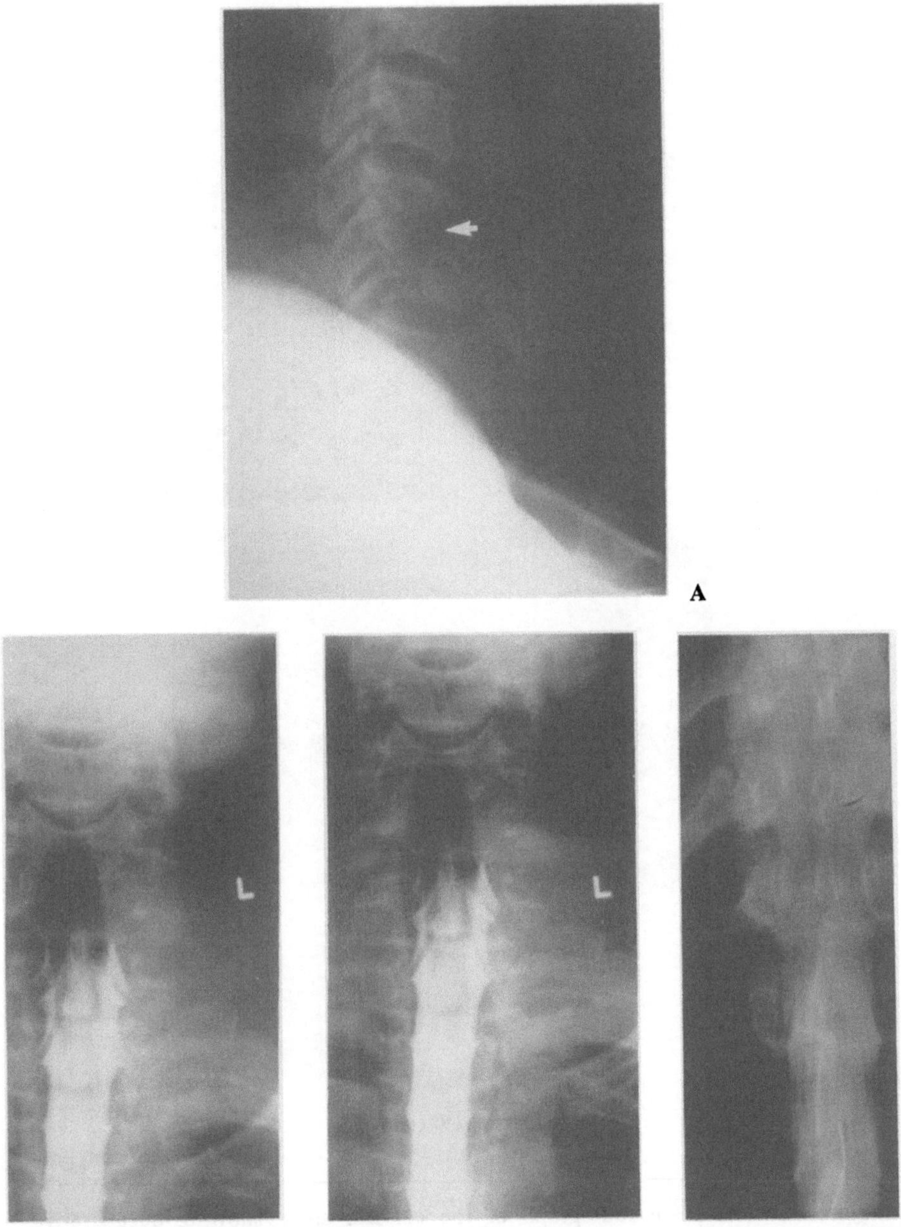

A

B

Figure 9.19. A: Plain radiograph demonstrated the C5-C6 subluxation and the intervertebral space showing bony changes compatible with osteomyelitis (*large white arrow*). **B:** High-grade myelographic block was seen at C5-C6. **C:** Halo-Vest fixation with "settling" and resubluxation (*large black arrows*). **D:** Progressive subluxation in the Halo-Vest during healing (*large black arrow*).

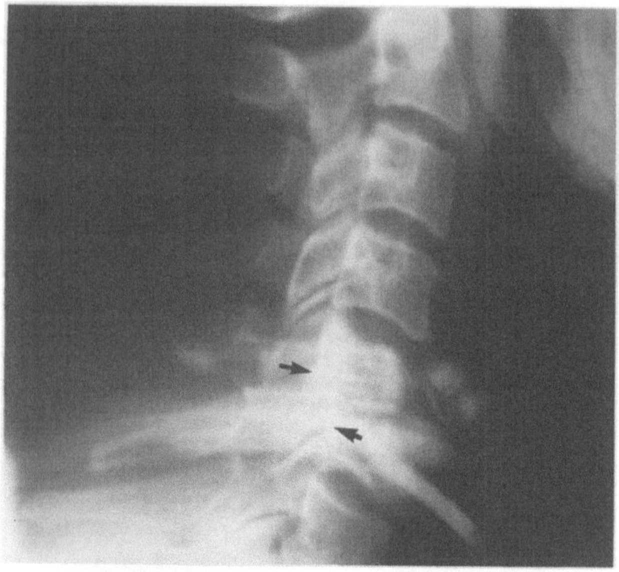

C

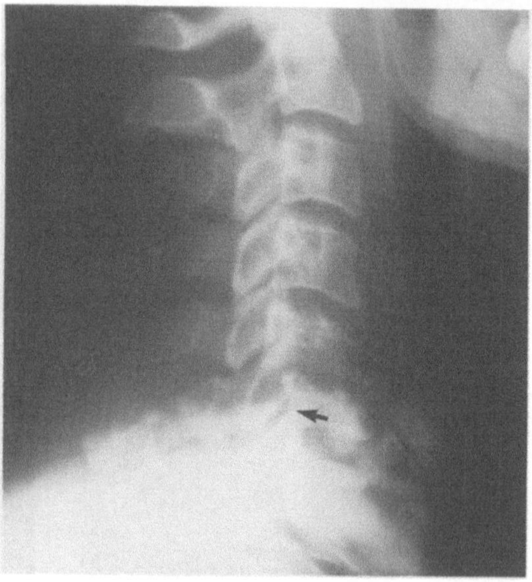

D

Figure 9.19. (*cont.*)

Figure 9.20. A: Plain radiograph of the cervical spine showing degenerative changes. **B,C:** One and one-half months later bony changes consistent with osteomyelitis were seen on plain films (*large white arrow*) and CT scanning. **D:** Needle aspiration for an ongoing ostomyelitic process was performed (*large white arrow*). **E:** MRI with T2-weighted images showed moderately severe spinal cord compression. **F:** Postoperative film documenting the C4-C7 iliac bone strut graft fusion (*large white arrows*).

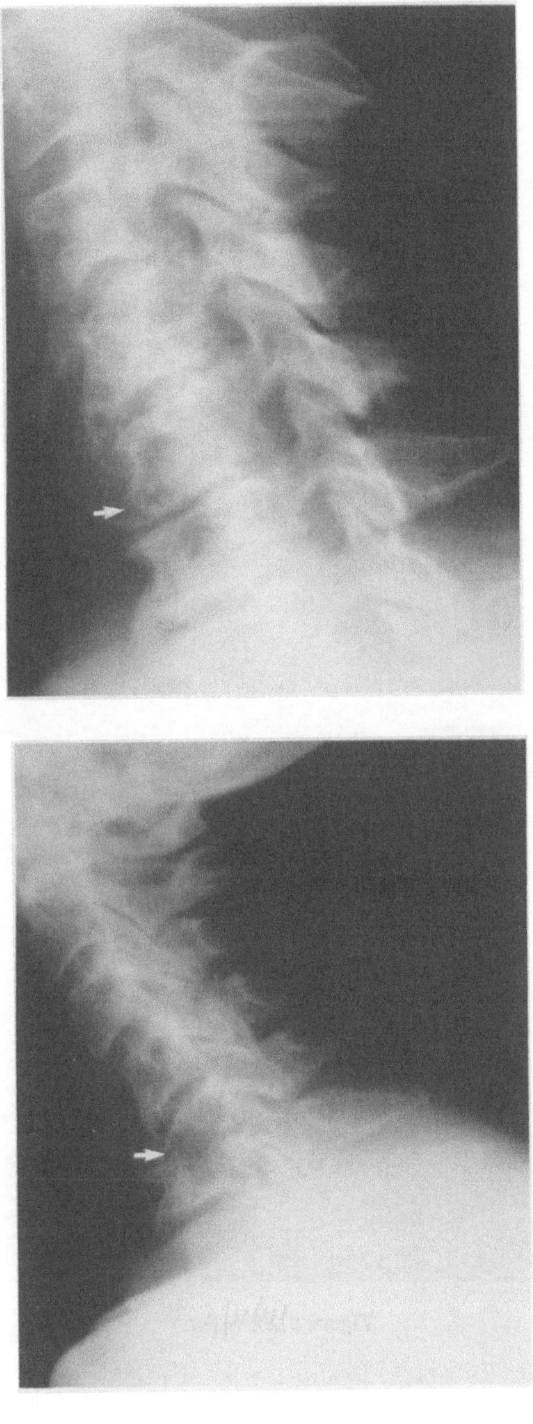

A

B

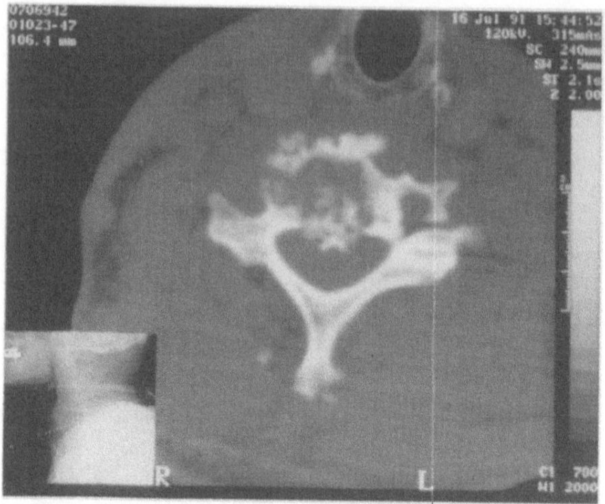

C

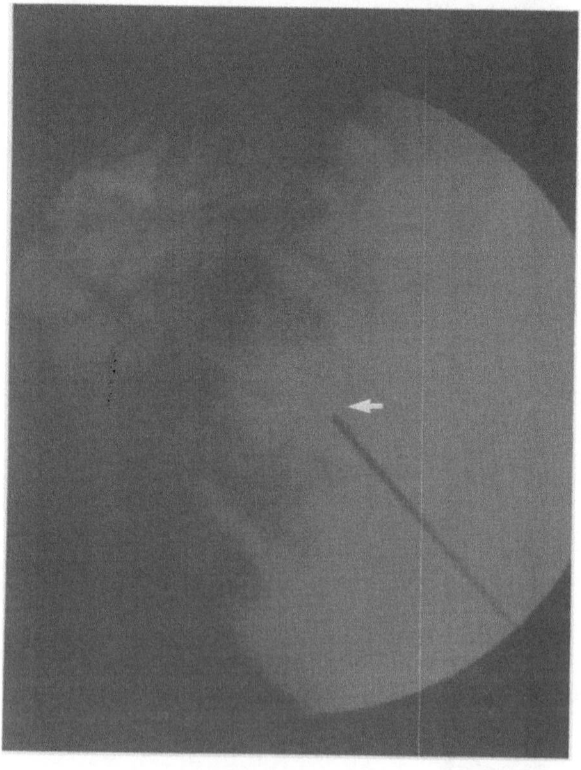

D

Figure 9.20. (*cont.*)

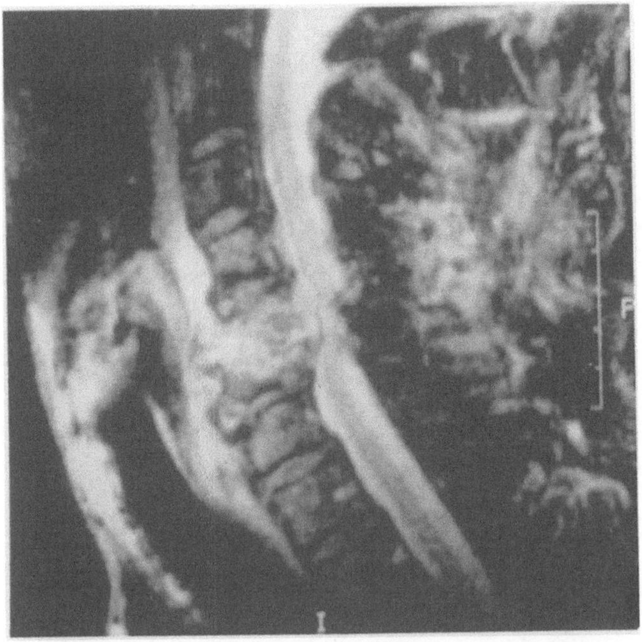

E

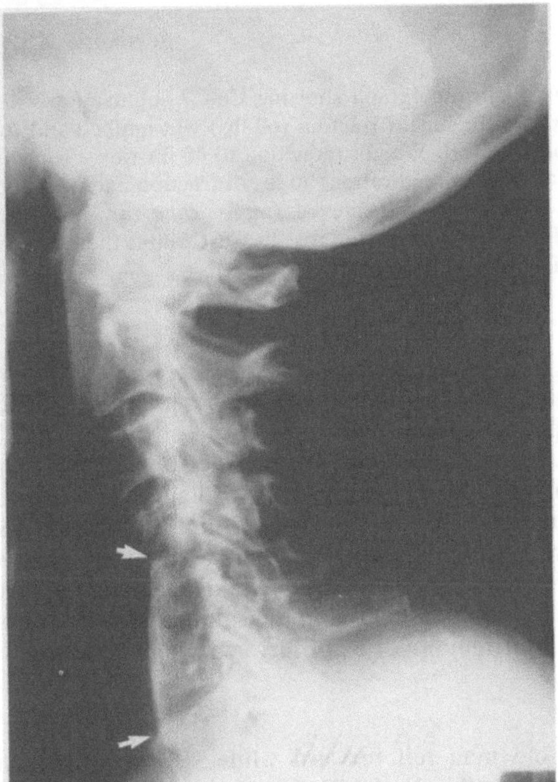

F

Figure 9.20. (*cont.*)

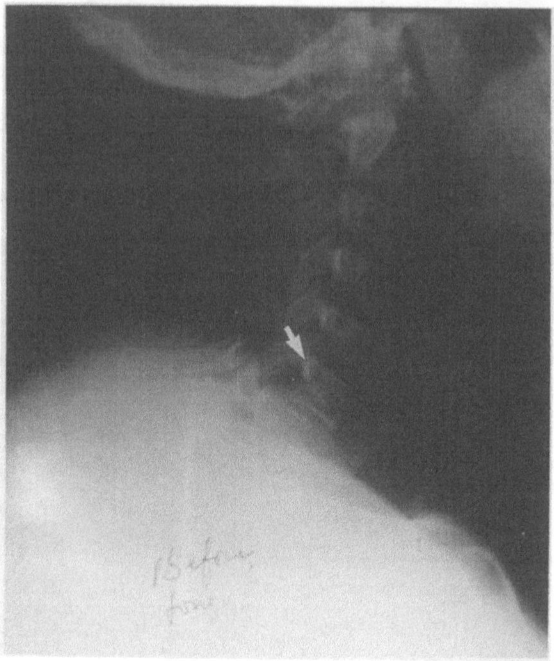

A

Figure 9.21. **A:** Plain radiograph showing C6-C7 subluxation with locked facets (*large white arrow*). **B:** Linear traction (60 lbs) was applied and rotation resulted in unlocking of one facet. Weight reduction to 40 lbs (*large white arrow*). **C:** The following day after Halo application, 70 lbs of traction and neck rotation and flexion complete reduction was achieved (*large white arrow*). **D,E:** T1- and T2-weighted MRIs suggest a herniated disc at CS-C6, but there is no cord compression or distortion at C6-C7 (*large white arrows*).

shoulders, and pain and numbness in her right arm and a transient Lhermitte's phenomenon. Plain radiographs showed a C6-C7 subluxation (Fig. 9.23A). Halo traction to 45 lbs achieved a reduction (Fig. 9.23B) and Vest fixation was added. At 2 months a plain radiograph demonstrated forward angulation of C6 on C7 with a 3-mm subluxation and collapse of the interspace compatible with "settling." The Halo was removed at 3 months, whereupon flexion-extension films demonstrated a solid fusion without motion (Fig. 9.23C,D) and the subluxation. She returned to work at 5 months. Her right upper extremity symptoms remitted.

Case 24

This 26-year-old man fell forward while skiing, striking his head and somersaulting onto his back. There was no loss of consciousness. On

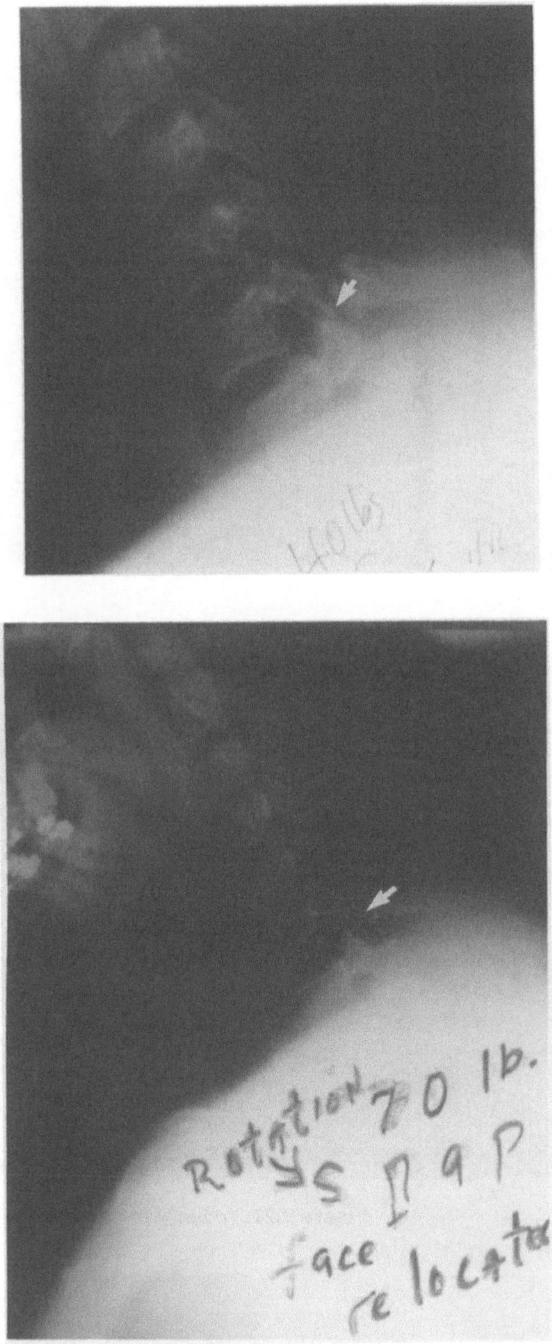

B

C

Figure 9.21. (*cont.*)

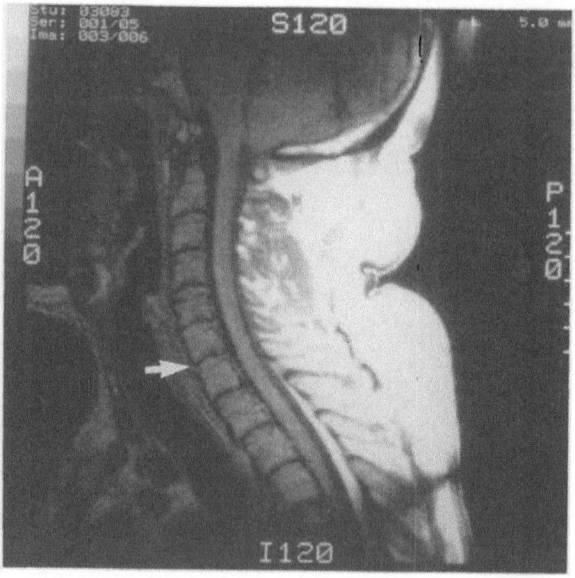

D

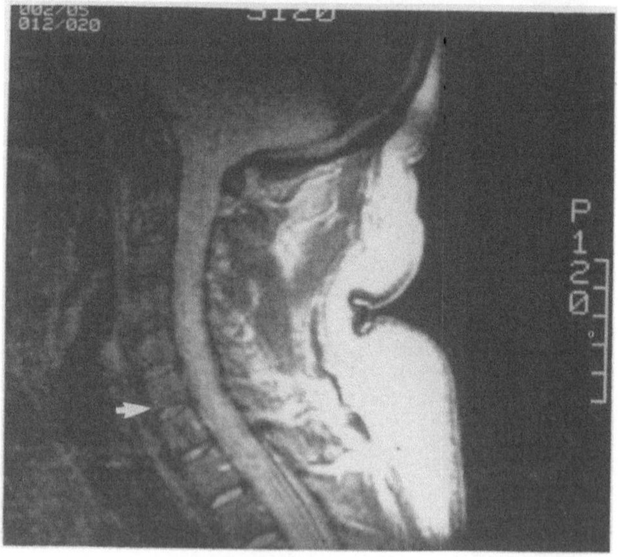

E

Figure 9.21. (*cont.*)

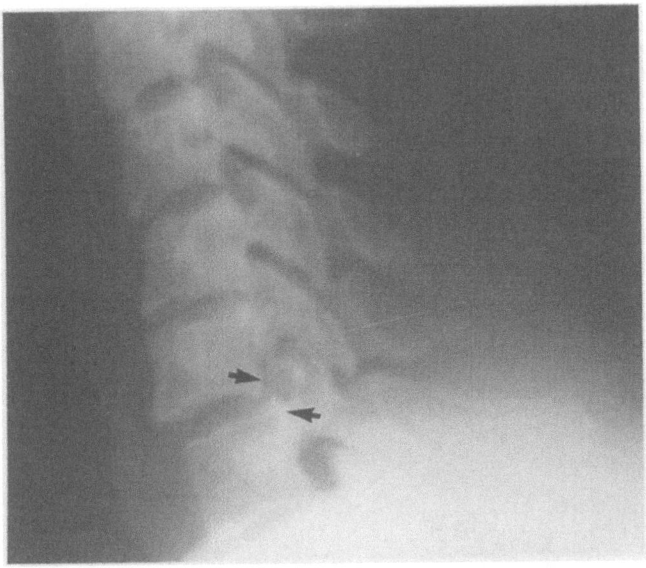

A

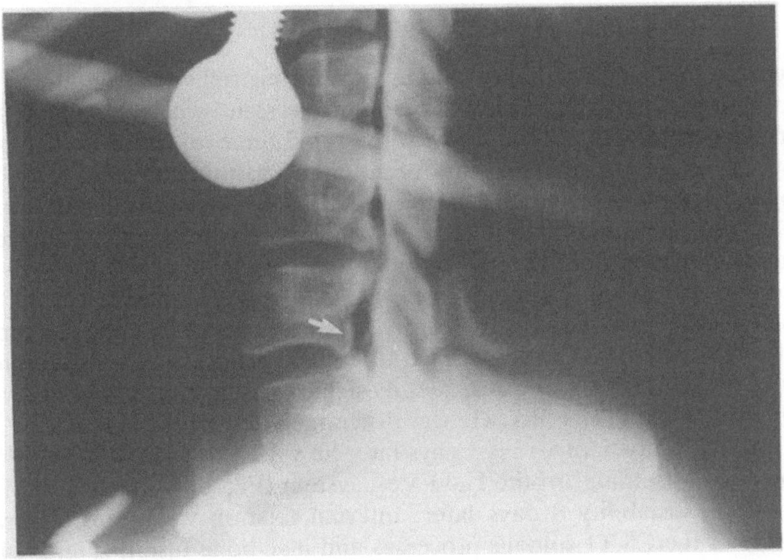

B

Figure 9.22. **A:** Plain radiograph shows C6-C7 subluxation (*large black arrows*). **B:** Myelogram after Halo stabilization shows no evidence of spinal cord compression. A 2-mm subluxation persists (*large white arrow*). **C:** Good alignment is seen after Halo removal (*large black arrow*).

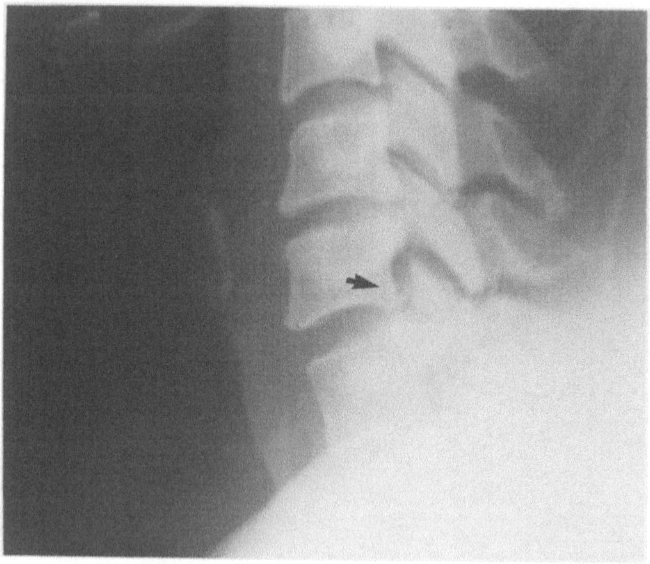

C

Figure 9.22. (*cont.*)

the slopes he was transiently unable to move his right arm. Following immobilized transportation he was permitted to stand whereupon he felt interscapular and chest pressure with the rapid onset of inability to coordinate his right upper and lower extremities and painful paresthesias in both upper extremities. Examination showed C6 and C7 radiculopathies, more so on the right, and bilateral Babinski signs. Plain radiographs showed a 5-mm subluxation of C6 on C7 with anterior wedging of C7 and an anterior teardrop fracture (Fig. 9.24A). A Halo ring was positioned and reduction achieved with 30 lbs (Fig. 9.24B). Dramatic remission of upper extremity numbness accompanied the disappearance of the Babinski signs. Vest fixation was subsequently achieved and x-rays demonstrated full reduction and stability. He was discharged home fully ambulatory and on routine outpatient x-rays 3 days later he was seen to have a resubluxation due to "settling" of the Halo-Vest system (Fig. 9.24C). In view of the persisting instability 8 days later, internal fixation was performed with wiring of the C5-T1 spinous processes and iliac bone fusion (Fig. 9.24D).

Figure 9.23. A: Plain radiograph shows a C6-C7 subluxation (*large white arrow*). **B:** Reduction with 45 lbs using the Halo (*large white arrow*). **C,D:** After 3 months in the Halo "settling" occurred with a 3-mm subluxation that was stable on extension (*large white arrow*) and flexion views.

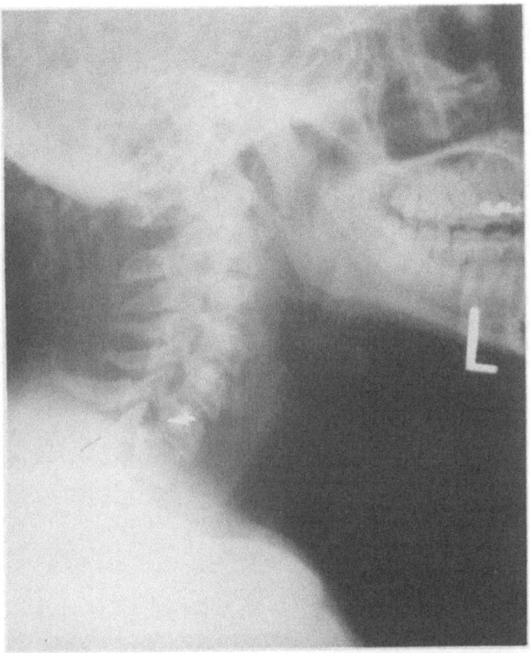

A

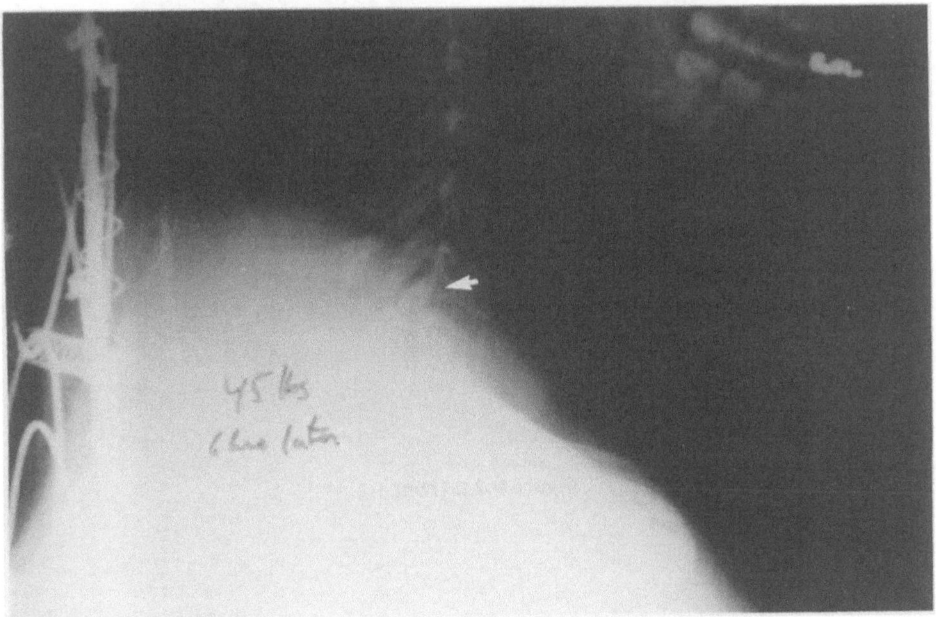

B

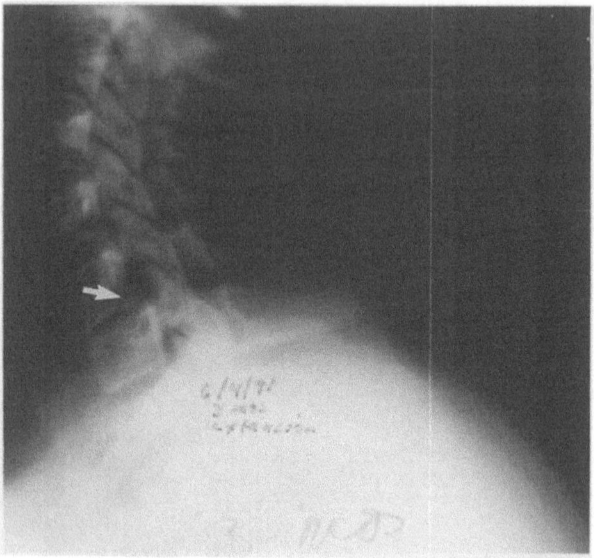

C

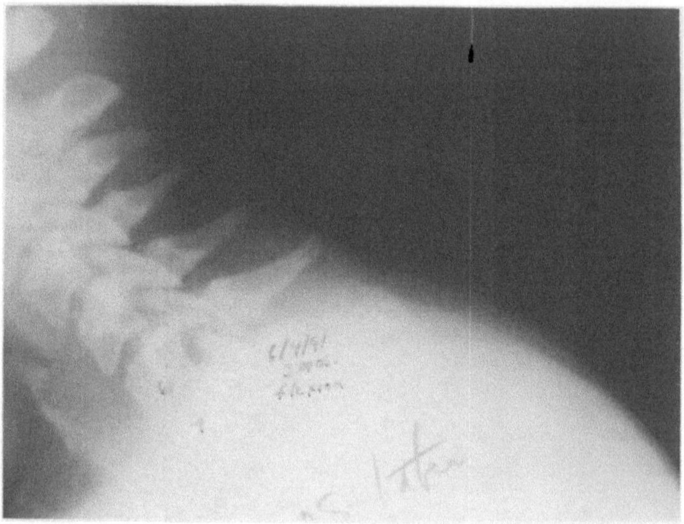

D

Figure 9.23. (*cont.*)

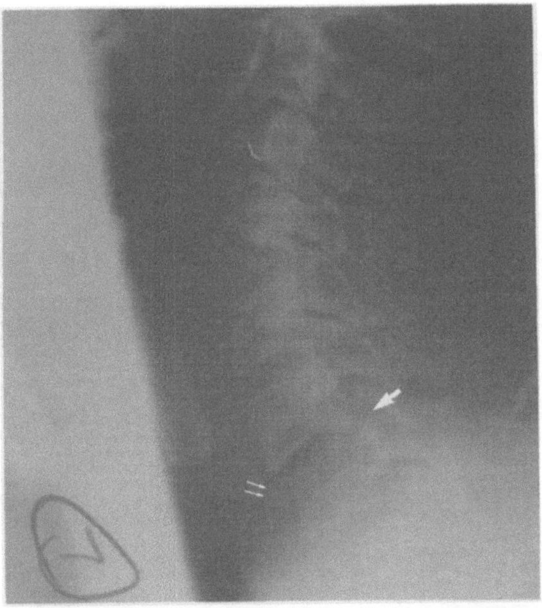

A

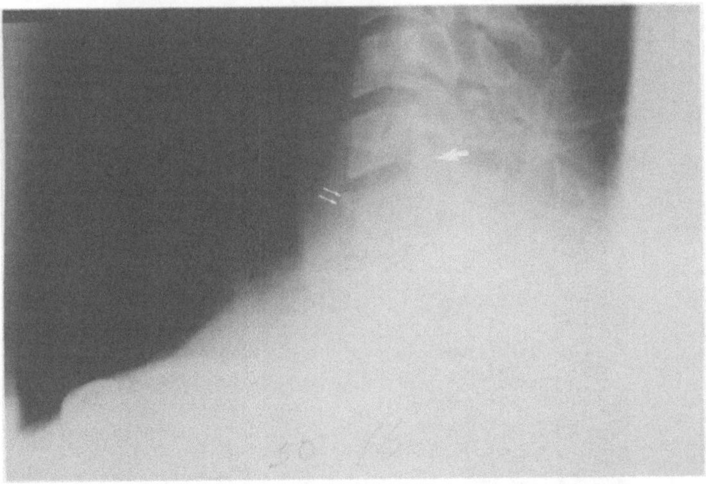

B

Figure 9.24. **A:** Plain radiograph demonstrates the C6-C7 subluxation (*large white arrow*) and the anterior teardrop fracture from the upper margin of C7 (*two small white arrows*). **B:** Reduction of the subluxation with 30 lbs of traction (*large white arrow*). The teardrop fracture is better seen (*two small white arrows*). **C:** Resubluxation in the Halo after 3 days due to "settling" (*large white arrow*). **D:** Reduction and internal fixation with spinous process wiring and iliac bone graft fusion (*large white arrow*).

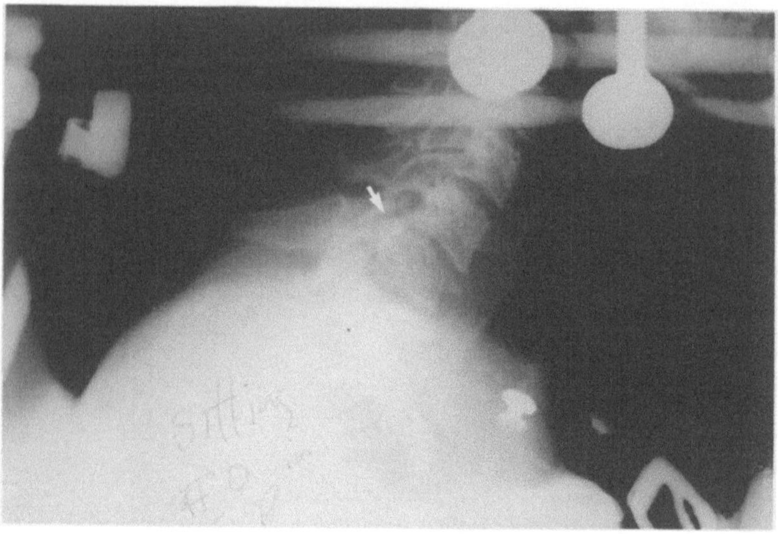

C

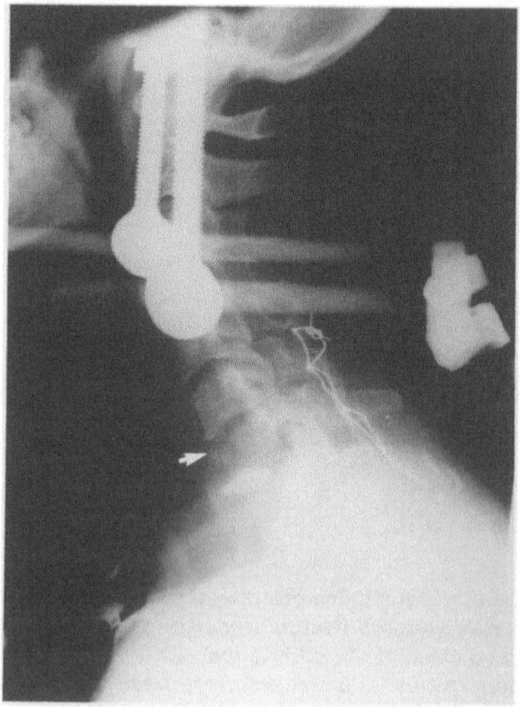

D

Figure 9.24. (*cont.*)

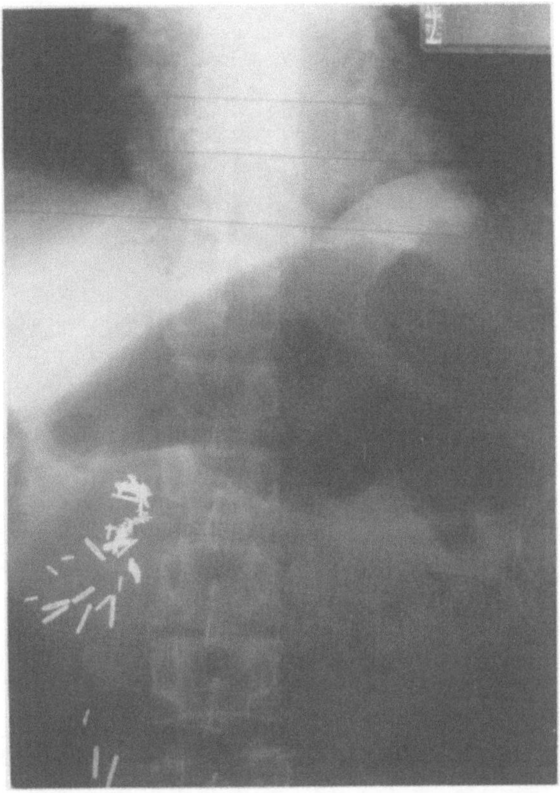
A

Figure 9.25. **A:** Flat plate of the abdomen showing clips in the area of the previously resected right hypernephroma. **B:** Complete myelographic block at C7 due to extradural metastatic compression. **C:** Bone destruction of the posterior and lateral elements at C6-C7 (*large white arrow*). **D:** Tomographic highlighting of the bony destruction (*two large white arrows*).

His recovery was progressive with full return of strength including the right triceps, such that he could return to competitive sculling.

Case 25

This 54-year-old man with a previously resected right hypernephroma (Fig. 9.25A) presented with a severe quadriparesis and complete myelographic block at the C7 level with bone destruction involving the posterior elements of C6 and C7 (Fig. 9.25B,C). Tomograms highlighted the extent of bone involvement (Fig. 9.25D). An emergency decompressive laminectomy confirmed the suspicion of metastatic hypernephroma. Radio-

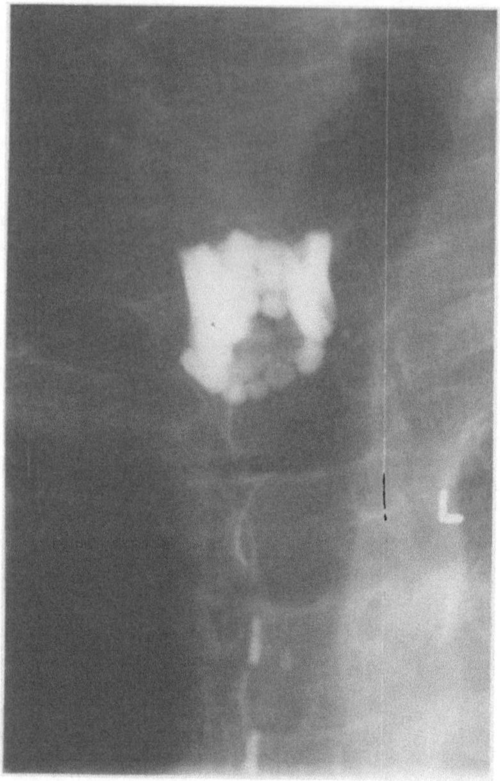

B

Figure 9.25. (*cont.*)

therapy was administered for a total of 3,000 R. The patient had a good recovery and regained the ability to ambulate independently, but remained with a residual C7 radiculopathy bilaterally. He was readmitted 1 year later with severe cervical pain and received an additional course of radiotherapy. Throughout this period his sole stabilization consisted of a Philadelphia collar. He succumbed $1\frac{1}{2}$ years later to generalized metastatic disease.

Case 26

This 20-year-old man experienced severe neck, arm, and leg pain and left arm paresthesias following a dive into a pool. X-rays showed a collapsed C7 vertebra (Fig. 9.26A). C1 scan demonstrated the fracture without paravertebral mass (Fig. 9.26B). He was maintained in Halo-Vest stabilization for 3 months. Neurological examination was unremarkable. Bone scan showed an uptake, but was not diagnostic of neoplasm (Fig.

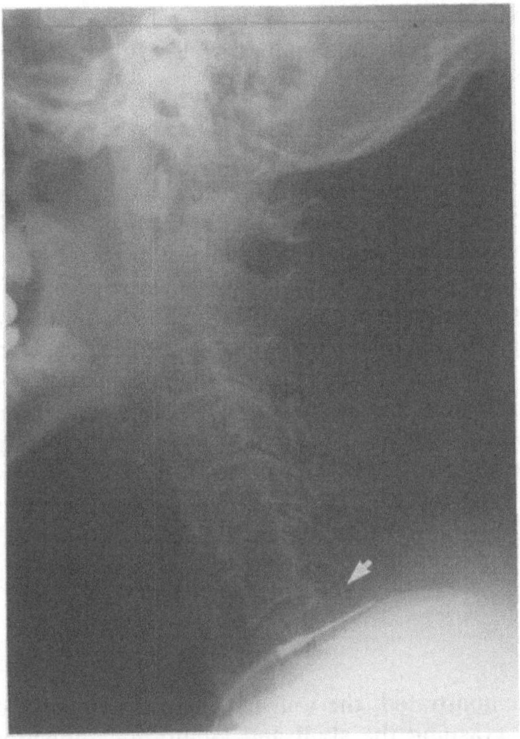

C

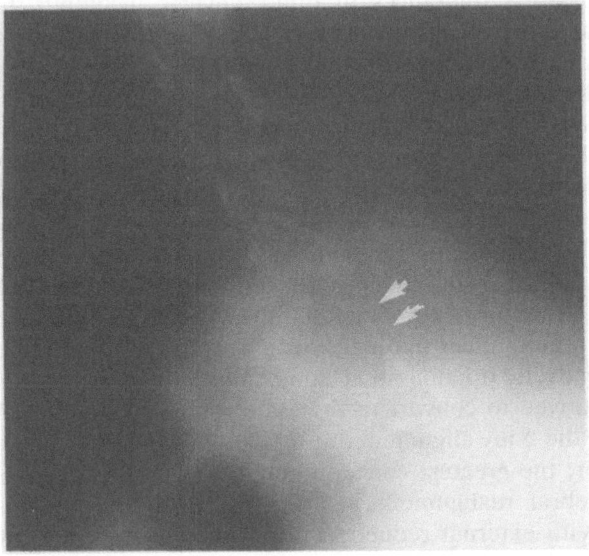

D

Figure 9.25. (*cont.*)

9.26C). Flexion-extension films taken at 3 months demonstrated stability (Fig. 9.26D,E). The patient remained well without change of the radiographic profile at 6 months (Fig. 9.26F).

Case 27

This 68-year-old man presented in the emergency room after a fall with his head retroflexed and quadriplegic at the C5/C6 level. He was fully awake and had difficulty breathing. Plain radiographs demonstrated the open fish-mouth fracture at C6 and ankylosing spondylitis (Fig. 9.27A). The Halo ring was applied and gentle flexion without traction afforded reduction (Fig. 9.27B). His respiratory pattern was largely diaphragmatic, but it improved. There was no change in his quadriplegia. Vest fixation was instituted. Large doses of Decadron were administered without effect. He remained in the intensive care unit, developed pneumonia and underwent tracheostomy. Despite this, he expired 2 weeks later from overwhelming sepsis. An interim CT scan showed laminar fractures and laminar bone in the vertebral canal (Fig. 9.27C).

Discussion

As has been demonstrated, the four-pin Halo ring is an excellent mechanical device for grasping the skull and facilitating reduction of a cervical subluxation. This is particularly true when the traction weight required exceeds the stress tolerances of other devices including the Gardner-Wells, Vincke, and Crutchfield tongs. Vest fixation affords stabilization and permits early mobilization, gratifying from the standpoints of the patient and the spine surgeon. However, significant interim and residual problems were noted that must be addressed in assessing the usefulness of external stabilization in general and in the selection of appropriate spine-injured patients for external stabilization as opposed to internal fixation and fusion.

Initially the risks facing the spine surgeon relate to placement of the Halo ring and pins and then to reduction of the subluxation. Radiographic confirmation of an intact skull devoid of fractures or metastatic lesions that would affect pin placement integrity is wise. In addition, the patient already in traction is at some jeopardy if that traction system must be removed to convert to the Halo system. Care must be given to maintaining the bony alignment during the conversion.

Thereafter, the greatest concerns relate to the adequacy or perfection of the vertebral realignment and the means by which this has been achieved. With external reduction in an awake patient there must be a continual monitoring of the patient's neurological condition during the application of weight to scrupulously avoid the possibility of overdistrac-

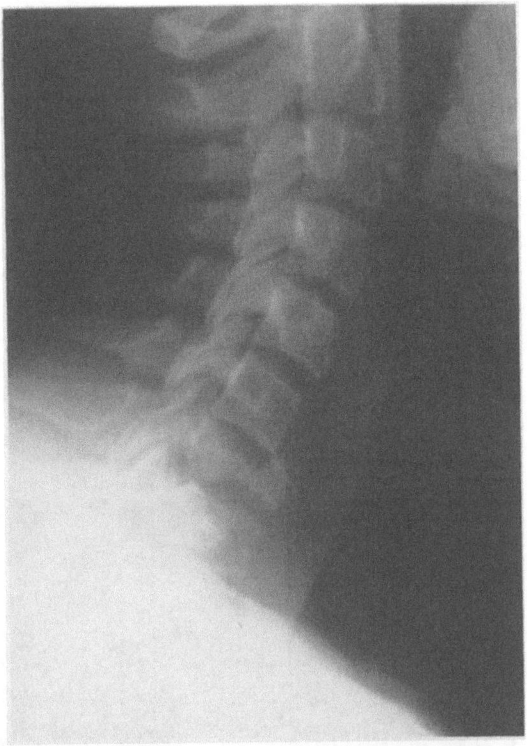

A

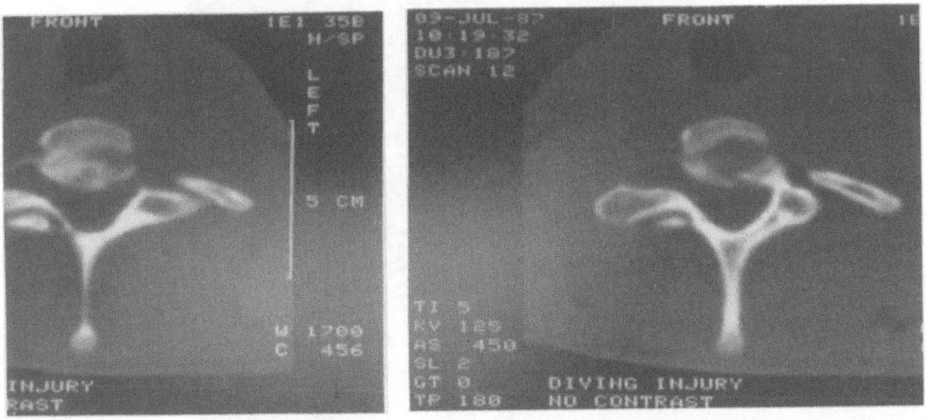

B

Figure 9.26. **A:** Plain radiograph shows compression fracture of the C7 vertebra. **B:** CT scan in axial view showing the fracture without paravertebral mass. **C:** Bone scan demonstrates dye uptake not characteristic of tumor. **D,E:** Flexion-extension views at 3 months demonstrate stability. **F:** No change at 6 months.

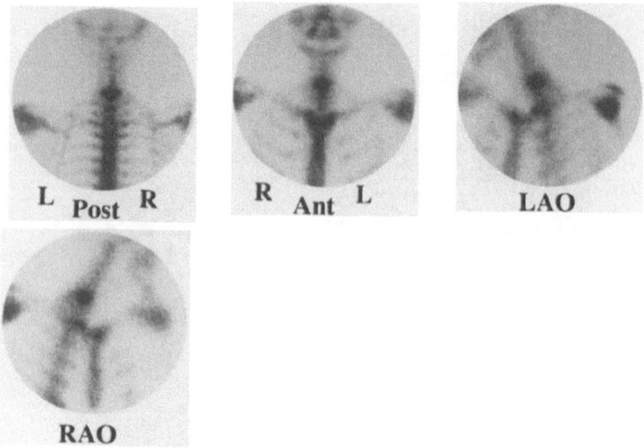

C

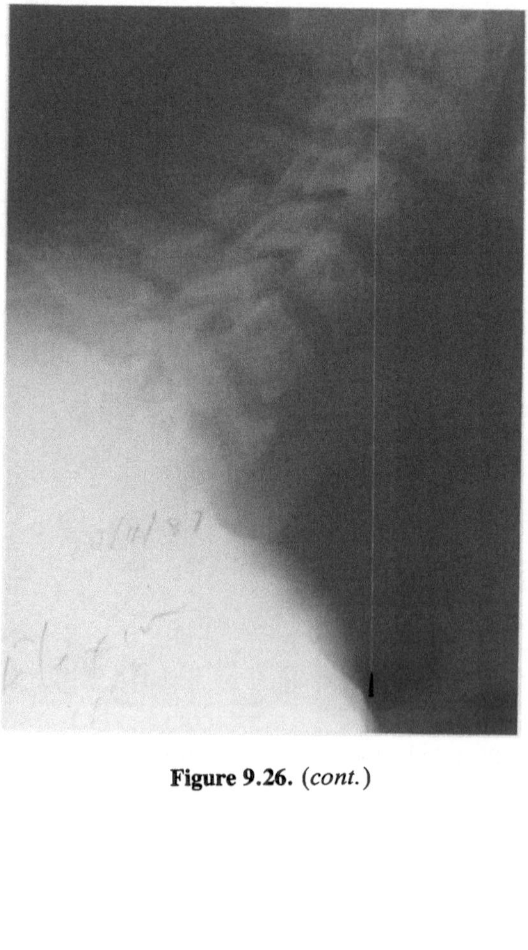

D

Figure 9.26. (*cont.*)

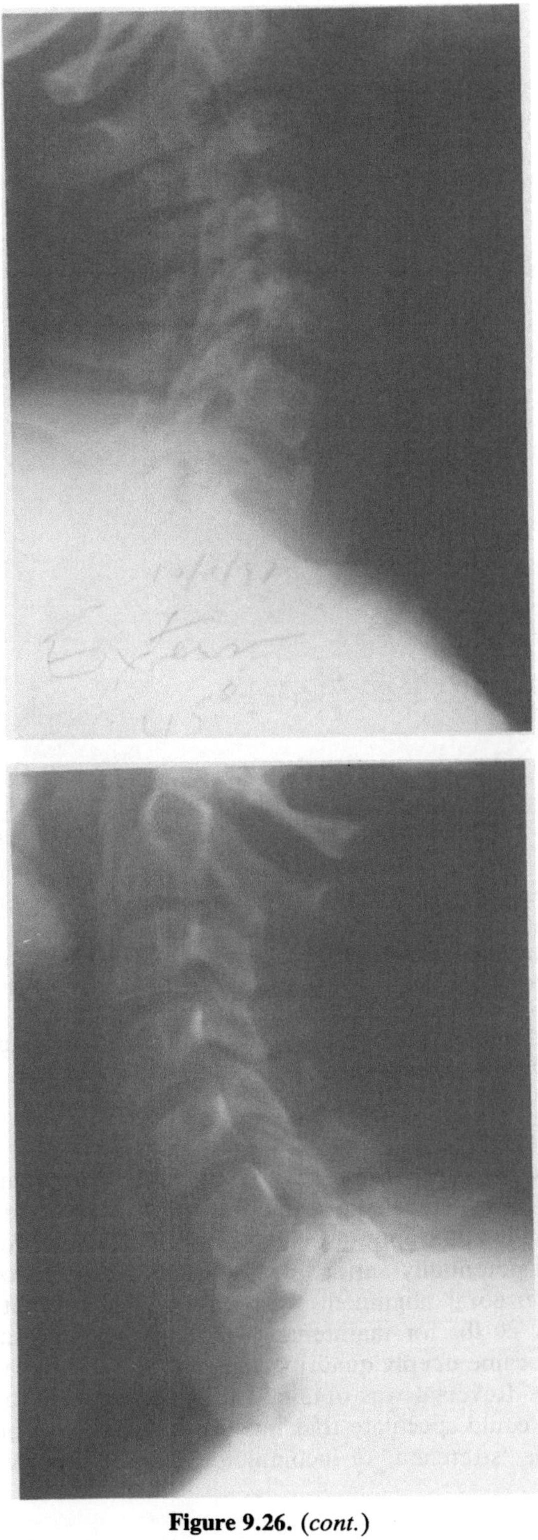

E

F

Figure 9.26. (*cont.*)

A

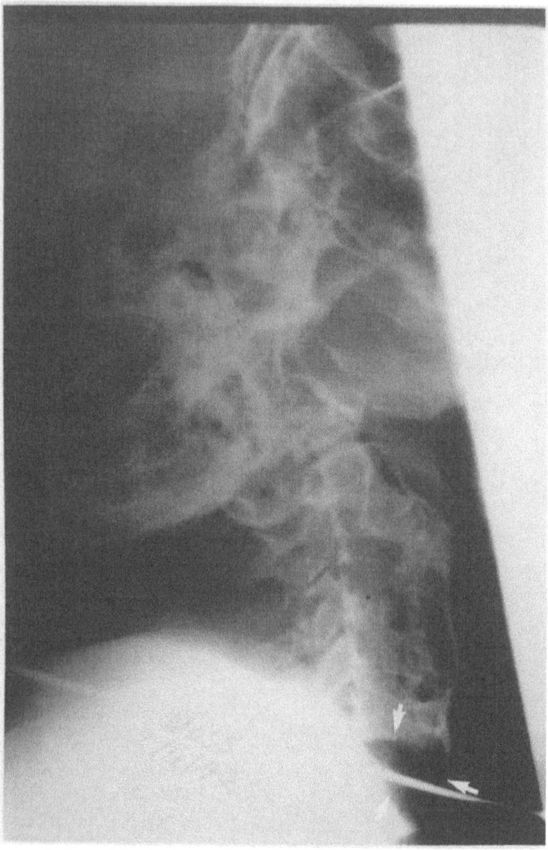

Figure 9.27. **A:** Plain radiograph of ankylosing spondylitis with an "open fish-mouth" fracture at C6 (*large white arrows*). **B:** Reduction of the fracture after Halo application and flexion without traction (*large white arrows*). **C:** CT scan demonstrating laminar fracture (*large white arrow*) and laminar bone in the vertebral canal (*large white arrow*).

tion. Similarly the surgeon must weigh the risks of intubation and positioning of the anesthetized patient using the least potentially traumatic methods, namely, fiberoptic awake intubation and positioning while in traction. One potentially serious and unusual problem occurred in this series after vertebral alignment was achieved and weight reduction to approximately 20 lbs for maintenance traction was instituted (case 17). The patient became deeply quadriparetic, and she lost her voice and ability to breathe. Reversal was obtained with the reinstitution of 40 lbs of traction. One could speculate that this event might have been related to buckling of the "stretched" or incompletely disrupted posterior longitudi-

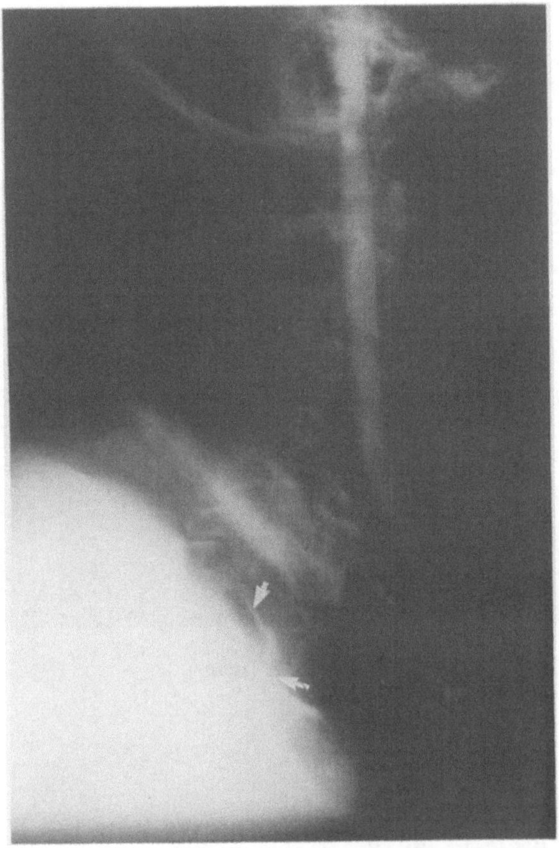

B

Figure 9.27. (*cont.*)

nal ligament in conjunction with the preexisting spinal stenosis, causing spinal cord compression, or to buckling and subsequent ischemia of the stretched spinal cord. Whatever the mechanism, the phenomenon is worrisome and points out that great care must be paid to the patient at these times.

Thereafter, problems arise concerning the maintaining of a reduction once it has been achieved either surgically with instrumentation and bony fusion or by external means such as the Halo-Vest device. With the latter, the phenomenon of "settling" with resulting partial resubluxation has been encountered on a number of occasions (cases 7, 10, 11, 12, 19, 23, and 24). Settling may be related to the direction of axial loading in the upright posture and to the associated shear forces inherent in the lordosis that normally exists in the cervical spine. It was seen in instances in which there was only one level involved (cases 7, 10, 11, 19, 23, and 24) and

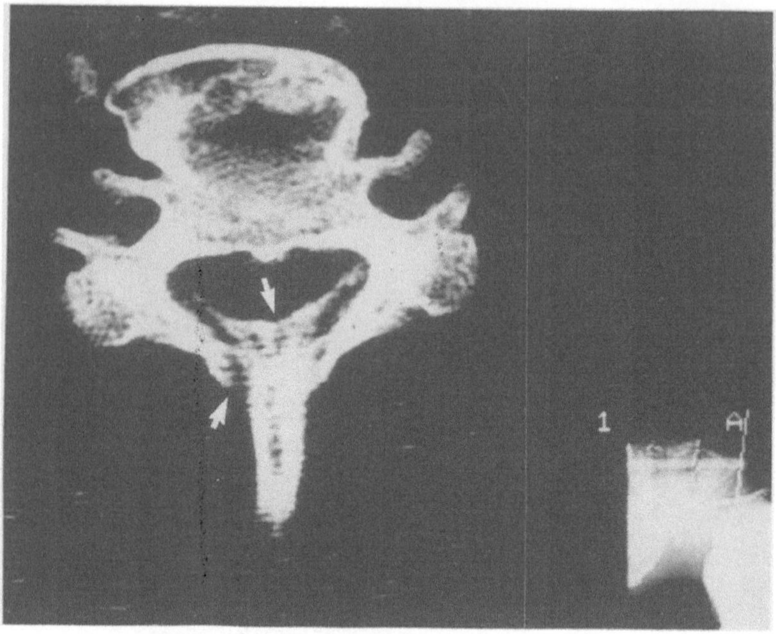

C

Figure 9.27. (*cont.*)

where more than one level of instability existed (case 12). It occurred in the elderly individual with ligamentous weakening and superimposed acute trauma (cases 9 and 11). It was seen in C1-C2 subluxations with odontoid fractures (case 7) and in trauma and osteomyelitis where the patients were noncompliant with external stabilization, removing or disrupting their Halo-Vests during the healing period (cases 15 and 19). Certainly, it could be argued that early surgical fixation and fusion might prevent settling and considerable thought must be given to this when entertaining external stabilization as the sole therapeutic modality.

The third major problem surrounds the failure of fusion despite an adequate period of immobilization. This was demonstrated unequivocally in cases 11 and 12 and must be contrasted with the rapid fusion and healing in cases 23 and 7 and with the long immobilization period required for case 1. There is no immediate explanation and therefore no strictly predictable index as to which cases will undergo spontaneous fusion. Age is not the sole factor since case 1 showed evidence of fusion after 6 months in the Halo. Neither is the presence or absence of a vertebral body or arch fracture. Three months has been accepted as adequate immobilization, but certainly there are factors that are not absolutely recognized that lead to spontaneous fusions, and others that abort that process.

Using the new Halo-Vest apparatus with locking bolts on either side of each pin averted the problem of *pin dislodgment* after initial tightening. *Pin infection* was a problem in two instances (cases 1 and 12), and could be treated for a time locally and with pin replacement. It should be borne in mind that *Candida albicans* may be implicated in some of these infections (case 12). *Confinement psychosis* was a problem with only one individual (case 13) and *pressure sores* occurred in two cases both treated successfully with conservative measures (cases 7 and 9).

Medical-legal concerns are raised in an instance such as is seen in case 9 where the C3-C4 subluxation may have been related to chronic changes associated with spondylosis rather than the traumatic event. Some credence may therefore be given to considering such an instance a "subtle instability" and managing it solely with a Philadelphia collar. In view of the motion demonstrated on flexion-extension views, it may in some communities be deemed suboptimal not to treat with rigid stabilization in these marginal instances.

The surgical cases in this series are summarized as follows: one patient underwent cervical laminectomy for postreduction spinal cord compression documented by cervical puncture myelography (case 17) and four patients underwent internal fixation procedures for problems related to external stabilization; one patient for multiple disruptions of the Halo ring (case 2); one patient for failure of fusion despite immobilization (case 12); one patient whose osteoporotic and rheumatoid spine gave the impression that its atlantoaxial instability would not respond to external rigid immobilization alone (case 6); and one operation was performed to protect against future extreme exertion and sports-related trauma (case 24).

Despite these problems, all patients were stabilized in external devices and those surviving the acute insult, excluding cases 4 and 27, experienced recovery of neurological function during the period of wearing the apparatus.

On the basis of this experience the Halo-Vest represents a logical option for immediate nonsurgical reduction in almost all cases of subluxation or fracture dislocation. In this series it was used exclusively in instances: in three for extreme age (cases 1, 13, 17); in one for severe osteoporosis (case 7); in three for medical factors precluding surgery combined with age (cases 3, 9, and 10); in one who refused surgical intervention (case 11); in five who were treated initially in facilities without equipment for optimum surgical intervention early in the series (cases 8, 14, 22, 23 and 26); in one who expired from sepsis shortly after the reduction (case 27), and in one patient who had the Halo applied for reduction of locked facets (case 21). Although some surgeons may elect to reduce locked facets surgically on an emergency basis it is demonstrated that this is eminently possible to achieve nonsurgically utilizing as much as 70 lbs of traction should that be required (case 21).

Subsequent Vest fixation allows for early mobilization of the patient, but frequent monitoring is required to identify such problems as "settling" and attempt to correct them with Halo-Vest readjustment or, if that fails, surgical internal fixation (cases 2, 12, and 24). In addition, efforts must be directed to better understand the spontaneous fusion processes and to heed them such that the most effective fusion, ultimately a bony fusion, along with bony and ligamentous healing of fracture sites can restore a semblance of natural stability to the disrupted spinal mechanism.

Acknowledgments. The author wishes to thank Drs. Jacob Graham, Louis Lombardi, and Patrick O'Leary for their involvement in some of the cases presented and for the opportunity to present those cases.

Bibliography

Bucholz RD, Cheung KC. Halo Vest versus spinal fusion for cervical injury: Evidence from an outcome study. *JNS.* 1989;70(6):884–892.

Hadley MN, Dickman CA, Browner CM, Sonntag VKH. Acute axis fractures: A review of 229 cases. JNS. 1989;71(5):642–647.

Hadley MN, Sonntag VKH. *Acute Axis Fractures. Contemporary Neurosurgery.* Vol. 9. Baltimore: Williams & Wilkins; 1987:2.

Garfin SR, Botte MJ, Waters RL, Nickel VL. Complications in the use of the halo fixation device. *J Bone Joint Surg.* 1986;68-A(3):320–325.

Waters RL, Adkins RH, Nelson R, Garland D. Cervical spinal cord trauma: Evaluation and nonoperative treatment with halo-vest immobilization. *Contemp Orthop.* 1987;14(1):35–45.

Whitehill R, Richman JA, Glaser JA. Failure of immobilization of the cervical spine by the halo vest. A report of five cases. *J Bone Joint Surg.* 1986;68-A(3):326–332.

II. CLINICAL ASPECTS OF INSTABILITY

B. OPERATIVE MANAGEMENT: THE PEDIATRIC SPINE

CHAPTER 10

Instability of the Spine Secondary to the Treatment of Intraspinal Tumors in Children: Diagnosis, Cure, and Prevention

Jean Dubousset

Pediatric oncology has made tremendous progress in the cure of tumors, particularly malignant tumors, during these last 30 years. The result was a higher and higher rate of children surviving with a complete cure of their tumor disease, although with some sequelae, sometimes very mild and negligible, and sometimes very important, creating a secondary pathology during their growth.

During the last 15 years, we have been able to study, follow, and treat more than 300 such patients; 127 of them underwent spinal fusion with or without instrumentation for the treatment of their deformity, and they represent the data for this work.

Etiology

For the *etiology* of a spinal deformity, we must distinguish deformities arising at the lesional zone of the primary tumor from those arising in the underlying part of the spine, which can be involved in a secondary manner in relation with paralysis or general growth hormonal disturbances.

We can distinguish four groupings of primary tumor location: extra-, juxta-, and intraspinal, and a combination of these (Fig. 10.1):

Extraspinal means away from the spine itself with no direct anatomical relationship, as in Wilms' tumor, for example (33 cases).

Juxtaspinal means outside of the spinal canal but with a close relationship between the tumor and the bony or soft tissue of the spine itself, as in some neuroblastomas or rhabdomyosarcomas (20 cases).

Intraspinal means inside the spine itself (45 cases), either in the bony structure (bone tumors) (20 cases) or in the nervous structures (25 cases), tumor of the cord, or the roots of the meninx.

Combined locations include juxtaspinal tumors growing inside the canal through the foramen, as in the dumbbell tumor in neuroblastomas (29 cases).

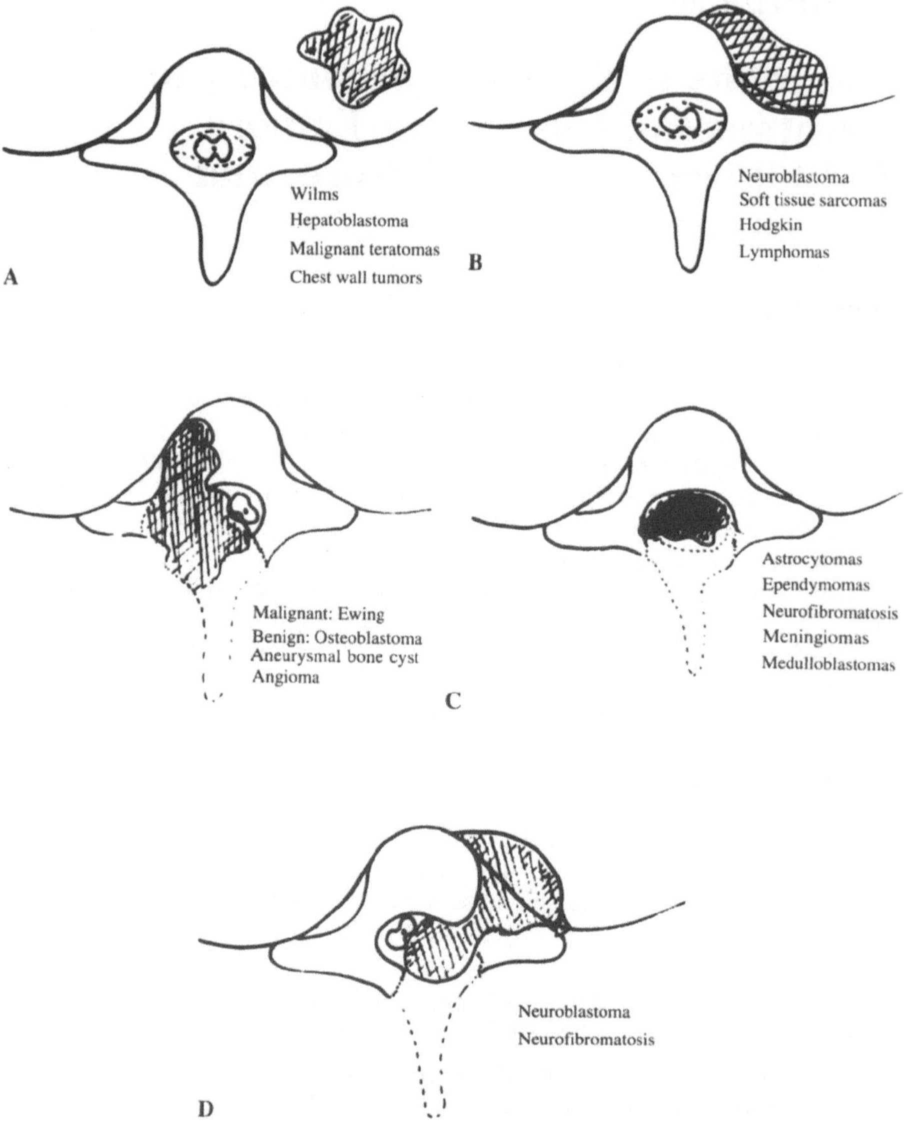

Figure 10.1. Our classification of tumors involving the spine in children. **A:** Extraspinal: away from the spine itself with no direct anatomical relationship (Wilms' tumors, for example). **B:** Juxtaspinal: outside of the spinal canal but with closed relationship between the tumor and the bony or soft tissue elements of the spine itself (neuroblastoma, for example). **C:** Intraspinal: the tumor arises inside the spine itself on the bony and ligamentous structures (posterior arc or body) or in the nervous structures: cord, roots, meninges. **D:** Combined: when a juxtaspinal tumor grows inside the spinal canal through the foramen (dumbbell tumors or neuroblastoma, for example).

Table 10.1. Tumors involving the spine in children spinal fusion with or without instrumentation: 127 cases.

Etiology	No. of cases	
Extraspinal	33	
Juxtaspinal	20	
Intraspinal		
Bone	20	74 (58%)
Nerve / Cord	25	
Combined	29	
Total	127	

Table 10.2. Secondary local deformities according to the etiology.

	Total	Kyphosis	Scoliosis
Extraspinal	33	19	14
Juxtaspinal	20	9	11
Intraspinal			
Bone	20	18	2
Nerve / Cord	25	24	1
Combined	29	25	4
Total	127	95	32

The treatment of the primary tumor is sometimes the only surgery in cases when the tumor is benign, but there is always an association of complete or partial surgical removal of the tumor and adjuvant therapy, either chemo- or radiotherapy, or both for the malignant one.

For our 127 cases, we found that 58% of the lesions developed more or less inside the spinal canal and so they required treatment involving a more or less extensive surgery inside the spinal canal (Table 10.1). After such an approach, as was expected, a kyphosis deformity was predominant in 90% of the cases (Table 10.2). In addition, 17 cases presented paralytic spine sufficiently large to be treated surgically below the lesional zone.

The Pathogenesis at the Lesional Area

We see first a direct lesion of the spinal structure coming from the tumor itself, including destruction of body, pedicles, and facets.

A direct lesion may arise from the surgical approach for removing the

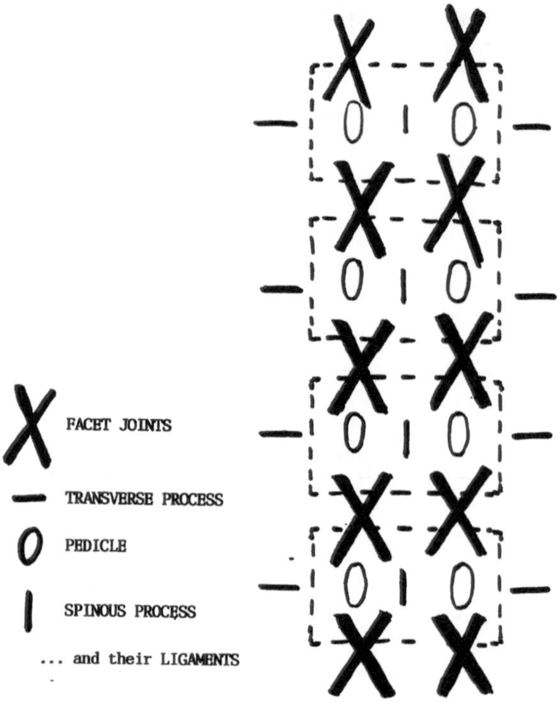

A

Figure 10.2. Postlaminectomy mechanical failure. **A:** Schematic drawing of the posterior spinal stability; 2-year-old patient 6 months after laminectomy for neuroblastoma (direct drawing from x-rays). Notice the bilateral removal of facets and posterior arch at the thoracolumbar junction. Bilateral removal at one level of the elements of the posterior arc always results in a kyphotic instability and deformity in the growing child. The more major the removal, the worse the instability. The younger the patient, the worse the deformity. **B:** Postlaminectomy instability for neuroblastoma. Notice that bilateral complete removal of the facet joints (X) with or without the pedicle (O) leads to kyphotic deformity exactly centered at the level of the missing elements.

tumor. A tumor involving the spinal canal, as in an intraspinal lesion, is the main problem for which a laminectomy is performed in children. We were able to demonstrate in 1971 at the first European Congress on Neurosurgery that a bilateral facet-joint removal at one level of the growing spine always results in a kyphosis (Fig. 10.2).

This tumor progresses in relation with age, and the younger the patient the more severe the deformity.

Regarding the level of the tumor in the cervical spine, kyphosis and instability never result if only the posterior arch of C1 is removed, but there

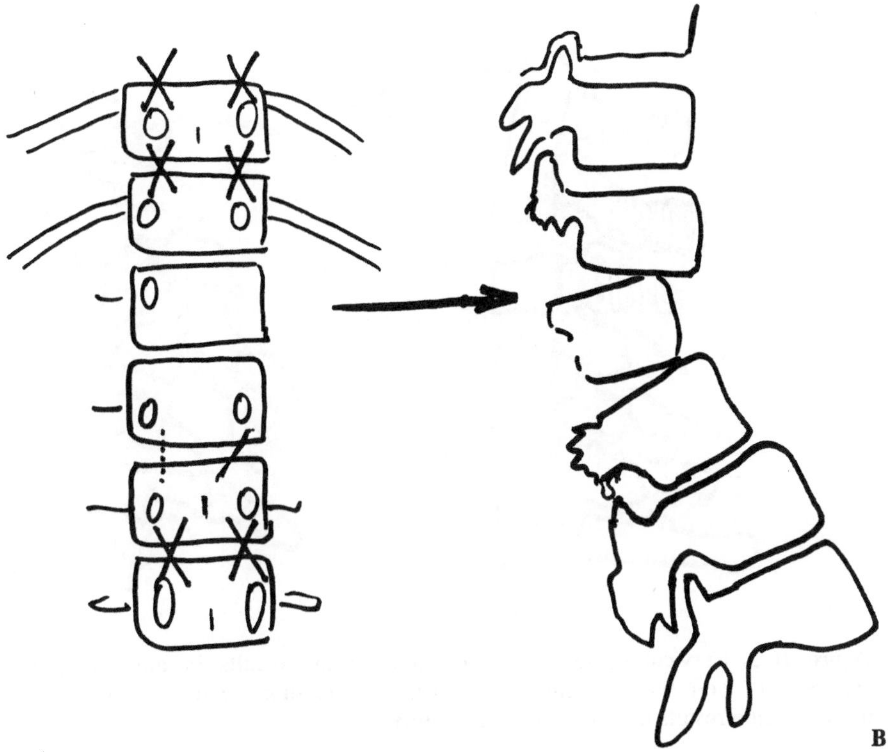

Figure 10.2. (*cont.*)

is a 25% chance of kyphosis and dislocation if C1 and C2 posterior arches are removed, and so on progressing to a 100% chance if laminectomy is extended to C7. Kyphosis can appear at every level of the spine, but the greatest frequency is in the cervicothoracic and thoracolumbar areas. When laminectomy is done in the lower lumbar spine, which is spontaneously and normally lordotic, there is less of a chance to develop kyphosis.

The relation of the tumor with the amount of posterior destruction, with emphasis on the ligamentum flavum, has been demonstrated experimentally. Interspinous ligaments are a very strong structure and their removal is sufficient to initiate the kyphosis. The wider the removal, the worse the instability and deformity. If we can keep one-half of the posterior arch intacts such as by performing a hemilaminectomy even at several consecutive levels, we can prevent a kyphosing deformity. The difference is clear at the cervical spine level between acute kyphosis for short laminectomy and swan neck for long laminectomy (Fig. 10.3).

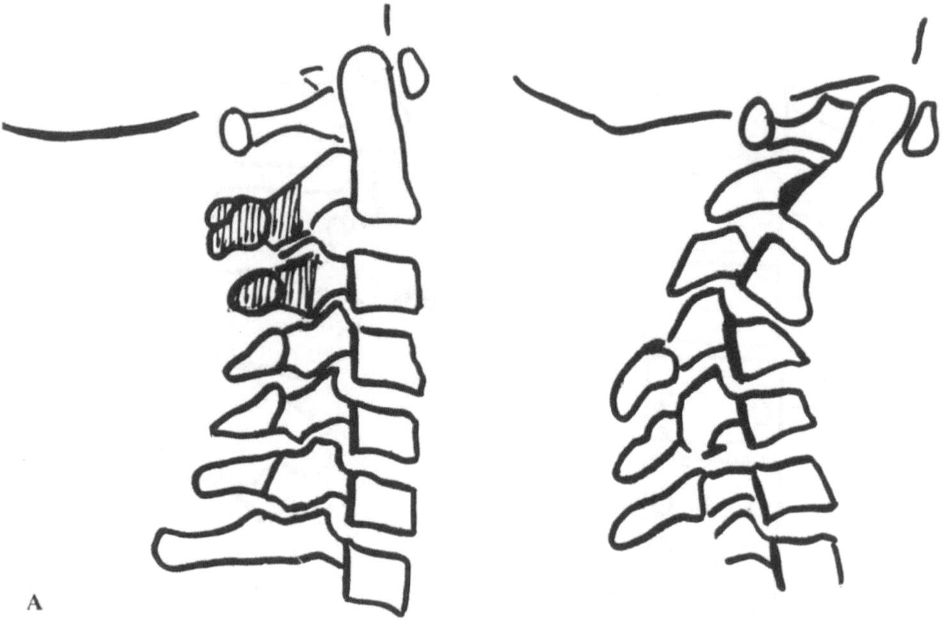

Figure 10.3. Cervical spine. **A:** Short laminectomy results in angular acute kyphosis. **B:** Long laminectomy down to the cervicothoracic junction or upper thoracic spine results in a swan neck deformity.

The surgical approach and removal of the tumor can also damage the soft tissues surrounding the spine and resulting in a direct or indirect lesion of the spine.

For the completely extraspinal lesion, such as Wilms' tumors even away from the spine, the more extensive the surgery the more severe was the deformity, especially when radiation therapy was given soon after surgery. In such cases, it is interesting to note that the concavity of the deformity was always on the side on which the surgery was done.

For juxtaspinal tumors and especially for neuroblastomas involving the thoracic area with or without invasion of the spinal canal, we have generally seen that the side of the thoracotomy, and therefore the side of the surgery, was located on the *convexity of the deformity*, whether or not radiotherapy was used in addition. Among 27 patients with a purely thoracic neuroblastoma, 25 patients had the convexity of their curve on the same side as the thoracotomy. We were able to demonstrate that this was secondary to the ligation of the intercostal vessels and nerve bundle, and we performed curettage of the foramen to completely remove the tumor. Doing so for a unilateral and isolated lesion of the posterior column of the cord can lead to a problem with the proprioception conduction and

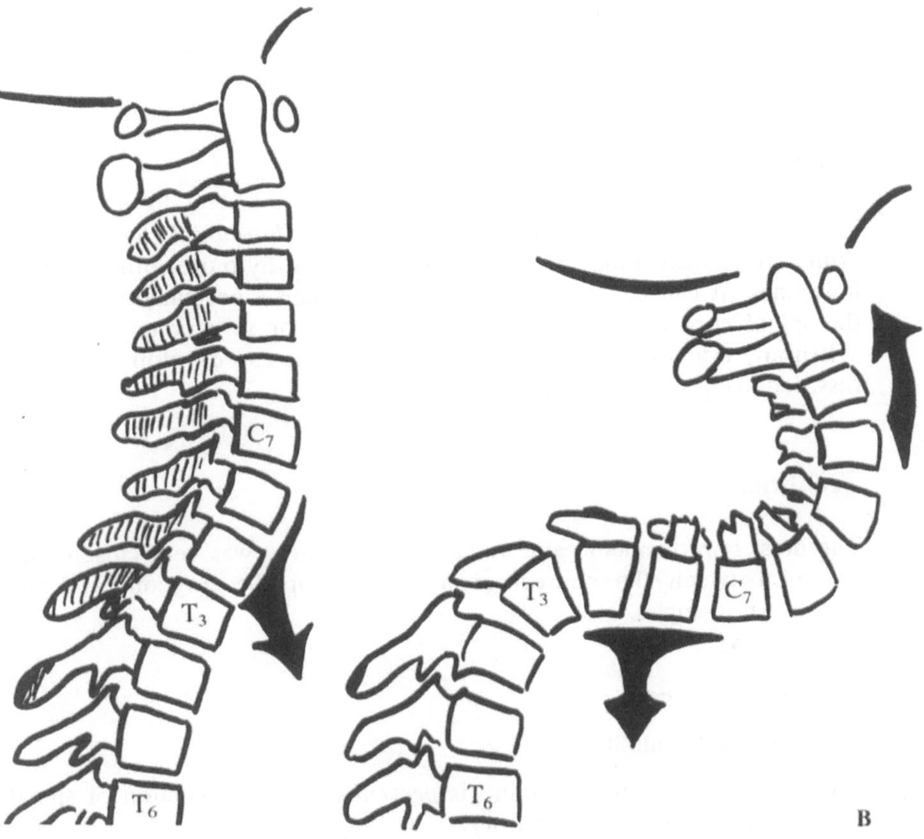

Figure 10.3. (*cont.*)

result in deformities such as those demonstrated experimentally by many authors.

Moreover, it is also possible to observe and record some asymmetrical paralysis of paravertebral posterior muscles of the spine. This very important point was confirmed also by the group of intra- and juxtaspinal tumors with progression, with the importance of age always evident in these cases without any radiation therapy. Finally, direct lesions result from radiation therapy, not only with sclerosis of the soft tissues but also with damage of the growth plates of the vertebrae.

The dosimetry of the radiation when observed in three dimensions, explains the deformities with anterior wedging and the kyphosis with lateral wedging and scoliosis. With new radiation, the dosimetry is related to the age of the patient who is followed until maturity. For similar doses, the younger the patient the worse the deformity, with a clear increase at puberty. For example, a patient receiving 4,500 rad at age 5, may have a 20° kyphosis at age 10, and a 70° Kyphosis at age 17.

The Extra or Infralesional Area

The damage can be secondary to *radiation of the hormonal glands* (lower skull and cervical spine), leading to deficiency in thyroid or other growth hormones. It can be secondary to *paralysis* when a permanent lesion of the spinal cord or the roots is treated by tumor surgery or radiation. When any asymmetry exists, a paralytic scoliosis can develop and progress, requiring specific treatment.

Treatment

The most improvement came in cases where there was very close cooperation between the neurosurgeon, the orthopedic surgeon, and the pediatric oncologist.

The Lesional Area

The Cure for Instability

The best approach to instability is *prevention*, and protection of spinal cord function is always mandatory.

In the past, when orthopedic work was delayed because of neurosurgery, we had to distinguish between immediate and potential instability at the level of the laminectomy. *Immediate* means the visible, abnormal motion between two vertebrae, and *potential* means abnormal motion not demonstrable by dynamic x-rays but rather instability may be revealed by sudden injury or trauma, or a deformity gradually increases, generally with kyphosis at one specific level. All of these types of instability need immediate treatment.

If laminectomy for such a lesion is delayed, and if the lesion itself has interfered with posterior elements, leading to the initiation of an instability, then *posterolateral fusion*, with or without instrumention, is recommended.

In very young children, under age 4 or 5, we can expose and decorticate the remaining posterior elements (transverse process and part of the remaining facets, and fuse the laminectomized part one or two levels above and below).

It is mandatory to have a good postoperative external fixation with the cast or halo cast in a correct posture. It is equally important to have a

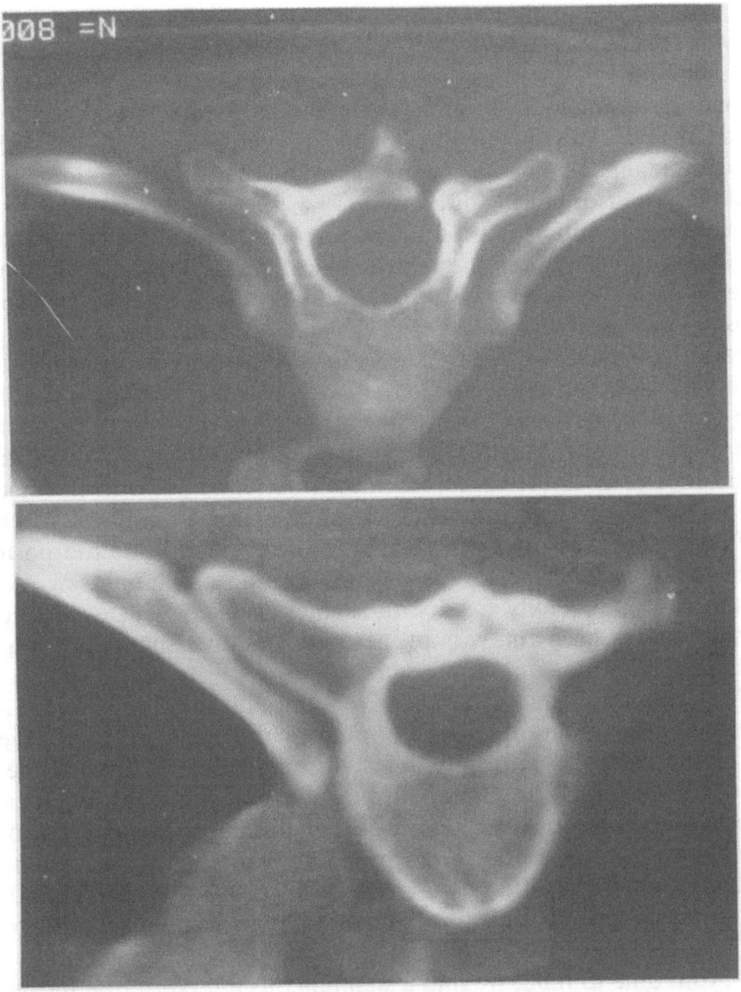

A

B

Figure 10.4. Laminotomy with reinsertion of the posterior arch; 4 months post-operative, the CT scan control demonstrates the fusion of the divided posterior elements (**A**,**B**).

simultaneous anterior interbody fusion as soon as there is any damage to the anterior column or disc space, or a large amount of kyphosis at the beginning, or any amount of kyphosis remaining after the correction. If any kyphosis exists, this will place the posterior fusion under permanent stress and lead to stress fracture at the apex of the kyphos.

If the patient is over age 4 or 5 or a teenager, it is advisable to use Cotrel-Dubousset (CD) instrumentation in addition to the posterior fusion, with a combination of claw and hooks at the upper and lower level, and even a pedicular screw when the thoracolumbar or lumbar area is addressed. This helps in avoiding postoperative cast immobilization if the bone metal junction is solid. The same recommendation applies for anterior fusion. This is the recommended management at the lesional area when a laminectomy has been performed or when the lesion has destroyed the posterior bolting of the spine.

However, prevention is preferable, for example, doing the stabilizing work at the same time as the neurosurgical work. When the lesion has affected a more or less extensive part of the posterior arches, or when the neurosurgeon can do nothing but perform a laminectomy, then the posterolateral fusion as previously described is best done at the same time, even if radiation therapy is used afterward. It has been shown that bone fusion can occur perfectly, even after a radiation dose of 45 Gy is delivered postoperatively. But for intraspinal lesions without involvement of the posterior arch of the spine, it is much better to perform laminotomy removing en bloc all the posterior "tap" as a roof or tilting it laterally. Many neurosurgeons prefer to remove completely en bloc the posterior part of the spine after a careful division with an oscillating saw. At the end, the roof is carefully fixed with segmental fixation at each level on both sides and at each end with proper postoperative immobilization with cast, brace, halo cast, etc.

If there is not adequate postoperative immobilization, the patient is exposed to the possibility of nonunion and to the recurrence or development of the kyphotic deformity. This is similar to a fracture of the leg, which need postoperative immobilization and a good posture to avoid kyphosis. The time for adequate fusion of the bony element is 2 or 2.5 months maximum in a child, and probably 3 months for an adult. We keep the patient in a good posture cast or brace for this time period. We can control the good fusion postlaminotomy with computed tomography (CT) scan checking clearly at each level the quality of the fusion (Fig. 10.4). From time to time, we find a spontaneous intervertebral fusion.

Achieving postoperatively the immediate, correct posture is very important. Neurosurgeons in France used to treat an upper cervical laminectomy at the C1-C2 level in conjunction with surgery of the posterior fossa, performing this surgery with the patient in a sitting position. The head was strapped in a flexed position to the operating table frame and the closure of soft tissue was then performed. Many of these patients later developed an acute upper cervical kyphosis. In such cases, it is recommended that the head not be strapped but rather placed in extension, when rebuilding the soft tissue in the extension of the neck and to suturing the nuchal ligament to the skull. It is also advisable to place a collar, keeping the head in extension, and to start head and neck exercises as soon as possible.

The Cure for Asymmetrical Growth Disturbance

We have tried to treat asymmetrical growth disturbance, secondary to irradiation in three cases, by early posterior fusion done at a young age. This was a mistake, because the growth potential of the irradiated growing cartilage of the vertebrae in the front was low, leading to failure. For example, one 4-year-old patient with deformity secondary to Wilms' tumors was almost completely corrected and fused posteriorly only at the level corresponding to the irradiated spine. Good fusion resulted, but stress fractures occurred within 2 years postoperatively, and the final correction was obtained by the addition of an anterior interbody fusion. So if it is possible, it is better to wait until maturity to perform the fusion of the entire lesion. But if for some reason, necessity requires that it be done early, it is advisable to perform a front and back fusion.

We believe that bracing is useful in the thoracic area while considering surgical intervention with the aim of preventing an increasing deformity. In a few cases it may provide definitive treatment for a mild lumbar curve until the end of the growth phase.

Final Treatment

The final treatment of these deformities when growth is completed was realized in three ways:

1. *Posterior fusion alone without instrumentation* was used in the oldest cases. The treatment was very long and needed almost 1 year of casting and bracing, always with the possibility of secondary pseudarthrosis. That is why we now always try to instrument the spine in order to give a better correction and to reduce the time of external immobilization. CD is good for that, and is used without anterior fusion when only rotational pseudokyphoscoliosis exists. When a kyphosis exists, anterior fusion in addition is always required.
2. *Anterior fusion alone* was used without instrumentation in very few cases. For example, when there is a patient with very poor skin associated with a clear swan neck deformity secondary to wide laminectomy at the cervicothoracic junction and high-dose radiation therapy, then in such cases posterior instruments will bulge under the skin, with a high risk of infection. Anterior fusion alone, with a strut palisade graft, can give a very good and stable result when sufficient postoperative external immobilization is achieved (Fig. 10.5).
3. *Anterior and posterior fusion* performed simultaneously or at an interval of 8 days was the most commonly used technique. (Fig. 10.6).

In order to decide which is the first stage of this circumferential fusion, we use both the sagittal bending and the direct stretching x-rays. If a good amount of flexibility is demonstrated with hyperextension x-rays, we start

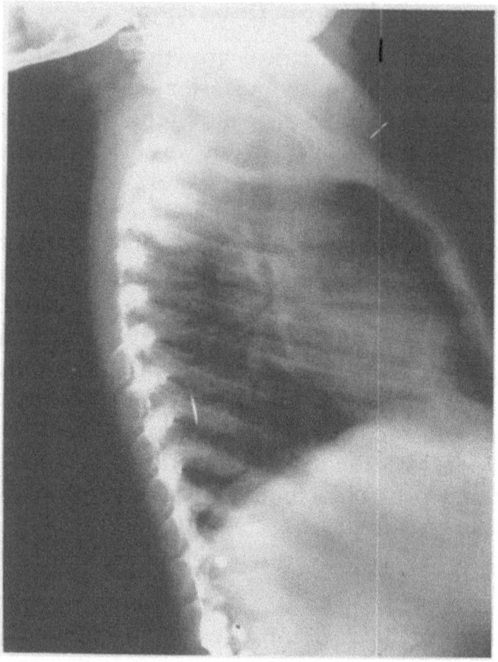

Figure 10.5. A: Swan neck deformity secondary to wide laminectomy done at age 9 months with additional radiation therapy. **B:** Age 9 years; clinical aspect of a swan neck deformity. **C:** (*Left*) Correction with anterior palisade interbody fusion. (*Right*) Clinical aspect, age 12.6 years.

with posterior instrumentation when possible. Then, the anterior fusion is performed. If the curve is demonstrated to be rigid, we do the reverse, starting with the anterior and continuing with the posterior.

Remarks

In postlaminectomy cases with a wide loss of bone, there may be some difficulty instituting posterior instrumentation, particularly when we are not confident with the bone metal interface. Therefore we do not hesitate to use a postoperative cast or brace, even with CD instrumentation, for some weeks or months.

When we have to bypass the level of laminectomy with rods that are attached above and below the laminectomized site, the anterior interbody fusion of this site is mandatory. This is true as well for kyphosis of any etiology corrected from a posterior approach leaving a real potential "empty space in the front."

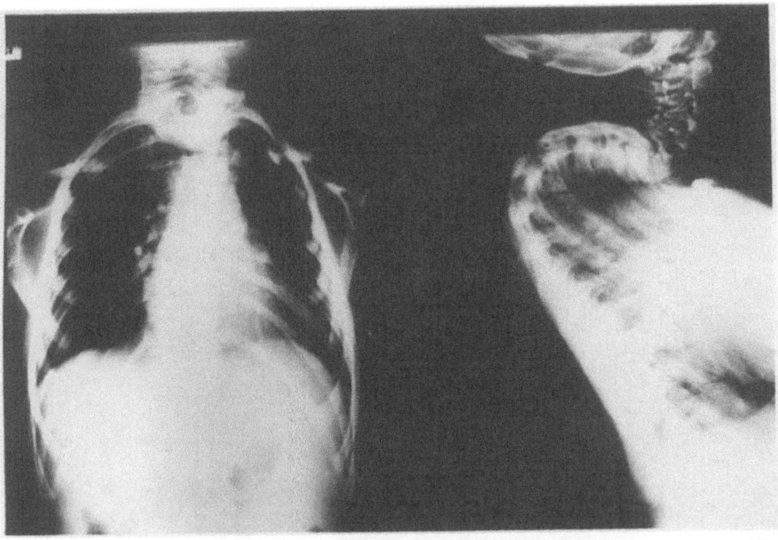

B

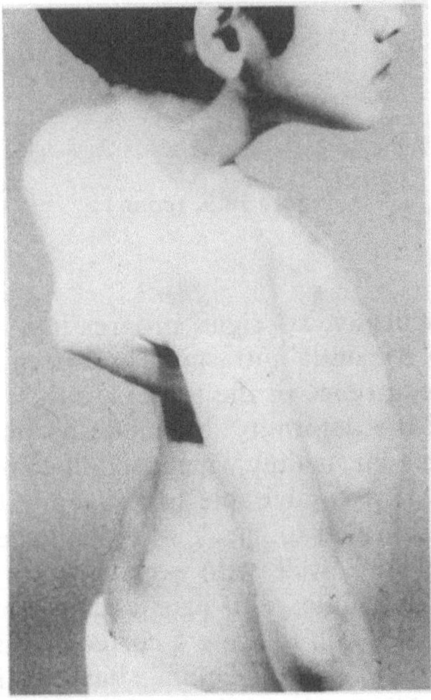

B

Figure 10.5. (*cont.*)

C

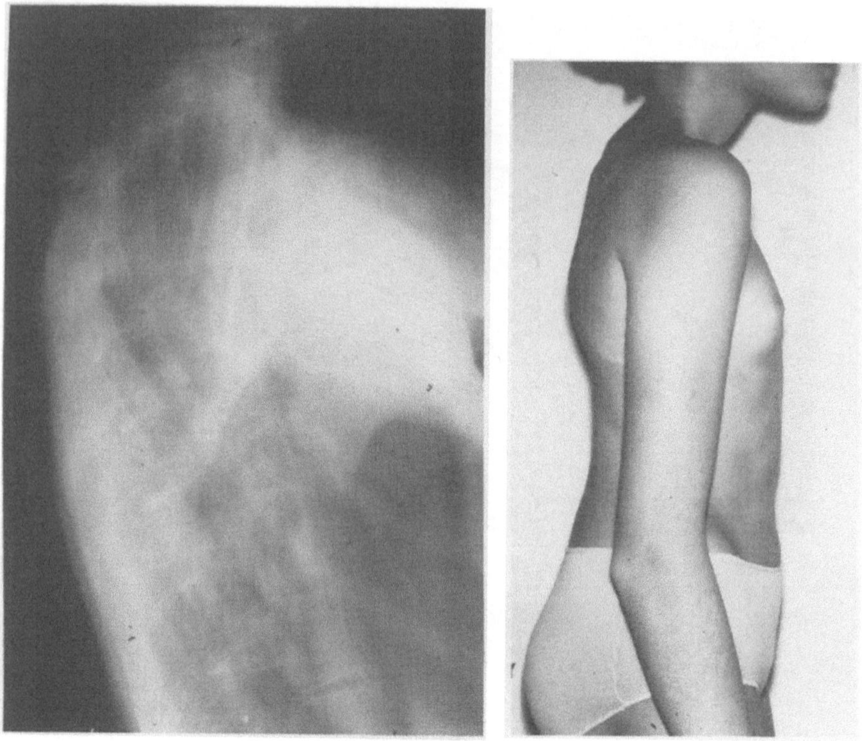

Figure 10.5. (*cont.*)

When we have neurological signs progressing, for example, some months or years after the initial intraspinal approach, we never know if it is secondary to the recurrence of the tumor, to the radiation therapy, or to the progression of the deformity. Magnetic resonance imaging (MRI) and CT scan can help a bit, mainly when used in conjunction with gadolinium. With such cases, it is advisable to try gentle but permanent traction with hyperextension and to check what is happening for the neurological signs, clinically as well with somatosensory evoked potential (SSEP) monitoring. Sometimes, the signs decrease and disappear as the SSEP also improves. This will indicate a correction and fixation from the orthopedic point of view without coming back again inside the canal, where repeated fibrotic scars on such multioperated spinal cords are not beneficial.

Each time we can get a strong internal instrumentation, no matter how great the neurological difficulty, is a benefit for the patient because we can avoid a postoperative brace or cast, which is always difficult to use on

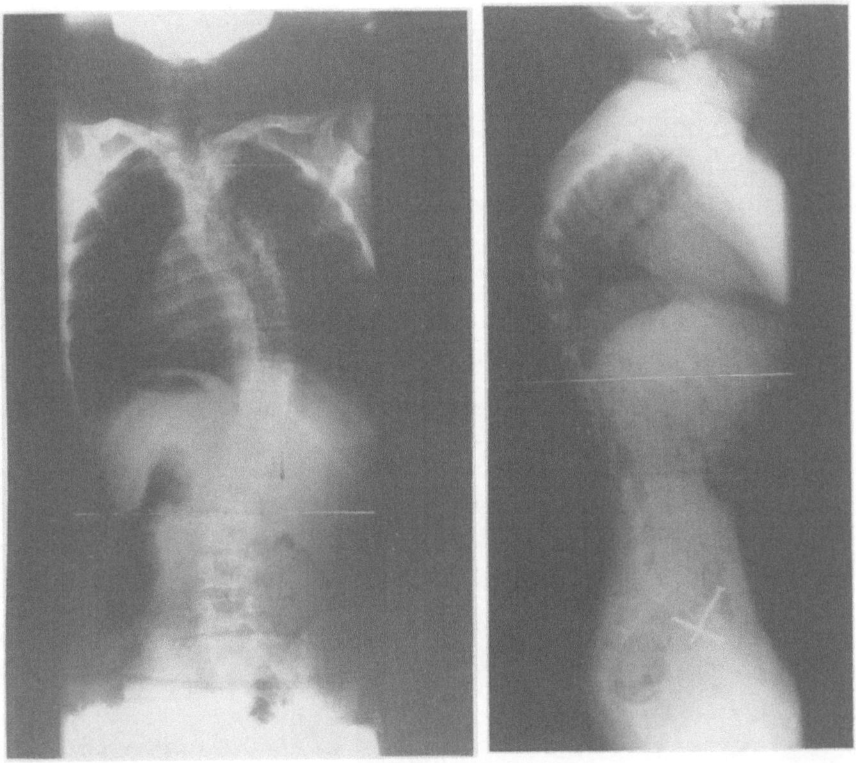

A

Figure 10.6. A: Sagittal pelvic obliquity with paralytic spine and upper thoracic postlaminectomy kyphosis. B: Halo traction and preoperative planning of position instrumentation. C: Correction with anterior fusion of the kyphosis and post–CD instrumentation down to the sacrum.

paralytic patients who have sensory and skin trophic problems. For these difficult problems, we analyze our series so that we can demonstrate that for the nonlaminectomyzed patients as well as for the intraspinal lesion patients, the best result and least loss of correction is obtained when front and back surgery are performed.

The Infralesional Area

When a paralytic spine existed below the lesion, the management of the spinal deformity was done at the same time as the lesional level using subcutaneous rodding and bracing during the years of growth. After the completion of growth, the fusion of the paralytic spine was performed down to the sacrum, because the main problem was pelvic obliquity (Fig. 10.6).

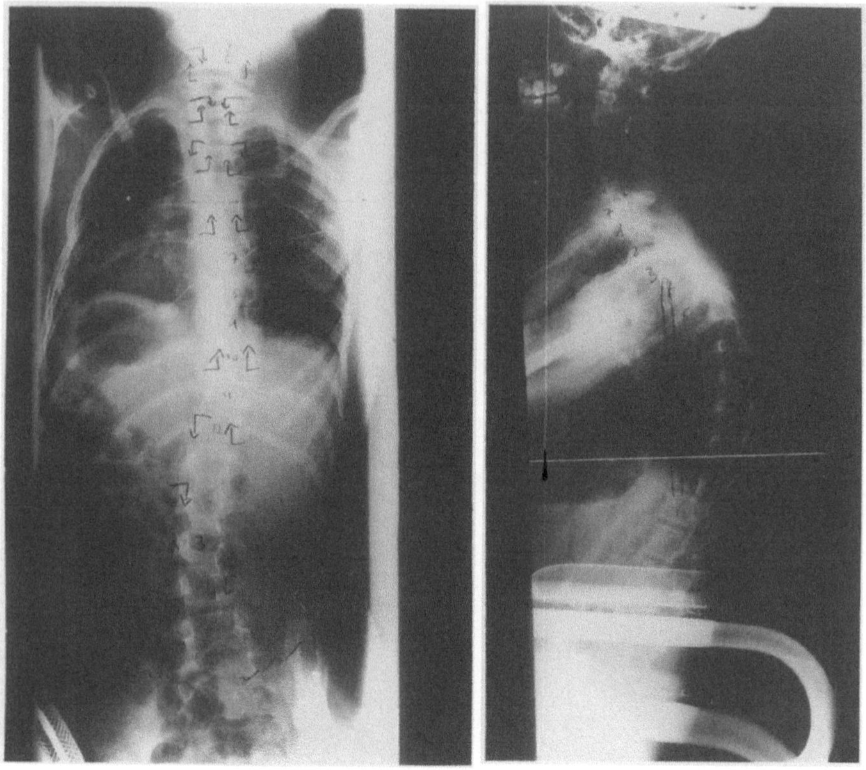

B

Figure 10.6. (*cont.*)

Complications

In patients treated with radiation with or without persisting neurological trouble, complications were observed in about 15% (Table 10.3).

Infection is the first complication, and it is mandatory to have good postoperative suction drainage, especially when the CD system is used. This is true because of the dead space existing below the metallic transverse system when the patient has poor skin or atrophic muscles. This can result in the complication of skin breakdown. If infection does not occur, delayed skin breakdown may not be disastrous for the simple reason that after 1 year a good fusion is formed which is generally capable of maintaining a good correction following the removal of the instrumentation. Only one fracture due to major trauma involving an anterior and posterior fusion was observed, and it was cured by a vascularized rib graft.

The main difficulty was respiratory problems, especially when the thoracic cage was irradiated with high doses when the patient was young.

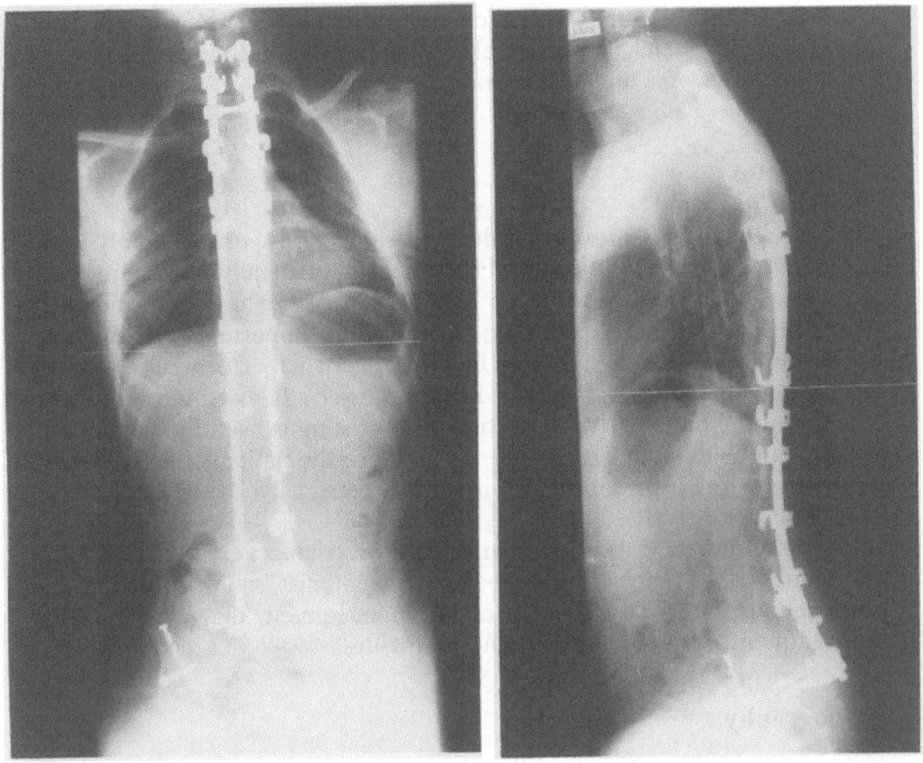

C

Figure 10.6. (*cont.*)

Table 10.3. Spinal deformities secondary to tumors involving the spine: 127 spinal fusions

Complication	No. of cases
Fracture of anterior and posterior fusion	1
Stress fracture of posterior fusion	1
Extension of kyphosis above and below an early fusion	2
Pseudarthrosis	2
Infection	1
Skin necrosis	1
Duodenum compression	1
Instrument dislodgment	3
Bulging instruments under skin	2
Loss of vital capacity (after anterior and posterior fusion)	5
	19 (15%)

These patients present poor lung function, which is sometimes worse after anterior surgery. This is why we always choose the anterior approach on the side of the worse lung when irradiation is necessary.

Conclusion

The best approach is prevention during laminectomy, or preferably laminotomy if possible. Good postural treatment immediately postoperative is mandatory. The use of lower and lower doses of radiation and the early treatment of respiratory problems is of primary importance. Lung cells do not multiply after age 8. The best treatment is performing a circumferential fusion front and back if kyphosis exists. If for some reason fusion had to be done early, protection with bracing is useful in some cases throughout childhood. Finally, we must advise the patients that extension might have to be performed at maturity, especially if neurological sequelae occur.

The main lesson of this work in France was that a very close cooperation must exist between the pediatric oncologist, neurosurgeon, and orthopedic surgeon at each step of the management: diagnosis, strategy for treatment, active treatment, and follow-up.

Bibliography

Dubousset J. Cyphose et cyphoscolioses angulaires chez l'enfant. In: *Skoliose und Kyphose*. Vol. 1. Stuttgart: Hippokrates Verlag; 1978:146–161.

Dubousset J. Deformations rachidiennes post radiothérapique après traitement du nephroblastome chez l'enfant. *Rev Chir Orthop*. 1980;66:444–451.

Dubousset J, Cotrel Y. Application technique of Cotrel-Dubousset instrumentation for scoliosis deformities. *Clin Orthop*. 1991;264:103–110.

Dubousset J, Guillaumat M, Mechin JF. Retentissement rachidien des lamminectomies chez l'enfant. In: Rougerie J, ed. *Compression Medullaires Non Traumatiques de l'Enfant*. Vol. 1. Paris: Masson; 1973:185–193.

Dubousset J, Herring JA, Shuffleburger H. The crankshaft phenomenon. *J Pediatr Orthop*. 1989;9:541–550.

Dubousset J, Rabet AM. Spinal deformities due to tumors in children. Pathological considerations and treatment. Presentation at the Scoliosis Research Society, Toronto; 1987.

CHAPTER 11

Spinal Trauma in Children

Gerard Bollini, J.L. Jouve, and J. Cottalorda

Clinical instability is defined as the loss of the ability of the spine under physiological loads to maintain relationships between vertebrae in such a way that there is neither damage nor subsequent irritation to the spinal cord or nerve roots and in addition, there is no development of incapacitating deformity or pain from structural changes.

A.A. White and M.M. Panjabi, Update on the evaluation of instability of the lower cervical spine *American Academy of Orthopaedic Surgeons*, Instructional Course Lecture XXXVI, St. Louis, C.V. Mosby, 1987, 513–520.

This definition used for posttraumatic spine instability in adults can be extended to children if the following conditions are considered: Relationships between vertebrae allow a wider range of motion in children than in adults. Physiological limits of displacement have to be assessed before speaking of instability in children. Damage to the spinal cord may occur without evidence of spinal instability. This is due to greater elasticity in the "discovertebroligamentous complex" than in the spinal cord. Immediate posttraumatic instability in relation to end-plate fractures has a good chance of healing under immobilization with subsequent stability of the spine. Subsequent irritation to the spinal cord or nerve roots after spinal trauma in children can be the consequence of worsened kyphosis or of kyphoscoliosis that started at the site of the initial trauma in relation to damage to the growth structures in very young children. Incapacitating deformity can be correlated with paralytic scoliosis, kyphosis, or lordosis occurring below the site of the damaged cord together with tetraplegia or paraplegia.

According to Ruge et al. (Pediatric spinal injury: The very young. *J Neurosurg*. 1988;68:25–30) spinal trauma in children represent 1% to 10% of all spinal trauma. This relative rarity has led to a general lack of knowledge about the specific presenting features and appropriate treatments. We have chosen, in presenting our series of 118 patients, to stress the problems of posttraumatic spinal instability in children. This is why we have preferred to develop the specific characteristics and their effect on stability for each type of fracture presented rather than discussing the results of our cases at the end of the chapter.

Cervical Spine

In our series of 118 patients, 39 showed a severe traumatism of the cervical spine; 17 were male and 22 female. Although the average age of our patients is 10 years (ranging from newborn to 15 years 7 months in age), the lesions of the higher cervical spine (occipito–C2) concerned younger children, whereas those involving the lower cervical spine affected the older age group. This can be explained by the higher weight of the head in relationship to that of the rest of the body in the younger child together with a lesser development of the cervical spinal muscles. Another explanation comes from the fact that the orientation of the upper cervical articular facets with regard to the horizontal increases from 30° in the newborn child to 60°/70° in adults, whereas that of the lower cervical spine develops to a lesser degree (55° at birth to 70° at adult age). The younger child is therefore more prone to lesions of the higher cervical rachis (occipito–C2). We shall only describe the traumas that were observed in our series.

The circumstances leading to the trauma in our 39 patients were in 18 cases road accidents (11 passengers, two pedestrians, three bikes, and two not stated); four falls from a substantial height; seven dives; one roll; one discus throw; one ski accident; one obstetrical traumatism; one case of child beating; and one accident with an agricultural machine. (Causes for the remaining four patients are unknown.) One type of neurological involvement was found 17 times, that is to say in 44% of the cases.

Medullary involvement was complete 11 times, partial four times. Two children had radicular involvement. Three patients died, the remaining 14 remain unchanged, after a mean follow-up of 4 years, as far as the complete medullary involvement was concerned, apart from a few who regained function one or two metameres above the level of injury. Two of the four partial medullary involvements have improved as have the two radicular ones. On the contrary to what is sometimes written, neurological do not in children do not have a better prognosis than those in adults.

Fracture of the Odontoid

Our series included 11 fractures of the odontoid, in 3 boys and 8 girls, average age 6 years (1 year 14 months to 14 years 2 months). The fractures of the odontoid show the specificity of fractures in children by their relationship with growth zones. We formed three groups of children. The first group consisted of five children, aged respectively 1 year 4 months, 1 year 4 months, 2 years, 2 years 4 months, and 3 years. All of these patients showed growth plate separation of the odontoid process at its base, slightly set into the body of the axis. One of these patients who, in addition, had a dislocation of C2-C3 with complete paraplegia, died. The other four patients, without neurological symptoms, had their fractures consolidated by 8 weeks' immobilization with the neck in hyperextension in a cervical support collar.

A slight defective callus of the odontoid, anteriorly tilted with regard to the body of C2, was present in two cases after an average follow-up of 2 years. The immediate instability of the spine in this type of fracture does not last. Immobilization in a corrective position for 8 weeks is enough to stabilize the spine. Maintaining traction on the cervical spine can be dangerous in the case of associated dislocation at occipito–C1 or at lower levels since we know that some of these dislocations that affect the end plates of the vertebral bodies are not always visible on the initial x-rays.

The second group of patients included three older children (8 years, 13 years 10 months, and 14 years 2 months). These children showed a fracture of the base of the odontoid similar to those seen in adults: in one of these patients flaccid paraplegia was associated with an undisplaced fracture of the odontoid, and myelography showed blockage of the contrast medium at T10. A laminectomy that was carried out showed medullary atrophia.

These three fractures consolidated with the use of a cervical collar for 3 months. Here again, immediate instability did not lead to any secondary instability after this orthopedic treatment.

The third group of patients perfectly illustrates the problems of secondary instability of the spine linked to the growth zone in the young child. Three children, aged respectively 4 years 8 months, 5 years 11 months, and 6 years at the time of the traumatism (three road accidents), experienced instability at C2 afterward; two of these were discovered 1 year and 4 years after the trauma. For the third, instability occurred immediately after the traumatism. In this series of three, the intermediary portion of the odontoid process was found to have disappeared in two of the cases.

These three patients underwent C1-C2 posterior arthrodesis, two of which did not result in stabilization for technical reasons (case history available). One patient had lasting residual hemiparesia in spite of stable arthrodesis. Paraparesia appeared in another patient after progressive recovery following a coma and this led to the discovery of instability.

Our proposal concerning this type of secondary instability is the following: Certain traumatisms cause a fracture of the point of the odontoid when it is still cartilaginous. The transversal odontoid ligament may then rupture, leading to immediate instability. When this ligament is intact there is immediate C2 stability, but the lack of immobilization resulting from this leads to pseudarthrosis between the point and the rest of the body of the odontoid.

As a result of the combined effects of pseudarthrosis and the stresses caused by the transversal ligament of the acetabulum, the intermediary part of the odontoid undergoes a process of lysis until it no longer acts as a brake to the transverse ligament. The instability then shows up together with the discovery of a pseudo-odontoid bone.

This secondary instability is therefore to be suspected in the case of a pseudo-odontoid bone. It is much more difficult to identify in cases where there is separation of a purely cartilaginous point of the odontoid, which will become ossified secondarily. The magnetic resonance imaging (MRI) will perhaps be a solution for early diagnosis.

Before instability occurs, a 3-month orthopedic immobilization should be attempted in case of fracture of the point of the odontoid. Once secondary instability occurs, only a C2 posterior graft will allow stabilization.

Rotatory Dislocation at C1-C2

Four children, aged respectively 13 years 9 months, 7 years 2 months, 12 years 3 months, and 5 years 6 months, showed a rotatory dislocation at C1-C2 (one fall from a bicycle, one gym accident, and two road accidents, one of which was a pedestrian). A patient with a rotatory dislocation type C, checked by computed tonnography (CT) scan (with rupture of the transverse ligament) died with signs of flaccid tetraplegia. Another patient without neurological symptoms, with a rotatory type D dislocation (posterior dislocation of a joint surface of C1 in relation to C2) underwent reduction under general anesthesia followed by 2 months with a cervical support collar. A year after removal of the collar, reduction was maintained with normal stability of C1-C2.

A third child with rotatory dislocation type A (dislocation of both articulating surfaces of C1, one anterior, one posterior) without any neurological symptoms, underwent two attempts at reduction under general anesthetia: this changed the rotatory dislocation from type A into type D (reduction of only one of the two articulating surfaces), requiring a posterior C1-C2 arthrodesis with stability in this reduced position 1 year later. The fourth child had a later diagnosis of rotatory dislocation from case history (x-ray and CT scan). It is impossible to diagnose the type of rotatory dislocation for this type of old case without CT scan. The patient had hemiparesis and was treated by traction and cervical collar for 3 months.

With 16 years' follow-up, only a deficit in dorsiflexion of the left foot persists. Therefore, these rotatory, dislocations show immediate instability, which can be treated by reduction under general anesthesia and support. The irreducible forms, or those which remain unstable after reduction, require C1-C2 posterior arthrodesis in the best possible position between C1 and C2. In the absence of diagnosis, C2 becomes fixed in a deformed position leading to an incapacitating deformity that comes under the definition of spinal instability in its widest sense. Such a deformity requires a C1-C2 posterior arthrodesis in the best possible corrective position. As we have no documented case history of C1–occiput instability, it will not be discussed.

Fracture of the Posterior Arch of the Atlas

We have only one case of this type of fracture: a girl of 12 years 6 months, victim of a road accident (passenger), treated by immobilization in a cervical collar for 6 weeks. This fracture does not lead to either immediate or secondary instability. It is, however, difficult to diagnose in children by default because it is difficult to see without a CT scan, or by x-ray, since the synchondroses of the posterior arch of C1 can be mistaken for a fracture.

Bipedicular Fractures of C2

We have three cases of this type of fracture: a child of 2 years who was beaten, a child of 10 years 9 months who had a seat belt injury, and a child of 14 years 11 months who after a fall from a substantial height, experienced resolving unilateral anesthesia in the area of C5. In these "hangman" fractures the forms with C2-C3 corporeodiscal integrity should be distinguished from those where there is dislocation associated to a greater or lesser degree with a C3 anterior corporeal compression.

In 2 of our cases there was no immediate instability. Two unnecessary pedicular screws were used as these fractures always heal with a cervical collar. These two spines are perfectly stable with an average follow-up of 2 years. The third case (case history available), the child who was beaten, had a bipedicular C2 fracture and anterior C2-C3 dislocation without any neurological symptoms. Immediate instability was evident and was likely to develop into secondary instability without any treatment. The C2-C3 dislocation responsible for the instability represents a epiphyseal detachment of the end plates of the vertebral bodies, which can heal with orthopedic treatment, thus reestablishing spinal stability.

Fractures of the Rachis Under C2

We have 14 patients with this type of fracture. Apart from two patients, a newborn child with obstetrical trauma and a child of 2 years (passenger of a vehicle), the other 12 patients had an average age of 14 years (11 years 10 months to 15 years 7 months). This confirms that the older the patient, the more predominantly cervical lesions are found in the distal part of the cervical rachis. Eight children had complete initial medullary involvement; two died and the remaining six only recovered function at best one or two metameres above. Two children, one with partial medullary involvement and the other with radicular involvement, returned to a subnormal neurological status. No patient without initial neurological lesions had any secondary neurological problem.

The types of accident for the 12 older children were six diving accidents, one bike accident, three road accidents (passengers), and a fall from a substantial height (the remaining type of accident is unknown). Two main elementary lesions were found:

Segmentary dislocations between two vertebrae for which the separation zone was not through the disc but at the corporeal growth plate. This anterior segmentary dislocation was mostly coupled with a dislocation or more rarely with a dislocated fracture of the back joint surfaces.

Anterior corporeal compressions concerning one or several vertebrae, mostly adjacent. These two elementary lesions may be associated. Some cases showed sagittal fractures of the vertebral bodies, or frontal fractures of these bodies with segmentary dislocation of the anterior part of the body, whereas the posterior wall remained intact; fractures of the pedicles were also seen.

Seven segmentary dislocations were found, twice on the C3-C4 level, three times on the C5-C6 level, and twice on the C6-C7 level, all with neurological complications except in one case with dislocation of the anterior part of the vertebral body of C6 on C7 but with the posterior wall remaining intact.

There were six compression fractures concerning one vertebra three times, two vertebrae twice, and three vertebrae in one case affecting mainly C5. Three of these six patients had complete medullary involvement; the other three had no neurological lesion. Among the 12 patients with fractures below C2, seven were operated: four isolated anterior arthrodeses and three posterior and anterior arthrodeses. Two children had to be reoperated because of instability that was more extensive than the initial zone of arthrodesis.

With an average follow-up of 2 years 4 months, two having died, the 12 remaining patients have a stable cervical spine with a loss of physiological lordosis but with no kyphosis. As long as the deformation is reducible, the immediate instability of segmentary dislocations is quite likely to heal with orthopedic treatment. Compressions of the vertebral bodies in small children are also likely to be corrected with growth.

The prognosis of these instabilities depends above all on posterior elements, a posterior ligamentary involvement being no more likely to heal in children than in adults. In cases of irreducible anterior dislocation, or of severe corporeal compression in older children, a reduction with anterior arthrodesis is justified. In cases of posterior ligamentary involvement, a posterior arthrodesis in a corrective position is indicated. Anterior and posterior arthrodesis is only justified in complex forms and in the very young child, any isolated anterior or posterior arthrodesis being dangerous because of the epiphysiodesis effect it leads to.

Severe Dislocations

Four children, aged respectively 9 years 2 months, 14 years, 14 years 4 months, and 15 years, were seen for a severe dislocation of the cervical spine consequent to a diving accident, throwing of the discus, and an agricultural machine accident. The cause for the fourth child was unknown. Only one patient had neurological involvement, a purely motor diplegia of the upper limbs.

One patient showed instability that was initially estimated to originate from the C2-C3 level. After arthrodesis limited to this level, C3-C4 and C4-C5 instability appeared. The patient (case history available) was not followed up. The second patient underwent anterior C2-C3 arthrodesis for segmentary instability limited to this level. The third patient, who was treated by traction followed by immobilization with a cervical collar, developed C3-C4 angular kyphosis at 45°. He underwent C3-C4 anterior and posterior arthrodesis. We saw him again after 3 years' evolution; the spine is straight and stable. The last patient underwent C2-C3 anterior arthrodesis, which complemented secondarily anterior C3-C5 and posterior C2-C7 arthrodeses. With a follow-up of 8 years, the spine is straight and stable. The patient's motor diplegia has disappeared.

These four case histories illustrate clearly the difficulty in analyzing the levels of instability that justify arthrodesis. The assessment of such patients should be carried out by analyzing the state of their discs with the help of MRI. If the disc signals show that they are intact, which is mostly the case in children, isolated posterior arthrodesis is indicated on all levels where capsuloligamentary instability, appreciated by dynamic x-ray, is found.

Fractures of the Cervical Spinal Process

There were two cases with fractures of this type in our series, a child of 2 years 8 months, a passenger in a car crash, and a patient of 14 years 4 months, a victim of a ski fall. These two patients had no sequelae after immobilization in a collar for a month. It should, however, be noted that our younger patient had pseudarthrosis of the C2 spinal process after a 13-year follow-up.

Spinal Cord Injury Without Radiographic Abnormality

Eight children, three boys and five girls, were seen for this type of lesion. As far as age is concerned, they form two groups:

a group of five younger children (ages 7 months, 8 months, 1 year 8 months, 2 years 8 months, and 3 years 5 months), a group of three older children (ages 9 years, 13 years 5 months, and 14 years).

The circumstances of onset were a fall from a substantial height, an obstetrical accident, five passengers of car accidents, and one who was run over by a car.

A case of neonatal hypotonia with blockage of the myelography at C7 to T2 died. Out of the other seven patients, five had complete medullary lesions and two had incomplete medullary involvement. The five patients with complete medullary involvement had blockage on the myelography, which was found for four of them to be at the cervicothoracic junction and for the fifth at the thoracolumbar junction. None of these patients showed any marked neurological improvement. The two patients with incomplete neurological involvement had a normal myelography; they returned to a subnormal neurological status.

The neurological lesions are not related to an instability of the spine that is unable to protect the spinal cord, but to a very great difference in elasticity between the discovertebroligamentary complex, which is highly elastic, and the spinal cord, which has low elasticity.

Thoracic Spine

Our series includes 41 fractures of the dorsal spine that we have subdivided into four groups, as discussed in the following subsections.

Corporeal Compression Fractures

We found 35 such cases (17 boys and 18 girls) whose average age at the time of the traumatism was 11 years 3 months (6 years 4 months to 15 years 2 months), with a mean follow-up of 3 years 6 months (3 months to 12 years). The causes of these trauma were as follows: 16 falls, nine road accidents (three car passengers, four pedestrians run over, two bike accidents), nine sports accidents (three ski accidents, four falls from the bar in gymnastics, and one case each of falls from horseback, from a beam, and from a skateboard), and a corporeal compression fracture occurred in one child following a fit of opisthotonus. None of these 35 patients had neurological symptoms. On average two vertebrae were involved (one to five in the series), mostly contiguous, but sometimes at a distance.

The two vertebrae that were the most often affected were T5 and T6 (13 times for each), followed by T11 and T12 (11 times for each). In six cases the thoracic and lumbar spine were the seat of compression fractures. The treatment in all cases was orthopedic, with immobilization in a plaster or a corset for 1 to 6 months, according to the degree of compression. The compression of vertebral bodies is often clear but sometimes less obvious. In these latter cases it is difficult to distinguish such a deformity from spinal growth dystrophia.

The use of bone scintigrams does not add to the diagnosis; however, MRI seemed to us to be an indispensable examination. Apart from the fact that it shows up the fracture zone as a change of signal, it also provides information on the discal condition and on the presence or absence of a "fracture line" concerning the posterior ligamentary elements.

What is the outcome of spinal instability in terms of evolutive kyphosis in this type of fracture? Six patients in the series of 35 were affected afterward by thoracic kyphosis. In three cases this was a regular kyphosis, measured respectively at the last checkup at 40°, 43°, and 53°, and in three cases an angular kyphosis, respectively at 20°, 40°, and 47°.

There are two opposite situations: On the one hand there are stacked anterior compressions with an MRI examination showing integrity of the disc and posterior ligamentary structures; either the child is close to being fully grown and the gain on lesional kyphosis will be that obtained at the end of the orthopedic treatment, or the child still has a substantial growth potential and a spontaneous improvement can be expected when the growth process resumes—guided, if necessary, by an orthopedic treatment. On the other hand there are cases in which the MRI examination shows disc involvement and/or posterior ligament involvement. These are angular kyphoses, which are potentially likely to become worse and should be treated orthopedically on a long-term basis, sometimes with secondary indication for correction by posterior arthrodesis.

In the frontal plane, vertebral compressions may be asymmetrical and generate scolioses. In our series of 35 patients, this type of scoliosis occurred, but it never had the evolving nature of real scoliosis insofar as the vertebral rotation remained moderate and Cobb's angle never exceeded 20°.

There are rare cases in which, although there are no associated discoligamentary lesions, evolutive kyphosis occurs. It should then be considered that the growth structures are involved.

Complete Segmentary Dislocations

Four cases in our series had this type of injury. These were road accidents involving children of 14 and 15 years. The level of the lesions was T6 and T7 in two cases, T8 and T9 in one case, and T9 and T10 in one case. Three of these children showed complete flaccid paraplegia upon admission and did not improve. The fourth with initial paraparesia improved and recovered autonomous walking. This last, very old, case only had orthopedic treatment, whereas the other three cases underwent posterior instrumented spinal arthrodesis after surgical reduction, with additional anterior arthrodesis in two cases. One of the patients with flaccid paraplegia developed major sublesional paralytic hyperlordosis, which led to stabilization by the Luque-Galveston procedure.

Dislocation of the Dorsal Spine

A child of 6 years 10 months who had tried to hold back a heavy, falling door, was seen with a pure dislocation at T11-T12, together with dislocation of the articulating surfaces with no neurological symptoms. Surgical reduction by a posterior approach together with a graft and T10-L1 instrumentation was carried out, associated with an anterior graft of the same levels because of the young age of the patient; at 3 years' follow-up the spine is stable.

Separation of the Neurocentral Growth Plate

A baby of 9 months, passenger in a car in his mother's arms, was seen for T12 level paraplegia following a car accident. The myelography showed a medullary lesion with no apparent bone lesion, which could have led us to classify this case in the SCICOWRA (spinal cord injury without any radiologic abnormalities) category. In fact, the CT scan showed disjunction of the right neurocentral growth plate of T12. No neurological improvement was seen in this patient.

We have individualized the main types of dorsal spinal trauma in children. Obviously, close analysis by CT scan enables us to find other elementary lesions at this level and in the adjacent vertebrae, particularly in segmentary dislocations, that we cannot detail here.

Lumbar Spine

Thirty-one patients presented a lesion concerning only the lumbar spine. We divided these into three groups, as described in the following subsections.

Corporeal Compressions

This type of injury affected 25 patients of an average age of 11 years 9 months (3 years 1 month to 16 years) at the time of their traumatism and the mean follow-up was 3 years (6 months to 10 years 9 months). The causes of the traumatism were 10 falls from a window, six road accidents (two car passengers, two pedestrians run over, two bike accidents), three falls from a substantial height, and six sports accidents (skiing, horseback riding, diving, and pole vaulting). Apart from one case of acute bladder retention, none of these patients had neurological complications.

An orthopedic treatment with a corset in hyperlordosis for 3 months was mostly prescribed. Four patients with lesional kyphoses underwent arthrodesis: two isolated anterior arthrodeses and two anterior and posterior arthrodeses. None of the patients treated by orthopedic means had kyphosis greater than the loss of physiological lordosis. The lumbar spine does not undergo the same kyphotic stresses as the dorsal spine during growth and is probably more likely to recover anterior vertebral growth after compression fracture as long as the remaining growth potential is substantial.

No evolving scoliosis was noted in asymmetrical lumbar compressions in the frontal plane. A 20° lesional scoliosis in a child aged 5 years 2 months at the time of injury, treated with an orthopedic corset for 12 months, disappeared almost completely after 11 years' evolution.

Fracture of the Isthmus and the Pedicle

A child of 2 years 9 months complaining of lumbalgia after a fall was found to have a fracture of the isthmus of L5. Treatment with an orthopedic corset for 3 months allowed consolidation to be obtained. A boy of 13 years 7 months with lumbalgia after a football match was found to have a fracture of the right pedicle of L4. A bone graft allowed this lysis to consolidate. The reality concerning traumatic lyses of the isthmus in children remains controversial. The age of our first patient and the fact that we obtained consolidation by immobilization sustain the hypothesis that it was in fact a traumatic lysis of the isthmus.

Rim Fracture

Four patients, aged respectively 10 years 5 months, 11 years, 12 years 1 month, and 13 years 7 months, were seen, in three cases for L5 sciatica and in the fourth case for cruralgia. The CT scan and MRI examinations showed a fracture of the vertebral rim. The symptoms disappeared in three of these patients who underwent surgery. The fourth patient had L5 and S1 right motor paralysis after surgery and is in the course of recovery.

Conclusion

Stability of the spine in children demonstrates the role played by the growth zones both in the onset of immediate instability and in the possibilities of rapid secondary stabilization. Concerning evolving spinal deviations after fracture, lesional deformities whose departure point is at the fracture site should be distinguished from sublesional spinal deviations consequent to neurological involvement in growing children. These sublesional deformities can be seen as scolioses, kyphoses, or hyperlordoses. The higher the spinal injury is, the higher the risk of lesional or sublesional deformity occurring.

Discussion

Circumferential Fusion

Dr. Floman asked: When you have had the occasion to perform a 360° fusion in children, what happens to the vertebral canal? Do you have a smaller canal later on and does it affect the child?

Dr. Bollini responded: The transverse growth of the vertebral canal is dependent on the growth of the neurocentral growth plate and we must be careful when performing an arthrodesis. On the posterior aspect it is quite impossible to fuse the neurocentral end plate. On the anterior aspect, in the very young, we must avoid fusing the neurocentral growth plate and then the vertebral canal can grow.

Dr. Neuwirth commented: If you fuse the posterior elements of a young child the anterior column continues to grow and the spine will rotate around a solid posterior tether. Dr. Kostuik emphasized that that occurs only in very young children. Dr. Neuwirth added that if there is sufficient growth taking place over enough levels you will get a deformity as though the child was born with a congenital lordosis.

Ring Apophysis Fracture

Dr. Floman commented on the ring apophysis fracture that in his experience was a very common occurrence not only in children but in adults, and we have published a series of about 40 cases in the journal *Neuroradiology*. We believe it is an analogue of a posterior Schmorl's node. The relationship to trauma is not certain at all since we have seen cases where there was no history of trauma in those patients. Dr. Bollini indicated that in a number of his cases there was a history of trauma, but he could not have an opinion since he was not absolutely certain of the traumatic etiology.

Adult Shoulder Harness Seat Belts, Odontoid Fractures, and Decapitation

Dr. Neuwirth stated that a picture of a child was shown with an odontoid fracture who was seated in his car seat at the time of injury. Everyone recommends facing rearward in the seat for a young child. For the child aged 3 and older, the adult-size shoulder harness has been implicated in instances of decapitation. It is a legal problem, and better seating must be devised with a shoulder harness that restrains the chest but does not slip upward and cause decapitation.

Spinal Cord Injuries with an Intact Vertebral Column

Dr. Sonntag inquired about the treatment of spinal cord–injured patients without vertebral abnormalities. You had approximately six complete and two incomplete spinal injuries. How do you treat them, especially the incomplete ones? What external orthosis, if any, do you use?

Dr. Bollini replied: At first we perform a myelogram. If the myelogram is normal there is nothing additional for us to do from the surgical standpoint. I don't believe a Minerva jacket or cast is necessary. It is important to try to avoid laminectomy and to permit the patient to rest for at least 2 months. Dr. Sonntag agreed with that protocol. He continued: Dr. Dachling Pang from Pittsburgh also agreed with our conservative management, but noted that one-third of the individuals suffered repetitive injuries after recovery, so that he now advocates some sort of external orthosis to prevent such a recurrence, and he so advises the families.

The Need for Screws to Incorporate the Posterior Cortex in Children

Dr. Sonntag noted that in some of Dr. Bollini's cases the screws did not incorporate the posterior vertebral cortex. Dr. Bollini indicated that this has been his method and he has not encountered any problems even in the thoracic and lumbar spine.

Dr. Kostuik added that in children you are going to get a good bite on the screw and in the young adult you probably will get a good bite as well without incorporating the posterior cortex. However, in the elderly patient and in the setting of rheumatoid arthritis the situation is substantially different and incorporating the posterior cortex is more important. A sound internal fixation is also achieved by use of the Morsher system.

The Question of Os Odontoideum

Dr. Kostuik felt that it was time to introduce the subject of os odontoideum, which is seen both in children and in adults. This has evoked a great deal of controversy among the subspecialties and also from the medical-legal point of view. I believe it was Fielding in New York who is on record as saying that all os odontoideum seen in New York City should be strongly considered to be posttraumatic. I don't know whether that is true or not.

Dr. Bollini said that he believes there is first a fracture through the odontoid cartilage. The tip of the dens has separated from the base and pseudarthrosis occurs. Over the ensuing months and years there is growth at the C1-C2 level and you have this relative change and at some point in time delayed instability is discovered. The transverse ligament is now higher than the intermediate part of the dens. There is in my opinion no embryologic explanation for an os odontoideum.

Dr. Sonntag said: I totally agree. I think all os odontoideum are traumatic in origin. Dr. Fielding pointed out in his elegant papers that there are three germinal centers: the os ossicle, the os, and the body of C2. If the os odontoideum is congenital then on the AP film we should see a divot into the body of C2 because that germinal center goes into it. It makes sense to me that the apical ligament pulls it apart, but I am not certain why it becomes unstable. Even if the transverse ligament is not opposite the odontoid, and given that the remaining portion of the cruciate ligament which is the vertical portion of the transverse ligament is not as strong, I am still not sure why these lesions become unstable.

Dr. Kostuik asked: Are we at least all in agreement with the recommendations of the Cervical Spine Research Society as to the indications of fusion in os odontoideum, which I believe is 7 mm of translation? What do we do for a patient who comes into the office with minimal to mild neck discomfort, no neurological deficits, and flexion-extension radiographs demonstrating 7 mm of translation? Prof. Louis said he would prefer to follow him for several months. Dr. Kostuik asked if there is any indication for prophylactic fusion? Dr. Louis said some of the cases with 7 mm of translation are still well 2 years later. Dr. Sonntag added that the number of 6 or 7 mm is a good guideline for fusion. Dr. Kostuik inquired: So you would recommend a fusion for an asymptomatic 26-year-old man with 6 or 7 mm of translational motion? Dr. Sonntag concurred, as did Dr. Floman. Dr. Bennett said he would be willing to individualize this recommendation, possibly excluding individuals not at risk. Dr. Kostuik emphasized that those are individuals who do not live in apartments with stairs, do not ski, and in general do not engage in stressful activities beyond reading books and watching television.

Anecdotally, Dr. Sonntag mentioned the case of a 28-year-old man who was beaten up in an alley, became quadriplegic and apneic. He was revived and recovered nicely. Radiographs showed only 6 mm of translational motion.

Rotational Subluxations

Dr. Holtzman inquired as to how Dr. Bollini was able to reduce the rotational subluxation at C1-C2. Dr. Bollini generalized, saying that if the injury was fresh it can be reduced under general anesthesia by rotation of the head and the application of traction. On the other hand, if the injury is a delayed one, then in my opinion reduction may be very difficult and the only possible option may be a posterior arthrodesis. Dr. Kostuik asked, Would you try a period of traction? Dr. Bollini replied, Of course we have, and in most instances simple traction was not successful. Dr. Kostuik added, In my experience I have been able to reduce them. Maybe I am seeing them at an earlier stage? Dr. Neuwirth asked, But have you maintained the reduction? The ones I have seen that are delayed, I have been able to reduce in traction, but I could not maintain the reduction. Dr. Neuwirth continued: I had a patient with a cervical deformity that I initially believed was a congenital anomaly. The history, however, indicated that she was normal 5 months previously and there was no mention of trauma. I had Dr. Fielding review the films and he diagnosed a rotatory subluxation. She was reduced completely in cervical traction over a 3- to 4-day period, but I could not maintain the reduction even in a Halo and finally with internal fixation she was stabilized.

Dr. Holtzman asked what period of time is the period of "stickiness" beyond which it becomes more difficult to reduce a rotational subluxation? No certain time period was given by any of the neurosurgeons or orthopedists.

Do Ligaments Stretch?

Dr. Holtzman said that earlier Dr. Kostuik indicated that ligaments do not stretch. Clearly this conference made up of orthopedic spine surgeons and neurosurgeons will address concepts where there are differences in definition and there is a sense among neurosurgeons that ligaments do indeed stretch. What therefore happens to a ligament that is subjected to ongoing trauma, pressure, and tears? Subsequently there is delayed instability. Does that imply that the ligament is longer than it was previously?

Dr. Kostuik replied: A classic example is the knee joint. If the ligament tears to the degree that there is instability demonstrated by physical examination, it signifies nonhealing. Ligaments always heal with scar tissue.

Dr. Holtzman continued: I have a sense that ligaments are not always totally disrupted in injuries, but that they may become less firm and somewhat attenuated and are more easily disrupted at a later time.

Dr. Kostuik said that even with burst injuries of the spine it is rare to see a complete tear of the anterior longitudinal ligament.

Dr. Holtzman continued: I agree with you about the anterior longitudinal ligament, but what about the posterior longitudinal ligament and structures such as the ligamentum flavum?

Dr. Panjabi said: I think your points are difficult to answer. You are referring to subfailure injuries of ligaments. We can determine what the failure load of a ligament is, but the threshold for microinjury with pressure deformation is unknown. The only biomechanics that have been done on ligaments are to see their end failure. There is no answer as to whether there is 40% stretching in microinjuries or 60% stretching or even 80% stretching.

Dr. Neuwirth indicated that a study had been performed at the Orthopedic Institute using MR imaging to evaluate knee ligament injuries, which demonstrated changes in the ligament during the healing period to the point where the knee was clinically stable. Dr. Kostuik added that those changes were probably related to water content of the ligaments. Clearly there are chemical and biological changes taking place in the healing ligament that may allow it to ultimately have a normal appearance on MRI, whether or not it functions normally.

Dr. Holtzman continued: In terms of the ligamentum flavum, with its high elastic fiber component, we often see redundancy in elderly people in the cervical spine. I suspect that may also be true of the posterior longitudinal ligament, particularly after disruption by a herniated disc.

The Use of Megadose Steroids in Pediatric Spinal Trauma

Dr. Sonntag inquired of Dr. Bollini whether he uses steroids in acute spinal injury. Dr. Bollini responded that he did not. He was uncertain of the basis for their use and suspicious that they did not change the outcome of acute spinal cord injury. Dr. Farcy supported their use.

The Burst Vertebral Fracture

Dr. Bennett asked about the flexion compression injury with wedging of the anterior aspect of the vertebral body, but the fracture extends back to the posterior cortex. Perhaps the distraction or the flexion deformities are greater than 30° and there is no bone in the vertebral canal. I have read that this fracture is classified as a two-column injury. Therefore, by definition it must be an unstable fracture. Is that a misinterpretation of the classification? Dr. Kostuik responded: I think the classification is based on engineering principles, based on looking at building bridges. It is unstable from that standpoint without taking into consideration the biological aspects. Dr. Larson said that it has been our experience that the burst fracture or the axial load fracture has an intact posterior ligamentous complex and does not need stabilization. The only indication for operation as I see it is neurological deficit.

Dr. Neuwirth described a presentation by Shannon Stoppler of a series of cases of burst fracture at the University of Southern Illinois. These were classic, usually two-column, even occasionally three-column, injuries. Dr. Kostuik interjected that there may be variations in the burst fracture; there can be flexion compression burst injury and flexion distraction burst injury. Dr. Neuwirth continued: These were flexion-compression, they were wedged anteriorly. The posterior body was ballooned out. The point was that he used criteria of less than 30° deformity and a stable or intact neurological examination for closed treatment. He treated these people in extension casts without surgery. I believe only two or three of the patients out of approximately 30 went on to progressive deformity. I now believe there is a significant number of these patients who do not need surgery. Dr. Larson added that if something is unstable it does not mean necessarily that it needs surgery, it just means that there is a need for immobilization.

Dr. Kostuik asked: What are the clinical and radiographic criteria for deciding that a burst fracture is unstable? Prof. Louis responded: I do not operate if there is no spinal cord or cauda equina compression and if there is no deformity in the coronal and sagittal planes. I perform a perfect reduction in the scoliosis frame, which I have been doing for the past 20 years with CT or MRI control to check the vertebral canal. I prefer a plaster cast for 3 months and the patient is able to ambulate the next day.

Dr. Kostuik asked: What if there is an angulation of 30°? Prof. Louis responded that this was an indication for surgery particularly since without repair of the anterior column by bone graft there might be a future risk of kyphosis. That to me is an indication for surgery. He then asked: Dr. Kostuik, how do you measure the 30° angle? For in my practice the 30° is the angle between the end plate above the lesion and that below, not the curve.

Dr. Farcy interjected saying that he has a prospective study that has continued over the past 6 years about the sagittal index showing the deformity at the level of injury or the end plate to end plate. I started the prospective study with a number of 15° on the sagittal index, which means the deformity of 15° at the thoracolumbar junction, but a deformity of 20° above and only 10° or 5° below because I add the normal lordosis and the normal scoliosis. So this sagittal index was started for the prospective study of about 15°. Returning to the numbers of the fractures I have analyzed I can say that I have an absolutely constant result with 25°.

Dr. Kostuik replied: You mean that everyone under 25° does not require surgery? Dr. Farcy answered: Yes, and everyone 25° and higher must be operated upon. And I have noted that everyone above 35° sagittal index needs both anterior and posterior fusions.

Dr. Bennett inquired about the presence or absence of spread pedicles. My impression is that in those patients who do not have posterior element fractures and had a two-column injury with a normal interpedicular distance, no angulation and neurologically intact pedicle will do better than those with spread pedicles. Dr. Kostuik said he was not certain that that was a burst fracture.

Dr. Bennett continued: What would you call a fracture with loss of vertebral height, but without angulation? Dr. Kostuik said an axial compression fracture. Dr. Bennett continued: Rather than a burst fracture as described by Holdsworth? Dr. Kostuik said: I don't think that Holdsworth's classification holds nowadays.

Dr. Neuwirth said: The key to the definition of the burst fracture is the integrity of what Dennis calls the middle column. There may be a hairline of difference between an axial compression injury and a burst fracture which involves perhaps an impaction or a crack through the posterior cortex, but by definition that is a burst fracture.

Dr. Kostuik continued: So everyone agrees that 25° to 30° of angulation is tolerable. No controversy there. Now, what about loss of anterior column height? The literature that states that 50% of loss of anterior height will lead to chronic instability. That is a pretty gross statement. Dr. Neuwirth said that number is probably too high. Dr. Farcy added: If there is no deformity such that the alignment is perfectly preserved I would not agree with that number.

Dr. Kostuik said: What if the anterior column has 50% loss of height and the posterior cortex is of normal height? Dr. Farcy said: So you have angulation. Dr. Kostuik continued: Yes, maybe not; do you think that angulation is more important than loss of height? Dr. Farcy said: But we have to check that on the CT scan after reduction.

Prof. Louis said: If there is no continuity, i.e., a lot of gap, between the fragments you need to operate. If there is good continuity, i.e., a line that might fuse within a few months, then it may not be necessary to operate. Therefore we cannot have fixed ideas, we need to know all criteria.

Dr. Kostuik said: Tell us about the criteria. What are the other criteria? Prof. Louis said: The criteria for me are the functions of the spine namely: (a) stability, (b) continuity, (c) balance in the sagittal plane, and (d) canal patency.

Dr. Kostuik said: Okay, let's stop right there. What about canal stenosis? When CT scans first came out in the 1970s, I was one of the big proponents of decompressing the vertebral canal. I used to preach that endlessly and I was wrong. How much canal stenosis is permissible? Is there any consensus on that? The long-term studies from Iowa were not done prospectively and showed that canal fragments absorb. Obviously it does not happen all of the time because some studies show that between 8% and 18% of people who have had a burst fracture develop late neurological problems due to spinal stenosis. What percentage of canal stenosis will the cauda equina tolerate? I am not talking about the spinal cord.

Prof. Louis said: Less that one-half, but that is related to the neural syndrome. If you have no neural syndrome you might accept a narrow canal. Otherwise you might have to decompress.

Dr. Sonntag said: I think anytime there is a neurological deficit accompanied by bone fragments in the canal I would like to have that canal decompressed. The controversy revolves about the typical L1-L2 burst fracture with a fragment of bone in the canal and a neurologically intact patient. The immediate reaction is "How can this patient be neurologically normal and what is to be done for him?" Dr. Sonntag continued: There are two points here; one regards decompression of the vertebral canal and the relates to fusion. Dr. Farcy stated that in neurologically intact individuals his efforts would be more directed to correcting the spinal deformity than to the capacity of the canal.

Dr. Kostuik asked: If the patient is unstable, neurologically intact, and has a lot of bone in the canal do you take the bone out of the canal, or do you just fuse it? Dr. Farcy said: Since I am there performing a fusion I would also remove the bone. Dr. Floman said: I don't think you necessarily have to decompress the canal. If you realign the spine in the sagittal plane and do a follow-up CT scan you will have a clearing of the canal with a residual 20% stenosis and patients can live with that.

Dr. Rydevik said: I think we should remember that there is an optimum time frame between 3 and 5 days to achieve a reduction of fragments in the canal with indirect surgery in the presence of an intact anterior longitudinal ligament. Distraction with posteriorly placed Harrington rods may achieve this end. Dr. Kostuik agreed that this must be achieved within 5 days, after which this is not possible. Dr. Rydevik continued: I just want to emphasize that there is a reserve space for the cauda equina which is normally about 50% of the vertebral canal.

It was agreed that in the patient with a partial neurological deficit and bone in the canal an anterior decompression should be accompanied by the removal of the bony fragments. In the neurologically intact patient with bone in the canal short segment fixation posteriorly can reduce the stenosis of the canal from 50% to 20% if it is done in the first 5 days after injury.

Dr. Hughes inquired: How much instability in the posterior column is tolerable to permit proceeding with anterior fixation primarily? Dr. Kostuik responded: In the very beginning, in the 1970s, we just used anterior fixation. When we reviewed our first 100 cases we had a 4% incidence of nonunion. These involved patients with significant posterior laminar destruction. Nowadays, we would perform anterior and posterior fixation and fusion on the same day. Kaneda's incidence of pseudarthrosis with his device was also 4% in his first 100 cases.

II. CLINICAL ASPECTS OF INSTABILITY

C. OPERATIVE MANAGEMENT: THE ADULT SPINE

CHAPTER 12

Operative Management of Occipitocervical and Atlantoaxial Instability

Volker K.H. Sonntag and Curtis A. Dickman

The biomechanical and anatomical properties of the occipitoatlantoaxial complex predispose this area to instability due to a variety of pathological processes. The alterations of the normal architectural and functional relationships must be analyzed critically to plan rational treatment strategies. The skull base, atlas, and axis are intimately interrelated by a complex network of important osseous and ligamentous structures. The loss of integrity of specific bony and ligamentous structures determines the site of instability. The motions of the occiput–C1-C2 region are complex; this region provides an important supportive role and a transition between the rigid skull base and the mobile cervical spine.

A variety of operative approaches and internal fixation techniques are available to treat instability of the craniovertebral junction and upper cervical spine. Alternative anterior and anterolateral operative approaches include transoral arthrodesis, facet screw fixation of C1-C2, screw fixation of the odontoid, and plating with screw fixation of C2-C3. Posterior surgical approaches offer a wide variety of methods for fixation and provide a better means of including the occiput in a fusion. Alternative posterior operative techniques for occipitocervical fusion, atlantoaxial fusion, and upper cervical (C1-C2-C3, C2-C3) fusions are available, employing a variety of hardware (e.g., pins, rods, plates, screws, clamps, and hooks) and wiring techniques. This chapter presents the relative merits, limitations, indications, and complications of these specific operative techniques.

Osseous Anatomy of the Craniovertebral Junction (12)

Occipital Condyles

The broad, paired, shallow occipital condyles anchor the basal surface of the occiput firmly to the atlas. The condyles are oval-ellipsoids directed anteromedially along the anterior margins of the foramen magnum (Fig. 12.1). The hypoglossal canal traverses the occipital bone above and ante-

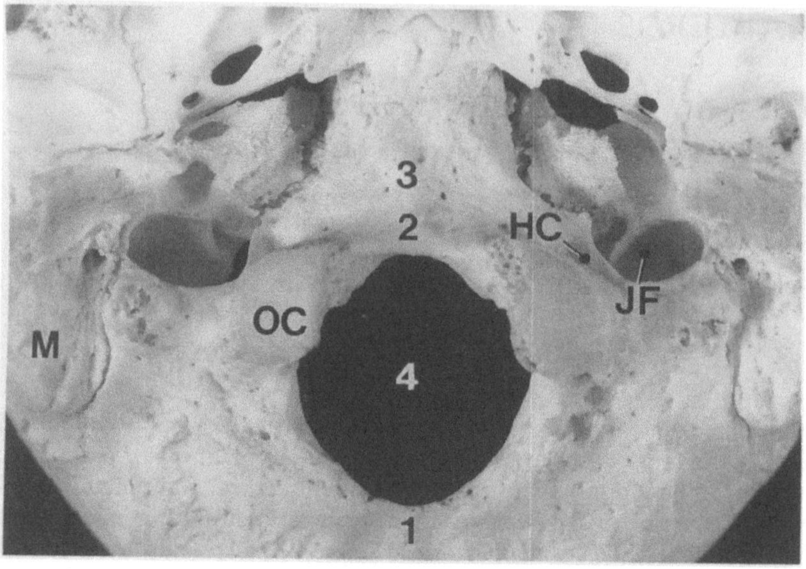

Figure 12.1. Occipital condyles and basal skull surface: (1) opisthion, (2) basion, (3) clivus, and (4) foramen magnum. OC, occipital condyle; HC, hypoglossal canal; JF, jugular foramen; M, mastoid process.

rior to the condyles. The basion represents the anterior margin of the foramen magnum (formed by the inferior clivus), which bears a close relationship to the apex of the dens and has a tubercle for attachment of the apical dental ligament. The opisthion is the middle point on the posterior margin of the foramen magnum, formed by the occipital bone. The dorsal margin of the foramen magnum is formed by a thickened lip of the occipital bone posterior to the occipital condyles. The foramen magnum has an oval shape.

Atlas

The atlas is a unique, modified ring-shaped vertebra that lacks a vertebral body. The anterior and posterior arches blend into two stout, wide lateral articular masses. These lateral masses are wedge-shaped from an anterior view (Fig. 12.2). The convex, kidney-shaped superior facets face upward

Figure 12.2. Anterior (**A**), superior (**B**), and inferior (**C**) views of the atlas or first cervical vertebra: (5) anterior arch, (6) posterior arch, (7) lateral mass, (8) tubercle for transverse ligament attachment, (9) anterior tubercle, (10) posterior tubercle, (11) foramen transversaria, (12) transverse process, (13) superior articular fossa, (14) inferior articular fossa, and (15) groove for vertebral artery.

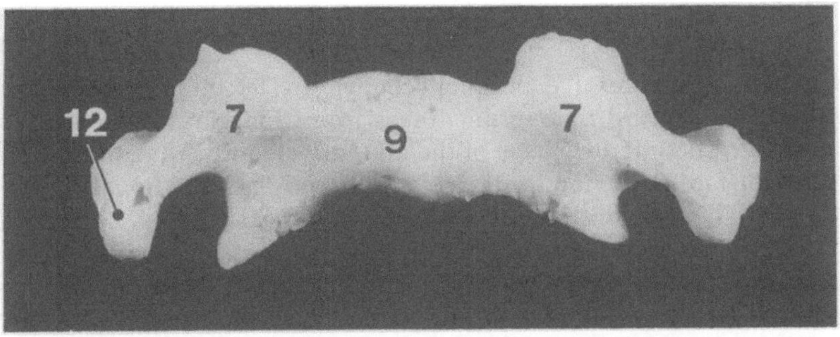

A

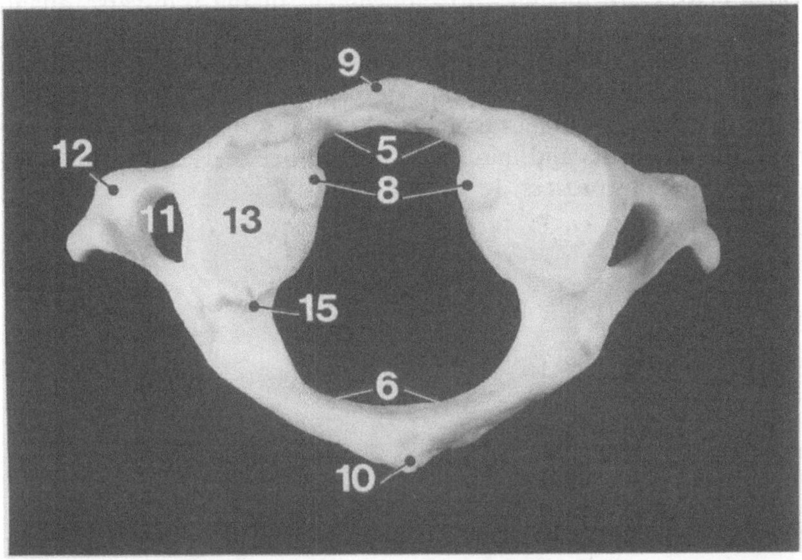

B

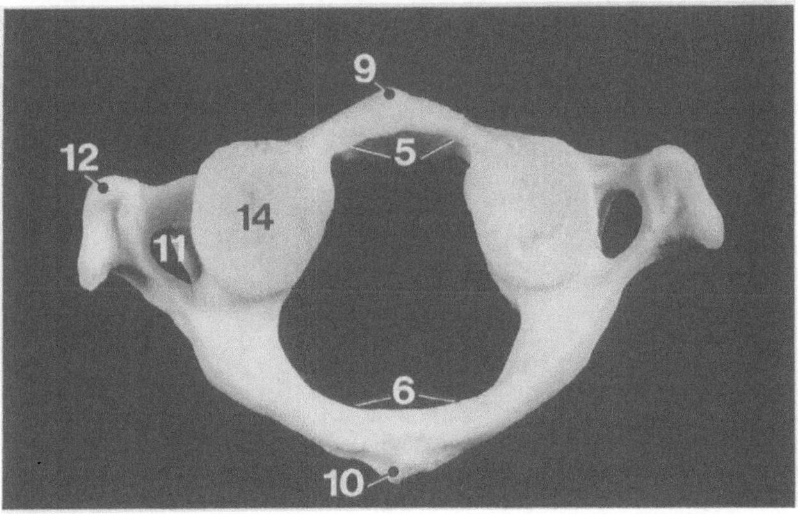

C

and inward to support the occipital condyles. The inferior facets face downward and inward to transmit forces from the atlas to the superior facets of C2. The inferior facets of the atlas are smoother and flatter than the superior facets; the inferior facets are the primary rotational surfaces for C1.

Transverse processes extend laterally from the articular masses of the atlas. These serve as sites of muscular and ligament attachment and contain the foramina transversaria, through which the vertebral arteries course lateral to the atlas (Fig. 12.3). On the medial surfaces of the articular masses are tubercles for attachment of the transverse atlantal ligament.

The posterior arch of the atlas is grooved superiorly just dorsal to the lateral masses where the vertebral artery passes over the C1 ring. The anterior and posterior arches contain tubercles in the midline for attachment of the ligaments and muscles. Unlike other cervical vertebrae, the atlas has no spinous process.

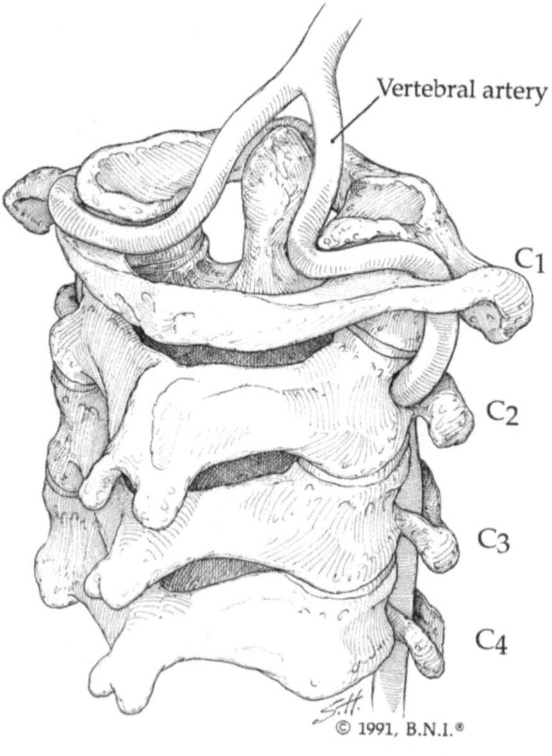

Figure 12.3. The relationship of the vertebral artery to the atlas and axis. (Reprinted with permission of Barrow Neurologic Institute.)

Axis

The axis (C2) also has a unique structure although it more closely resembles a typical cervical vertebrae than does C1 (Fig. 12.4). The odontoid process or dens is the most distinctive feature of C2; it projects superiorly from the vertebral body of C2. Embryologically, the dens was the vertebral body of C1 that was incorporated into the structure of the axis rather than C1. The odontoid process originates from the body of the axis and extends upward to reach the anterior lip of the foramen magnum. The odontoid is surrounded by synovium at its base; the dens articulates anteriorly with the anterior arch of C1 and posteriorly with the transverse ligament (Fig. 12.5). The waist of the dens is narrowed where the transverse ligament passes posteriorly. The dens then widens above this point and abruptly tapers to its apex.

The superior facets of the axis are broad, horizontal portions of the upper body that slope outward to articulate with the broad articular surfaces of the lateral masses of the atlas. The transverse processes of C2 are attached to the body laterally and contain the foramina transversaria for the vertebral arteries. The inferior facets of C2 are more vertical than the superior facets, and they are positioned posteriorly in continuity with the pars interarticularis of the neural arch. The inferior portion of the axis resembles the vertebrae of the lower cervical segments. A prominent, usually bifid, spinous process is in continuity with heavy, strong laminae.

Ligamentous Anatomy

The spinal ligaments are critical structures that provide spinal stability. They maintain anatomic relationships, both permit and restrict motion, and protect the spinal cord during trauma. The primary ligamentous structures stabilizing and integrating this osseous complex are the transverse atlantal ligament and the alar ligaments (15,17,19,61). The transverse ligament is the thickest and strongest ligament stabilizing the upper cervical spine (15,17). This structure is actually the transverse portion of the cruciate ligament, which also contains ascending and descending bands (Figs. 12.5 and 12.6). The transverse ligament extends between the lateral masses of C1 behind the base of the odontoid process and serves to prevent anterior subluxation of the atlas (15,19). It also provides an axis of rotation for the atlas and skull about the dens (17,34). The alar ligaments (also called check ligaments) extend from the occipital condyles to the dens and connect the skull base to C2 (Fig. 12.6). The alar ligaments limit rotation of the atlas and skull and entrap the atlas between the occipital condyles and axis (17,34).

The remaining ligaments of the craniovertebral junction (Fig. 12.7) include the accessory, capsular, and apical odontoid ligaments; the

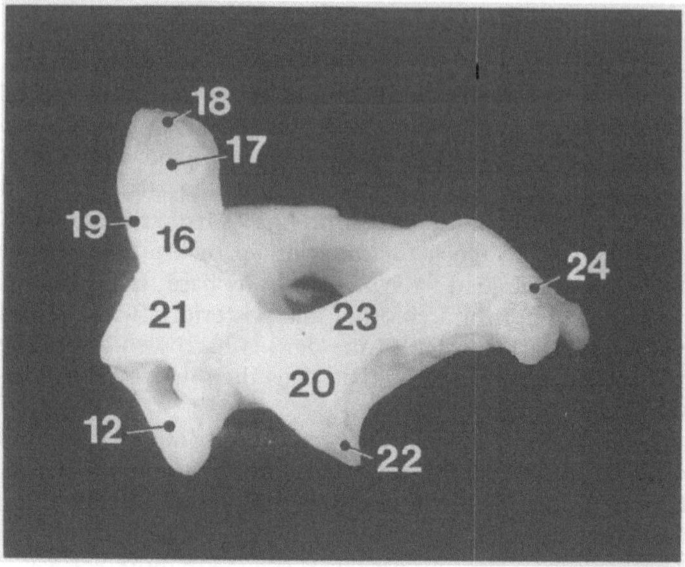

A

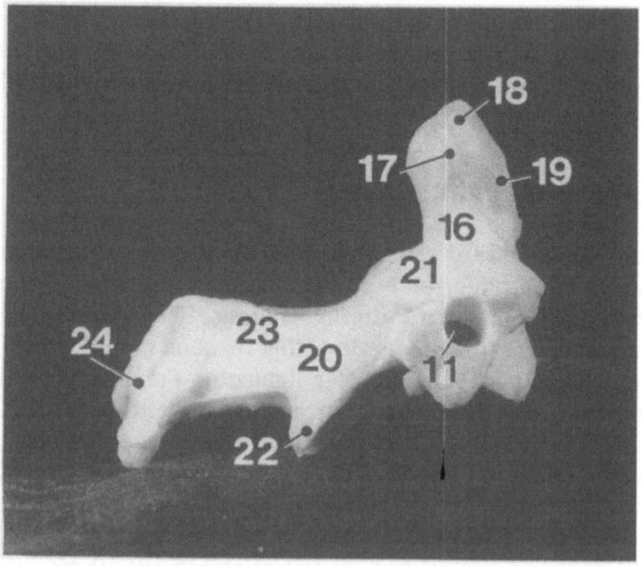

B

Figure 12.4. Oblique (**A**), lateral (**B**), and anterior (**C**) views of the axis or second cervical vertebra: (16) odontoid process (base), (17) attachment of alar ligament, (18) apex of dens, (19) articular surface of dens, (20) pars interarticularis, (21) superior articular facet surface, (22) inferior articular facet, (23) lamina, (24) spinous process, and (25) vertebral body.

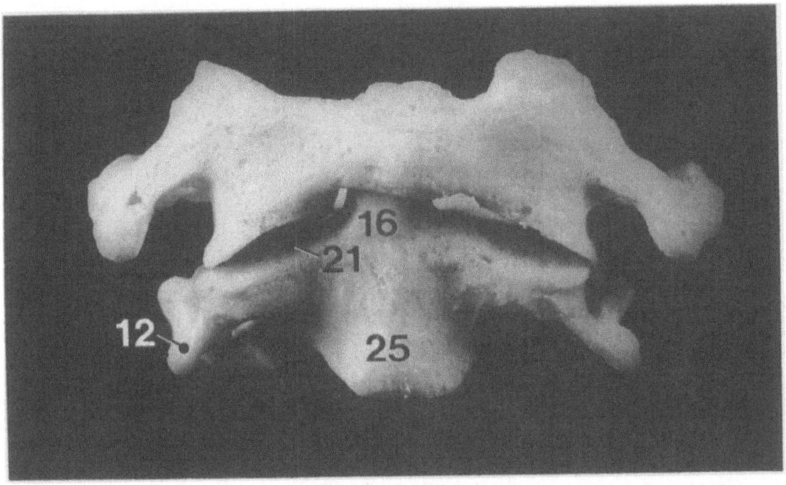

C

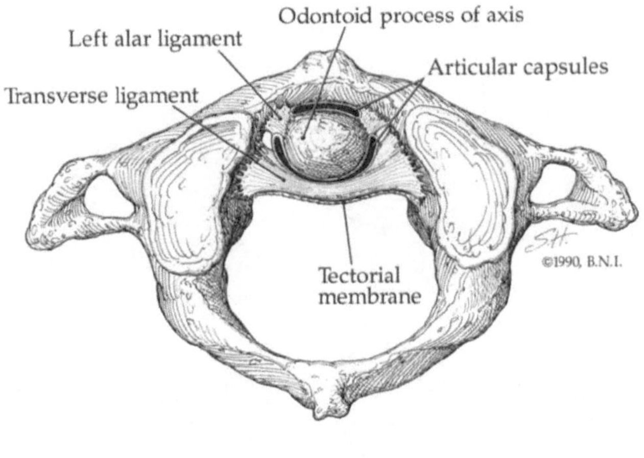

Figure 12.5. Superior view of transverse atlantal ligament. (Reprinted with permission of Barrow Neurologic Institute.)

ligamentum flavum; the anterior and posterior longitudinal ligaments; the tectorial membrane; and the anterior and posterior atlanto-occipital membranes. These ligaments provide a secondary support as they are weaker than the transverse and alar ligaments (15,19). Once the primary ligaments (transverse and alar) are disrupted, the secondary ligaments are susceptible to injury and stretch with relative ease (12,17,19,20).

The secondary ligaments reinforce the primary ligaments and also have

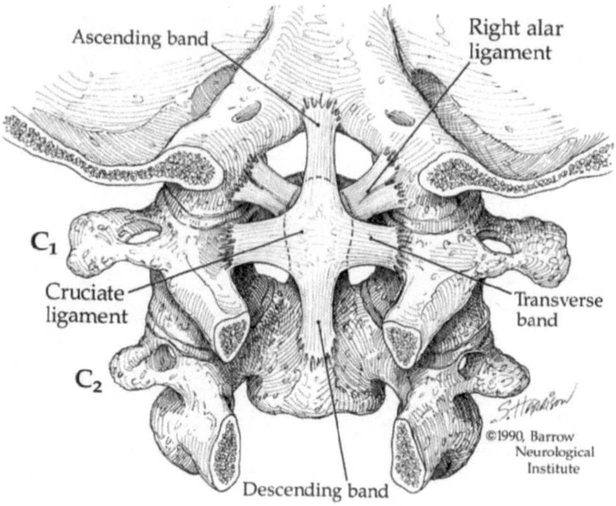

Figure 12.6. Dorsal view of the alar and transverse ligaments. (Reprinted with permission of Barrow Neurologic Institute.)

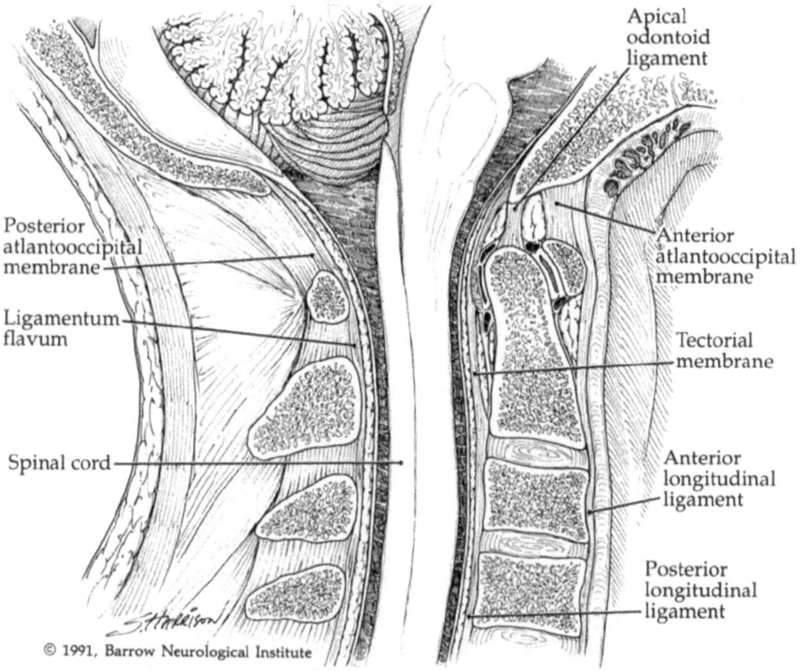

Figure 12.7. Lateral view of the secondary ligaments of the craniovertebral junction. (Reprinted with permission of Barrow Neurologic Institute.)

specific functional capabilities (46,60). The anterior longitudinal ligament and its upper continuation, the anterior atlanto-occipital ligament, prevent hyperextension. The apical ligament connects the dens to the anterior lip of the foramen magnum and also prevents hyperextension. In comparison, the posterior longitudinal ligament and its rostral continuation, the tectorial membrane, prevent hyperflexion of the cervical spine. The capsular ligaments connect the facets together and limit distraction, rotation, and hyperflexion. The interspinous and supraspinous ligaments, the ligamentum flavum, and the posterior atlanto-occipital ligament limit hyperflexion.

Biomechanics and Kinematics

The occipitoatlantoaxial complex is unique in that it serves as a transition zone from the immobile skull base to the mobile cervical spine. It is the most complicated series of articulations in the human being (12,60). Due to the lack of discs within the occiput–C1-C2 complex, the normal motions and stabilizing features depend upon the arrangements of the bones and ligaments (12,17,60). The range and types of movements within the occiput–C1-C2 complex have been well delineated (Table 12.1) (60). The skull base is relatively immobile in its relation to the atlas; in contrast, C1 is extremely mobile at the atlantoaxial articulation. The skull base and C1 tend to move as a unit in relation to C2 (17,34,42,46,60).

The unique osseous and ligamentous interrelationships of this region provide the basis for extensive functional flexibility: flexion, extension, and rotation are all prominent motions. The broadest range of motion within the cervical spinal occurs with rotation at the atlantoaxial articulations (34,42). This motion accounts for half of all of the rotation of the entire cervical spine (34,42). In contrast, minimal rotation occurs between the occiput and C1 (34,42). The atlas also functions to absorb or buffer forces and to integrate and control motion between the occiput and axis.

The transverse atlantal ligament is one of the strongest and thickest ligaments of the spine (15,19). It is inelastic and limits flexion, extension,

Table 12.1. Normal motions of the craniovertebral junction.

Cervical level	Unilateral axial rotation	Combined flexion-extension	Unilateral lateral bending
Occipitoatlantal (occiput–C1)	5°	25°	5°
Atlantoaxial (C1-C2)	40°	20°	5°

Data are from refs. 19, 34, 42, 60.

and horizontal translation of C1 (15). It both limits and facilitates rotation of C1 on C2. In contrast, the alar ligaments are relatively elastic and function to limit rotation by tethering the occipital condyles to the dens. The stability of the entire occipitoatlantoaxial complex depends principally upon the integrity of the transverse and alar ligaments (15,19,20,33,46).

The motions of the individual segments within the occipitoatlantal complex do not occur in isolation; instead, they are coupled. Coupling refers to simultaneous motions that are linked, such as when translation or rotation occurs simultaneously along and about their respective axes, or when movement about one axis is associated with movement about a secondary axis (34,42,60). Multiple types of motion occur in the cervical spine independent of induced motions (34,60). For example, axial rotation usually is coupled with lateral bending, rather than isolated movement of one joint occurring. Together, individual and coupled motions interact to provide three-dimensional movement of the craniovertebral junction.

Surgical Indications and Spinal Instability

Current definitions of instability are based upon clinical, biomechanical, and functional applications (46,54,60). Many useful concepts have emerged for practical application. White and Panjabi have provided a broadly practical definition of spinal instability based upon damage or irritation of the spinal cord or nerve roots, or upon the development of incapacitating deformity or pain due to structural changes (46,60). The radiographic appearance, mechanisms of injury, extent of osseous and ligamentous injury, and neurological status are the most prominent features for assessment of spinal stability.

Although occipitoatlantoaxial region instability can occur suddenly from violent traumatic forces, it can also develop in a slow, progressive fashion as occurs with congenital abnormalities, infections, neoplasms, or rheumatoid arthritis. In certain instances, spinal components may fail along a continuum; anatomic changes can appear long before pathologic motion develops (42).

Neurological dysfunction due to spinal instability is the most urgent indication for arthrodesis. Mechanical compression of neural structures can present with occipital radicular pain, myelopathy, cranial nerve deficits, nystagmus, and bulbar dysfunction. Sudden death has been reported with occiput, C1, and C2 subluxations (13,19,33,45,47,48). Subluxations of the craniovertebral junction may also present with vertebrobasilar insufficiency from vertebral artery compression.

In the absence of neurological deficits, specific pathological and clinical features become crucial to consider in determining the need for internal fixation. Patients who are at high risk for nonunion of fractures (1,3,14,27,28,44), those at risk of developing neurological deficits from compression or progressive subluxations (13,15,16,47), or those with predominantly ligamentous injuries (15,19,21,45,48) may be considered for arthrodesis. However, the decision for internal fixation must be individualized based upon the patient's neurological status, age, and medical condition and upon the extent of subluxations, the type of pathology, and the level(s) of instability.

Operative Approaches

Principles of Selection (18,21,26,36,54)

The effective treatment of upper cervical and craniovertebral instability depends on a thorough knowledge of the normal and pathological anatomical and biomechanical features of each patient. This information is the basis for rationally planning a single operative approach or combination of approaches for neural decompression and internal fixation. Operative strategies are directed at decompressing neural structures, fixating unstable segments, attaining an osseous union, and preserving as much normal cervical mobility as possible (Table 12.2).

Table 12.2. Operative techniques for internal fixation of the occipitoatlantoaxial complex.

Type of fixation	Anterolateral and anterior approaches	Posterior approaches
C1-C2	Transoral arthrodesis Ventral dens screw fixation Ventral atlantoaxial facet screw fixation	Onlay bone grafts Wiring/bone grafts Interspinous Gallie Brooks Halifax clamps Posterior C1-C2 screw fixation Methylmethacrylate fixation
Occipitocervical	Transoral arthrodesis Retropharyngeal arthrodesis	Onlay bone grafts Wiring/bone grafts Steinmann pin fixation/ arthrodesis Ransford loop fixation/ arthrodesis Metal plate and screw fixation Methylmethacrylate fixation
C2-C3	Osteosynthesis with metal plates and screws Ventral interbody fusion (Cloward, Smith-Robinson)	Wiring/bone grafts Interlaminar clamps Hook-plate fixation Plate-screw fixation

Ideally, a single operative approach should be sought to achieve neural decompression and internal fixation. However, a combination of ventral and dorsal surgical strategies are often required. This is a common scenario with instability associated with basilar invagination of the dens. Transoral surgery provides an excellent decompression, but transoral grafts are inadequate for rigid internal fixation; therefore, posterior fixation must also be performed (13,16,55). The operative approaches must be aimed at directly attacking the specific sites of compression *and* instability. In general, anterior operative approaches are best suited for decompression of anterior pathology but usually provide a less desirable means of internal fixation at the craniovertebral junction.

Posterior operative approaches provide a wide exposure of the osseous anatomy of the skull base and cervical spine. Such wide exposure offers more options for arthrodesis and for attaining optimal rigid internal fixation (10,13,16,32,41,50,52–54,59). Posterior decompression of dorsal pathology can be readily achieved; however, decompression of ventrally located pathology usually cannot be obtained by posterior approaches. Additionally, the visceral structures of the anterior neck (e.g., pharynx, larynx, cranial nerves, arteries, veins) are avoided by the posterior approaches.

When staged procedures are required, we suggest performing the decompressive operative procedure first. Instrumenting the vertebral column in the presence of a stenotic canal and neural compromise may create additional neural injury.

The use of the halo brace may be widely applicable for many cases of upper cervical spinal instability. This device is the best available form of rigid external cervical immobilization and carries a low risk to the patient if fitting and care are meticulous (11,35,39). The halo brace provides the optimal external milieu to maintain alignment and to allow healing. The halo brace is necessary for many fractures of the atlas or axis and is often the sole treatment (1,14,27,28). Additionally, we have also used the halo brace as a postoperative adjunct to internal fixation. The halo brace improves the rate of osseous union with wiring and bone graft techniques (13,16,18,36), possibly reflecting the supplemental immobilization of the spine. The halo brace may also be needed as an adjunct to internal fixation in patients with extensive injuries to multiple motion segments (11).

Internal fixation techniques can provide an alternative to halo immobilization when patients cannot tolerate the brace or its use is contraindicated. Among all the operative approaches for internal fixation, one must maintain stringent criteria for surgical selection and success. When surgery is indicated, one must employ methods that have the greatest likelihood of attaining internal fixation and fusion while minimizing the risk to the patient. This point cannot be overemphasized.

The goal of surgical strategies is initially to attain a stable internal fixation and subsequently to develop an osseous union or fusion. *Implants are only temporary measures* (e.g., wiring, instrumentation, plates, and screws) and cannot be depended upon solely for long-term stability because they loosen, fatigue, and may eventually break. Instead, an osseous union should be pursued. A successful arthrodesis ultimately depends on the long-term formation of an osseous union or fusion mass. The formation of a solid fusion mass can be maximized by segmentally decorticating the bone to be fused and covering the fusion site with generous amounts of finely morcellized cancellous bone fragments to supplement the initial internal fixation construct (18,21,36). Facet obliteration, posterior element decortication, thorough soft tissue removal, and precise instrumentation are the most important factors to avoid pseudoarthrodesis (36).

Whenever possible, normal cervical mobility should be preserved—more extensive fixation is not better! Specifically, occipitocervical fusion should be considered only if occipitoatlantal instability exists or if atlantoaxial instability exists where C1 cannot be incorporated into the fusion. Occipitocervical fusion has a higher pseudoarthrodesis rate and restricts additional motion compared to atlantoaxial arthrodesis (13,26,54,61).

Transoral Arthrodesis

The transoral operative approach to the craniovertebral junction and upper cervical spine has been employed since the 1950s for neural decompression or fusion (55). The anterior transoral interbody fusion has not gained widespread popularity. The transoral operative route has been primarily reserved for decompression of the ventral cervicomedullary junction and upper cervical spine. The lower third of the clivus to the C2-C3 interspace can usually be exposed transorally (55). When bone grafts are placed, they are seated into the lower clivus and upper cervical spine in a lock-and-key fashion (Fig. 12.8).

This technique is limited because fusion carries a risk of infection of the nonvascularized bone graft after it is placed through a contaminated field such as the oral cavity. Also, transoral fusion has not provided adequate biomechanical and structural fixation of the atlantoaxial complex and is not accepted as the sole means of fusing the craniovertebral junction. We do not routinely treat instability by transoral fusion. Instead, patients with atlantoaxial instability undergo staged operative procedures when a transoral decompression is indicated. Transoral decompression is performed first and the instability subsequently is treated by a posterior approach. The fusion is supplemented by transoral placement of bone grafts *if* extensive anterior osseous destruction of the craniovertebral junction is present.

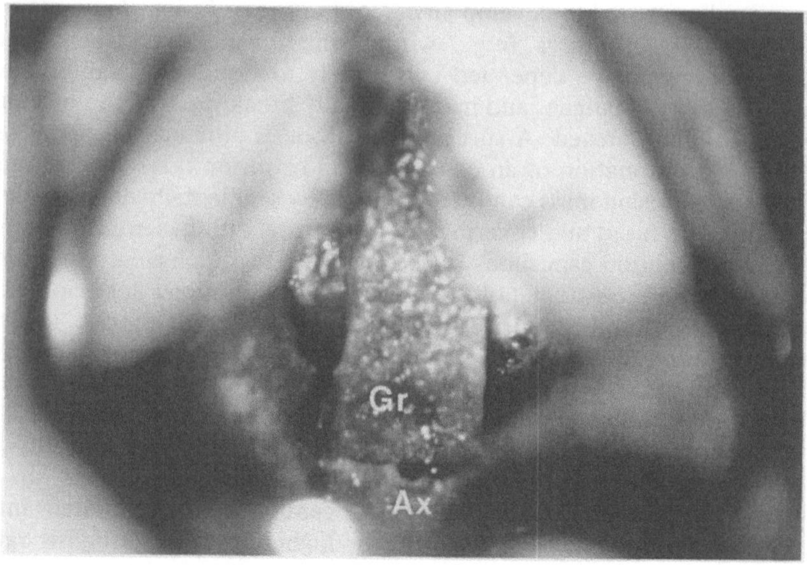

Figure 12.8. Intraoperative view of a transoral exposure with fusion. The bone graft (Gr) is placed in a lock-and-key fashion between the clivus and C2 (Ax).

Wiring and Bone Graft Constructs for Cervical Fusion

In 1910, Mixter and Osgood (44) described the first operative approach to atlantoaxial instability using internal fixation. They successfully treated a 15-year-old boy with a nonunion of an odontoid fracture and chronic C1-C2 subluxation by performing a posterior operative exposure of the atlantoaxial complex and by reducing the odontoid fracture transorally with a finger. The posterior arches of C1 and C2 were fixated with a heavy braided silk suture soaked in tincture of benzoin. Since this first treatment of an atlantoaxial instability, the posterior operative approach has remained the most popular and effective route for treatment of instability of the upper cervical spine; however, the surgical techniques have improved substantially.

The use of onlay bone grafts may be considered when there are no sites for placement of wires. However, onlay bone grafts do not provide a means of immediate internal fixation, and they must be supplemented with rigid external immobilization such as a halo brace. Wire provides only temporary fixation; they fatigue and break. Therefore, the use of wire without bone grafts is also to be avoided, especially in children. As children's bones mature and enlarge, wire will tear through incompletely ossified bone and prohibit osseous union. The optimal means of obtaining

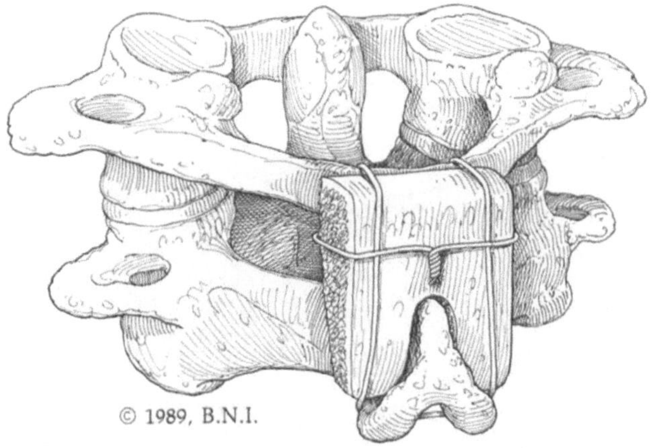

Figure 12.9. Gallie fusion technique. The bone graft is wired behind C1 with an "H" graft. (Reprinted with permission of Barrow Neurologic Institute.)

a successful arthrodesis using the posterior operative approach is with a combination of wiring or instrumentation and bone graft techniques.

Posterior Atlantoaxial Arthrodesis

Gallie (23) popularized posterior atlantoaxial arthrodesis in 1939. He referred to the general principle of obtaining internal fixation and fusion by passing a steel wire around the laminae of C1 and the spinous process of C2 and using bone grafts. This technique has been elaborated further (21,54): a midline posterior operative exposure of the atlantoaxial complex is obtained by dividing the suboccipital and paraspinous muscles in the midline plane with a sagittally oriented incision. The arches of the atlas and axis are exposed using subperiosteal dissection. After the atlantoaxial complex has been exposed, a wire loop is passed under the posterior atlantal arch and beneath the C2 spinous process. A unicortical iliac crest graft is notched into an "H" graft to conform to the spinous process of C2 and then placed posterior to the ring of C1. The wires are fixed behind the posterior arch of C1 and dorsal to the C2 arch securing the graft in position (Fig. 12.9). This fusion is supplemented with cancellous bone. This midline fixation technique is analogous to an onlay-graft technique and may be difficult to employ for posterior subluxations of the arch of C1, as seen with posteriorly displaced odontoid fractures.

The modified Brooks technique or wedge-compression method of atlantoaxial arthrodesis was initially popularized by Brooks and Jenkins (5) in 1978. This technique improved internal fixation of the atlantoaxial complex compared to the midline wiring method of Gallie. The "Brooks

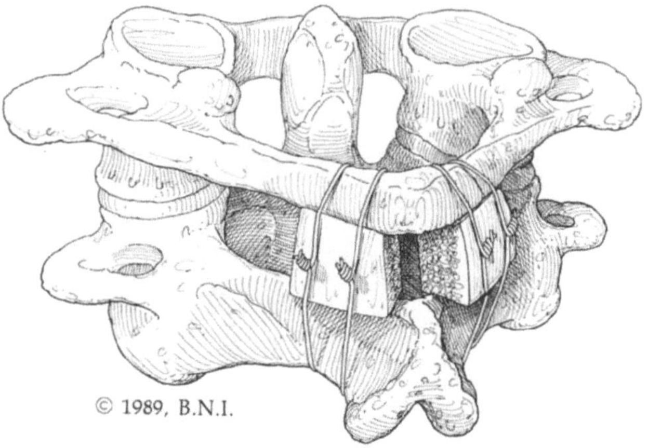

Figure 12.10. Modified Brooks technique. Wedges of iliac crest bone are secured with sublaminar wires at C1 and C2. (Reprinted with permission of Barrow Neurologic Institute.)

method" involves passing four sublaminar wires at C1 *and* C2. Two unicortical iliac crest wedge grafts are beveled to fit into the spaces between the arch of the atlas and the laminae of the axis. The grafts are fixed into the interlaminal space on each side, and the wires are tightened to secure the bone grafts (Fig. 12.10). This construct limits rotation. The sublaminar passage of the four wires creates the potential for neurological injury.

The interspinous method of atlantoaxial arthrodesis (16) is an alternative that employs a bicortical strut graft wedged between the posterior arch of C1 and the spinolaminar junction of C2 (Fig. 12.11). The graft is fixated with wire in a way that provides rotational and translational stability of the atlantoaxial complex and that provides a rigid means of obtaining immediate internal fixation. For this operative technique, the standard posterior exposure of the atlantoaxial complex is performed, and a tricortical bone graft approximately 4 cm long and 1 cm wide is taken from the patient's posterior iliac crest. The rounded cortical side of the graft is removed to create a two-sided bicortical curvilinear strut graft (Fig. 12.12). Additional cortical and cancellous bone is harvested from the iliac crest for onlay bone grafts. The iliac crest strut graft is positioned horizontally between C1 and C2 so that the concave cortical margin lies opposed to the dura and approximates the curve of the posterior ring of C1. A midline notch is fashioned in the inferior cancellous portion of the graft to match the contour of the spinous process of C2.

Once the graft has been shaped and fitted, it is removed to allow placement of wires. A 24-gauge, double-stranded, twisted wire (3 turns/cm) is halved, looped, and passed beneath the ring of C1 in the midline,

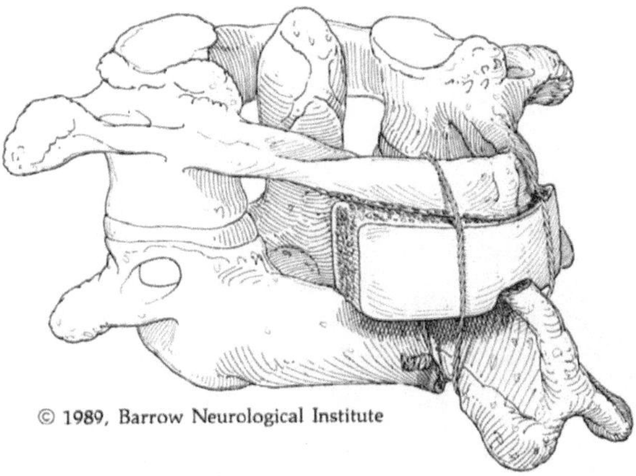

A

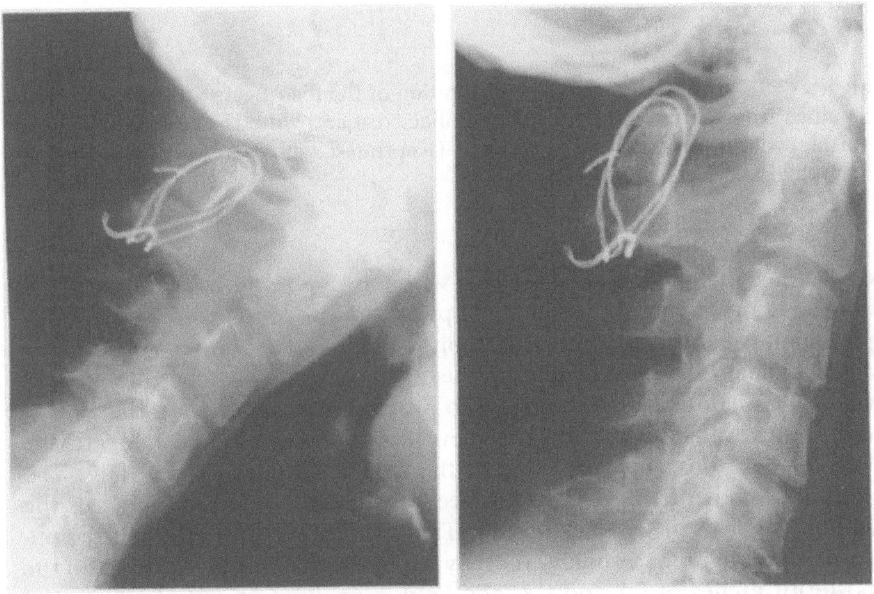

B

Figure 12.11. Interspinous technique. A bicortical iliac strut graft is fixed between C1 and C2 (**A**). Postoperative flexion and extension radiographs (**B**). (Reprinted with permission of Barrow Neurologic Institute.)

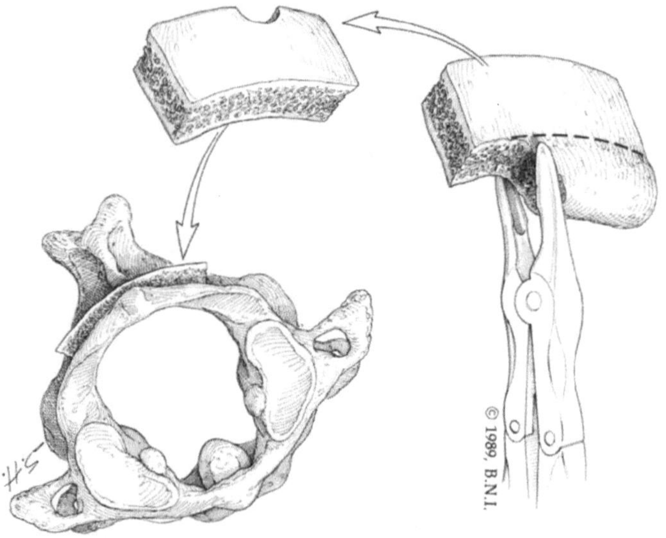

Figure 12.12. Interspinous fusion. Illustration of the bicortical strut graft, which is obtained from the curved portion of the iliac crest and "fitted" to approximate the dorsal contour of the atlas and axis. (Reprinted with permission of Barrow Neurologic Institute.)

directed cephalad (Fig. 12.13). This wire passage requires two hands and involves simultaneously feeding and pulling the wire to avoid anterior displacement of the wire. The wire loop is passed over the C1 ring and secured beneath the base of the spinous process of C2. Notches are created at the spinolaminar junction at C2 to provide slots for fixating the wire at the C2 level. The bone graft is then inserted and trapped beneath the loop of wire dorsally and beneath the free ends of wire ventrally. The ventral strands of free wire are placed around the inferior aspect of the spinous process of C2 and twisted. This maneuver allows the entire construct to be tightened snugly, thereby fixing the graft in place between the posterior arches of C1 and C2, and held in position by wire both ventral and dorsal to the graft (Fig. 12.11). The remaining exposed lamina of C2, posterior ring of C1, and the cortical portion of the graft are segmentally decorticated with a high-speed drill and covered with fragments of finely morcellized cancellous bone to complete the fusion procedure. The wound is closed in a routinely multilayered fashion.

Tensile tests have determined that the double-stranded, twisted, 24-gauge wire (3 turns/cm) provides both strength and malleability (56). This fusion construct provides an ideal means of immediately fixating the atlantoaxial complex. Precise fitting of the bone graft prevents overdis-

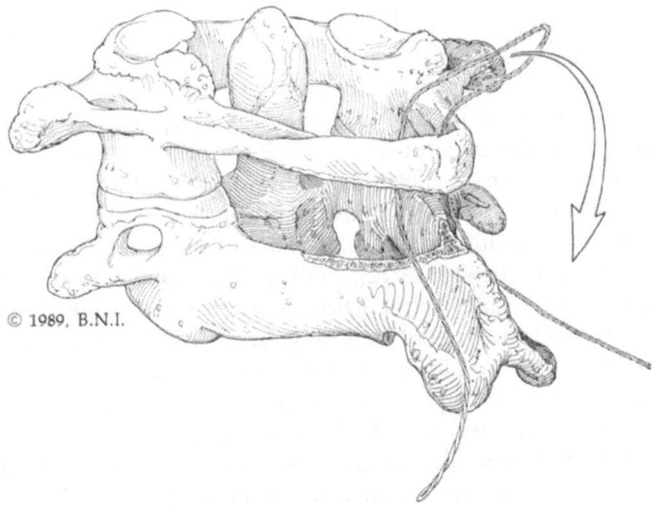

Figure 12.13. Interspinous fusion. The wire is halved and directed cephalad beneath the atlas. The loop of wire is brought dorsal to the bone graft, beneath the C2 spinous process. The free strands of wire are kept ventral to the bone graft and brought beneath the C2 spinous process and twisted together. (Reprinted with permission of Barrow Neurologic Institute.)

traction or overreduction of posteriorly displaced fractures and allows the maintenance of normal anatomical relationships. The technique also provides both translational and rotational stability. Furthermore, the wire passage carries less risk than the Brooks technique by avoiding sublaminar wire passage at C2. A 97% union rate has been obtained with this technique (16).

Occipitocervical Fusion

Occipitocervical fusion can be performed with ribs or iliac crest bone grafts or with metallic struts that are wired into the occipital bone and wired to the lamina or facets of the upper cervical spine (13,26,31,50,54,59,61). The use of metallic implants (to obtain immediate internal fixation), supplemented by bone grafts (to obtain osseous union), provides a preferential alternative for obtaining an extensive arthrodesis of the skull base and upper cervical spine (13). The primary indications for occipitocervical fusion are occipitoatlantal joint instability or atlantoaxial instability in the setting of a deficient posterior atlantal arch. An extensive fusion should be avoided for isolated atlantoaxial instability with an intact arch. Fusion of the occiput also restricts the range of motion of the cervical spine and results in a higher rate of pseudoarthrodesis compared with atlantoaxial arthrodesis.

A posterior operative approach is the most appropriate means of fixating the occipitoatlantal joint. No successful methods are available for anterior fixation of the occiput–C1 level. Posterior occipitocervical fusion can be performed using a large ($\frac{3}{8}$ inch) threaded Steinmann pin contoured in a U shape to fit the craniovertebral junction (13). This threaded pin prevents vertical subluxation and is wired in place by occipital and sublaminar or facet wires (Fig. 12.14) (13). The standard exposure of the atlantoaxial complex and occipital bone is performed using subperiosteal dissection. The rim of the foramen magnum is enlarged with a Kerrison rongeur to facilitate wire passage and to avoid dural injury. Bilateral burr holes are placed 0.5 cm superior to the rim of the foramen magnum for passage of wire. Wires are passed sublaminar at levels to be fused and between the burr hole and the foramen magnum. A U-shaped Steinmann pin is contoured and secured with wire. If an occipital or C1 decompression was performed, the dura can be covered with a unicortical iliac crest graft, which can be wired to the central portion of the construct (Fig. 12.15). The fusion site is segmentally decorticated with a high-speed air drill and covered with finely morcellized cancellous bone. Generous amounts of grafted bone are used to promote an osseous union.

Other technical innovations, such as contoured metal loops that are wired into place and supplemented with cancellous bone grafts, are available for occipitocervical fusions (31,50,54). These techniques are similar to the threaded Steinmann pin; however, they have the potential disadvantage of vertical translation or "settling" of the operative fusion construct. Occipitocervical fusion may also be performed with a metal plate and screw technique (53). Screw fixation of the occipitocervical junction is supplemented with cancellous bone grafts, but this technique has not gained widespread popularity.

Metallic Plate and Screw Systems

Metallic plate and screw systems have become popular for "osteosynthetic plate stabilization" of the upper cervical spine (58). Systems are available for anterior or posterior operative approaches. Contemporary surgical series have been described by Caspar (6–8), Roy-Camille et al. (53), Haid et al. (29), Cooper et al. (10), Papadopoulos et al. (49), and others (22,25,30,57,58).

Figure 12.14. Occipitocervical fusion utilizing a threaded Steinmann pin. Illustration (**A**) and postoperative lateral cervical radiograph (**B**). Reprinted with permission of Barrow Neurologic Institute.)

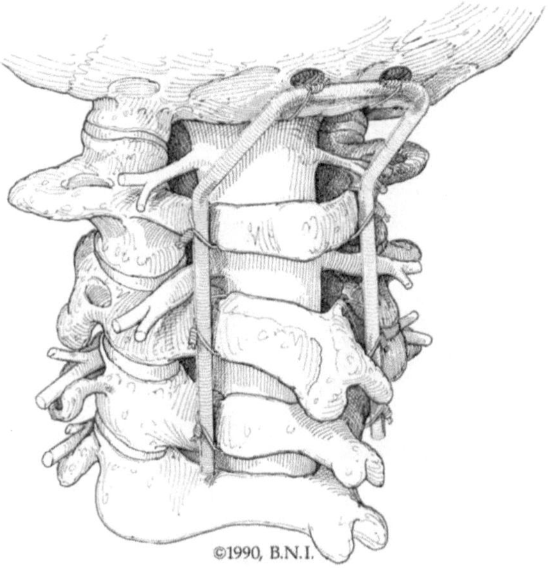

A

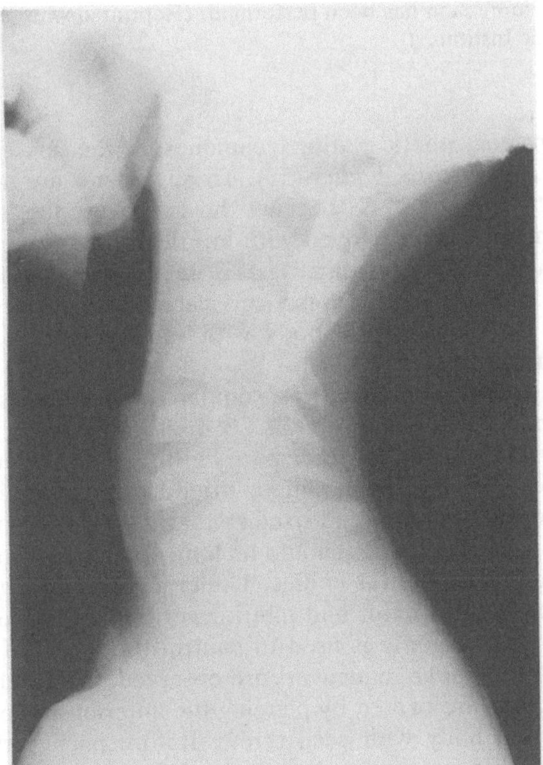

B

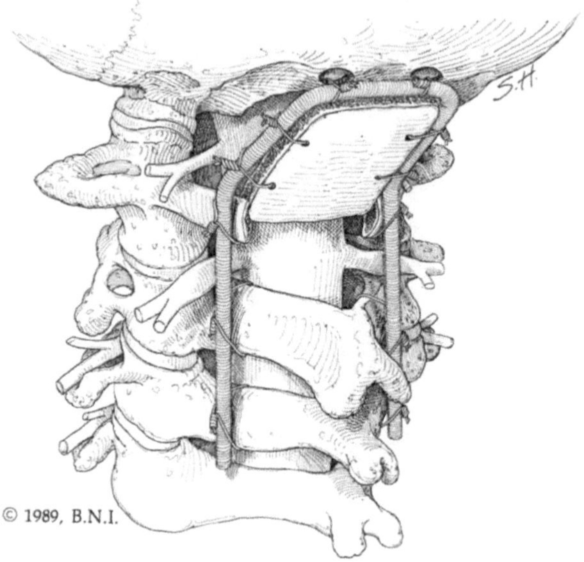

Figure 12.15. Occipitocervical fusion. An iliac crest graft is wired to the bone if a posterior decompression has been performed. (Reprinted with permission of Barrow Neurologic Institute.)

Anterior osteosynthetic plating techniques for the cervical spine are designed to fixate *vertebral bodies* (58). These systems are not designed for application to the arch of C1 because the screws are too large. However, these systems may be employed with injuries of C2 (i.e., C2 and C3 instability) when the anterior approach is needed for operative fixation as in complex fractures of the upper cervical spine involving anterior subluxation of the C2 vertebral body with spondylolysis, i.e., irreducible hangman's fractures (Fig. 12.16).

Operative access is obtained by a standard anterior transcervical operative approach (9). An anterior C2-C3 discectomy is performed, and a bone graft is placed into the interspace by the Smith-Robinson technique (7). A cervical osteosynthetic plate is fitted along the anterior portion of the C2-C3 vertebral bodies and sized so that it does not extend across the C3-C4 disc space. The plates should be long enough to allow screw placement into the midvertebral bodies. Under fluoroscopic guidance, holes are drilled into the superior and inferior vertebrae to accommodate fixation screws. A drill guide is used to control the depth of the advancing drill, and intraoperative maneuvers are observed under fluoroscopic guidance. The screws are fixated by piercing the anterior and posterior cortex of the vertebral body with each screw. Before placing the screws, the depth of the hole is measured, and the hole is tapped with a tapping screw of the appropriate length. The fixation screw is tightened into place, engaging both anterior and posterior vertebral cortices and securing the osteosynthetic plate into position. Fixation screws may also be placed into the graft to further secure the graft into position. The anterior osteosynthetic plating technique for internal fixation of the upper cervical spine has been a useful alternative when instability cannot be fixated by a posterior operative approach (e.g., posterior fractures of the atlantoaxial complex). This technique can be used for anterior fixation of C2 to C7 segments; however, it cannot be used to fixate C1. Access to upper cervical levels with a transcervical route can be difficult.

Posterolateral osteosynthetic plating of the cervical spine has been pioneered by Roy-Camille (53), Cooper (10), and Haid (29). Like the osteosynthetic plating systems for anterior fixation, these methods are not

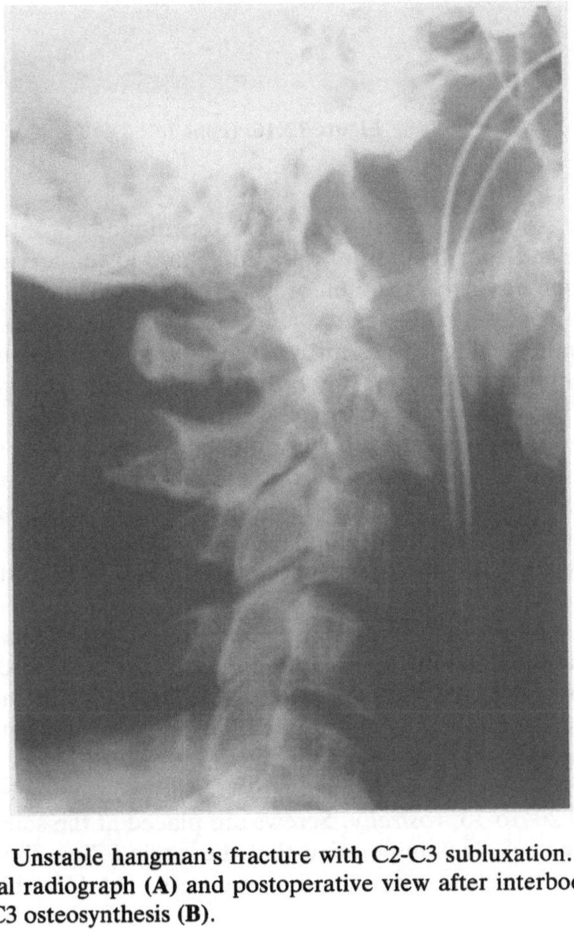

A

Figure 12.16. Unstable hangman's fracture with C2-C3 subluxation. Preoperative lateral cervical radiograph **(A)** and postoperative view after interbody fusion and anterior C2-C3 osteosynthesis **(B)**.

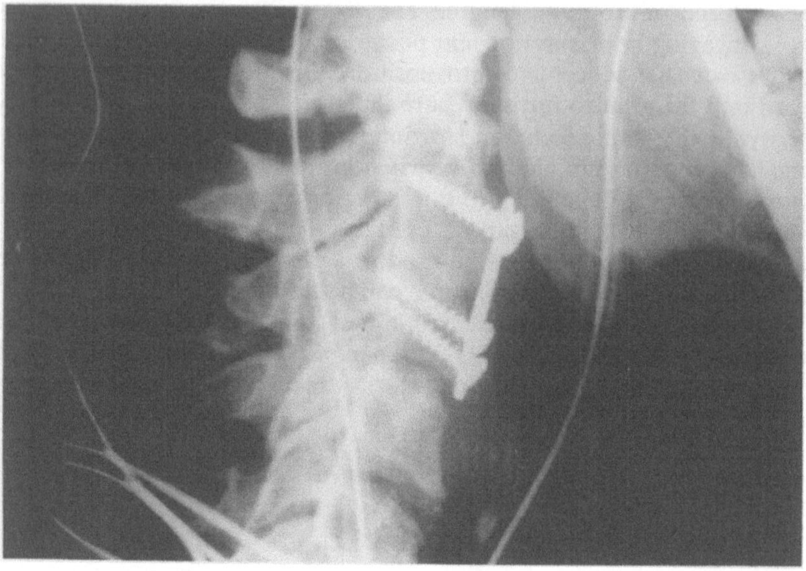

B

Figure 12.16. (*cont.*)

designed for fixation of C1 to C2. These techniques are intended for C2 and C3 fixation or for fixation of the middle and lower cervical segments. The technique involves fixation of the pedicle or lateral masses with osteosynthetic plates and screws (Fig. 12.17). The development of a curved titanium plate has improved the bone-to-plate interface that allows assumption of a normal cervical curvature with compression of the facet joint. The result is an improved anatomical fusion (29).

A standard midline posterior incision is performed with a subperiosteal dissection to the extreme edges of the lateral masses to be instrumented. Subluxations are reduced, and the synovial facet joints are curetted. Loose connective tissues are removed from the facets with curettes and rongeurs. Wedges of autologous cancellous bone are placed in the facet joints for fusion.

The center of the lateral mass is identified using the facet landmarks (the lateral and medial facet margins and the rostral and caudal aspects of the facets of the joint). Screw placement is begun 1 mm medial to the center of the lateral mass. An awl or drill tap is used to lightly pierce the cortical bone and to mark the drill starting point to insure a good drill purchase (Fig. 12.18). For C3 through C7 the drill is angled 20° to 30° *laterally* and 20° to 30° *rostrally*. Screws are placed at the same angles into the lateral masses. It is imperative that the angle follow these guidelines to avoid the vertebral artery and nerve root. At C2, the screws are

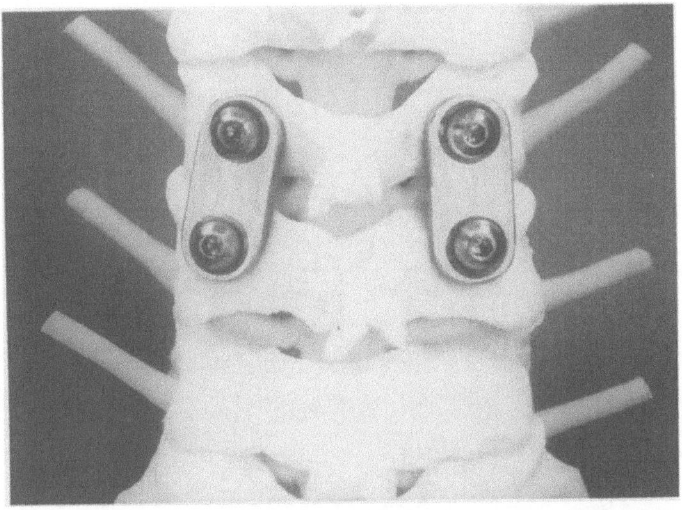

Figure 12.17. Posterolateral osteosynthetic plating in a spine model at C3 and C4.

directed into the *pedicle* by angling 20° to 30° *rostrally* and 20° to 30° *medially*. This distinction for C2 screw placement is of paramount importance. A preoperative axial CT scan is needed to determine if any anomalous features of the vertebral artery or vertebrae exist.

Subluxations are reduced, the lateral mass plates are fitted, and the drill holes are placed. The surgeon is able to "feel" the drill penetrating the bone cortex. The drill has a depth of 11 mm. Bicortical penetration is necessary to provide adequate screw fixation. The plates are placed over the drill holes. The screws are then placed in the same angle as the drilling and tightened sequentially. Self-tapping screws are used and should be "finger tight" (i.e., use two fingers for fixation). The screws should not be overtightened.

Like anterior systems, the posterior systems have a broad application to injuries of C2 through C7. Multiple-holed plates are available for instability of multiple motion segments. This type of posterior plate fixation can be considered for isolated unilateral facet injury, bilateral facet injuries, or isolated posterior element injury (such as lamina and spinous process fractures) with associated ligament instability (10,29,51–53).

Screw plate systems are also available for posterior internal fixation of the occipitocervical junction (Fig. 12.19) (51,52). Screws are placed in a similar fashion into the occipital bone and the cervical levels to be fixated. A hook plate system is also available for posterior stabilization of the cervical laminae and facets (Fig. 12.20) (41). Screws are placed into the

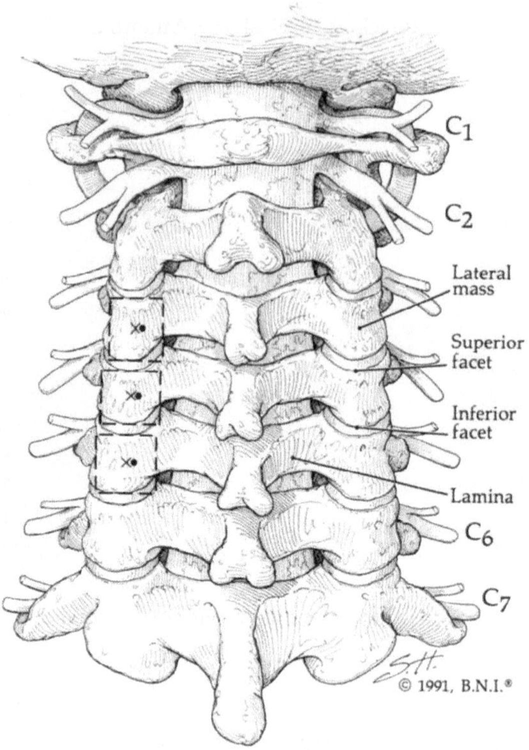
C1
C2
Lateral mass
Superior facet
Inferior facet
Lamina
C6
C7
© 1991, B.N.I.®

A

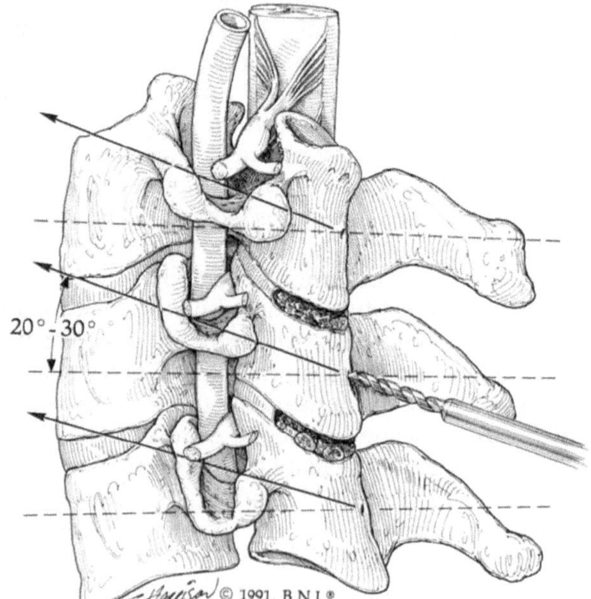
20° - 30°
© 1991, B.N.I.®

B

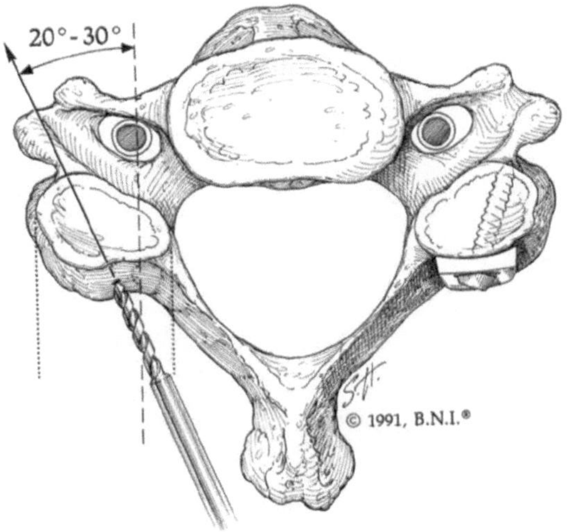

C

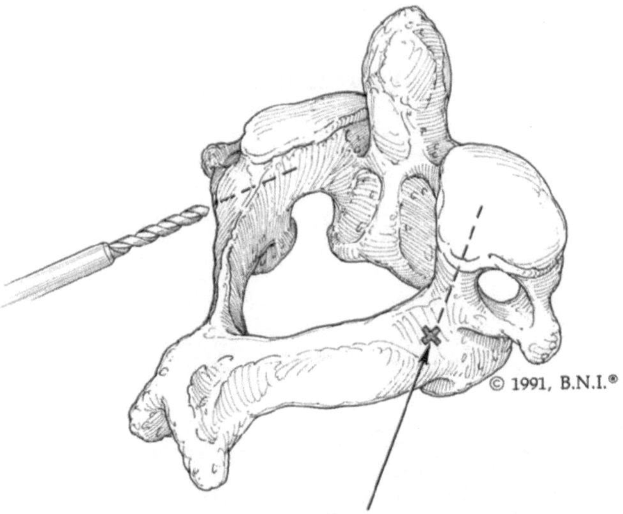

D

Figure 12.18. Posterolateral plating. Drill angles for C3 through C7 into the lateral masses, 20° to 30° rostral and 20° to 30° lateral (**A, B, C**) and for the C2 pedicle, 20° to 30° rostral and 20° to 30° medial (**D, E**). (Reprinted with permission of Barrow Neurologic Institute.)

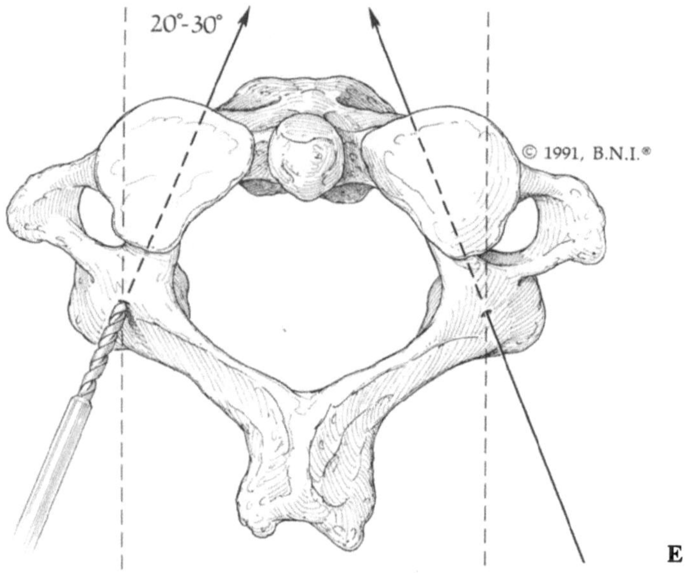

Figure 12.18. (*cont.*)

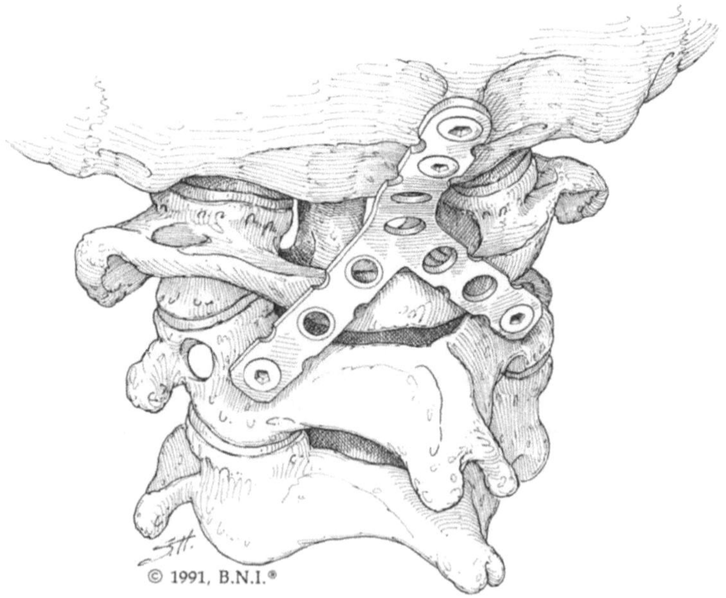

Figure 12.19. Occipitocervical screw-plate systems. (Reprinted with permission of Barrow Neurologic Institute.)

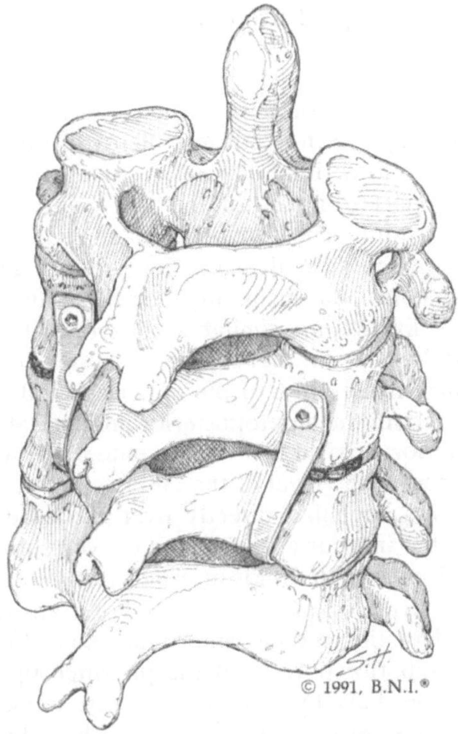

Figure 12.20. Hook plate system for posterior cervical fixation. (Reprinted with permission of Barrow Neurologic Institute.)

lateral masses, and the hooks are fixated under the lamina of the inferior level. This system requires an intact lamina for successful fixation.

These anterior and posterior osteosynthetic techniques using metallic plate and screw systems should be supplemented with grafted bone whenever possible to obtain an osseous union (36,58). The screws must be placed so that *bicortical* screw fixation is obtained, or the screws will loosen. If intraoperative loosening or stripping of a screw hole occurs, the hole can be filled with methylmethacrylate or cancellous bone to obtain an improved screw purchase. "Rescue screws," which have a larger bore than the regular screws, are available to obtain an improved purchase. The osteosynthetic plate systems are *not suited for soft or osteoporotic bone* (i.e., rheumatoid disease) (58). In all cases, the screws should be finger tight. Overtightening will strip the screw and result in a poor purchase, with a potential loss of internal fixation.

Odontoid Screw Fixation and Atlantoaxial Facet Screw Fixation (2,4,24,38,40)

These techniques provide alternatives to the posterior stabilization procedures if the posterior approach is not feasible or if a persistent posterior pseudoarthrodesis develops. In the presence of C1-C2 instability with a defective or absent posterior ring of the atlas, anterior screw fixation techniques can be useful. These techniques may be preferable to an occipitocervical fusion because they do not produce loss of motion of the occipitoatlantal joint. The techniques for the anterior transodontoid and transfacet screw fixation are similar in their operative approach. The procedures are performed in the supine position, under fluoroscopic guidance, to provide visualization of the upper cervical spine and craniovertebral junction in both the anteroposterior and lateral planes.

A transverse anterior cervical incision is made at the C5 level, and the dissection is deepened to the level of the anterior cervical vertebrae. The dissection is extended cephalad directly over the anterior longitudinal ligament to expose the inferior aspect of the C2 vertebrae. Under fluoroscopic guidance, a 2-mm width drill is inserted, parallel to the body of C2, beginning at the anterior inferior C2 body. For transodontoid fixation, the drill is directed in the midline and at an angle that will allow for penetration of the superior portion of the proximal tip of the odontoid process. Once the holes have been drilled, they are tapped with a 3.5-mm tap or K-wires. Two screws are inserted into the odontoid process to obtain rotational control (Fig. 12.21). Odontoid screw fixation can be used for odontoid fractures with atlantoaxial subluxations only if the transverse ligament is intact (15). The ligament is best assessed with MR imaging (Fig. 12.22). If the transverse ligament is disrupted, fixating the odontoid will not fixate C1. Rotation at C1 and C2 is preserved with this technique.

The C1-C2 transfacet screw fixation technique is essentially the same as odontoid screw fixation except the screws are directed laterally through the C2 body into the lateral masses of C1. The insertion of the drill begins at the anterior inferior aspect of the C2 vertebral body. The angle is adjusted in a superolateral direction that allows for passage of the drill through the lateral mass of C2, across the C1-C2 joint space (Fig. 12.23). Single 4.0-mm cancellous screws are passed under fluoroscopic guidance through each lateral C1-C2 joint space into the lateral mass of C1. The facet joints are decorticated with a curet before placement of the screws to enhance fusion. This technique stabilizes C1 and C2 but sacrifices rotation.

These techniques do not represent procedures of choice for atlantoaxial internal fixation; however, they do provide viable alternatives if posterior fixation cannot be performed. These anterior screw fixation techniques

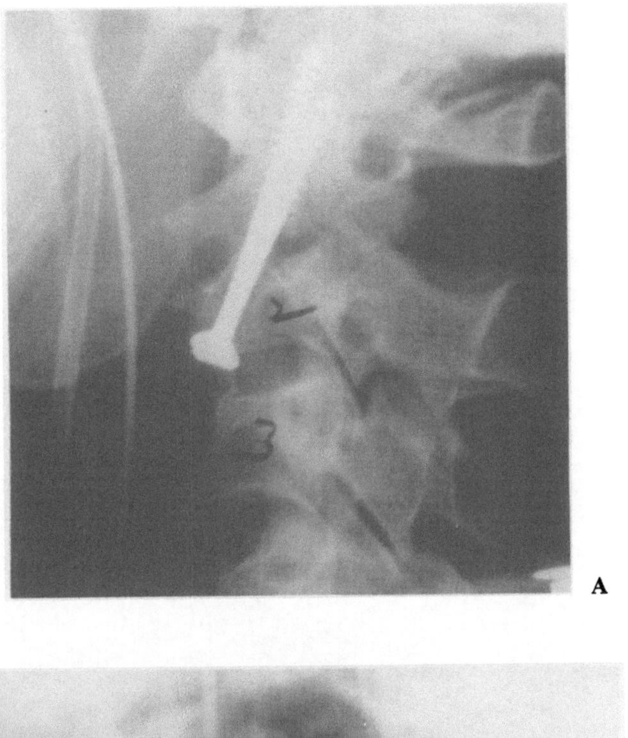

Figure 12.21. Odontoid screw fixation. Two screws are directed into the odontoid to obtain secure fixation. Lateral (**A**) and anteroposterior (**B**) radiographs.

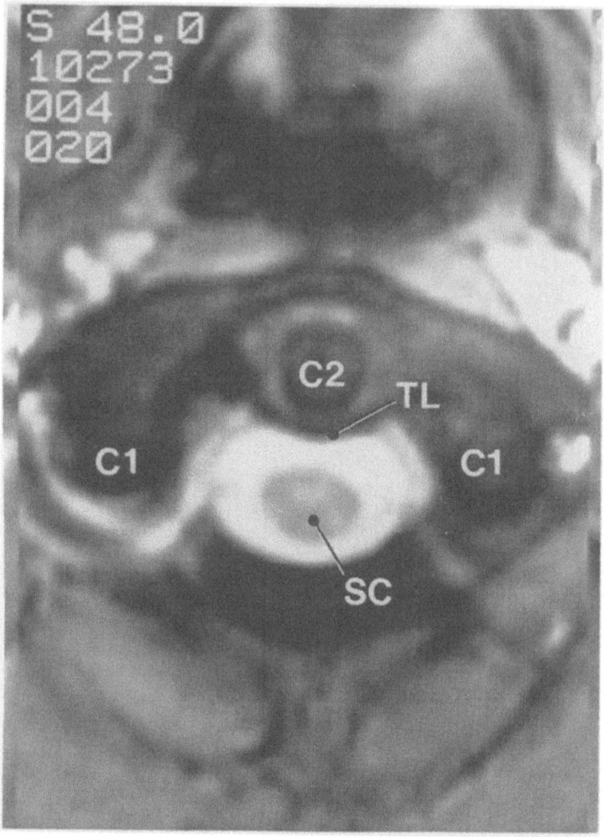

Figure 12.22. Axial-plane magnetic resonance imaging study at the C1 level. (TR: 800 msec, TE: 14, flip angle 20°). The transverse ligament (TL) appears as a band of homogeneous low signal intensity extending between the lateral masses of the atlas (C1) behind the odontoid (C2). The odontoid is surrounded by a circular rim of high signal intensity, which is the synovial space. SC, spinal cord.

are suited for patients with thin body habitus. The screw fixation techniques require a rather horizontal angle for correct placement of the screws. Barrel chests or short necks hinder operative access. Both the transodontoid and transfacet screw fixation techniques are limited by the inability to add bone grafts to enhance the fusion. Curets must therefore be used to decorticate the bone to promote fusion.

Figure 12.23. Transfacet atlantoaxial screw fixation. Single screws are directed anteriorly across the C1-2 facet joints. Lateral (**A**) and anteroposterior (**B**) radiographs.

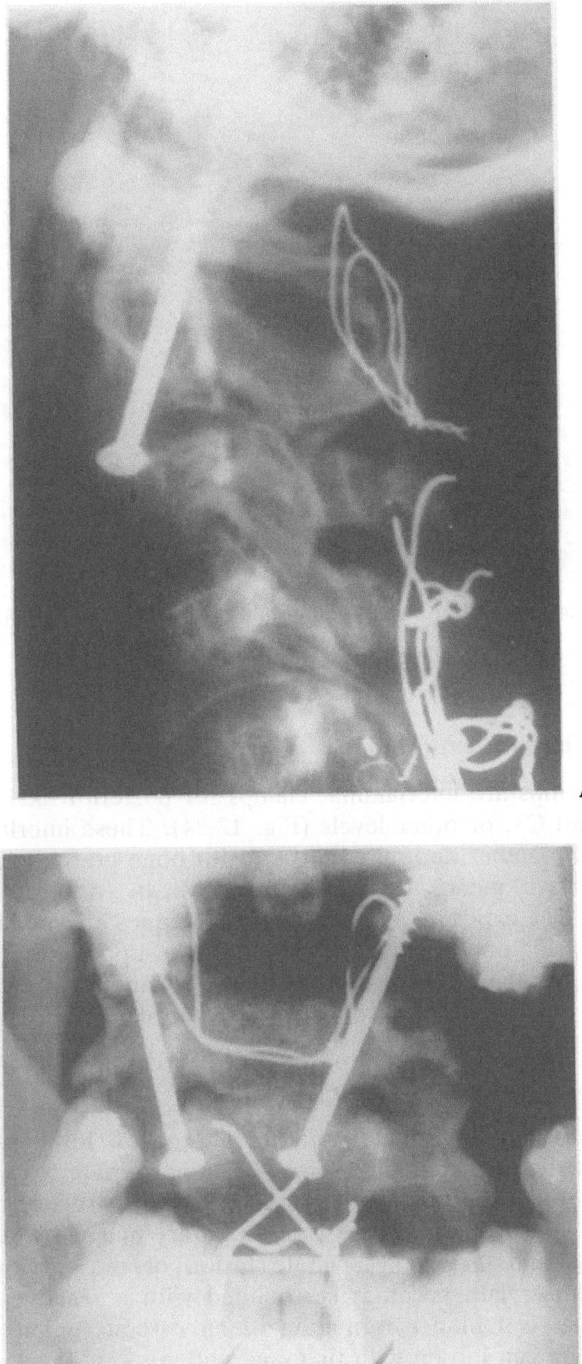

A

B

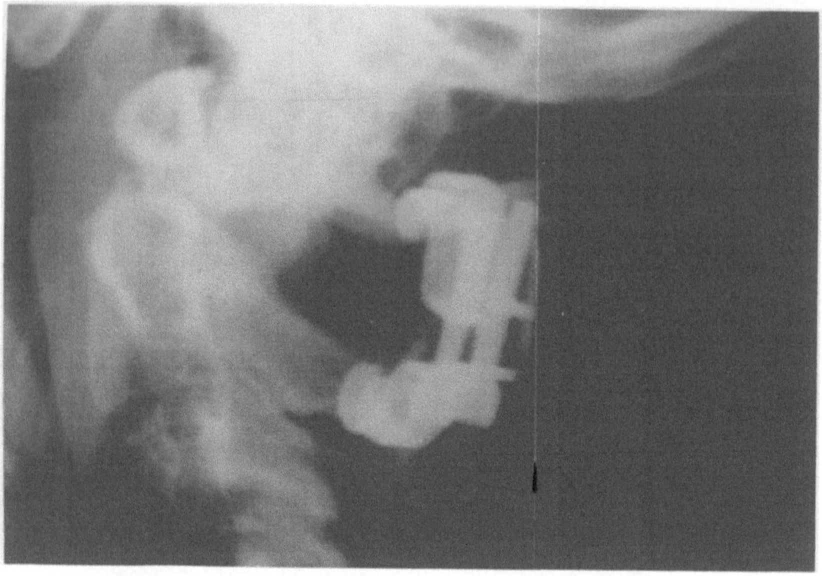

Figure 12.24. Lateral cervical radiograph of an interlaminar clamp fixation of C1-2.

Halifax Clamp Fixation (32)

Halifax clamps are interlaminar clamps for posterior fixation of C1 and C2, C2 and C3, or other levels (Fig. 12.24). These interlaminar clamps are bolted together and may be used with bone graft wedges to provide an alternative means of internal fixation by a posterior operative approach. The exposure and operative techniques are similar to the exposure for wiring and bone graft fixation of the upper cervical spine. This technique has the advantage of avoiding sublaminar wire passage, but it cannot be employed if the laminae are fractured.

Methylmethacrylate Fixation (37,43)

Methylmethacrylate provides another alternative for posterior internal fixation of the upper cervical spine. It is appropriate for patients with a decreased life expectancy or extensive bone destruction from tumoral processes. Methylmethacrylate is a temporary means of fixating the cervical spine and *does not* facilitate fusion of the cervical spine (43). Methylmethacrylate becomes surrounded with a reactive fibrous tissue capsule that can hinder formation of an osseous union (43). Methylmethacrylate can loosen with time and patients can develop a loss of internal fixation (43). Methylmethacrylate is not recommended for instability secondary to trauma, degenerative disease, or rheumatoid arthritis. These conditions have excellent outcomes when treated with conventional bone grafts. Methylmethacrylate should only be used as a salvage technique for spinal fixation in patients with a limited life expectancy (43).

If methylmethacrylate is needed, it should be supplemented with autogenous bone grafts and internally fixated with wire. If a wound infection develops, methylmethacrylate must be debrided and completely removed. Patients with methylmethacrylate augumentation of spine fusion must receive antibiotics during dental procedures or any procedures that could result in bacteremia.

Summary

A spectrum of new techniques and operative adjuncts has become available for internal fixation of the upper cervical spine. This expanding surgical armamentarium offers successful fusion, preserves normal motion, and protects neurological function.

References

1. Anderson LD, D'Alonzo RT. Fractures of the odontoid process of the axis. *J Bone Joint Surg*. 1974;56A:1663–1674.
2. Barbour JR. Screw fixation and fractures of the odontoid process. *South Austral Clin*. 1971;5:20–24.
3. Böhler J. Anterior stabilization for acute fractures in non-unions of the dens. *J Bone Joint Surg*. 1982;64A:18–27.
4. Borne GM, Bedou GL, Pinaudeau M, et al. Odontoid process fracture osteosynthesis with a direct screw fixation technique in nine consecutive cases. *J Neurosurg*. 1988;68:223–226.
5. Brooks AL, Jenkins EB. Atlanto-axial arthrodesis by the wedge compression method. *J Bone Joint Surg*. 1978;60A:279–284.
6. Caspar W. *Anterior Cervical Fusion and Interbody Stabilization with the Trapezial Osteosynthetic Plate Techniqe*. Tuttlingen, West Germany: Aesculap Wissenschaftl. Informationen, Aesculap-Werke AG: D-7200, 1986.
7. Caspar W. Anterior stabilization with trapezial osteosynthetic plate technique in cervical spine injuries. In: Kehr P, Weidner A, eds. *Cervical Spine*. New York: Springer-Verlag; 1987:198–204.
8. Caspar W, Barbier DD, Klara PM. Anterior cervical fusion and Caspar plate stabilization for cervical trauma. *Neurosurgery*. 1989;25(4):491–502.
9. Cloward RB. The anterior approach for removal of ruptured cervical disks. *J Neurosurg*. 1958;15:602–617.
10. Cooper PR, Cohen A, Rosiello A, et al. Posterior stabilization of cervical spine fractures and subluxations using plates and screws. *Neurosurgery*. 1988;23:300–306.
11. Cooper PR, Maravilla KR, Sklar FH, et al. Halo immobilization of cervical spine fractures. Indications and results. *J Neurosurg*. 1979;50:603–610.

12. de Oliveira E, Rhoton AL Jr, Peace D. Microsurgical anatomy of the region of the foramen magnum. *Surg Neurol.* 1985;24:293–352.
13. Dickman CA, Douglas RA, Sonntag VKH. Occipitocervical fusion: Posterior stabilization of the craniovertebral junction and upper cervical spine. *BNI Quarterly*. 1990;6(2):2–14.
14. Dickman CA, Hadley MN, Browner C, et al. Neurosurgical management of acute atlas-axis combination fractures: A review of 25 cases. *J Neurosurg.* 1989;70:45–49.
15. Dickman CA, Mamourian A, Sonntag VKH, et al. Magnetic resonance imaging of the transverse atlantal ligament for the evaluation of atlantoaxial instability. *J Neurosurg*. 1991;75:221–227.
16. Dickman CA, Papadopoulos SM, Sonntag VKH, et al. The interspinous method of posterior atlantoaxial arthrodesis. *J Neurosurg*. 1991;74:190–198.
17. Dvorak J, Schneider E, Saldinger P, et al. Biomechanics of the craniocervical region: The alar and transverse ligaments. *J Orthop Res*. 1988;6:452–461.
18. Fielding JW. The status of arthrodesis of the cervical spine. *J Bone Joint Surg*. 1988;70A:1571–1574.
19. Fielding JW, Cochran GVB, Lawsing JF III, et al. Tears of the transverse ligament of the atlas. A clinical and biomechanical study. *J Bone Joint Surg*. 1974;56A:1683–1691.
20. Fielding JW, Hawkins RJ. Atlanto-axial rotatory fixation. Fixed rotatory subluxation of the atlanto-axial joint. *J Bone Joint Surg*. 1977;59A:37–44.
21. Fielding JW, Hawkins RJ, Ratzan SA. Spine fusion for atlanto-axial instability. *J Bone Joint Surg*. 1976;58A:400–407.
22. Fuentes JM, Benezech J. *Les Osteosyntheses Rachidiennes en Neurochirurgie*. Montpellier, France: Centre de Neurochirurgie: Clinique Rech; 1989.
23. Gallie WE. Fractures and dislocations of the cervical spine. *Am J Surg*. 1939;46:495–499.
24. Geisler FH, Cheng C, Poka A, et al. Anterior screw fixation of posteriorly displaced type II odontoid fractures. *Neurosurgery*. 1989;25:30–38.
25. Goffin J, Plets C, Van den Bergh R. Anterior cervical fusion and osteosynthetic stabilization according to Caspar: A prospective study of 41 patients with fractures and/or dislocations of the cervical spine. *Neurosurgery*. 1989;25(6):865–871.
26. Grantham SA, Dick HM, Thompson RC Jr, et al. Occipitocervical arthrodesis. Indications, technic and results. *Clin Orthop*. 1969;65:118–129.
27. Hadley MN, Dickman CA, Browner CM, et al. Acute traumatic atlas fractures: Management and long term outcome. *Neurosurgery*. 1988;23(1):31–35.
28. Hadley MN, Dickman CA, Browner CM, et al. Acute axis fractures. A review of 229 cases. *J Neurosurg*. 1989;71:642–647.
29. Haid RW, Papadopoulos SM, Sonntag VKH. *Lateral Mass Plating for Cervical Instability (Instability)*. American Association of Neurological Surgeons. 1991;706:112.
30. Herrmann HD. Metal plate fixation after anterior fusion of unstable fracture dislocations of the cervical spine. *Acta Neurochir*. 1975;32:101–112.
31. Heywood AWB, Learmonth ID, Thomas M. Internal fixation for occipitocervical fusion. *J Bone Joint Surg*. 1988;70B:708–711.
32. Holness RO, Huestis WS, Howes WJ, et al. Posterior stabilization with an in-

terlaminar clamp in cervical injuries: Technical note and review of the long term experience with the method. *Neurosurgery*. 1984;14:318–322.
33. Jefferson G. Fracture of the atlas vertebra. Report of four cases, and a review of those previously recorded. *Br J Surg*. 1920;7:407–422.
34. Jofe MH, White AA, Panjabi MM. Clinically relevant kinematics of the cervical spine. In: Cervical Spine Research Society, ed. *The Cervical Spine*. 2nd ed. Philadelphia: JB Lippincott; 1989:57–69.
35. Johnson RM, Hart DL, Simmons EF, et al. Cervical orthoses. A study comparing their effectiveness in restricting cervical motion in normal subjects. *J Bone Joint Surg*. 1977;59A:332–339.
36. Kaufman HH, Jones E. The principles of bony spinal fusion. *Neurosurgery*. 1989;24:264–270.
37. Kelly DL Jr, Alexander E Jr, David CH Jr, et al. Acrylic fixation of atlantoaxial dislocations. Technical note. *J Neurosurg*. 1972;36:366–367.
38. Knoringer P. Double-threaded compression screws in osteosynthesis of acute fractures of the odontoid process. In: Voth D, Glees O, eds. *Disease in the Cranio-Cervical Junction*. Berlin-New York: de Gruyter; 1987:217.
39. Koch RA, Nickel VL. The halo vest. An evaluation of motion and forces across the neck. *Spine*. 1978;3:103–107.
40. Lesoin F, Autricque A, Franz K, et al. Transcervical approach and screw fixation for upper cervical spine pathology. *Surg Neurol*. 1987;27:459–465.
41. Magerl F, Grob D, Seemann P. Stable dorsal fusion of the cervical spine (C2-Th1) using hook plates. In: Kehr P, Weidner A, eds. *Cervical Spine I*. Wien-New York: Springer-Verlag; 1987:217.
42. Maiman DJ, Yoganandan N. Biomechanics of cervical spine trauma. *Clin Neurosurg*. 1991;37:543–570.
43. McAfee PC, Bohlman HH, Eismont FJ. Failure of methylmethacrylate stabilization of the spine: A retrospective analysis of 24 cases. In: Cervical Spine Research Society, ed. *The Cervical Spine*. 2nd ed. Philadelphia: JB Lippincott; 1989:838–849.
44. Mixter SJ, Osgood RB. Traumatic lesions of the atlas and axis. *Ann Surg*. 1910;51:193–207.
45. Pang D, Wilberger JE Jr. Traumatic atlanto-occipital dislocation with survival: Case report and review. *Neurosurgery*. 1980;7(5):503–508.
46. Panjabi MM, Thibodeau LL, Crisco JJ III, et al. What constitutes spinal instability? *Clin Orthop*. 1988;34:313–339.
47. Papadopoulos SM, Dickman CA, Sonntag VKH. Atlantoaxial stabilization in rheumatoid arthritis. *J Neurosurg*. 1991;74:1–7.
48. Papadopoulos SM, Dickman CA, Sonntag VKH, et al. Traumatic atlantooccipital dislocation with survival. *Neurosurgery*. 1991;28(4):574–579.
49. Papadopoulos SM, Sonntag VKH, Kalfas IH. *Caspar Plate Stabilization: Indications, Results, and Complications in 90 Consecutive Patients (Abstract)*. American Association of Neurological Surgeons. 1991;732:150.
50. Ranford AO, Crockard HA, Pozo JL, et al. Craniocervical instability treated by contoured loop fixation. *J Bone Joint Surg*. 1986;68B:173–177.
51. Roy-Camille R, Mazel CH, Saillant G. Treatment of cervical spine injuries by a posterior osteosynthesis with plates and screws. In: Kehr P, Weidner A, eds. *Cervical Spine I*. Wien-New York: Springer-Verlag; 1987:163.

52. Roy-Camille R, Saillant G. Chirurgie du rachis cervical. 3. Fractures complexe du rachis cervical inferieur. Tetraplegies. *Nouv Presse Med.* 1972; 1:2707–2709.
53. Roy-Camille R, Saillant G, Mazel C. Internal fixation of the unstable cervical spine by a posterior osteosynthesis with plates and screws. In: Cervical Spine Research Society, ed. *The Cervical Spine.* 2nd ed. Philadelphia: JB Lippincott; 1989:390–403.
54. Sherk HH, Snyder B. Posterior fusions of the upper cervical spine: Indications, techniques, and prognosis. *Orthop Clin North Am.* 1978;9:1091–1099.
55. Spetzler RF, Dickman CA, Sonntag VKH. The transoral approach to the anterior cervical spine. *Contemp Neurosurg.* 1991;13(9):1–6.
56. Taitsman JP, Saha S. Tensile strength of wire-reinforced bone cement and twisted stainless-steel wire. *J Bone Joint Surg.* 1977;59A:419–425.
57. Tippets RH, Apfelbaum RI. Anterior cervical fusion with the Caspar instrumentation system. *Neurosurgery.* 1988;22:1008–1013.
58. Weidner A. Internal fixation with metal plates and screws. In: Cervical Spine Research Society, ed. *The Cervical Spine.* 2nd ed. Philadelphia: JB Lippincott; 1989:404–421.
59. Wertheim SB, Bohlman HH. Occipitocervical fusion. Indications, technique, and long-term results in thirteen patients. *J Bone Joint Surg.* 1987;69A:833–836.
60. White AA III, Panjabi MM. The clinical biomechanics of the spine. *Clin Orthop North Am.* 1978;9:867–878.
61. Wiesel SW, Rothman RH. Occipitoatlantal hypermobility. *Spine.* 1979;4: 187–191.

Discussion

The Acute Management of Cervical Spine Disruption

At the Barrow Institute patients with cervical spine trauma are stabilized, x-rayed, and immediately reduced. They may arrive with halter traction, but after the initial x-rays are reviewed a decision is made regarding reduction and the use of internal fixation versus external immobilization. If a subluxation is less than 6 mm we utilize the Halo-Vest, which is available from a Halo-cart and applied by a Halo team. If the subluxation is greater than 6 mm we begin with the Halo and also arrange for surgery and internal fixation.

Dr. White asked: If your Halo systems are that available and you are using them to that extent and they do provide as good stabilization, why would you use internal fixation?

Dr. Sonntag answered: As I mentioned there are certain times when the Halo does not work. For example, we initially treated all our odontoid type II fractures in a Halo until we discovered that those subluxed more than 6 mm were not stable in the Halo. Similarly, the C2-C3 subluxations are not stabilized in a Halo, which is also true for the occiput–C1 disruptions. Clearly the Halo is good for certain types of injuries, but if one has any reservations internal fixation is required. Against the use of the Halo is the 12-week immobilization time and the scars on the forehead.

Dr. Kostuik raised the point about the need for Halo immobilization below C2 and whether a simpler device such as a Somi brace would not suffice for non-operative management. There are no studies to support that view and certainly the Halo is safe. Dr. Neuwirth added that 10 years ago it was shown that the Somi brace worked reasonably well below C2. My problem with those braces is that people take them off. Dr. Kostuik agreed and added that that is one of the problems with the Halo-Vest. Patients will relax the jacket straps and even remove the vests. This can even happen with a Halo-cast. I applied one to a motorcyclist with a hangman's fracture and he soaked it off in the bathtub.

Dr. White continued: If you are going to do a total corpectomy, two or three levels in the lower cervical spine anteriorly, will you use a Halo alone? Will you combine it with internal fixation? Or will you use internal fixation alone? Dr. Sonntag replied: Typically I'll do a corpectomy and put a Caspar plate on it without using the Halo. Dr. Kostuik said he no longer used the Caspar plates, rather he used the Morsher plates, which he felt were better biomechanically with the Halo, and a Philadelphia collar or a soft collar. Dr. Sonntag agreed. Dr. Neuwirth asked: Do you use internal fixation for a one-level corpectomy? Dr. Kostuik replied: It's controversial. I think it depends on whether the procedure is for tumor, in which case I would, or for spondylosis, in which case I would not. Dr. Sonntag concurred.

Dr. Kostuik asked if Dr. Sonntag agreed with the classification of hangman's fractures espoused by Loran. Dr. Sonntag said he definitely does.

Resorption of the Bone Graft

Dr. Kostuik said: The question of bone grafting and resorption of the grafts was raised. I believe kyphos is one of the factors contributing to bone resorption.

Another factor is movement. Dr. Neuwirth said: Grafts do heal in kyphosis. Dr. Kostuik said: Yes, they do, but they also resorb. Dr. Neuwirth countered, saying: Yes, but they heal also. I mean consider all the thoracic fusions done for idiopathic scoliosis. Dr. Kostuik responded: Those people are not kyphotic, they are lordotic. Dr. Neuwirth continued: Well, but one fuses them further than the apex of their scoliosis deformity, so you are fusing them through a junction of kyphos. I just don't think that kyphosis alone is sufficient reason for bone graft reabsorption. We all have experiences with patients whose lumbar spine is lordotic and whose bone grafts have been resorbed. Dr. Kostuik reiterated: I think that kyphosis is one factor in the problem with or without scoliosis. Panjabe and White have shown that a long fusion in kyphosis will work. Short fusions, on the other hand, do not work very well. This is one of the reasons why if you fuse a traumatic patient at the thoracolumbar junction in kyphosis they will have such a high incidence of nonunion. If you look at Sherman's problems long-term, a significant percentage that are solid at 3 to 4 years go on later in life to develop stress fractures.

Dr. Farcy said: The problem with long fusions in kyphosis and those with segmental kyphosis do not have the same mechanical implications. Dr. Neuwirth continued: I'm not saying that excessive kyphosis or abnormal sagittal deformity is not related to pseudarthrosis; clearly, that is not true. The Sherman ones I have done front and back and the thoracolumbar cases, if they cannot be reduced, I will do them front and back, but I think it is safe to say that the sagittal alignment is the prime cause, although there are nutritional and biochemical factors including, as Dr. Farcy indicated, smoking.

Some Aspects of Management of Upper Cervical Fusions

Dr. Kostuik addressed Dr. Sonntag saying, I noticed that you are using Bohler screws. How long have you been using them? Dr. Sonntag said: About 2 to 3 years. Dr. Kostuik said, I think there is a greater and greater tendency to do that. Are any other participants using anterior screws for odontoid fractures? Prof. Louis responded: I have my own technique. I use a screw plate for the dens by the transoral approach with two hooks for the lateral aspect of the odontoid and horizontal screws and two screws for the vertebral body of C2. When bone grafting is necessary I use iliac bone. I operate only for *unstable* dens fractures since the majority of them are likely to heal with conservative measures.

Dr. Sonntag indicated that his cases were done primarily under general anesthesia. Dr. Kostuik said his were done under local. Dr. Sonntag felt that the biggest danger may occur during turning of the patient and he wanted an external orthosis in place. Dr. Kostuik agreed and mentioned a second danger related to the passing of sublaminar wires.

CHAPTER 13

Surgical Stabilization for Tumors of the Thoracic Spine

Narayan Sundaresan, Alleyne B. Fraser, and George Krol

During the past decade, improvements in neuroradiological diagnosis by computed tomography (CT) as well as magnetic resonance imaging (MRI), together with the development of effective multidisciplinary treatment, have considerably expanded the role of surgery in the treatment of neoplasms of the spine (43,50,51,55). Primary tumors of the spine are rare and account for less than 10% of all bone tumors. By far the most common cause of neoplastic involvement of the spine is metastasis to the vertebral column, which outnumbers primary tumors by a ratio of more than 10 to 1 (3,6,42). Autopsy data indicate that approximately one in three patients dying of cancer has metastasis to the vertebral column (57), and thus spinal metastases represent a major cause of morbidity in cancer patients.

In the past, the goals of operation have been limited largely to providing tissue diagnosis, as well as palliation of pain and neurological deficit by decompressive laminectomy (13,15,59). Except in those instances where the tumor is located predominantly in the posterior elements of the spine, it is difficult to justify the routine use of laminectomy in all patients because the morbidity from this procedure does not justify the potential benefits; and yet, in the smaller community hospital in which the clinical syndrome of cord compression is frequently encountered, it is difficult to fault the neurosurgeon who is forced to "do something" for the deteriorating patient. With the radiological demonstration that the majority of tumors, both primary and metastastic, occur ventral to the cord, it is obvious that tumor resection requires exposures of the anterior spine that are only currently becoming in vogue (9,12,18,19,25,28,31,39,45,47). Historically, however, the principles of anterior spinal surgery were outlined by Hodgson (20) in their extensive experience with Pott's disease of the spine. The last decade might also properly be viewed as the beginning of a new era in spinal fixation, which has brought together a concentration of orthopedic and neurosurgeons focusing on a closer understanding of the response of neural, discoligamentous, and osseous elements of the spine in response to tumor and trauma.

To a certain extent, the modern concepts of spine fixation were developed along similar principles for long bone fixation in Europe over the past several decades. The widely accepted surgical principle that rigid internal fixation provides faster and more complete resolution of limb and joint function is now accepted as being applicable to the axial skeleton. Although this chapter concerns itself mainly with the current concepts of stabilization of the thoracic spine, the approaches outlined are applicable to all segments. Unlike trauma, where stability may be the predominant goal of treatment, the fundamental problem in managing tumors is essentially one of obtaining local control by operation. The concept of "cure" requires in addition a multidisciplinary effort to eradicate overt or silent metastases by systemic approaches, i.e., chemotherapy. Most radical tumor resections of the spine render the spine unstable, and reconstruction of the resected segment is necessary to restore stability. Resected segments may be stabilized either by polymethylmethacrylate (PMMA) and spinal instrumentation (5,14,39,46), or by bone grafts, which allow physiologic fusion. The major rationale for the use of spinal instrumentation is that it provides immediate support, can be used to correct deformities, and provides for load sharing. In addition, the reduction of motion across the resected segments reduces the incidence of nonunion. With the advent of effective instrumentation, it is technically feasible to remove an entire vertebra (spondylectomy) by either a staged or a single approach (44).

Incidence and Clinical Presentation

Approximately 1,000 bone tumors and 5,000 soft part sarcomas are diagnosed each year in the the United States, of which less than 10% involve the spine. However, involvement of the vertebral column is a relatively common feature of many solid tumors. Clinical data suggest that 20% to 70% of patients with metastatic disease from the breast, lung, prostate, and hematopoietic system will have involvement of the axial spine. Compression of the spinal cord results from extension of a focus within the vertebral body; other possible mechanisms include direct invasion of the spine from a paraspinal tumor, as well as extension through the intervetebral foramina along the perineurium or its lymphatics without bone involvement.

The typical clinical syndrome of neural compression should be easily recognized—more than 90% of patients present with back pain, which may be associated with a referred or radicular component. The median duration of pain is about 6 to 10 weeks, and may be followed by the development of neurological deficits. Unfortunately, the diagnosis of cord compression is still being misdiagnosed so that more than half the patients have severe deficits at initial presentation; approximately 10% of patients present with acute onset of weakness, whereas 10% to 20% of patients deteriorate either while or shortly after undergoing radiation therapy.

Early diagnosis is crucial, since results of treatment depend largely on pretreatment neurological status (1,15,35,39). Since spinal involvement may result in an array of clinical manifestations other than the classical presentation above, we believe it is useful to classify the various syndromes into four major categories. *Asymptomatic* patients are those with posterior mediastinal tumors (either neuroblastomas or neurofibromas) that have varying degrees of intraspinal extension that are generally detected during myelography or MRI scans. In patients with solid tumors, radionuclide bone scanning or MRI may identify spine involvement when performed as a routine staging procedure. Other patients may have *back pain* alone, with minor neurological deficits, i.e., radiculopathy. Frequently the back pain may resolve on high-dose corticosteroid therapy. Patients presenting with neurological deficits may be *ambulatory* or *nonambulatory*. We propose that neurological deficits be classified as *stable* or *unstable* on steroid therapy. Generally, patients who are stable on high-dose corticosteroids can be further evaluated by radiological studies, since it is the exceptional patient who requires emergency operation.

Radiological Evaluation

Accurate radiological assessment of the spinal segments involved, including bone and soft tissue components, as well as staging studies may require several days. To a large extent, the pace of radiological evaluation should be based on the urgency for treatment, but every effort should be made to complete the evaluation as quickly as possible. Plain radiography, preferably of the entire spine, should be the initial study. Classical signs of spinal tumor include (a) vertebral collapse, (b) destruction of the pedicle, (c) lytic destruction or focal osteopenia, and (d) malalignment of the spine. In patients with normal x-rays, the decision to perform the next procedure is generally based on the evolving neurological deficit—patients with paraparesis generally undergo myelography, whereas those with pain alone may be further evaluated by MRI, CT, or radionuclide bone scan. Radionuclide bone scans are particularly useful in demonstrating multifocal versus unifocal involvement.

Magnetic resonance imaging is the procedure of choice in evaluating patients with spinal tumors, although bone detail is better shown with CT scans (17,35,53). In patients presenting with an evolving deficit, myelography is recommended. Evaluation of the entire spinal axis is important because discontinuous epidural tumor may be seen in 10% to 30% of patients, especially those with breast or prostate cancer. Following myelography, myelo–CT is generally performed to outline the tumor extent completely. With the current emphasis on the use of instrumentation, follow-up of patients with MRI scans may be difficult. We generally recommend the use of myelo–CT scan at 6-month intervals to assess local tumor recurrence, and suggest that MRI-compatible implants be used whenever feasible. If a complete block is found, it is not uncommon for patients to deteriorate following lumbar puncture; therefore, all patients with epidural extension of tumor should be treated with a bolus of Decadron (dexamethasone 20 to 100 mg intravenously) after the procedure.

In patients with hypervascular tumors, spinal angiography may be indicated to diminish tumor vascularity, demonstrate feeding vessels, and determine the location of critical spinal arterial supply such as the artery of Adamkiewicz. Profuse bleeding may be encountered from a variety of metastatic tumors such as those from the kidney, thyroid, plasmacytoma, and other primary bone tumors such as aneurysmal bone cysts, hemangiomas, and giant cell tumors (22,41). For presurgical embolization, a variety of therapeutic agents may be used. Temporary materials (such as autologous clot, gelatin foam, and microfibrillar collagen) are easy to handle, associated with minimal risk of permanent damage, and are used for temporary embolization until operative resection is scheduled within several days. Permanent materials include polyvinyl alcohol foam (Ivalon) in particulate form, Silastic spheres, silicone polymers, and absolute alcohol. Particles of Ivalon (150 to 500 microns in diameter) are mixed with solutions of warmed saline and radiographic contract in a proportion designed to produce a liquid slurry of a concentration and viscosity appropriate to the lesion. If superselective catheterization can be achieved, absolute alcohol can be used for permanent tumor necrosis before surgery. The importance of this therapeutic maneuver is shown in our recent series of 52 operations performed for spinal metastases from kidney cancer (41). Excessive blood loss (defined as blood loss greater than 10 units with associated intraoperative hypotension occurred in 11 (37%) of 30 patients; nine episodes occurred in patients who did not have presurgical embolization (41). Our experience also suggests an association between surgical morbidity and blood loss during operation.

Indications for Surgery

Attempts to define absolute indications for surgery are hampered by the fact that treatment has to be individualized in most patients. A knowledge of important prognostic factors may be helpful in the decision-making process (1,38). The most important variables that affect outcome include biology of the neoplasm, pretreatment neurological status, and therapy used (38). More recently, Tokuhashi et al. (54) have developed a scoring system using several parameters: (a) general condition, (b) number of extraspinal metastases, (c) metastases to major organ systems, (d) primary site, and (e) severity of deficit. Each variable was given a scoring system ranging from 0 to 2; the major finding was that prognosis could not be inferred from any one variable, but depended on several of them. Tokuhashi et al. considered radical excisional operation the treatment of choice in patients with good scores (more than 9), and conservative operations in patients with scores less than 5.

We believe that, for optimum results, operations are indicated when patients are ambulatory or have moderate deficit; there is little justification in subjecting paraplegic or near-paraplegic patients to extensive surgery. Patients who have rapidly evolving deficits (less than 24 hours) probably are destined to have a poor outcome regardless of therapy, especially if the deficits progress on high-dose steroid therapy. Patients with structural abnormalities (instability, retropulsed bone fragments, acute collapse of the vertebral body) do not respond to radiotherapy (RT) alone, since compression of the neural elements results from bone. Although there is general acceptance of the concept that RT should be used initially in most patients with spinal metastases, current data clearly indicate a substantial increase in morbidity in patients who have received prior treatment (27,30,40). In the irradiated patient, postsurgical morbidity results mainly from sepsis and wound-related complications, especially if instrumentation is used.

We strongly advocate operation in good risk patients prior to RT, with the view that RT should be used as an adjunct to eradicate microscopic foci of residual disease. Although no prospective randomized studies are available, we believe that such studies are not feasible in view of the numerous variables, and the context in which spinal cord compression occurs. Several recent prospective studies have shown that the historically poor results of surgery could be attributed to the nonselective use of laminectomy in all patients regardless of the site of compression within the spinal canal; with proper tailoring of the operative approach to the site of compression, success rates of 70% to 80% can be achieved (32,37).

Our recently completed study of neoplastic cord compression of 54 de novo patients operated upon over a $4\frac{1}{2}$ year period showed a posttreatment ambulation rate of 100% in survivors, with a median survival of 2 years; ambulatory status was maintained in survivors in more than 90%, but repeat operations for local recurrences were required in 25% of the patients (49). In our view, the fact that more than 25% of patients undergoing de novo surgery and postoperative RT and chemotherapy required repeat operation is an indication that it is the extent of surgical resection that determines local recurrence, and that spondylectomy may be required in a greater portion of patients. Although multifocality within the spinal axis is thought to represent a relative contraindication to operation, it should be remembered that patients with purely osseous metastases have a favorable prognosis; we have operated on multifocal lesions (in stages) on patients with biologically slowly growing tumors (such as breast and thyroid cancer) with excellent long-term palliation. On the other hand, patients with advanced systemic cancer, with multiorgan metastases, and in poor performance status do not benefit from surgery.

Since the goals of therapy vary in any individual patient, we have classified indications along five major categories: cancer therapy, stabilization, neurologic palliation, tissue diagnosis, and pain relief.

Cancer Therapy

In patients with primary osseous neoplasms, localized paraspinal tumors with direct spine involvement, as well as those presenting with solitary rates of relapse, local treatment has a major bearing on overall survival. Other patients presenting with pathological compression fractures and radioresistant tumors such as kidney cancer with limited systemic disease also fall into this category. In these patients, the extent of epidural extension and the presence or absence of neurological deficit have little bearing on the timing of operation; rather the goal of operation should be maximal reduction of tumor bulk. As at other sites, the concept of resecting a solitary metastatic focus is equally valid for the spine.

Stabilization

A second but especially major goal of operation is the restoration or maintenance of stability of the spine involved by tumor (4,8,11,48). Patients with fracture-dislocations, localized kyphosis, or collapsed vertebra with retropulsion of a bone fragment require operative decompression in conjunction with RT. In these patients, the radiosensitivity of the primary tumor has little bearing on the indication for therapy. A major subgroup of patients in this category present with "segmental instability" of the spine. This is clinically manifest by pain aggravated by movement, and is usually seen after radiotherapy. Plain radiography may show progressive collapse of the vertebral bodies, or MRI may show retropulsion of bony elements with a local kyphosis. Stabilization across this motion segment will generally result in prompt relief of pain. This can be accomplished by anterior stabilization following vertebral body resection, or by posterior stabilization with instrumentation.

Neurological Palliation

In patients who present with acutely evolving deficit, surgery offers the potential of neurological palliation even though there may be little impact on overall survival. Similarly, patients who deteriorate while undergoing RT, or others who cannot receive further RT, may be relieved for several months by surgical decompression. In such patients, the goal of therapy is more limited, since it is being performed for salvage. Since these patients have received both RT and prolonged steroid therapy, morbidity from extensive operative procedures may be considerable, and more limited decompression by posterior or posterolateral approaches may be appropriate. Since posterolateral approaches offer less adequate exposure for tumor resection, local recurrences are high if the patient lives a year.

Tissue Diagnosis

With current radiological evaluation, the need for a major procedure to document a diagnosis of malignancy should be rare. Frequently the primary site may be obvious, i.e., on chest x-ray or abdominal CT, or a more accessible site for biopsy may be seen on radionuclide bone scan. If no site is evident, the diagnosis of malignancy can frequently be established by a CT-guided needle biopsy of the spinal lesion, especially if a paraspinal soft tissue mass is present (10). However, with current methods of immunohistochemistry, tissue testing for chemosensitivity, and the potential ability to predict tumor behavior by flow cytometry, adequate tissue sampling is important. For these reasons, we favor open biopsy, and stabilization of the spinal lesion whenever feasible. In our series of patients with "unclassified" malignancies involving the spine, the use of open biopsy and resection changed the diagnosis in 20% of the patients.

Another indication for operative intervention is to differentiate benign from malignant compression, e.g., disc disease versus metastatic tumor, since disc disease may simulate malignancy in some patients; surgery may also be required for the occasional intradural lesion in which distinction from a primary intraspinal tumor such as meningioma versus metastases must be made.

Pain Relief

In most patients, resection of tumor and restoration of stability frequently result in pain relief; exceptionally in patients with intractable pain either from local plexus or nerve root invasion, the goal of therapy may be pain relief even though motor deficits are permanent and irreversible. The roles of local rhizotomies, cordotomy, resection of lesions compressing the brachial plexus fall into this category.

Choice of Operative Approaches and Biomechanical Considerations

There are three basic approaches to the spine: (a) posterior approaches by laminectomy or pediculotomy, (b) posterolateral approaches by costotransversectomy (also called lateral rhacotomy or extracavitary approach), and (c) anterior (anterolateral) approaches by vertebral body resection (11,20,26,33,34,36,38,43). When both anterior and posterior elements are involved, staged or combined anterior-posterior approaches may be required. The choice of surgical approach should be based on the radiographic extent of tumor, the ability of the patient to tolerate the proposed operation based on clinical and laboratory criteria, as well as the desired goal of therapy. Indications for using the posterolateral approach instead of the anterior approach include (a) multiple levels of spinal involvement, (b) discontinuous levels of involvement, (c) three-column involvement, and (d) patient's inability to tolerate a thoracotomy (4).

Biomechanically, the thoracic spine is stiffer and less mobile than the other segments by virtue of the rib cage and costovertebral articulations. Since the thoracic vertebrae have a natural kyphosis, this segment is more likely to be unstable in flexion. Both the anterior and posterior longitudinal ligaments of the costovertebral articulation (costotransverse and radiate ligaments) offer considerable resistance against flexion, but postlaminectomy kyphosis is frequently seen after tumor resection by laminectomy approaches.

In the upper thoracic spine, the facets provide stability primarily against translation, whereas in the lower thoracic spine the joints are oriented in the sagittal plane and provide stability against axial rotation. Axial rotation is also resisted by the rib cage and costovertebral articulations, with the greatest stiffness occurring at the T1 level.

White and Panjabi (56) have shown that with all the posterior elements cut, the motion segment remains stable in flexion until the costovertebral articulation is destroyed. All anterior ligaments and one posterior component must be cut to cause failure in extension. The maximum physiologic sagittal plane translation was 2.5 mm, and the maximum sagittal plane rotation was 5°. Based on these considerations, they have proposed a checklist for the diagnosis of instability in the thoracic spine. Although these criteria may be helpful in the evaluation of the patient with spinal pain, determining instability in the tumor patient is more difficult.

Siegal et al. (39) have proposed several criteria that are useful: involvement of two or more adjacent vertebra, involvement of both anterior and posterior elements, loss of more than 50% of vertebral height, and combinations of the above. Since these criteria are acceptable to most surgeons, we advocate, similarly to DeWald et al. (9), prophylactic stabilization prior to the onset of neurological symptoms. Indeed, the finding of progressive collapse of the vertebral body is an indication of potential instability, and suggests the need for fixation.

The normal kyphotic curvature of the spine ranges from 20° to 50°, and any kyphosis measuring greater than 50° is likely to be progressive. Since the center of gravity of the thoracic spine is anterior to the body, the vertebral bodies are subject to compression and flexion forces, whereas the posterior elements are subject to tensile forces. Progressive kyphosis increases the moment arm, and this leads to more compression and tension.

Similarly, wedging or short angular kyphosis results in an increase in the lever arm with respect to the injured vertebra, with an increase in the flexion bending moment. The major goals in treating kyphosis are the following: (a) correct the deformity, (b) diminish the deforming forces, (c) provide neural decompression, and (d) achieve adequate fixation with implants and bone grafts (2). Posterior fusions are subject to tension and have a high incidence of failure. The proper surgical treatment includes anterior decompression, the use of a strut graft, followed by a second stage posterior fixation. Kostuik (24) has introduced the concept of anterior kyphosis correction with distraction screws, using a construct similar to the Kaneda system (21), which can be used with a standard Harrington set.

Vertebral Body Resection

In our experience, the anterior approach by vertebral body resection fulfills the basic requirements of tumor surgery; it provides extensive exposure, thus allowing complete resection of all gross tumor, and allows adequate access for anterior stabilization. In patients with neoplasms, the importance of immediate stabilization cannot be overemphasized. Stabilization allows immediate ambulation and minimizes pulmonary and embolic complications. In view of the limited life expectancy in the cancer patient, and the need for postoperative radiation therapy, we believe that polymethylmethacrylate (PMMA) as an immediate stabilizing agent allows major advantages over bone grafts. Polymethylmethacrylate is an acrylic polymer belonging to the polyolefin group of synthetic plastics. It is commercially available as a liquid monomer (40 ml), which is mixed with the powdered polymer (20 g). "Curing" or self-polymerization occurs through a self-catalytic process as well as with additives. During the heat of polymerization, intense heat is generated (80° to 100°C) for periods of 5 minutes.

The orthopedic PMMA is impregnated by 10% barium sulfate, and is available from three major sources: Howmedica, Zimmer, and Richards. There is no bonding at the bone-cement interface, and therefore the brittle acrylic has to be kept in place with additional instrumentation. Although McAfee et al. (29) have reported long-term failures with the use of PMMA, our data do not support their contention; a long-term analysis of anterior PMMA constructs used for vertebral body replacement showed no evidence of failure during follow-up times ranging from 2 to 7 years (23).

There are several techniques described in the literature to supplement PMMA fixation. All three techniques are relatively simple, easy to master, and should be part of the armamentarium of all spinal surgeons. In previous years, we used a simple technique using Steinmann pins impacted into healthy vertebra in the middle of the resected segment to provide a matrix for the cement. More recently, we have developed anterior spinal fixation system using titanium pins (called ATSS), which are superior to the previous pins. Proper placement of the pins within the vertebral axis so that the ends do not protrude has been one of the major difficulties with this technique. To facilitate proper placement, Arbit has designed washers for the system, which should be impacted into the end plates above and below the construct. The Arbit washers come in two-hole and single-hole models to accommodate either one or two pins. The pins are of three diameters—3 mm, 3.5 mm, and 4 mm—and come in precut lengths ranging from 60 to 130 mm. Their ends have trocar points, and their surfaces have been knurled to allow adequate gripping by drivers and needle holders. Excessive force on a Steinmann pin can result in stress lines that could lead to fatigue: fractures. The system comes with predesigned sets that allow tumor resection, and a variety of instruments are included for proper positioning of the pin within the vertebra.

The anterior spine requires a variety of approaches because of the complex soft part anatomy anterior to the prevertebral space. In this chapter, we will focus on the transthoracic approach, which will serve as the model for approaches to the other segments. An initial consideration is the side from which an anterolateral exposure should be performed. In the majority, the side that allows maximal tumor resection should be chosen. This can usually be ascertained by CT. If CT is not available, then the side of increased pedicle destruction or collapse, or the symptomatic side of radiculopathy or plexopathy, probably indicates the site of tumor compression. In equivocal cases, a right-sided approach is chosen for thoracic segments, and a left-sided approach for lumbar segments.

The upper two thoracic segments form the posterior border of the thoracic inlet; this region may be exposed by a direct anterior transsternal approach (52), or indirectly by a posterolateral thoracotomy with resection of the upper three ribs for extensive tumors with lateral extension. The transsternal anterior operation is performed in the supine position with the head extended. Prior to operation, the range of extension and flexion is tested with the patient awake. After induction of anesthesia, the image intensifier is positioned in place for intraoperative fluoroscopy. A T-shaped incision is planned. The horizontal limb of the T extends 1 cm above the clavicle, and extends past the sternomastoid on either side, and the vertical limb is carried down to the body of the sternum. The sternal and clavicular heads of the sternomastoid are detached from their bony origins by cautery and retracted superiorly and posteriorly. The inferior strap muscles (sternohyoid and sternothyroid) are sectioned inferiorly and retracted superiorly and medially. The sternal origin of the pectoralis major is cleared from the sternum, and the clavicle stripped subperiosteally. The medial third of the clavicle is sectioned with a Gigli saw, and the medial end disarticulated from the sternum. At this point, a decision may be made as to whether the sternum can be left intact, split completely, or a portion of the manubrium sterni removed. Using a high speed drill, the manubrium may be removed to provide access to the top of the second and third thoracic vertebra.

The innominate vein should be underneath the manubrium. The thymus and surrounding fat should be dissected and resected. The avascular plane between the trachea and esophagus medially, and the vascular sheath laterally, is developed. The recurrent laryngeal nerve should be identified. The prevertebral space is then opened in the midline, and the longus colli muscles stripped laterally with the periosteum. Intact discs above and below the level of involvement are identified. Self-retaining retractors are placed under the longus colli muscles. The involved vertebra is then resected piecemeal with curets, rongeurs, and osteotomes. If the bone is markedly sclerotic, a high-speed drill may be used. All involved bone and soft tissue tumor and devitalized tissues are removed down to the dura. Meticulous hemostasis is achieved with the bipolar current. After the dura is cleaned of all tumor, a sheet of Gelfoam is used to protect the dura. Reconstruction of the resected segments is then carried out using the clavicle as a strut graft by impacting it in place under gentle traction. Since there is a physiological curvature across the cervicothoracic junction, we generally do not advocate the use of cement; however, if the defect is small, methylmethacrylate reconstruction using either a small Harms basket or the ATSS pin is possible.

If a bone graft is used, we recommend the use of Caspar plates since the cervicothoracic segment cannot be immobilized completely in a Halo. Suction drains are placed, and the wound closed in layers. Postoperatively, a cervicothoracic orthosis is prescribed (either the Halo or a Philadelphia collar with thoracic extension). If a bone graft is used, RT should be delayed for 3 months. In our experience, if three-column instability was present, or if there was a kyphosis prior to surgery, patients require a second stage posterior fixation later. We generally use Luque rectangles or L-rods with sublaminar wiring using Songer cables for the cervicothoracic fixation. Using the Cotrel-Dubousset (CD) or Texas Scottish Rite Hospital (TSRH) system across the cervicothoracic curvature is more difficult, because it requires a combination of adult and pediatric implants.

The transthoracic approach is used for tumors below the third thoracic segment. Patients are positioned in the lateral position on an Olympic Vac-Pac unit, and general endotracheal anesthesia with a double lumen tube is used. A generous skin incision similar to a posterolateral thoracotomy is used, and placed below the scapula. The posterior incision should be parallel to the paraspinal muscles but not extend to the midline. After the skin incision is made, we use the electrocautery to cut through the chest wall muscles (trapezius, serratus, latissimus, and pectoralis major) to reach the rib cage.

When the interspace is entered, it should be above the body that one has to work on, since the ribs turn caudally proximal to the angle. In the lower thoracic segments, at least two spaces above the level of involvement are chosen because of the rising dome of the diaphragm. Only the posterior 5 to 10 cm of rib needs to be removed. The intercostal bundle should be carefully isolated with right-angle clamps, and cleanly ligated or clipped. During the initial phase of tumor resection, the head of the ribs overlies the pedicle and should be kept intact to prevent injury to the cord.

The anterior spine is then exposed by retraction of the lung, which can be gradually deflated if required. To expose the spine, the pleura is then reflected in the form of a window. Intercostal vessels (which are direct tributaries of the aorta or vena cava) are carefully identified, and ligated as well as clipped. This maneuver also allows mobilization of the major vessels over the surface of the vertebra. All soft tissues anterior to the vertebra are dissected off (including the sympathetic ganglia). The isolated segments are packed off with lap pads, and if a prevertebral tumor is identified, we can be reasonably sure of the proper location of the segment to be resected.

If no tumor is evident on the surface, it is important to establish the correct level not only by counting the ribs from within the chest, but also by an intraoperative radiograph. Before commencing work on the spine, the anterior surface of the vertebral body is cleared by periosteal elevators. Intact disc structures above and below the level of involvement are identified; the discs are incised with a No. 15 blade, and the vertebral segments removed with the use of rongeurs, curets, and osteotomes. Tumor resection should be complete, and the posterior longitudinal ligament should be removed.

In radiated patients, the bone and tumor may be fibrotic, and the posterior longitudinal ligament densely adherent to the dura. By tracing the epidural tumor posteriorly, it is possible to decompress the dura laterally and posteriorly by performing a facetectomy and removing the pedicle. To allow additional posterior decompression, a hemilaminectomy can be performed at this time. The anterior longitudinal ligament is left intact if it is not destroyed. A high-speed drill is then used to drill out the opposite half of the body until a thin cortical shell is left.

If a curative resection is contemplated, every effort must be made to remove all bone and soft tissue so that the spondylectomy can be completed by a second stage posterior approach. Following tumor resection, all soft tissues on the end plates above and below are removed to provide the broadest possible support for the construct. The construct may be a bone graft, or methylmethacrylate. If a bone graft is used, it can be impacted in place by manual pressure posteriorly, or else instrumentation is required. At present, anterior instrumentation for the thoracic spine requires the placement of cortical screws above and below the resected segment, with rods to keep the screws compressed to the bone graft; both the Kaneda and Kostuik-Harrington systems are now available, but their use in the high thoracic spine does not have FDA approval. If acrylic fixation is decided upon, the surgeon must be sure that all vertebral segments involved by tumor have been resected, since fixation of the acrylic to diseased vertebrae will result in postoperative displacement. In half the patients, more than one vertebra has to be removed; we have resected up to four vertebrae in the thoracic region with little morbidity.

Prior to stabilization, hemostasis must be secured, and all soft tissues in the region of the construct removed. The ATSS pins are selected based on the region involved, length of fixation required, and the quality of the recipient bone. Prior to pin insertion, the Arbit washers are positioned on the healthy end plates by gentle impaction. Using the distractors available, the washers are completely embedded in the healthy vertebra. Through the holes in the washers, the initial penetration of bone may be accomplished by bone awls or by a right angle drill. Predrilling allows easier passage of the washers. Prior to insertion, the pins are prebent using in situ benders. The pin is introduced with two smaller holders, or with the larger driver that allows proper grasping of the implant. Using gradual force, the pin is driven through the washer hole. If the distal end plate is encountered, the driver is used to penetrate the bone. By overdriving the pin, it can now be brought back into the caudal vertebra by bending it into the plane of the inferior washer hole. These pins should straddle the resected segments, and be securely in place to the vertebra above and below. Once the pins (generally two) are secured, their position should be checked by intraoperative fluoroscopy or x-rays.

Methylmethacrylate is injected into the resected space and molded to recreate the resected bodies. At the same time, Penfield dissectors and tongue blades are used to keep the hardening acrylic away from the dura, which is protected by strips of Gelfoam. During the heat generated by the polymerization process, copious saline irrigation is used to dissipate heat. The epidural space should be kept free of all trapped fluid, and no effort should be made to pack this space tightly. The resected rib may be placed adjacent to the bodies and tied in position with Vicryl sutures as a lateral fusion mass.

If a kyphosis is present, correction of the deformity requires distraction with screws, and the use of pins may be associated with pin penetration outside the vertebral bodies. The anterior distraction devices are then incorporated within the acrylic construct. More recently, Harms has introduced a titanium basket to contain the acrylic, or else bone chips may be used to fill the basket. These baskets are available in several standard lengths and diameters.

The chest cavity is drained by chest tubes, and the closure is that of a standard thoracotomy. Postoperatively, patients are kept in intensive care for a few days, and the chest tube drainage is monitored. When the drainage is less than 100 cc over 24 hours, it is removed. Extensive chest tube drainage over a week suggests a CSF leaf into the pleural cavity.

Anterior Approach to Lower Thoracic and Upper Lumbar Segments

A variety of approaches are available for the thoracolumbar region, because the diaphragm separates this region into two cavities. The lower thoracic approach may also be performed by a completely extrapleural procedure, but the widest exposures are obtained by a transthoracic approach with detachment of the diaphragm.

The diaphragm is a dome-shaped muscle that is muscular around its periphery and tendinous centrally. Anteriorly it arises from the xiphoid and cartilaginous portions of the lower six ribs, posteriorly it originates from the crura that are attached to the anterior longitudinal ligament; superiorly it arises from the medial and lateral arcuate ligaments, which are attached to the transverse processes of the first lumbar and the 12th rib. The widest exposures are obtained by resection of the 10th or 11th ribs, and by detaching the muscle from the costal articulations as well as the arcuate ligaments.

For the widest and most direct anterior exposure to the thoracoabdominal spine, a long skin incision centered on the 10th or 11th ribs is required. Posteriorly, the incision should extend to the paraspinous muscles. The latissimus dorsi and serratus anterior muscles are divided, and the ribs chosen for resection identified. The oblique muscles are detached from the rib with cautery, or cut in the intercostal space. The endothoracic fascia and parietal pleura are opened, and the ribs spread. The diaphragm is then put on tension by retraction, and circumferentially detached toward the arcuate ligaments. The retroperitoneal space is gradually enlarged by blunt dissection, and the spleen retracted downward. The sympathetic trunk and the areolar tissue around the aorta are cleared. Segmental intercostal vessels are carefully ligated and cut. The anterior surface of the thoracolumbar spine is then exposed and the soft tissues cleared to expose the cortical surface. Tumor resection then proceeds as described in the thoracic segments. Following tumor resection and stabilization, repair proceeds by closure of the diaphragm and insertion of chest tubes. The muscles and skin are then closed in routine fashion.

The Kaneda system is useful for the thoracolumbar junction, especially if a bone allograft is used. Although indicated primarily for trauma, we have found it useful for anteriorly located tumors as well.

Posterolateral Approaches with Stabilization

A variety of posterolateral approaches (4,8,20,26,29) have been described in the literature for the thoracolumbar segment. These allow decompression of neural structures, and are better tolerated by poor-risk patients.

An excellent description of this operation is provided by Yonenobu et al. (58). The patient is positioned in the lateral decubitus or three-quarter prone position. The skin incision may be paramedian or centered two ribs above the affected segments. It begins in the posterior midline and extends to the anterior axillary line. The rib is exposed subperiosteally and resected from its anterior angle. After thoracotomy, the parietal pleura overlying the vertebral bodies is incised, and the exposing segmental vessels are ligated. Three or four vertebral levels in continuity are exposed subperiosteally, and tamponades are placed along the anterior portion of the vertebral bodies to protect the major vessels. The exposed rib is disarticulated from its costovertebral joint, and the cranial and caudal adjacent ribs can be cut close to their costovertebral joints to obtain a wider exposure to the posterior elements. The paraspinal muscles are incised for the same reason. In addition to the transverse process, the pedicle, articular facets, and part of the lamina are resected to expose and decompress the lateral and posterior portions of the spinal cord. These bony elements are initially nibbled by rongeurs and then made thin enough by an air drill to be removed. The intercostal nerve and its origin is used as a guide to the spinal canal. Continuous irrigation is used to prevent thermal damage to the neural tissue and the steel burr of the air drill should be changed to a diamond one to prevent minor trauma to the spinal cord when the lamina becomes thinner. After exposing the lateral and posterior portions of the spinal cord, the compressive lesion can be removed.

The next stage of the procedure is carried out by drilling down the posterior portions of the exposed vertebral bodies parallel to the posterior cortex, which is also the anterior wall of the spinal canal. Care should be taken to avoid penetration to the canal. About 40% of the involved vertebral bodies and the intervertebral disc material then are resected to obtain a working area for the excision of the space-occupying lesion.

If there are adhesions between the dura and the lesion, a gentle pulling and displacement of the dura will help removal of the lesion. If necessary, one or two segmental nerves emerging from the affected spinal cord segment are sacrificed in the thoracic region to manipulate the dura theca. The pathology is excised under direct visualization of the spinal cord, and the offending mass can be pushed away from the dura in this manner.

The disc material and the osseous end plates of the adjacent vertebrae are removed to prepare anchoring holes for a fibula or rib graft, to obtain intervertebral fusion. Instrumentation is not necessary to obtain stability in this procedure.

For more radical resections, and stabilization of the posterior thoracic spine, we prefer the use of CD (7) or TRSH instrumentation. In most patients, a simple claw construct superiorly and inferiorly will suffice; pedicle screws are only used in the lower thoracic and lumbar segments. In all patients, we believe that posterior instrumentation without providing for anterior stability will result in failure over the long term.

In our view, the major morbidity from posterior operations result from wound breakdown and infections; incidences as high as 20% have been reported in heavily irradiated patients. In addition, posterior instrumentation is time-consuming, and involves considerable "fiddling" with the implants that may contribute to infections. However, the posterolateral approach can be used for palliation of poor-risk patients who cannot tolerate transthoracic resection.

References

1. Barcena A, Lobato RD, Rivas JJ, Cordobes F, De Castro S, Cabrera A, Lamas E. Spinal metastastic disease: analysis of factors determining functional prognosis and choice of treatment. *Neurosurgery*. 1984;15:820–827.
2. Bohm H, Harms J, Donk R, Zielke K. Correction and stabilization of angular kyphosis. *Clin Orthop*. 1990;258:56–61.
3. Boland PJ, Lane JM, Sundaresan N. Metastatic disease of the spine. *Clin Orthop*. 1982;169:95–102.
4. Bridwell KH, Jenny AB, Saul T, Rich KM, Grubb RL. Posterior segmental spinal instrumentation (PSSI) with posterolateral decompression and debulking for metastatic thoracic and lumbar spine disease: Limitations of the technique. *Spine*. 1988;13:1383–1394.
5. Clark CR, Keggi KJ, Panjabi MM. Methyl methacrylate stabilization of the cervical spine. *J Bone Joint Surg*. 1984;66(A):40–46.
6. Constans JP, De Vitiis E, Donzelli, Spaziante R, Meder JF, Haye C. Spinal metastases with neurological manifestations. *J Neurosurg*. 1983;59:111–118.
7. Cotrel Y, Dubousset J, Guillaumat M. New universal instrumentation in spinal surgery. *Clin Orthop Rel Res*. 1988;227:10–23.
8. Cybulski GR, Von Roenn KA, D'Angelo CM, DeWald RL. Luque rod stabilization for metastatic disease of the spine. *Surg Neurol*. 1987;28:277–283.
9. DeWald RL, Bridwell KL, Prodromas C, Rodts MF. Reconstructive surgery as palliation for metastatic malignancies of the spine. *Spine*. 1985;10:21–26.
10. Dollahite HA, Tatum L, Moinuddin SM. Aspiration biopsy of primary neoplasms of bone. *J Bone Joint Surg*. 1989;71A:1166–1169.
11. Faccioli F, Lima J, Bricolo A. One stage decompression and stabilization in the treatment of spinal tumors. *J Neurol Sci*. 1985;29:199–205.
12. Fiedler MW. Anterior decompression and stabilization of metastatic spinal fractures. *J Bone Joint Surg*. 1986;68B:83–90.
13. Findlay GFG. Adverse effects of the management of malignant spinal cord compression. *J Neurol Neurosurg Psychiatry*. 1984;47:761–768.

14. Flatley JJ, Anderson MH, Anast GT. Spinal instability due to metastastic disease. *J Bone Joint Surg*. 1984;66(A):47–52.
15. Gilbert RW, Kim JH, Posner JB. Epidural spinal cord compression from metastastic tumor; diagnosis and treatment.
16. Godersky JC, Smoker WRK, Knutzon R. Use of magnetic resonance imaging in the evaluation of metastastic spinal disease. *Neurosurgery*. 1987;21:676–680.
17. Hagenau C, Grosh W, Currie M, Wiley RG. Comparison of magnetic resonance imaging and myelography in cancer patients. *J Clin Oncol*. 1987; 5:1663–1669.
18. Hall MW, Webb JK. Anterior plate fixation in spine tumor surgery: Indications, techniques, results. *Spine*. 1991;16:80–83.
19. Harrington KD. Anterior cord decompression and spinal stabilization for patients with metastastic lesions of the spine. *J Neurosurg*. 1984;61:107–117.
20. Hodgson AR, Stock FE, Fang Hsy et al. Anterior spinal fusion. The operative approach and pathological findings in 412 patients with Pott's disease of the spine. *Br J Surg*. 1960;48:177–178.
21. Kaneda K, Abumi K, Fujuja M. Burst fractures with neurological deficits of the thoraco-lumbar spine: results of anterior decompression and stabilization with anterior instrumentation. *Spine*. 1984;9:788–795.
22. King GJ, Kostuik JP, McBroom RJ, Richardson W. Surgical treatment of spinal metastases from renal cell carcinoma. *Spine*. 1991;16:265–271.
23. Ko K, Sundaresan N. Long term stability of methylmethacrylate constructs in cancer patients: a clinical study. *AANS Abstract*. 1991;724.
24. Kostuik JP. Anterior Kostuik-Harrington distraction systems for the treatment of kyphotic deformities. *Spine*. 1991;15:169–181.
25. Kostuik JP, Errico TJ, Gleason TF, Errico CC. Spinal stabilization of vertebral column tumors. *Spine*. 1988;13:250–256.
26. Lesoin F, Rousseaux M, Lozco G. Postero-lateral approach to tumors of the dorsolumbar spine. *Acta Neurochir*. 1986;81:40–44.
27. Macedo N, Sundaresan N, Galicich JH. Decompressive laminectomy for metastastic cancer: what are the current indications? *Proc Am Soc Am Oncol*. 1985;4:278.
28. Manabe S, Tateishi A, Abe M, Ohno T. Surgical treatment of metastastic tumors of the spine. *Spine*. 1989;14:41–47.
29. McAfee PC, Bohlman HH, Ducker T, Eismont FJ. Failure of stabilization of the spine with methyl methacrylate: A retrospective analysis of twenty-four cases. *J Bone Joint Surg*. 1986;68A:1145–1157.
30. McDonald DJ, Capanna R, Gherlinzoni F, Bacci G, Ferruzi A. Influence of chemotherapy on perioperative complications in limb salvage surgery for bone tumors. *Cancer*. 1990;65:1509–1516.
31. Miles J, Banks AJ, Dervin E, Noori Z. Stabilization of the spine affected by malignancy. *J Neurol Neurosurg Psychiatry*. 1984;47:897–904. *Ann Neurol*. 1978;3:40–51.
32. Moore AJ, Utley D. Anterior decompression and stabilization of the spine in malignant disease. *Neurosurgery*. 1989;24:713–717.
33. Overby MC, Rothman AS. Anterolateral decompression for metastastic epidural spinal cord tumors. *J Neurosurg*. 1985;62:344–348.
34. Perrin RG, McBroom RJ. Anterior versus posterior decompression for symptomatic spinal metastasis. *Can J Neurol Sci*. 1987;14:75–80.

35. Rodichok LD, Harper GR, Ruckdeschel JC. Early detection and treatment of spinal metastases: the role of myelography. *Ann Neurol*. 1986;20:696–702.
36. Shaw B, Mansfield FL, Borges L. One stage postero-lateral spinal decompression and stabilization. *J Neurosurg*. 1989;70:407–410.
37. Siegal T, Siegal T. Surgical decompression of anterior and posterior malignant epidural tumors compressing the spinal cord: a prospective study. *Neurosurgery*. 1985;17:424–432.
38. Siegal T, Siegal T. Current considerations in the management of neoplastic spinal cord compression. *Spine*. 1989;14:223–229.
39. Siegal T, Tikva P, Siegal T. Vertebral body resection for epidural compression by malignant tumors. A series of 47 consecutive cases. *J Bone Joint Surg*. 1985;67A:375–382.
40. Suit HD, Mankin HJ, Wood WC, Proppe KH. Preoperative, intra-operative and post operative radiation in the treatment of primary soft tissue sarcoma. *Cancer*. 1985;55:2659–2667.
41. Sundaresan N, Choi IS, Hughes JEO, Sachdev V. Surgical treatment of spinal metastases from kidney cancer by presurgical embolization and resection. *J Neurosurg*. 1990;73:548–554.
42. Sundaresan N, DiGiacinto GV, Hughes JEO: Surgical treatment of spinal metastases. *Clin Neurosurg*. 1986;33:503–522.
43. Sundaresan N, DiGiacinto GV, Hughes JEO. Surgical approaches to primary and metastastic tumors of the spine. In: Schmidek HH, Sweet WH, eds. *Operative Neurosurgical Techniques: Indications, Methods, Results*. Vol. 2. Orlando, Grune & Stratton; FL:1988:1525–1537.
44. Sundaresan N, DiGiacinto GV, Hughes JEO, Krol G. Spondylectomy for malignant tumors of the spine. *J Clin Oncol*. 1989;7:1485–1491.
45. Sundaresan N, Galicich JH, Bains MS, Martini N, Beattie E. Vertebral body resection in the treatment of cancer involving the spine. *Cancer*. 1984;53: 1393–1396.
46. Sundaresan N, Galicich JH, Lane JM. Harrington rod stabilization for pathological fractures of the spine. *J Neurosurg*. 1984;60:282–286.
47. Sundaresan N, Galicich JH, Lane JM, Bains M, McCormack P. Treatment of neoplastic epidural cord compression by vertebral body resection and stabilization. *J Neurosurg*. 1985;63:676–684.
48. Sundaresan N, Galicich JH, Lane JM, Scher H. Stabilization of the spine involved by cancer. In: Dunsker SB, Schmidek HH, Frymoyer J, Kahn III, eds. *The Unstable Spine*. Orlando, FL: Grune & Stratton; 1986:249–274.
49. Sundaresan N, Hughes JEO, DiGiacinto G, Cafferty M. Surgical treatment of neoplastic cord compression: Results of a prospective study. *Neurosurgery*. 1991;29:645–650.
50. Sundaresan N, Krol G, Hughes JEO. Treatment of malignant tumors of the spine. In: Youmans J, ed. *Neurological surgery*. Philadelphia: WB Saunders; 1987.
51. Sundaresan N, Schmidek H, Schiller A, Rosenthal A, eds. *Tumors of the Spine*. Philadelphia: WB Saunders; 1990.
52. Sundaresan N, Shah J, Feghali JG. A trans-sternal approach to the upper thoracic vertebra. *Am J Surg*. 1986;148:473–477.
53. Sze G. Magnetic resonance imaging in the evaluation of spinal tumors. *Cancer*. 1991;67:1229–1241.

54. Tokuhashi Y, Matsuzaki H, Toriyama S, Kawano H, Ohsaka S. Scoring system for the preoperative evaluation of metastastic spine tumor prognosis. *Spine*. 1991;15:1110–1113.
55. Weinstein JN, McLain RF. Primary tumors of the spine. *Spine*. 1987;12:843–851.
56. White AA III, Panjabi MM. *Clinical Biomechanics of the Spine*. 2nd ed. Philadelphia: JB Lippincott; 1990.
57. Wong DA, Fornasier VL, MacNab I. Spinal metastases: the obvious, the occult, and the impostors. *Spine*. 1990;15:1–4.
58. Yonenobu K, Korkusuz F, Hosono N, Ebana S, Ono K. Lateral rhacotomy for thoracic spinal lesions. *Spine*. 1991;15:1121–1125.
59. Young RF, Post EM, King GA. Treatment of spinal epidural metastases. Randomised prospective comparison of laminectomy and radiotherapy. *J Neurosury*. 1980;53:741–748.

Discussion

Methylmethacrylate and Metal

Dr. Kostuik began by saying that the orthopedic literature supported the use of polymethylmethacrylate. The problem with McAfee's work was that he used methylmethacrylate without metal reinforcement. We have been using methylmethacrylate with metal for more than 15 years with very, very few failures. I would say none except in the cervical spine that were related to unsatisfactory pin placement. In addition, we have not experienced pin breakage perhaps because we are using bigger pins. In both the lumbar and thoracic spine we have used short Harrington distraction rods and in the cervical spine we have used the heavy threaded Harrington compression rods, which we feel avoids that complication.

In addition we are frequently faced with the patient who presents with acute paraparesis or quadriparesis without a known primary lesion. Based on statistical evidence these are going to be metastatic, but frequently they turn out to be lymphoma or myeloma. We will use methylmethacrylate initially and then if their prognosis looks good at 1 year we will add a secondary posterior fusion prophylactically. In any case we have had people live many years with reinforced polymethylmethacrylate without loosening of the structure. Our experience parallels that of Dr. Sundaresan.

From a purely technical standpoint we use a variety of angled curets. I make a hole into the end plate of the vertebral body and pass the curet up or down as far as required. There is some positive feedback since you can feel the posterior cortex. We then insert the pins, push them up and down, remove them, and then put methylmethacrylate into the vertebral body above and below, and then reinsert the pins and fill the gap with methylmethacrylate. That technique is very simple and does not cost more than $100.

My last comment has to do with the Kostuik-Harrington system which, incidentally, was never named that by myself, and has been available since 1975 and it is just known as spinal screws. They are FDA approved and always have been available though I have never marketed them.

The Two-Team Approach to Combined Anterior and Posterior Approaches

Dr. Farcy indicated that when combined approaches are required he employs the two team approach simultaneously. I achieve my decompression and place the bone graft, allograft, cement, or the cage in front, and in the back I have loose instrumentation. I compress or distract to the degree that yields a perfect contour, the perfect jamming, and the perfect stability front and back. We jam everything together and then close the two wounds. This type of surgery takes $2\frac{1}{2}$ hours. The blood loss is minimal and I believe it is the way to go.

Dr. Kostuik agreed that a two-team approach for that sort of thing works well. We do that for our spinal osteotomies for major deformities as well and the morbidity has been shown to be significantly less for combined approaches as opposed to staged approaches in terms of nutrition, wound infection, thrombophlebitis, pulmonary embolism, and wound healing.

Prof. Louis said: I do not agree because I have more than 20 years of experience performing two-staged combined approaches. I have operated such cases often 1 week apart. It is comfortable both for the patient and for the surgeon. I perform the anterior approach, which usually lasts between $2\frac{1}{2}$ to 3 hours, and 1 week later the second stage posterior approach, which lasts $1\frac{1}{2}$ to 2 hours. My patients suffer no morbidity.

Dr. Kostuik said: I used to do the staged procedures and I have stopped. For the past 5 years I do most of them on the same day simply because the morbidity is less.

Anterior versus Posterolateral Approaches

Dr. Larson said he would just mention the approach described in this text by Dr. Paul McCormick, namely the posterolateral approach that was developed by Kapener primarily for Pott's disease. This approach has the advantage of a one stage procedure for instrumentation, vertebral body resection, and graft using the lateral extension, with a bilateral simultaneous lateral approach including incisional biopsy of the vertebral body by passing a malleable retractor around the vertebra, separating it from the great vessels, cutting the pedicles, cutting the discs, and ultimately delivering the vertebral body as a wide specimen.

Dr. Kostuik agreed that that approach has certainly been well described. I, however, would concur with Dr. Sundaresan that the anterior approach is better and my reasoning is derived from my experience, which began coincidently at the time an article was published in *Trauma* by Erickson and Bradford in the late 1970s on the so-called posterolateral approach for canal intrusion with associated posterior stabilization, just as you did. At that time I was doing anterior approaches for burst fractures. Bradford indicated that the anterior approach was too complex and unnecessary. I spoke with him later and said to him go back and CT scan your patients on whom you have performed posterolateral approaches and tell me whether you have been able to remove all the bone. From my experience as a visiting professor at Duke University I knew there was often difficulty with complete removal of bone and in fact when Bradford rescanned his patients he said there was indeed residual bone in the canal. I am not at all suggesting that that is your experience. I am pointing out that that was the experience at Duke.

Dr. Larson said that he found that once he got across the pedicle, and it is possible to do that routinely with a little care, then bone could be removed from the ventral dural surface without difficulty. A dental mirror was sometimes helpful and one could see across to the far side of the canal. Clearly until you see that you have not gotten an adequate resection. We have been able to use this technique from T3 to the sacrum.

Dr. Kostuik said that the dental mirrors are quite helpful and that they may be of use in the sacral area. As to the posterolateral approach I never liked it. It was too bloody and too hard for me.

Morbidity and Mortality

Dr. Holtzman said: Dr. Sundaresan must be commended for his work. I have had the privilege to observe his efforts for more than 5 years at Harlem Hospital. The great difficulty convincing neurologists that patients with cancer of the vertebral column should undergo decompression and stabilization was due to several articles in the literature indicating that there was little difference in mortality and morbidity from surgical intervention as opposed to radiotherapy provided there was a tissue diagnosis. These reports argued from the surgical standpoint of laminectomy and excepted instances of multiple myeloma, which was and is still considered to be highly radiosensitive. Dr. Sundaresan was able to overcome those arguments demonstrating the effectiveness of anterior approaches and the simplicity and effectiveness of the stabilizing combination of Steinmann pins and methylmethacrylate.

At the present time we have more universal agreement among neurologists as to the efficacy of anterior decompression when the spinal cord is threatened by intrusion of neoplasm into the vertebral canal. Of course we concur with the additive benefit of postoperative radiation therapy.

I wonder now that you have accumulated a large experience with these tumors and have a more extensive retrospective view of this situation are we correct in saying that the longevity of these patients is increased? And has the overall neurological morbidity decreased by urgent surgical intervention and stabilization?

Dr. Kostuik replied: I don't think longevity is increased.

Dr. Sundaresan said: I would disagree with that very strongly. One of the problems with cancer is its multifaceted nature. The only way you can compare whether your treatment is making a difference in survival is by observing a large pool of cancer patients and separating out those groups of patients that manifest themselves with localized sites of metastatic spread and then comparing your therapy with radiation. The problem exists when you intervene in patients with widespread disease; whether you give radiation or steroids probably does not make a difference at that point. It is in instances of localized disease that surgical intervention has its greatest efficacy. I have looked at the cases from Memorial–Sloan Kettering Hospital since I was part of their group. We reviewed the patients who were radiated first and then operated upon and we reviewed the patients who were operated upon and then received radiotherapy. We looked at the incidence of local recurrence. I would say that if the surgeon is aggressive enough at the present time the survival rate exceeds 2 years. Dr. Kostuik just published an article on metastatic renal cell tumors with an average survival of 14 months. The problem is that many patients actually die of local recurrence because the local treatment is ineffective and the ensuing paraplegia and its complications hasten the patient's demise.

Dr. Kostuik continued: The longevity of our patients with a single spinal metastasis on imaging was much longer than those individuals who also had a lesion in the proximal femur. More importantly the quality of the survival was tremendously improved. Dr. Bertle Steiner from Sweden believed in performing en bloc resections of renal cell spinal metastases if it could be demonstrated that there were no problems elsewhere. That was in the pre-MRI era. He claimed a very significant longevity.

Dr. Sunderesan said: I think that using kidney cancer as a model it is possible, if the surgeon is radical enough, to get 5-year survivals. I have already a 15% and 20% rate of 5-year survival. There is no doubt when you compare today's results to the old pacifist nihilistic approach to patients considered to be dying within 6 months that the latter argument is no longer valid. In fact most patients come to me wanting to live 2 to 5 years and willing to submit to aggressive therapy. What I have learned is that in the beginning very often I was not radical enough.

The Question Regarding Multilevel Surgery for Cancer of the Spine

Dr. Holtzman said: In the past we would be reluctant to operate if there was more than one level of vertebral involvement with spinal cord compression and myelographic block. Dr. Kostuik said: We have operated at all levels and I have operated on patients the same night at three and four levels, anywhere where there was a major neurological problem or an impending neurological problem based upon imaging studies showing evidence of major dural compression.

These were not necessarily all anterior approaches. It is very difficult to do them all anteriorly if you have a lesion here and a lesion there. What I have done in those cases is to do an extensive posterior sublaminar wiring with Luque rods and a posterolateral decompression. The thoracic spines were easy for a posterolateral decompression, cutting the nerve roots all on one side, rotating the cord, evacuating all the tumor necessary anteriorly and stabilizing with methylmethacrylate anteriorly if you want. The only proscription is not to sever roots bilaterally as that may lead to paraplegia. Our results on multiple level surgery are in the literature.

Prof. Louis said he presented 63 cases of total vertebrectomy for metastatic breast cancer with 8-year survivals. In addition I have 11-year survivals following vertebrectomies for malignant giant cell tumors and 3- to 4-year survivals for sarcoma. Dr. Kostuik said: I have a sarcoma with a 12-year survival, another with a 5-year survival, and one that died at 2 years. They are different. Primary tumors are different from metastatic.

Surgery for Spinal Metastasis from Cancer of the Prostate

Dr. Kostuik said that all cancer of the prostate is going to be curable within 5 years. We are very close to it now. Prof. Louis said: When the lesions are confined to one or two vertebrae I perform a resection. When the lesions are diffuse and multiple I perform only palliative surgery with a posterior decompression and stabilization.

Dr. Holtzman said: I think that this may be our aim now. We have reached the point where the technology of decompressing vertebral canal and stabilizing the spine is sufficient to allow for prolonged survivals and aggressive chemotherapy and radiotherapy as is tolerated.

Dr. Kostuik added: With prostatic cancer and the new techniques of radical prostatectomy that does not leave the patient impotent along with the new oncogenic therapies it appears that this will be a curable disease much like the leukemias. This will certainly be good for all the men here since 85% us will have cancer of the prostate by the time we are 85 years old.

CHAPTER 14

Surgical Treatment of the Unstable Thoracic Spine in Trauma and Infection

James E.O. Hughes

St. Luke's–Roosevelt and Harlem Hospital Centers in New York serve the Upper West Side of Manhattan and Harlem. In this urban setting injuries to the spine from falls are more common than from high-speed motor vehicle accidents. A high incidence of intravenous drug addiction has afforded us considerable experience with osteomyelitis and tuberculosis of the spine. Our interest in spinal stabilization has intensified over the past 10 years as the methods available for treatment have rapidly evolved with new techniques and instruments available. The posterior instrumentation has been developed specifically for scoliosis, whereas most of the anterior implants have been developed specifically for traumatic burst fractures with canal compromise.

Fractures and dislocation of the thoracic and thoracolumbar spines are typically separated into mechanisms of injury and anatomical type of fracture.

Axial compression causes either wedge compression fractures or burst fractures. In the wedge compression fracture the bone is impacted anteriorly or laterally with loss of body height. The disc is not driven into the body as it is in the burst fracture. In burst fractures, usually the upper third of the body at the level of the pedicles explodes circumferentially. Frequently a posterior portion is extruded into the canal. The amount of acceleration-deceleration of the axial compressive force is probably what determines whether the patient will suffer a burst fracture or a simple compression fracture (19). In addition to the bursting of the upper third of the body there is frequently a sagittal split (cleavage) in the lower two-thirds of the vertebra. This may extend into the lumina and posterior spinous process.

If in addition to axial loading there is flexion or rotation, there will be injuries to the pedicles, facets and ligaments, usually causing a much more serious burst fracture. Flexion injuries cause a loading force to be applied to the spine with compression loading anteriorly and tensile loading posteriorly, resulting in varying degrees of vertebral body fracture and facet capsule disruption, i.e., fracture dislocation or a flexion rotation injury (10).

Dennis describes three types of *fracture dislocation* (2):

1. *Flexion rotation*—There is complete rupture of the posterior and middle columns under tension and rotation. There are usually multiple transverse process fractures and multiple rib fractures.
2. *Shear*—There is an extension type of force with disruption of the anterior longitudinal ligament. According to Edwards (9) 2% to 3% of major spinal fractures are shear injuries. These result from a sustained translational force (severe low to the back) that ruptures the anterior ligament annulus or vertebral body, and fractures one or both facets. Shear injuries generally show both sagittal and coronal displacement without significant fracture of either vertebral body. Patients with ankylosing spondlylitis often present with shear injuries because when their calcified ligaments and disc spaces fracture, they are left without ligamentous support. Because shear injuries leave the spine unstable in all directions, further neurologic injury is likely upon rough transfer or with surgical manipulations.
3. *Flexion distraction* (seat belt or Chance fracture)—There is disruption of both posterior and middle columns under tension plus a tear of the anterior annulus fibrosis allowing stripping of the anterior longitudinal ligament during subluxation or dislocation. There is horizontal splitting of the vertebral body and neural arches throughout the pedicles with intact posterior ligaments. Edwards estimates that these injuries make up 12% of major injuries to the thoracolumbar spine. McAfee and his associates (15) reviewed 100 patients and tabulated the frequency of different types of spinal injury:

73 axial compression,
15 axial distraction,
12 translation in the transverse plane.

Spinal stability in part depends on who is asking. The emergency medical team (EMT) loading a patient onto a stretcher at the scene of the accident is asking a different question than the construction worker or professional athlete who wonders if he will be able to go back to work. A wedge compression fracture of over 50% loss of height or >20% kyphosis has a significant chance of developing into a painful kyphosis and would certainly be meaningful to the construction worker or athlete. Similarly a burst fracture with 50% canal compromise but no acute neurológical signs or symptoms may cause future symptoms (18).

Whitesides (20) characterized a stable spine as one that can withstand stress without progressive deformity or further neurologic damage.

Dennis (3) described three degrees of instability:

1. First-degree mechanical instability, which includes severe compression fractures (>50% wedging with posterior ligamentous injury) and seat belt injuries.

2. Second-degree neurological instability, which includes burst fractures with or without neurologic deficit.
3. Third-degree, which has both mechanical and neurological instability. This includes fractures, dislocations, and severe burst fractures with three-column involvement.

Inherent in Dennis's concept is that the greatest danger from spinal instability is neurological injury: therefore, any patient who has a neurological deficit or canal compromise has to be considered to have an unstable injury. This is not always true from a strictly mechanical sense in that there are certainly burst fractures with canal compromise but no injury to the pedicles or facets that others have characterized as a stable burst fracture.

Dennis's concept of the three-column spine is key to any discussion of spinal instability. As pointed out by McAfee (15), the anterior column resists compressive forces. The posterior column has a stabilizing function resisting tensile forces. The middle column (posterior cortex of the body, posterior longitudinal ligament, and annulus fibrosis) is the transition between the other two. This osteoligamentous complex is the key to the need for surgical stabilization. If the middle column has not failed, fixation is not necessary. The only exception is multiple anterior wedge compression fractures. The middle column fails in *axial compression*—burst fractures; in *tension*—flexion distraction (seat belt) and flexion dislocation; and in *translation*. In any injury where all three columns are involved there is marked instability, i.e., fracture dislocation.

Spinal stability can be evaluated very well with plain x-rays in the case of fracture dislocation and seat belt injuries. Computed tomography (CT) scan alone in these cases might miss the malalignment; hence, the CT terms "double body" and "naked facets" to denote axial dislocation seen in the transaxial scan. The burst fracture lends itself very nicely to CT scanning because the pathology causing canal compromise is in the transaxial plane. On plain x-rays these changes had to be deduced by narrowing of the disc space, fracture of the superior cortical plate or pedicle widening.

Surgical Treatment

The goals of surgical treatment of thoracic fractures are (a) restoration of vertebral height, (b) restoration of anatomical contours, and (c) decompression of a compromised canal. The timing usually depends on the patient's neurological status. The only absolute indications for emergent surgical treatment are the following (9):

1. Progressive neurological deterioration,
2. Acute spinal dislocation with residual function.

We recently had a patient with a fracture dislocation without neurological deficit. Posterior stabilization could not be done because of severe lung contusion. On the 10th day after injury while on a respirator he sat up on the edge of the bed and became paraplegic. He died suddenly 48 hours later.

Surgical decompression of the canal has raised many questions (13,21). There are patients with severe canal compromise at T12-L1 with surprisingly little deficit, and similarly patients who have recovered significant function without adequate decompression (6). McEvoy and Bradford (17) found greater improvement in patients decompressed anteriorly than in those decompressed posteriorly, which they attributed to a more complete decompression.

However, articles have been written that point out that recovery of function has not been proven to be related to complete removal of all compressing bone fragments (8,14). Most authors agree that decompression of the compromised canal is useful with neurological deficit. Jelsma et al. (11) reviewed the literature, showing that even late decompression of the spinal canal can help improve function.

Some authors feel a posterolateral decompression through either a transpedicular or costotransversectomy approach is simple and adequate (1). We do not agree. We have tried it and have not been satisfied, ending up doing a secondary anterior approach to completely decompress the canal. We have not tried intraoperative ultrasound or flexible scopes to evaluate the adequacy of the posterolateral approach as reported by others (5).

Like others we have treated burst fractures with Harrington distraction systems, intraoperative myelograms, posterolateral attempts to push the burst fragment out to the canal, and a second anterior approach.

More recently, until we started using the Kaneda system we were doing a posterior Cotrel-Dubousset (CD) fixation followed by an anterior decompression and iliac crest fusion.

The spinal surgeon will find indications to use both posterior and anterior instrumentation. Presently there are clinical fractures where one approach is clearly better than another and many situations where experienced surgeons will disagree. I will describe the posterior approach using CD rods and the use of the Kaneda system anteriorly.

The CD system is replacing Harrington rods as the preferred posterior approach. With it you can achieve segmented stabilization. It can be used in the distraction or compression modes. Any combination of laminar, transverse process, or pedicle hooks can be used as necessary. They can be clawed to prevent lateral rod displacement. Cross-linkage gives added rotation stability. Pedicle screws are available and are particularly useful in the lumbar area.

A good recent review of this system's use in trauma is by McBride (16) from Orlando, Florida.

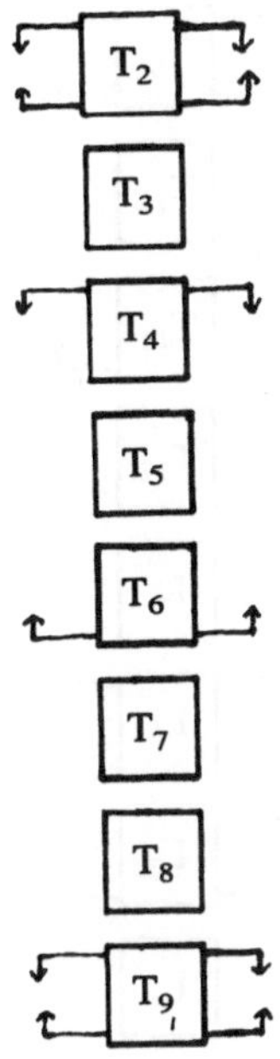

Figure 14.1. Compression construct.

In the thoracic region, fixation is three levels above and two levels below the unstable segment. The uppermost vertebral segment is clawed between the transverse process and pedicle hooks to prevent lateral rod displacement. A claw configuration at the lowest segment is also recommended. This allows switching from distraction to compression at the fracture site, allowing realignment of the spine with the distraction and compression to promote healing of the realigned fracture. There are two different configurations for the distraction and compression modes. Flexion distraction and seat belt injuries are treated with the compression mode (Fig. 14.1). Here, hooks above the unstable segment claw with the hooks below.

In situations where the middle column fails with compression, such as unstable burst fractures and common fracture dislocation, the distraction mode is used (Fig. 14.2). Here the fixation points above are pedicle hooks and the fixation points below are supralaminar hooks. This allows distraction of the compressed vertebra. When fixation extends to the lumbar region pedicle screws are used.

If we elect to use the CD system on a burst fracture with significant posterior column instability and canal compromise, we will do a secondary anterior decompression and fusion.

The burst fracture has occasioned the most controversy over treatment. The inability of posterior distraction to decompress the spinal canal with-

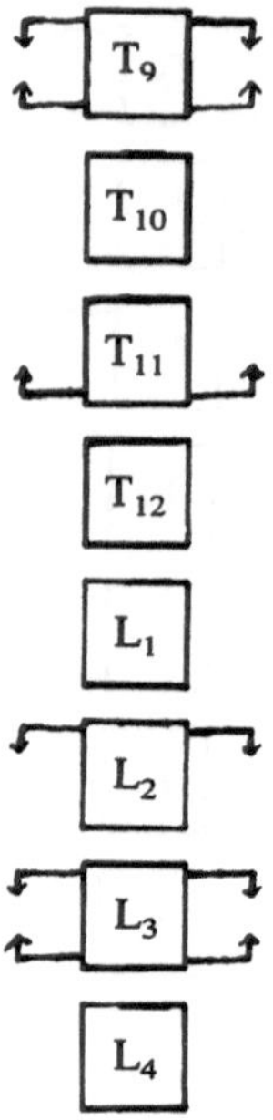

Figure 14.2. Distraction construct.

out anterolateral or anterior surgical decompression has encouraged investigators to produce an anterior device that will allow anterior decompression and instrumentation at the same time. Dunn's original device reported in 1978 had a single threaded rod (4). His last device had two curved collars connected by two threaded screws fixed to the vertebra by staples and screws (4) (Fig. 14.3). This device was withdrawn by the manufacturer after some rare late vascular complications were reported.

Kostuik et al. (13) have reported on their extensive experience with anterior fixation devices in burst fractures. They feel that unless there is severe posterior column instability, no additional posterior fixation is necessary. With their device, after doing an anterior dural decompression, the vertebra above and below are distracted with a short Harrington rod fixed with lateral transvertebral screws (Fig. 14.4).

After an appropriate iliac crest graft is placed the two vertebrae are compressed with a heavy Harrington compression rod fixed again with Kostuik spinal screws.

In 1984, Kaneda et al. (12) published the use of their low profile anterior device in 15 patients (Fig. 14.5). Since then, they have used it in over 250 patients with burst fractures. Vertebral plates are fixed to the lateral portion of the vertebral body with tetra spikes. These plates help stabilize the entry point of the four transvertebral screws that go through the cortex of the other side of the vertebra. A spreader is placed in the screw

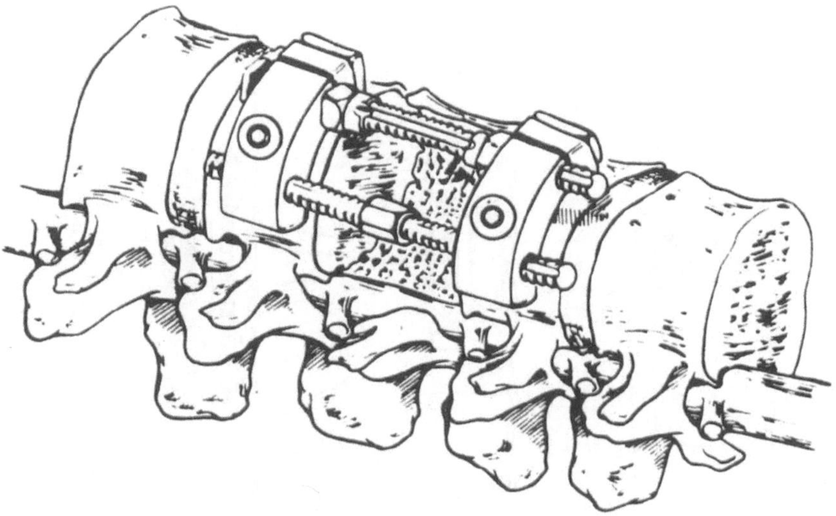

Figure 14.3. Dunn type III device. (Reprinted with permission from ref. 4.)

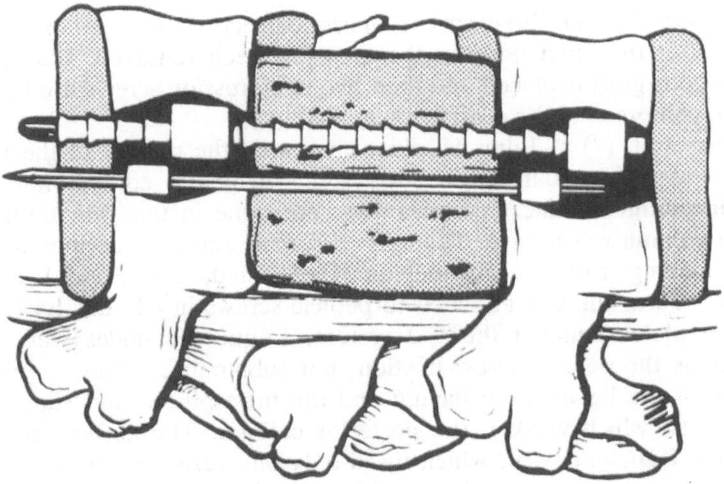

Figure 14.4. Kostuik device. (Reprinted with permission from ref. 13.)

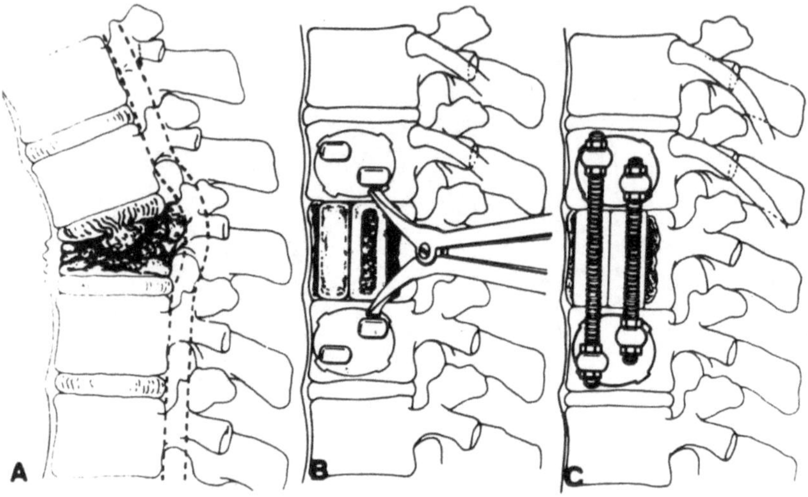

Figure 14.5. Burst fracture with anterior decompression and stabilization and anterior instrumentation using the Kaneda device. (Reprinted with permission from ref. 12.)

heads and the vertebrae spread apart, correcting the kyphosis. This is done after the burst body in the area has been removed. Iliac crest or autologous graft is placed and then two compression screws are tightened down, compressing the graft.

Gurr et al. (7) at Johns Hopkins compared the rigidity of the Kaneda device to the standard posterior systems in an L3 corpectomy model. Laminectomies or facetectomies were not done in this calf model (posterior column was intact). The excised spinal segment was studied during axial loading, rotation, and flexion. The Kaneda device (L2-L4) was as strong as was the CD attached to pedicle screws in L1, L2, L4, and L5. Steffee plates equaled the CD system. Luque rectangles were not as strong as the pedicle screw fixation, but sublaminar wiring required removal of the ligamentum flavum and the infraspinous and supraspinous ligaments, which weaken the posterior column. The authors concluded that the Kaneda device, which fused only one vertebra above and below the corpectomy, compared favorably with the CD and Steffee posterior systems, which included two additional motion segments.

This model does not answer relative strengths in disruptions of all three columns. Zdelblick et al. (22) have published another series of experiments where a dog model with three-column instability (excision of most of the L5 body and adjacent discs, L5 laminectomy, and partial facetectomy were treated with the Kaneda device, a strut graft alone, or an inert polymer spacer, with seven dogs per group). Five of the dogs in the Kaneda device group had two-level fusions and two had single-level fusions. The strut graft group produced four single-level fusions, and the control group (inert polymer spacers) two paraplegic animals. This study was designed to show the Kaneda device's ability to produce a strong fusion.

We have carefully followed the technique as outlined by Kaneda:

1. Approach the fracture from the left side unless more extensive exposure on the right is necessary.
2. L1 is exposed through the bed of T10 or T11. This is best determined by the rib that overlies the vertebra to be decompressed.
3. After adequate exposure of the fracture and the vertebral above and below, the two discs are completely removed and two-thirds of the fractured vertebra is removed. Some of the anterior vertebra on the opposite side is left to promote osteogenesis. The canal is then carefully decompressed, usually with a high-speed drill and curets.
4. Using biplanar imaging the implant tetraplates are tapped into place making sure the spikes are in the body and not in the disc.
5. The transvertebral screws are selected to make sure they just penetrate the contralateral cortex. Their final position is confirmed by the AP image.
6. The implants are now distracted using a laminar spreader on the most anterior screw heads.
7. After the kyphosis is corrected the tricortical iliac crest graft is inserted.
8. The two anterior paraspinal rods are then tightened to effectively compress the graft.
9. Two transfixing devices are added to create the desired rectangular biomechanical construct.
10. If the chest has been entered, a chest tube is placed. We also place a separate retroperitoneal drain.
11. We allow early ambulation in a thoracolumbar spinal orthosis (TLSO).

We have used the Kaneda device in a variety of burst fractures, including in a patient who was in her 70s.

The Kaneda device, like other anterior devices, cannot be used alone in burst fractures with significant posterior facet injury and posterior column instability.

Our group at St. Luke's–Roosevelt and Harlem Hospital Centers has operated on 85 patients with osteomyelitis of the spine. Nineteen of these patients have had osteomyelitis of the thoracic spine. Sixteen presented with cord compression and myelopathy. One patient had severe spine and radicular pain after an unsuccessful attempt at transthoracic debridement at another hospital. Two other patients had only severe spine pain and nondiagnostic needle biopsies. Seventeen patients had transthoracic exposure and complete removal of involved bone, discs, and granulation tissue. The dura is always decompressed, the kyphosis corrected, and interbody fusions done. In the thoracic area we almost always use a left thoracotomy, removing the rib above the infected disc space.

It is rare to encounter much real pus. Paraspinal abscesses are very unusual. Free pus, however, is no contraindication to fusions.

Fourteen patients were fused with pieces of the removed rib. Two patients were fixed with iliac crest grafts. Usually the first piece of rib is tightly wedged in the distracted decompression site. The other pieces of rib are wedged adjacent to the first rib. We usually bundle the ribs together with an absorbable suture. We have had no graft displacement during the hospital stay and know of no late pseudarthroses. However, these patients, many of whom are drug addicts, do not lend themselves to good long-term follow-up.

The thoracotomy patients are nursed in the semi-Fowler's position and are allowed to dangle without braces. We try to have a polyethylene TLSO ready for the patient when they are able to ambulate. Uncooperative patients frequently ambulate when the chest tube is out, whether the brace is available or not. We have had no instances of increasing neurologic deficit due to increasing angulation postoperative in the thoracic patients. This is a constant problem in cervical cases where uncooperative patients have removed their halos or tongs.

We have not used anterior instrumentation in any thoracic case. We are very reluctant to consider implants in addicts. We have used the Kaneda device once successfully in a non-drug addict with osteomyelitis at L2-3.

Two patients had thoracic disc space debridement through a transrib approach (Fig. 14.6). The CT scan demonstrates if the head of the rib articulates with the pathology. In the upper thorax the head of the rib articulates across the disc space. After the correct rib has been identified by image, a 3-inch skin incision is made over the rib about 2 inches off the midline. After the dorsal surface of the rib is exposed, a high-speed drill is used to get inside the center of the rib. The center of the rib is cored out until the spine is encountered. The intercostal artery and its foraminal branches are easily avoided. The exposure allows insertion of pituitary rongeurs into the disc space or vertebra (Fig. 14.7). We have usually done this procedure under local anesthesia; AP and lateral imaging assure accurate and safe instrument placement.

We have operated on 25 patients with Pott's disease. Most of these patients have had neurologic deficits or Pott's paraplegia. In the thoracic area we have always gone transthoracically when there is cord compression. As in the osteomyelitis cases, we completely remove the infected bone, granulation tissue and granuloma. The normal disc (acid-fast bacteria does not stimulate dissolution of the disc) is also removed. The posterior longitudinal ligament is removed. We never open the dura.

We have operated on patients transthoracically who have had previous

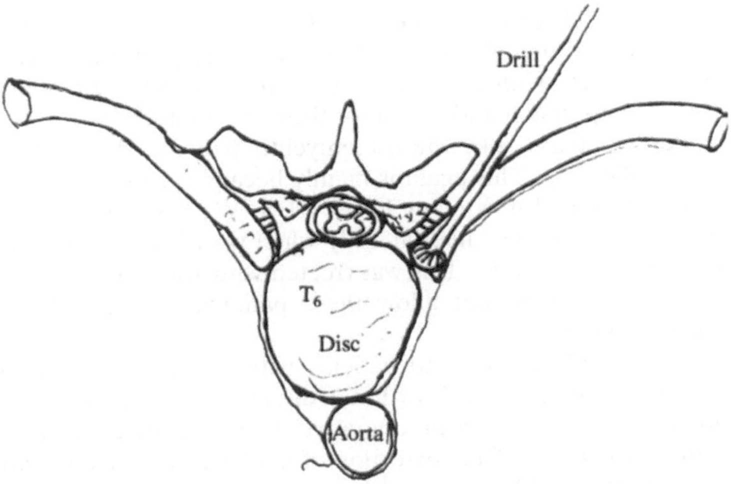

Figure 14.6. Transrib vertebral approach.

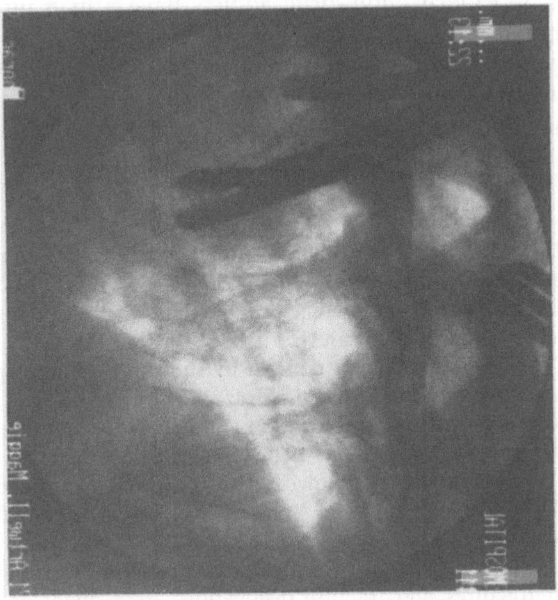

Figure 14.7. Transrib vertebral biopsy.

laminectomies. These patients eventually fuse but have to be nursed in bed for prolonged periods of time. We now would instrument this type of patient posteriorly with a CD compression construct after doing transthoracic decompression and fusion for the cord compression.

Our Pott's patients, like the osteomyelitis patients, do not have good long-term follow-up. This again is mainly because many of these patients are drug addicts and now many have AIDS. We have one Pott's patient with rib grafts who angulated laterally when we tried to sit her up in the first week postoperatively. This was treated with 1 month of bed rest with a good result. We do not allow these patients out of bed without a polyethylene TLSO.

As our surgical approach to patients with thoracic cord compression due to pyogenic osteomyelitis or Pott's disease is essentially the same, we are not concerned about a preoperative diagnosis. In either case, complete dural decompression, correction of kyphosis, and fusion with rib or iliac crest graft would be performed.

Excised material is cultured and examined by Gram stain and acid-fast techniques. Most pyogenic cases have been due to *staphylococcus aureus* in drug addicts. Elderly, non–drug addicts have a high incidence of urinary tract organisms.

If no pyogenic organism is seen on Gram stain and the bacterial culture is negative, the patients have been treated with AMT (antimicrobiol therapy) until the TB cultures are reported as normal.

References

1. Abitbol JJ, Garfin SR. Posterolateral spinal canal decompression for traumatic injuries. *Semin Spine Surg*. 1990;2(1):35–40.
2. Dennis F. The three column spine and its significance in the classification of acute thoraco lumbar spinal injuries. *Spine*. 1983;8:817–831.
3. Dennis F. Spinal instability as defined by the three-column spine concept in acute spinal trauma. *Clin Orthop Rel Res*. 1984;189:65–76.
4. Dunn HK. Anterior spine stabilization and decompression for thoracolumbar injuries. *Orthop Clin North Am*. 1986;17(1):113–119.
5. Eismont FJ, Green BA, Berkowitz BM. The role of intra operative ultrasonography in the treatment of thoracic and lumbar spine fractures. *Spine*. 1984;9:782–787.
6. Gaines RN, Humphreys WG. A plea for judgement in management of thoracolumbar fractures and fracture dislocation. Assessment of surgical indications. *Clin Orthop Rel Res*. 1984;189:36–42.
7. Gurr KR, McAfee PC, Shik C. Biomechanical analysis of anterior and posterior instrumentation systems after corpectomy: A calf-spine model. *J Bone Joint Surg*. 1988;70-A:1182–1191.
8. Haas N, Blauth M, Tschome H. Anterior plating in thoracolumbar spine injuries. *Spine*. 1991;16(suppl 3):5100–5111.
9. Hanley EN, Simpkins A, Phillips ED. Fracture of the thoracic thoracolumbar

and lumbar Spine: Classification basis for treatment and timing of surgery. *Semi Spine Surg*. 1990;2:227.

10. Jacobs RR, Asher MA, Snider RK. Thoracolumbar spinal injuries: a comparative study of recumbent and operative treatment in 100 patients. *Spine*. 1980;5(5):463–477.
11. Jelsma RK, Rice JF, Jelsma LF, Kirsch PT. The demonstration and significance of neural compression after spinal injury. *Surg Neurol*. 1982;18:79–92.
12. Kaneda K, Abumi K, Fujiya M. Burst fractures with neurologic deficits of the thoracolumbar spine: results of anterior decompression and stabilization with anterior instrumentation. *Spine*. 1984;9(8):788–795.
13. Kostuik J, Huler RJ, Eases SI. Thoracolumbar Spine Fracture. In: Frymoyer JW, ed. *The Adult Spine: Principle and Practice*. New York: Raven Press; 1991.
14. McAfee PC, Bohlman HH, Yuan HA. Anterior decompression of traumatic thoracolumbar fractures with incomplete neurological deficit using retroperitoneal approach. *J Bone Joint Surg*. 1985;67A:89–104.
15. McAfee RG, Yuan HA, Fredrickson BE. The value of computed tomography in thoracolumbar fractures. *J Bone Joint Surg*. 1983;65A:461.
16. McBride GG. Surgical stabilization of thoracolumbar fractures using Cotrel-Dubousset rods. *Semin Spine Surg*. 1990;2(1):24–30.
17. McEvoy RD, Bradford DS. The management of burst fractures of the thoracic and lumbar spine. Experience in 53 patients. *Spine*. 1985;10:631–637.
18. Trafton PG, Boyd CA. Computed tomography of thoracic and lumbar spine injuries. *J Trauma*. 1984;24:506.
19. Watkins RG. Decision making in thoraco-lumbar and lumbar fractures. In: Cauthen JC ed. *Lumbar Spine Surgery—Indication, Techniques, Failures, and Alternatives*. Baltimore: Williams & Wilkins; 1988:273–331.
20. Whitesides TE. Traumatic kyphosis of the thoracolumbar spine. *Clin Orthop*. 1977;128:78–92.
21. Whitesides TE, Shak SG. On the management of unstable fractures of the thoraco lumbar spine. Rationale for the use of anterior decompression and fusion and posterior stabilization. *Spine*. 1976;1:99–107.
22. Zdelblick TA, Shirado O, McAfee PC, Degroot H, Warden KE. Anterior spinal fixation after lumbar corpectomy: A study in dogs. *J Bone Joint Surg*. 1991;73-A(4): 527–534.

Discussion

The Recrudescence of Tuberculosis

Dr. Kostuik said: There is no doubt that TB in the so-called Western world is increasing. It appears to be reaching the incidence levels of 40 to 50 years ago in metropolitan areas such as New York. The reasons include immunosuppression with the AIDS epidemic, drug abuse with malnutrition, diabetes mellitus, and different immigration patterns. I think it is particularly acute in New York City as compared to the rest of continental North America. We are seeing much more of it than in Chicago, Philadelphia, or Toronto, though I don't know about Los Angeles yet.

The only thing I would add to Dr. Hughes's comments is that in older people, in order to enhance their rehabilitation, we will take them either the same day or at a staged procedure to the operating room for a posterior stabilization to allow them to get up out of bed and get going, particularly because older people do not tolerate orthoses or casts well. Dr. Hughes completely concurred with these remarks.

Dr. Neuwirth said: I have had a couple of cases of osteomyelitis with tremendous amounts of bone destruction. These were cases of bacterial osteomyelitis, not tubercular. They were kyphotic and very, very sick. Since the osteomyelitis was in their midthoracic spines, I was concerned about opening their chests. I did bilateral costotransversectomies, reached with my hand around the front of the vertebral column, thoroughly decompressed the canal, stabilized them posteriorly, and they healed perfectly well.

Dr. Kostuik said: Sure, you can get away with it, but someday you will have a problem with one of the radicular arteries and the patient will become paraplegic. That has happened to me.

Dr. Farcy said: We, too, are seeing a great deal of Pott's disease including abscesses containing enormous amounts of pus. Some of the tuberculous strains that we are encountering are resistant to all antibiotics. Some may be partially susceptible to ethambutol in combination with newer antimycobacterial agents. Dr. Harold Neu at Columbia-Presbyterian recommends not beginning treatment without a positive culture. Dr. Neuwirth emphasized that in many of these cases you can submit large amounts of necrotic material to the laboratory and not have any bacterial growth. Dr. Farcy continued: Since we have been under pressure from our colleagues, we have been more careful not to begin antibiotic therapy until open biopsy is performed. Consequently our outcome in terms of identifying organisms has remarkably improved.

Lastly, Dr. Sonntag pointed out that there is a considerable delay in the time frame from presentation to actual diagnosis and treatment. This may be, in some cases, a period of months. Dr. Kostuik noted that in his experience the average time from onset of symptoms, including pyrexia, is about 16 weeks.

Factors Related to Bony Union in Osteomyelitis

Dr. Farcy said: In the low thoracic and thoracolumbar regions I have had better results with vascularized rib grafts. I am not certain whether it is the direct perfusion of the area with intravenous antibiotics or other factors. Dr. Kostuik said that in his experience nonunion has never been a problem. The problem with rib grafts in older people is that they may be very soft and not offer sufficient support.

Several additional points are worth making concern the use of instrumentation and the possibility of it loosening some time later. In relation to CD fixation no matter which mode you want to use, the distraction mode or the compression mode, if you decide to go two levels above and two below, put a claw on, either a pedicle hook claw or a hook-hook claw and it will be possible to perform any distraction or compression that is required since you have a doubly stable fixation. Dr. Kostuik concurred, saying that often occurred with the use of bilateral Harrington distraction rods. You would distract one side and the other side would loosen.

Similarly, Dr. Farcy continued, when one puts screws in the apex of a curve such as the lumbar curve your screws must be positioned in a divergent manner since they carry and bear the load better. Dr. Kostuik said: That is one of the big advantages of the AO fixator compared to the CD system, which in my opinion is far superior. Dr. Farcy said double threaded screws can achieve the same result as the AO fixator.

CHAPTER 15

The Lateral Extracavitary Approach to the Thoracic and Lumbar Spine

Paul C. McCormick

In many cases of spinal instability, there coexists encroachment of the spinal canal with spinal cord or nerve root compression. Depending on etiology and clinical circumstances, consideration must be given not only to spinal stabilization but decompression or reconstruction of the spinal canal as well. These requirements can create a management dilemma because although most spinal instrumentation systems are applied posteriorly, spinal cord compression is most often ventral in origin. Many solutions to this problem have been offered. Examples include simultaneous operative exposure, anterior instrumentation systems, and a variety of indirect or blind posterior reductions/decompression techniques. The advantages and limitations of these procedures are well known.

This chapter describes the lateral extracavitary approach to the thoracic and lumbar spine, which can be quite useful when extensive exposure of the spine is required. This approach, originally described by Capener (2) and more recently popularized by Larson et al. (3), allows simultaneous dorsal and ventral exposure for decompression and circumferential bone/instrumentation stabilization to be achieved through a single "hockey stick" incision (Fig. 15.1).

Operative Procedure

Routine induction and intubation of the patient are performed. An arterial line and large bore intravenous access, usually central, is recommended because of the potential for prolonged operative duration and substantial blood loss associated with this procedure. Under appropriate circumstances preoperative autologous blood donation, cell saver, and isovolemic hemodilution prior to induction, may reduce the reliance on banked blood. The ideal banked product, in our opinion, is single donor whole blood that is reconstituted (fresh frozen plasma plus packed red blood cells) on the day of the surgery.

The patient is carefully turned into the prone position with the arms

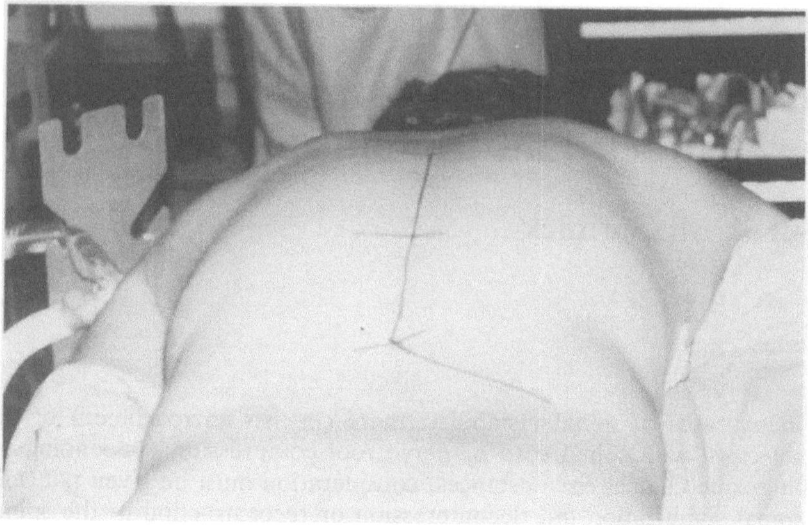

Figure 15.1. Operative photograph demonstrates skin incision for lateral extracavitary approach. The crosshatch at the center of the midline incision is centered over the pathology. Note the oblique angle of the lateral limb portion of the incision.

tucked in at the sides, which diminishes the risk of brachial plexus or ulnar nerve palsies that may be associated with prolonged operations with the arms held in an abducted position. Although any of the "knee-chest" frames are acceptable, we prefer standard chest rolls with care taken to minimize abdominal and chest compression. A smaller roll is placed on the side opposite the planned exposure (Fig. 15.2). This allows greater tilting of the table for a true three-quarter prone view during the ventral decompression. Benzel (1) has described this approach of the patient in a standard three-quarter prone position, which allows better ventral visualization and less intra-abdominal venous pressure. However, this position may be somewhat awkward when applying posterior instrumentation. Positioning and maintaining this position may be hazardous to the patient with a highly unstable spine. A brachial plexus palsy in the dependent arm may also occur in this position. However, by placing the patient on a smaller chest roll, the surgeon is able to perform the operation and alternate between a standard position for the initial exposure and placement of spinal instrumentation with the three-quarter prone exposure, which is employed by tilting the table during the time of ventral decompression.

A hockey stick incision is planned with a long limb centered over the level of pathology in the midline. The short limb is gently curved laterally

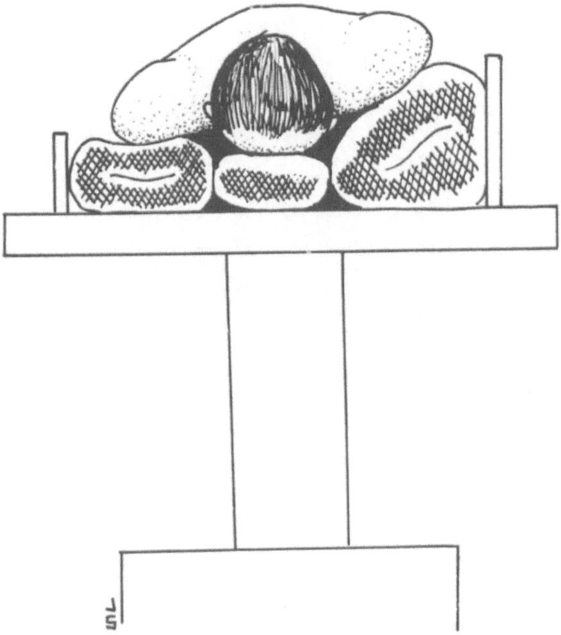

Figure 15.2. Schematic diagram of operative position showing the uneven sizes of the chest rolls.

about 10 to 12 cm off the midline (Fig. 15.1). An acute 90° angle often results in skin necrosis and slough in the corner of the wound. The midline portion of the wound is opened first and a standard subperiosteal exposure of the posterior elements is performed. Since the skin incision cannot be lengthened caudally following opening of the lateral limb, the spinal levels must be checked to assure that enough caudal exposure has been obtained for the instrumentation prior to lateral extension limb incision. In the lumbar region, the incision is carried down through the thoracodorsal fascia, which represents the medial extension of the latissimus dorsi muscle (Fig. 15.3). Medially, this fascia is fused to the paraspinal muscle fascia at their common spinous process insertion. This connection is divided sharply along the entire longitudinal extent of the midline incision. This creates a skin/subcutaneous tissue/thoracodorsal fascia flap, which is retracted laterally to expose the longitudinally oriented paraspinal (i.e., erector spinae) muscles on one side (Fig. 15.3). Previous reports described a skin/subcutaneous flap to be developed superficial to the thoracodorsal fascia with a separate T-shaped fascial incision at the level of the pathology (1,3). This has been modified to include the fascia in the flap because a separate dissection does not aid the exposure, and trouble-

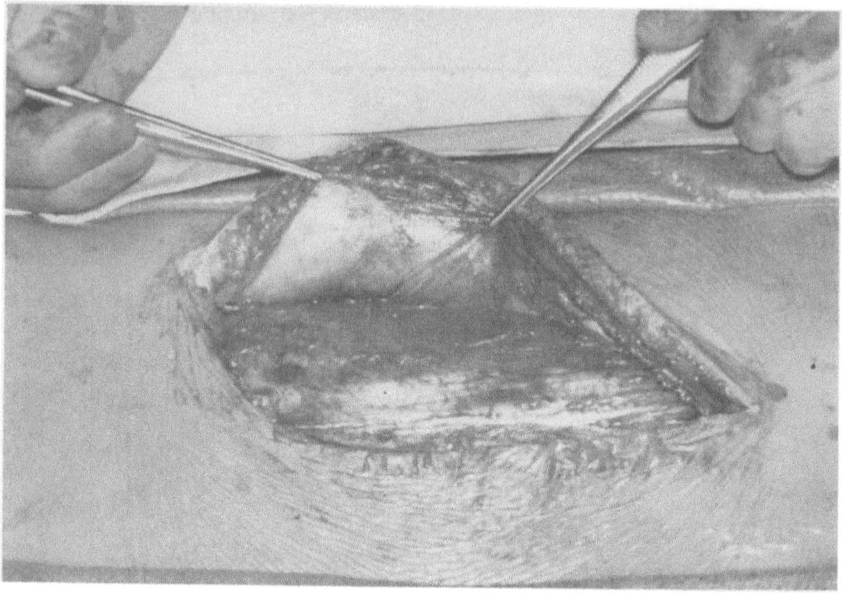

A

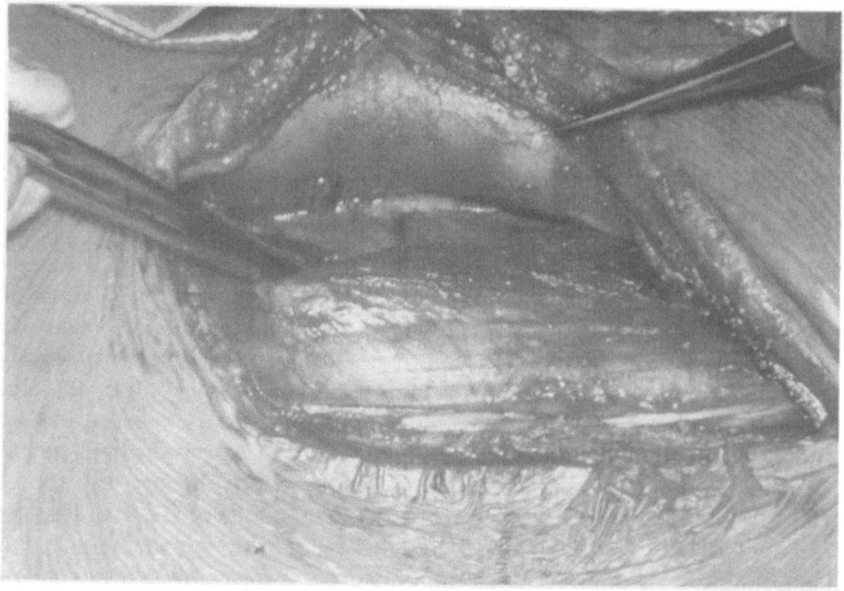

B

Figure 15.3. **A:** Operative photograph of initial exposure. The skin subcutaneous tissue and thoracodorsal fascia have been raised laterally to expose the longitudinally oriented paraspinal muscles. **B:** The lateral border of the paraspinal muscles is elevated and displaced medially. This exposes the quadratus lumborum muscle in the lumbar region and the ribs at the thoracic level. **C:** Operative photograph of medially directed view following elevation of the paraspinal muscles. The transverse processes of L1 and L2 can be seen and have been freed of their attachments. This is shown schematically in **D**.

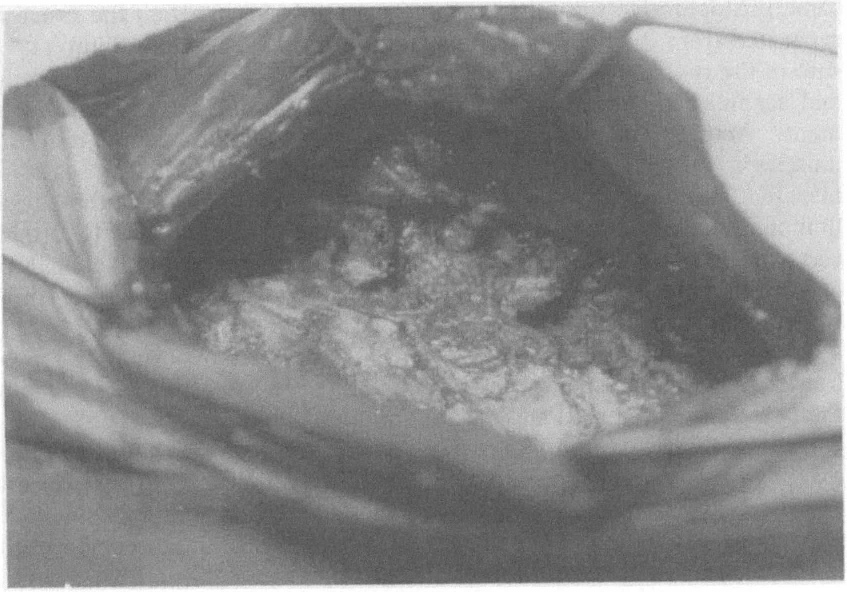

C

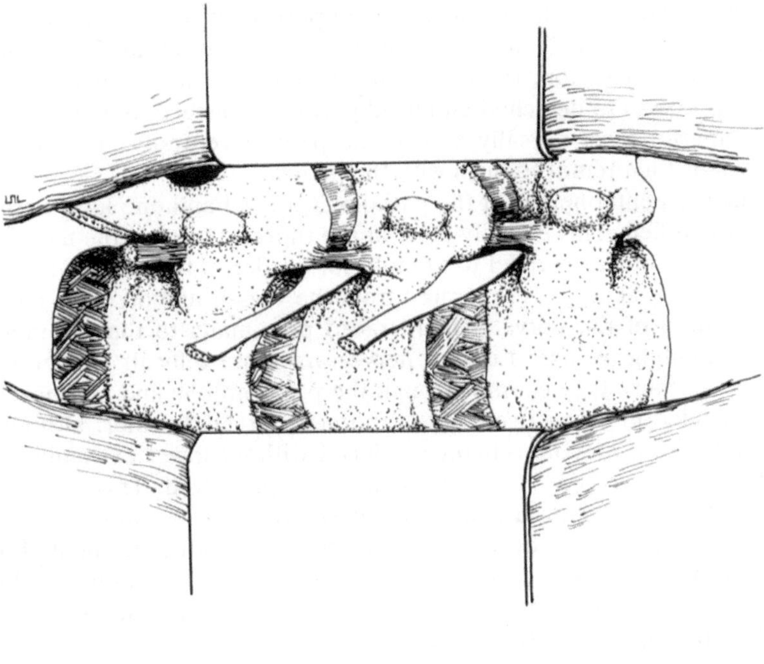

D

some postoperative wound seromas consistently occur when the fascia is separated from the overlying subcutaneous tissue. The lateral limb exposure in the thoracic region is complicated by the presence of the trapezius and scapular muscles, and the ribs and their associated muscle attachments. Actually, the exposure of thoracic region is quite simple if all the muscles superficial to the longitudinally oriented paraspinal muscles are elevated laterally with the skin flap. Depending on the level of the lateral limb incision, all muscles at this level above the paraspinal muscles are incised, in line with the skin incision. This applies even in the higher thoracic levels because the longitudinally oriented paraspinal muscles are a constant landmark throughout the thoracic and lumbar spine.

Irrespective of level, the flap is elevated laterally to exposure the lateral border of the paraspinal muscles (Fig. 15.3). The paraspinal muscles are then easily elevated medially off the quadratus lumborum and psoas muscles in the lumbar region and ribs in the thoracic region. The longitudinal extent of this mobilization must be adequate so that the paraspinal muscles can be retracted medially up over the facet joints at at least one level above and below the pathologic vertebral segment. In the thoracic region, a subperiosteal exposure of the ribs to be resected is performed. This usually includes the rib at the involved level as well as one level above and below. If necessary, the upper rib can be preserved as can most of the lower rib except for its most medial portion at the disc space, but this will limit exposure. Transverse processes at these levels are also removed. At the lumbar region, the musculoligamentous attachments to the transverse process are detached and a subperiosteal dissection is performed to the superior facet dorsally and to the pedicle ventrally. The transverse process is then removed flush with the pedicle.

The segmental nerves at the pathological level and one level above are then identified. This is easily done at the thoracic level as the neurovascular bundle courses parallel to the inferior border of the corresponding rib. The intercostal nerve is separated from the vessels and divided. The proximal stump of the nerve is then traced proximally to the foramina and corresponding pedicle. Lumbar nerves are more difficult to identify and dissect because they course through the psoas muscle and are more vertically angled in comparison to the thoracic nerves. Further, although the L1 nerve root may be reliably sacrificed without lower extremity deficit, the remainder of the lumbar roots must be preserved. This creates some difficulty because the surgeon must work around (i.e., above and below) the nerve during the decompression and bone graft placement. For this reason, the nerve should be dissected over a generous extent to allow for greater mobilization of the nerve during dissection. This decreases the risk of postoperative stretch palsy. An occasional consequence of root resection between T10 and L1 is the development of a postoperative abdominal hernia. These are usually asymptomatic and create a cosmetic inconvenience but occasionally may be quite painful. Once the nerve root at the level of pathology and one level above have been dissected to the corresponding foramina, the entire lateral aspect of the vertebral body and intervening discs are exposed. The pleura and the thoracic region and psoas muscle at the lumbar levels are displaced ventrally. This is performed with a periosteal elevator directly on the bone to prevent pleural entry or injury to proximal segmental vessels at the midbody level. Attachments tend to be more tenacious at the disc spaces, which require sharp dissection.

It is at this point that the table can be tilted away from the surgeon to allow a three-quarter prone exposure. The pedicle is identified between the two segmental nerves and resected with a Kerrison punch. A parallel view of the ventral canal/dural interface is now achieved. Visualization is improved if the lateral margin of the overlying facet joints, pars, and lamina are also removed. The discs are sharply incised, curetted, and removed. The corpectomy is then performed using any variety of rongeurs, high-speed drill, and curets. The most troublesome aspect of the decompression is the epidural bleeding, which may become profuse once the epidural space is decompressed. This is minimized by performing a generous corpectomy and thinning of the intracanal fragment prior to canal decompression. The final step of the decompression is to push the intracanal pathology (e.g., bone fragment) down into the corpectomy defect. Reverse angle curets are best suited for this maneuver. The canal is thus quickly decompressed and epidural bleeding is controlled with Gelfoam. The retractors are removed and the patient is turned back into a prone position. Midline retractors are placed to expose the posterior elements and the selected spinal instrumentation is placed.

Following instrumentation, the patient is placed back into the three-quarter prone position for placement of the interbody bone graft. Either rib, iliac crest, or allograft (e.g., femoral head), may be used depending on bone quality, spinal level, clinical circumstance, and surgeon preference. In the vast number of healthy patients, we have found that two or three pieces of rib autografts provide adequate support at all levels. Small troughs may be cut into the adjacent vertebral bodies to prevent graft migration. Some surgeons, however, prefer not to violate the adjacent end plates to minimize "pistoning" of the bone graft into the cancellous bone of the adjacent vertebrae. Once the graft has been placed, the nerve roots that have been sacrificed are clipped proximal to the dorsal root ganglion to prevent a painful postoperative neuralgia. The pleura is inspected and small holes are repaired with suture. If large pleural defects exist or if there is an air leak, a chest tube should be placed. Otherwise, a suction drain alone in the paraspinal space is sufficient. The lateral border of the paraspinal muscles is loosely tacked down with suture. The remainder of the wound is closed in layers.

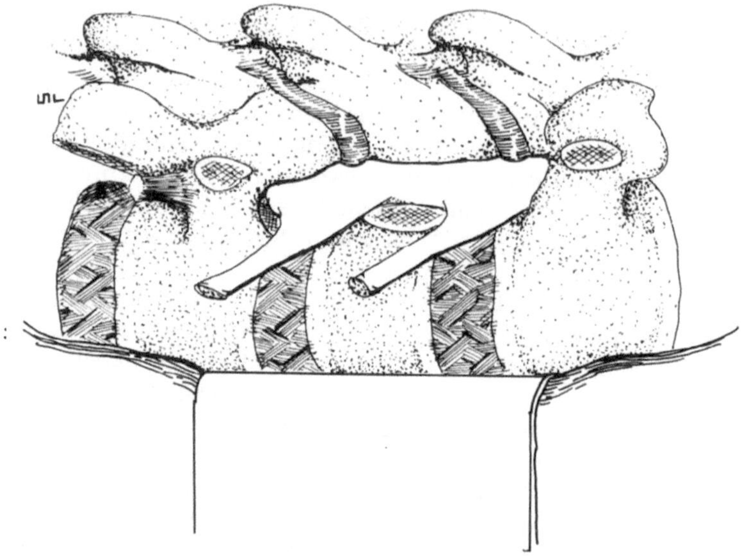

A

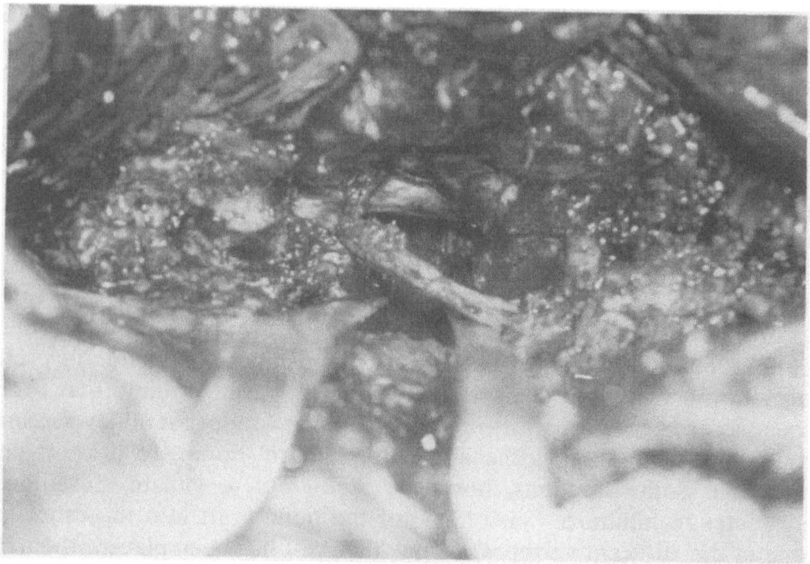

B

Figure 15.4. **A:** Schematic diagram demonstrates initial portion of bony removal to include transverse processes, facet joint, and pedicle at the involved level. **B:** Operative photograph following partial corpectomy and discectomy at the L1-2 level. The corpectomy defect is easily appreciated ventral to the dural sac. The L1 nerve root with its corresponding ganglion can be seen coursing obliquely across the operative field. **C:** A bone graft has now been placed in the corpectomy defect with preservation of the L1 nerve root. This can be seen schematically in **D**.

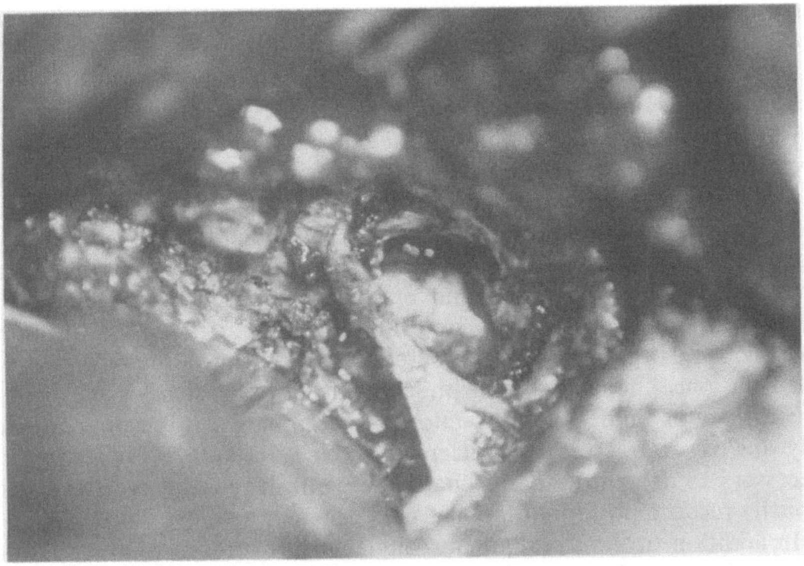

C

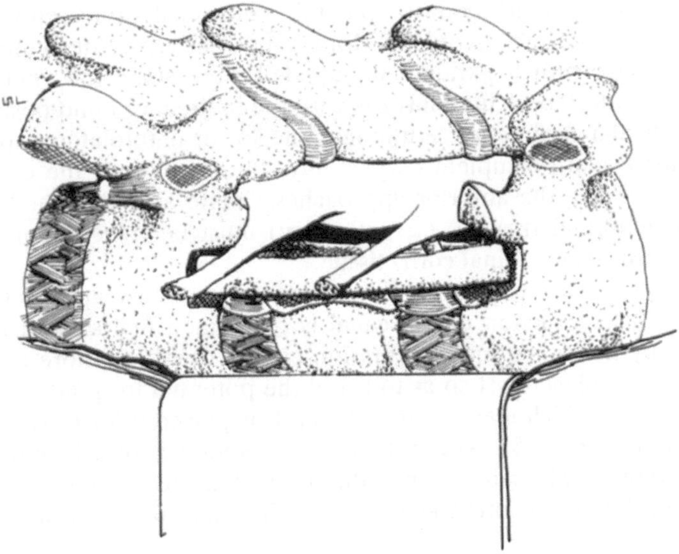

D

Figure 15.4. (*cont.*)

Discussion

The lateral extracavitary approach has been extremely useful for traumatic, neoplastic, inflammatory, or degenerative conditions of the spine in which simultaneous dorsal and ventral exposure is required. The ability to perform a near-complete corpectomy and decompress the entire transverse width of the spinal canal fundamentally differentiate this approach from the standard costotransversectomy. Dumbbell tumors with both intraspinal and extraspinal extension, even with an intradural component, are also adequately exposed and removed through this exposure (Fig. 15.4) (4). This approach may be utilized from T2 to L5. At the upper thoracic levels the exposure is limited somewhat by the narrow thoracic inlet, but once the medial attachment of the scapular muscles are divided, as with any midline spinal dissection, the scapula is easily retracted laterally and ventral access is sufficient. At the L4-5 and L5-S1 levels, it is necessary to detach the paraspinal muscles from the iliac crest and occasionally resect a portion of the iliac crest for adequate exposure.

In addition to the simultaneous single-stage exposure that can be performed by a single surgical team with the patient in a safe and neutral position, there are other advantages to this approach. The potential for morbidity or complications of pleural, peritoneal cavity entry and diaphragm division are avoided. More importantly, the decompression is done directly with a parallel, unimpeded view along the ventral–dural pathology interface. This contrasts with the indirect or blind posterior and transpedicular techniques. Although anterior or anterolateral approaches allow for a more complete corpectomy, the location of the canal is not apparent. Thus, the anterior approaches violate a fundamental principle in that abnormal tissue (i.e., pathology) must be traversed in order to reach normal (i.e., spinal cord) tissue.

The operative sequence of the lateral extracavitary approach is quite logical. Reconstruction of the canal is performed first so that any force applied by the spinal instrumentation can be delivered more safely. The bone graft is placed last so as to avoid the potential for graft dislodgment or loosening, which may occur if the graft is placed prior to spinal instrumentation (Fig. 15.5). The potential disadvantages of this approach are considerable. This can be an arduous, technically difficult exposure of long duration and is often associated with significant blood loss. Even in

→

Figure 15.5. **A:** Postmyelogram CT shows a burst fracture of L1 with retropulsion of bony fragments into the spinal canal. There is compression of the spinal cord. **B:** Operative photograph of medially directed view following decompression and instrumentation. The paraspinal muscles have been elevated dorsally. The psoas muscles are depressed with a malleable retractor. The T12 and L1 nerve roots have been cut and are suspended by suture ligatures. The corpectomy defect has

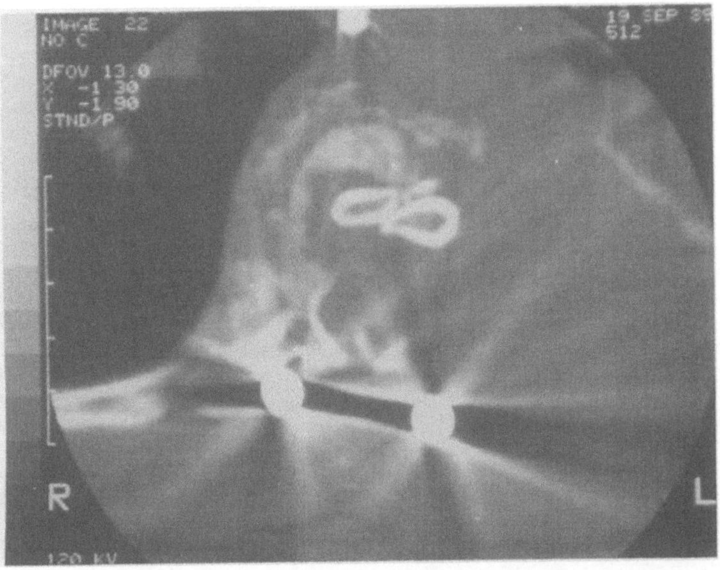

A

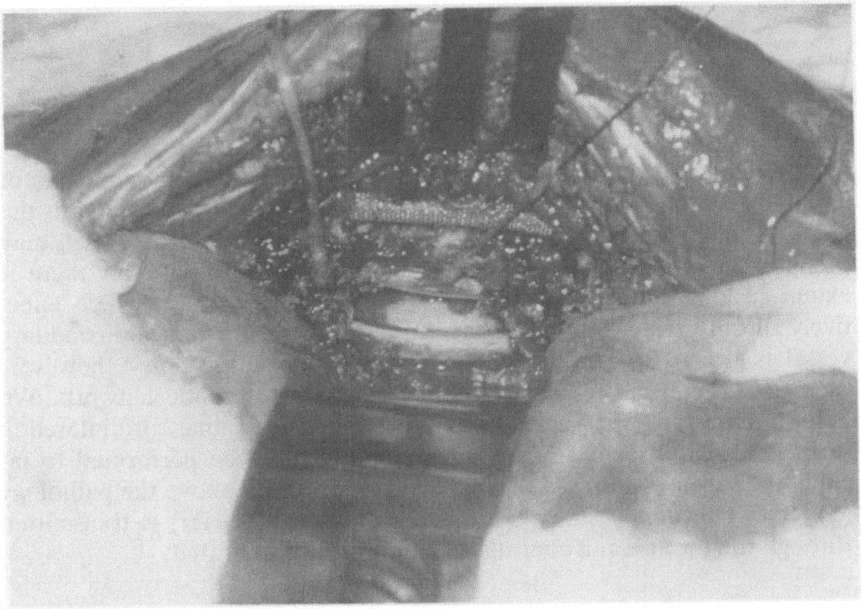

B

been filled with two rib struts. The spinal instrumentation with Cotrel-Dubousset rods can also be appreciated. **C:** Postoperative CT scan demonstrates extent of corpectomy. A nearly complete corpectomy has been performed with decompression of the spinal canal across to the contralateral pedicle. The two rib struts are in good position, well away from the spinal canal.

C 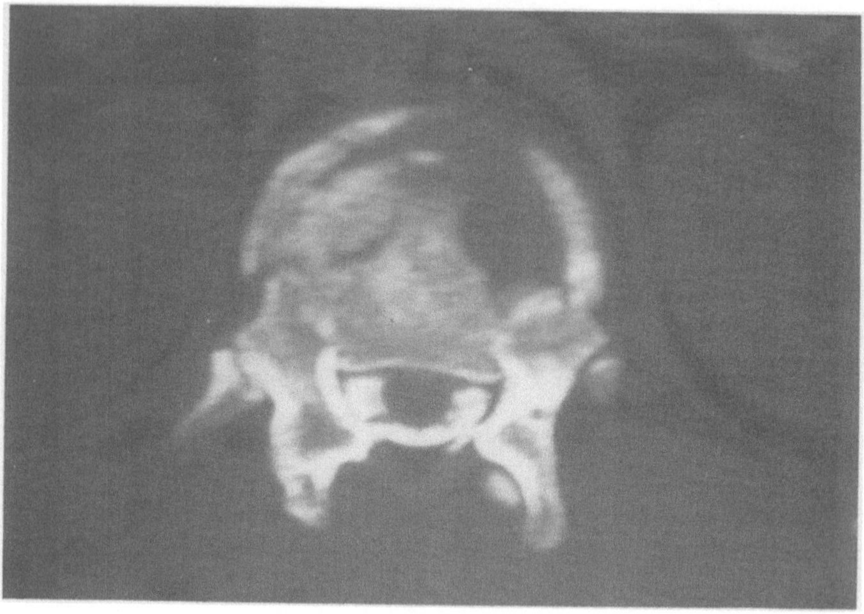

Figure 15.5. *(cont.)*

experienced hands, an operative time of 5 to 6 hours with an average blood loss of 1,500 to 3,000 ml can be anticipated. Since it is a transforaminal approach, consideration must also be given to the consequences of radiculomedullary vessel occlusion. Abundant clinical evidence with the anterior and anterolateral approaches suggests that segmental vessels may be ligated without the risk of spinal cord ischemia. Presumably there is extensive longitudinal and transverse muscle anastomoses, which effectively distally reconstitute the ligated vessel. When a radiculomedullary vessel is ligated distally (i.e., foramen) near its dural entry, however, there exists only an unpredictable intradural anastomotic network. We believe, therefore, that since there may be a risk of spinal cord infarction in these cases, selective spinal angiography should be performed to include the segmental vessels at the level and one level above the pathology (5). If a radiculomedullary (e.g., artery of Adamkiewicz) is transmitted through the foramina, a contralateral approach is indicated.

References

1. Benzel EC. The lateral extracavitary approach to the spine using the three-quarter prone position. *J Neurosurg*. 1989;71:837–841.
2. Capener N. The evolution of lateral rhachotomy. *J Bone Joint Surg [Br]*. 1954;36:173–179.

3. Larson SJ, Holst RA, Hemmy DC, et al. Lateral extracavitary approach to traumatic lesions of the thoracic and lumbar spine. *J Neurosurg*. 1976;45:628–637.
4. McCormick PC, Post KD, Stein BM. Intradural extramedullary tumors in adults. *Neurosurg Clin North Am*. 1990;1(3):591–608.
5. McCormick PC, Stein BM. Functional anatomy of the spinal cord and related structures. *Neurosurg Clin North Am*. 1990;1(3):469–490.

Discussion

Dr. Sonntag inquired as to the source of bone for grafting. Dr. McCormick replied that both rib and tibial allograft have been used.

Dr. Hughes was very pleased with this approach and acknowledged that in the case presented it was ideal since the tumor could not have been removed in its entirety from either an anterior or posterior approach. The lack of need for two surgical teams also makes it appealing. The only question to be raised is, How many of these cases will fit as perfectly as this one has?

Dr. Bennett said: Dr. McCormick, certainly one has to individualize approaches, but this should be in the armamentarium of all spine surgeons and it is for that reason that I have emphasized it. He also mentioned that spinal angiography is performed for all of these cases and there is at present the unanswered question of muscle atrophy due to the exposure.

CHAPTER 16

Lumbar Spine Instability

Patrick F. O'Leary

This chapter addresses the biomechanical principles of spinal instability and their practical application. For this purpose some simplified concepts of instability are suggested and supported by specific case studies. These concepts include *longitudinal instability* (L)—manifested by disc space collapse in disc degeneration and in the postdiscectomy syndrome; *translational instability* (T)—exemplified by spondylolisthesis; *angular instability* (A)—as is seen in the kyphotic deformity with wedge fractures; *rotational instability* (R)—exemplified by scoliosis; and *complex instability* (C)—which is a combination, either (T + L) or (T + L + R).

Case Reports

Longitudinal Instability

1. This 35-year-old woman presented with mechanical symptoms consisting solely of low back pain. Magnetic resonance imaging (MRI) demonstrated L5-S1 disc degeneration and a midline herniated disc (Fig. 16.1A). She was treated with discectomy and a posterior intertransverse fusion with a good outcome (Fig. 16.1B).
2. This patient in the mid-40s age group presented with mechanical low back pain without sciatic or neurological signs. Treatment consisted of facet screw fixation and posterior intertransverse fusion with a good outcome (Fig. 16.2).
3. This patient presented with mechanical low back pain without sciatica or neurological findings. An MRI and plain radiographs showed marked degenerative disc disease at L4-L5 and to a lesser extent at L5-S1. Treatment consisted of double level facet screw fixation and intertransverse fusion (Fig. 16.3).
4. This 45-year-old woman with a 20-year history of mechanical low back pain presented with 2 years of progressive pseudoclaudication symptomatology without neurological deficits. A myelogram showed

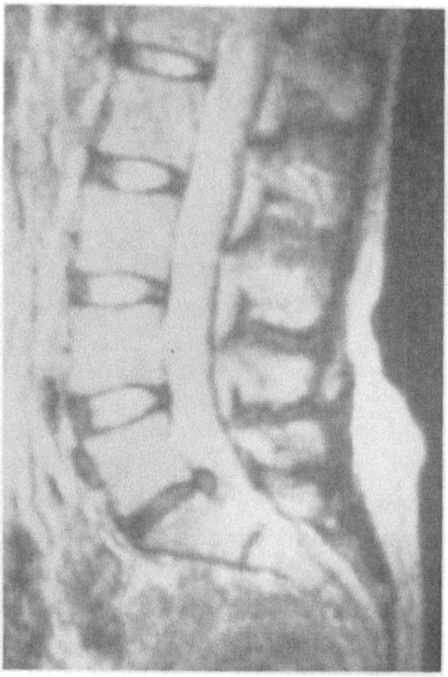

A

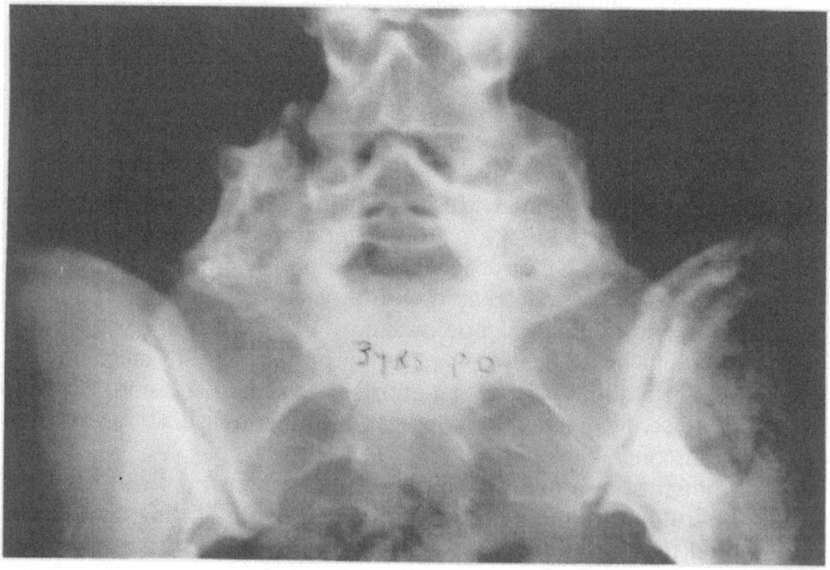

B

Figure 16.1. **A:** Lateral MRI demonstrating degenerative disc at L5-S1 with a midline herniation. **B:** Three years postoperatively demonstrating the posterior intertransverse fusion.

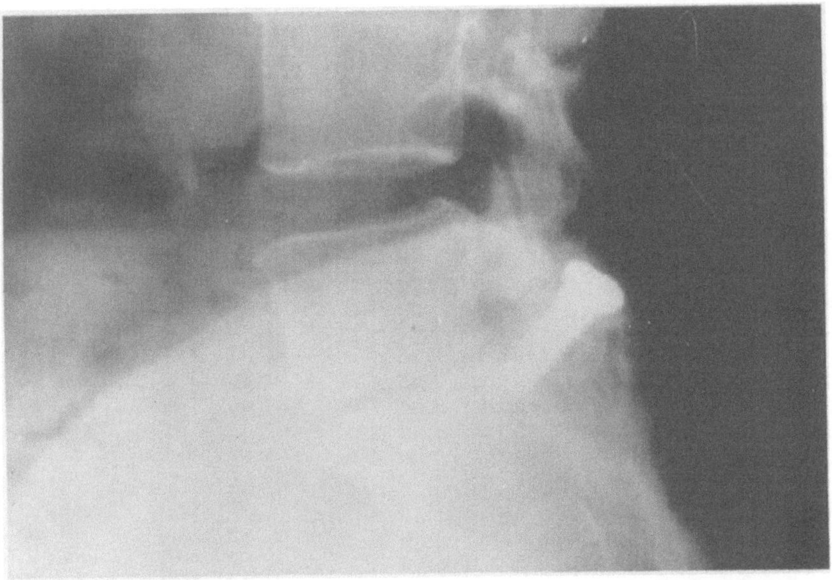

A

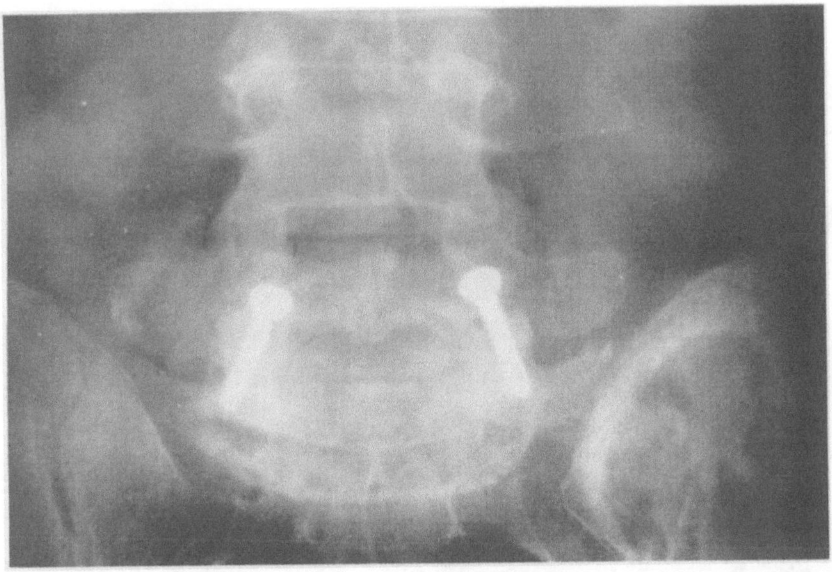

B

Figure 16.2. **A:** Lateral radiograph demonstrating marked L5-S1 disc space collapse and sclerosis with facet screws. **B:** Anteroposterior (AP) view demonstrates the facet screws and the bilateral intertransverse fusion.

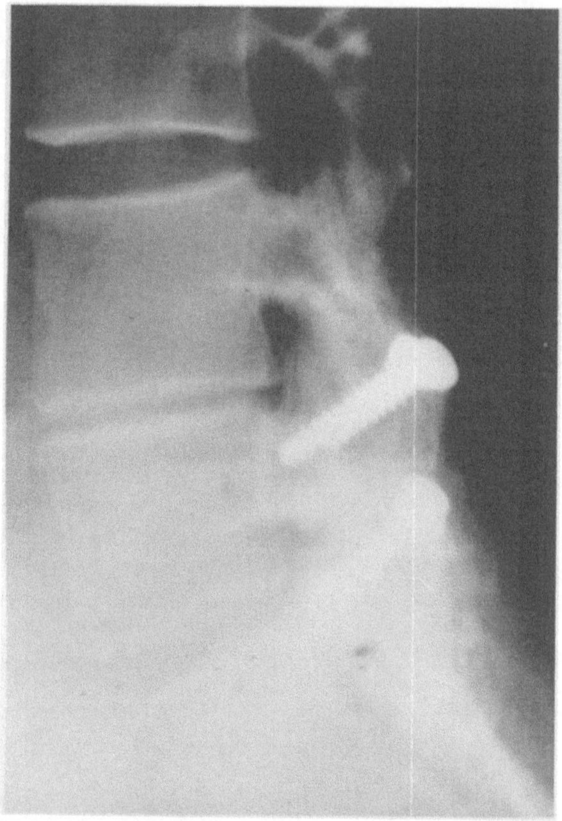

A

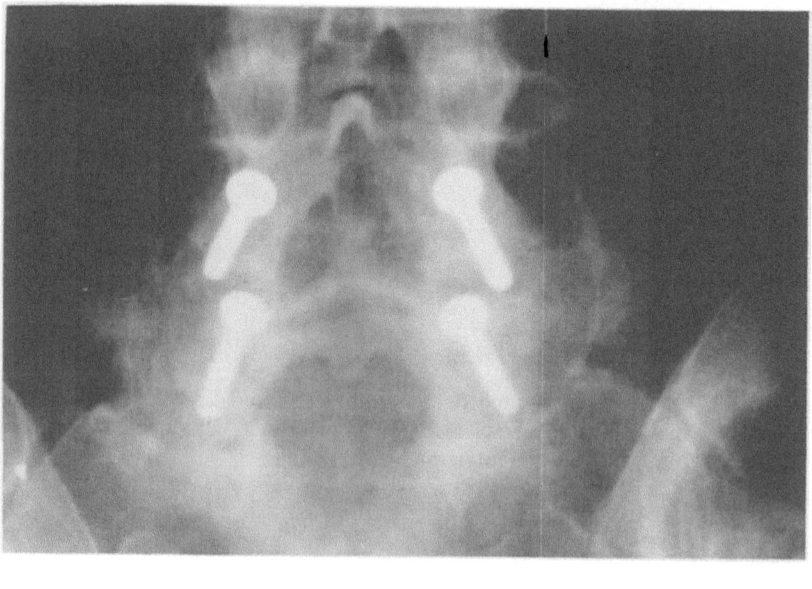

B

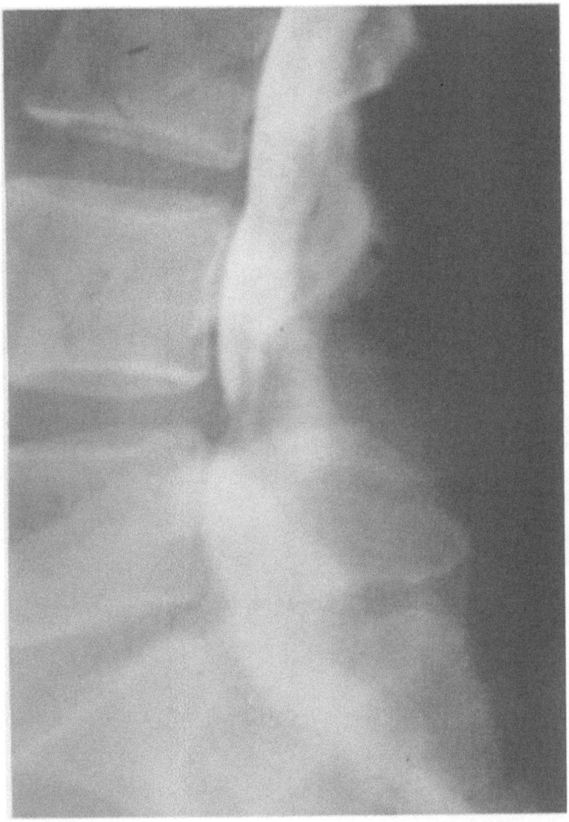

A

Figure 16.4. **A:** Metrizamide myelogram demonstrating a high-grade stenosis at L4-L5. **B:** Lateral radiograph postoperatively showing anterior interbody fusions L4-L5 and L5-S1; CD pedicle fixation L4 to the sacrum, coupled with laminotomies and intertransverse fusion from L4 to the sacrum.

high-grade obstruction at L4-L5 compatible with the diagnosis of spinal stenosis (Fig. 16.4A). She underwent anterior interbody fusions using bank bone at L4-L5 and L5-S1 and pedicle fixation from L4 to the sacrum using the CD system. This was coupled with laminotomies and intertransverse fusion from L4 to the sacrum using autogenous iliac bone grafts (Fig. 16.4B) with a good clinical outcome.

5. This 70-year-old woman fell, sustaining a burst fracture of T12 with retropulsion and a combined spinal cord and conus medullaris syn-

Figure 16.3. **A:** Lateral view showing marked disc space collapse at L4-L5 treated with a double level intertransverse fusion and facet fixation. **B:** AP view of the same.

B
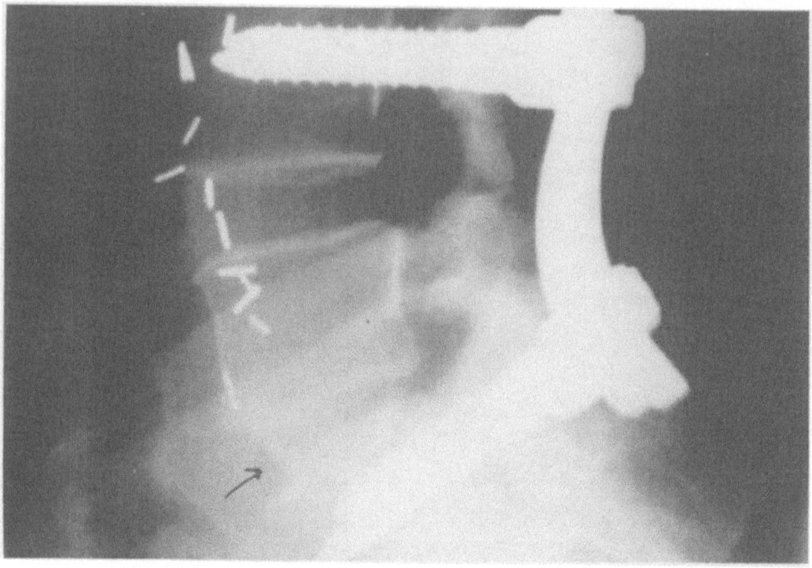

Figure 16.4. (*cont.*)

A
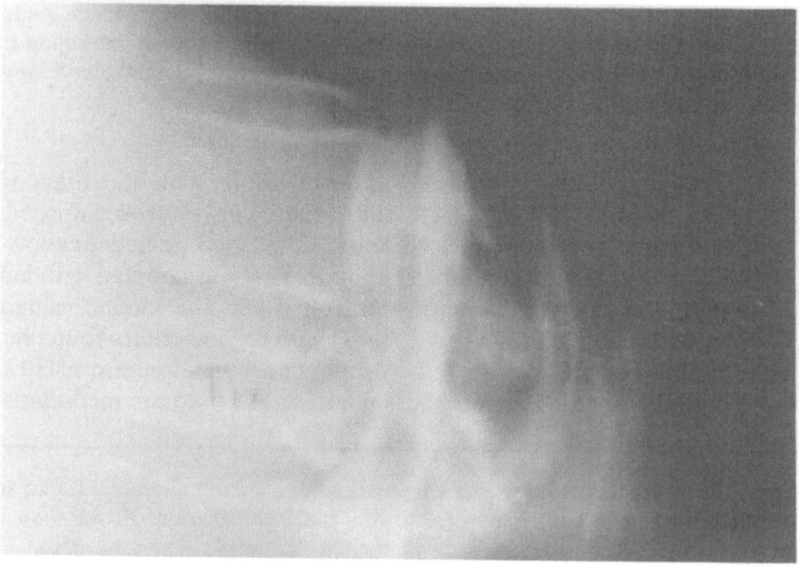

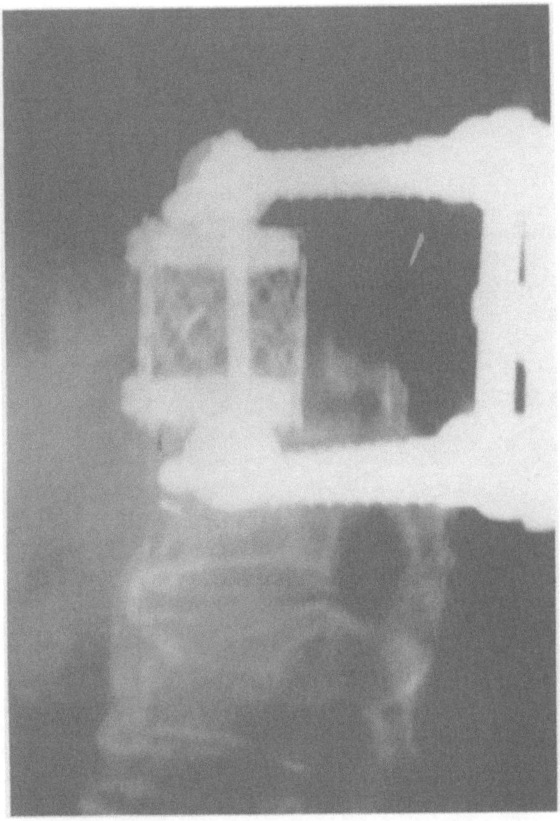

B

Figure 16.5. (*cont.*)

drome characterized by an incomplete paraparesis, a neurogenic bladder with an 1,800-cc capacity, overflow incontinence, and a flaccid anal sphincter. A myelogram showed the fracture and spinal cord compression (Fig. 16.5A). She underwent resection of the T12 vertebra with decompression of the vertebral canal and spinal cord and insertion of a Harms cage filled autogenous bone graft along with posterior CD pedicle fixation (Fig. 16.5B). She experienced a full recovery of bowel and bladder function along with lower extremity strength at 6 months. A mild exertion-related fatigue persisted.

Figure 16.5. A: Lateral myelogram demonstrating the T12 fracture and spinal cord compression. **B:** Lateral view postoperatively showing resection of the T12 vertebra, insertion of the Harms cage filled with autogenous bone, and the CD pedicle fixation.

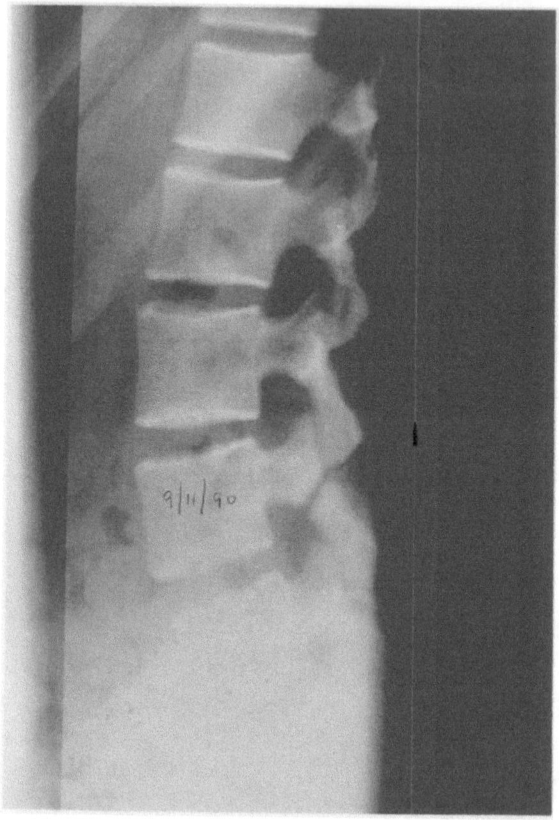

A

Figure 16.6. **A:** Lateral radiograph showing bilateral spondylolysis at the L4 neural arch. **B:** Lateral view 5 months later after brace management with evidence of healing.

Translational Instability

6. This 17-year-old female athlete presented with sports exertion-related mechanical low back pain without sciatica. There were no neurological deficits. Plain radiographs demonstrated bilateral spondylolysis at the L4 neural arch (Fig. 16.6A). She was treated conservatively with brace management for 6 months to allow for healing with a good outcome and returned to competitive swimming. The plain radiograph at 5 months illustrates the healing of the spondylolysis (Fig. 16.6B).
7. This 20-year-old man presented with stress-related mechanical low back of 1 year's duration without sciatica or neurological deficits. He was noted to have a unilateral spondylolysis at L5 (Fig. 16.7A), which failed to respond to conservative management with a lumbar

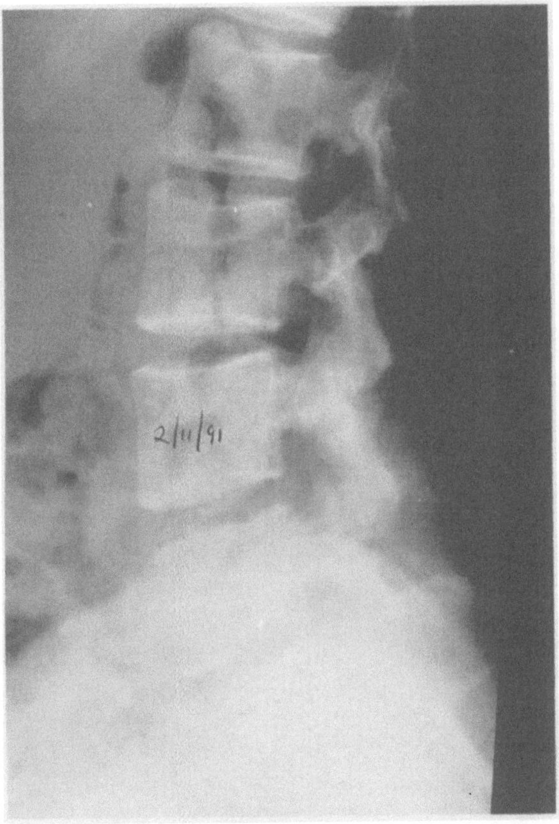

B

Figure 16.6. (*cont.*)

brace during that time period. He was treated with a translysis fixation and facet fixation along with a bilateral intertransverse fusion at L5-S1 (Fig. 16.7B) and experienced a good postoperative outcome.

8. This 40-year-old man presented with mechanical low back pain without sciatica or neurological deficits. Plain radiographs demonstrated degenerative discs with disc space narrowing at L4-L5 and L5-S1 and bilateral spondylolysis with minimal spondylolithesis (Fig. 16.8A). He was treated with an in situ intertransverse fusion L4 to the sacrum using autogenous iliac bone graft (Fig. 16.8B) with a good outcome.
9. This 35-year-old woman presented with mechanical low back pain and some radicular symptoms, but no neurological deficits. Plain radiographs demonstrated a grade II spondylolisthesis at L5-S1 (Fig. 16.9A). She was initially treated conservatively with physical therapy and a brace. In view of the incomplete response to therapy she underwent a posterior in situ intertransverse fusion from L4 to the

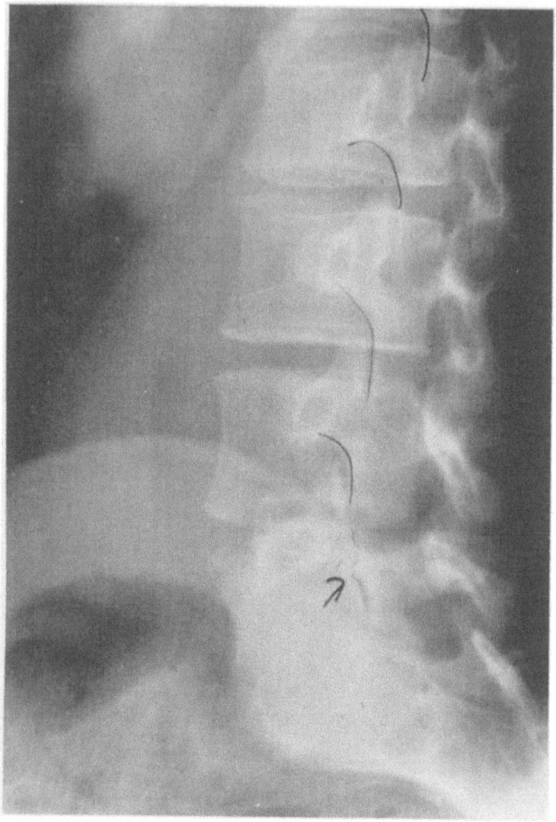

A

Figure 16.7. A: Lateral radiograph showing a unilateral spondylolysis at L5. **B:** Postoperative lateral view showing translysis fixation and facet fixation along with a bilateral intertransverse fusion L5-S1.

sacrum using autogenous iliac bone graft (Fig. 16.9B). Her outcome was fairly good with resolution of her radicular pain, but a persistent low back discomfort remained.

10. This 35-year-old mother of two failed to respond to surgical management of grade I spondylolisthesis consisting of posterior in situ intertransverse fusion. She presented with mechanical low back pain without sciatica and without neurological deficits. Plain radiographs demonstrated the postoperative in situ fusion with pseudarthrosis and instability (Fig. 16.10A). She was treated with reduction, interbody bank bone grafting, pedicle fixation with CD screws, and repeat intertransverse fusion at L5-S1 using autogenous iliac bone graft (Fig. 16.10B). The clinical outcome was good.

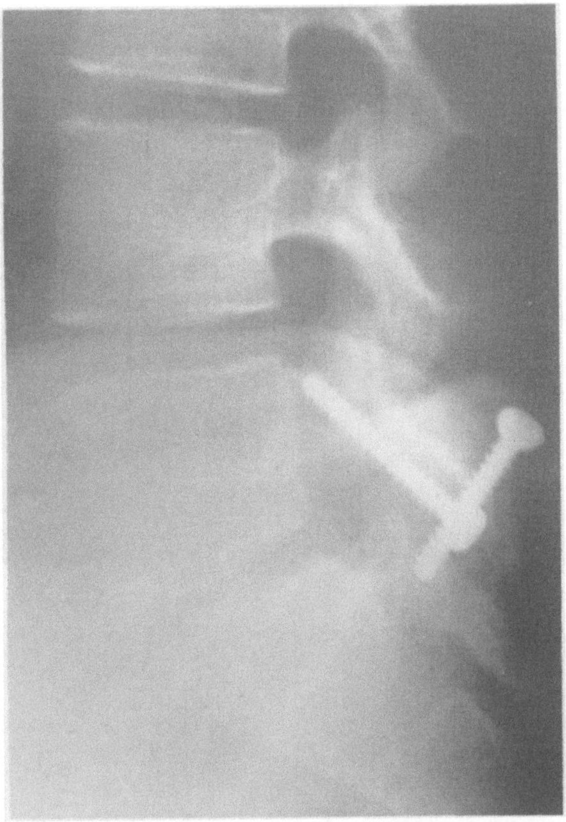

B

Figure 16.7. (*cont.*)

Angular Instability

11. This 45-year-old woman was involved in a motor vehicle accident and developed mechanical upper lumbar pain with a radicular component without neurological deficits. Plain radiographs showed a wedge compression fracture of L1 and angular instability (Fig. 16.11A). She was treated with anterior discectomy and fusion at T12-L1 and posterior pedicle fixation and in situ fusion at T12-L1 (Fig. 16.11B).
12. This 20-year-old male student suffered major abdominal injuries requiring a laparotomy following an automobile accident. He was later seen for a kyphotic angular deformity with a Chance fracture of L2, and midlumbar pain. There were no radicular symptoms and no neurological deficits. The preoperative plain radiographs showed the kyphotic deformity and L2-L3 disc space collapse (Fig. 16.12A). He

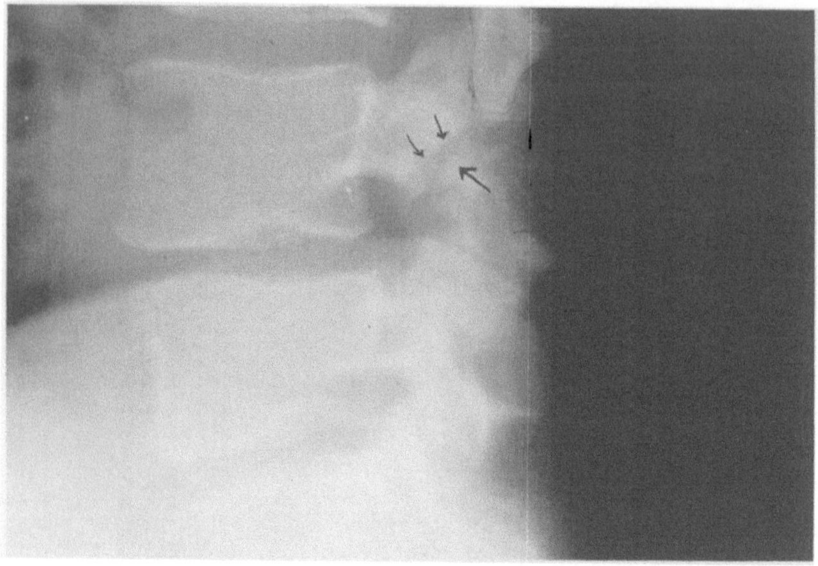

A

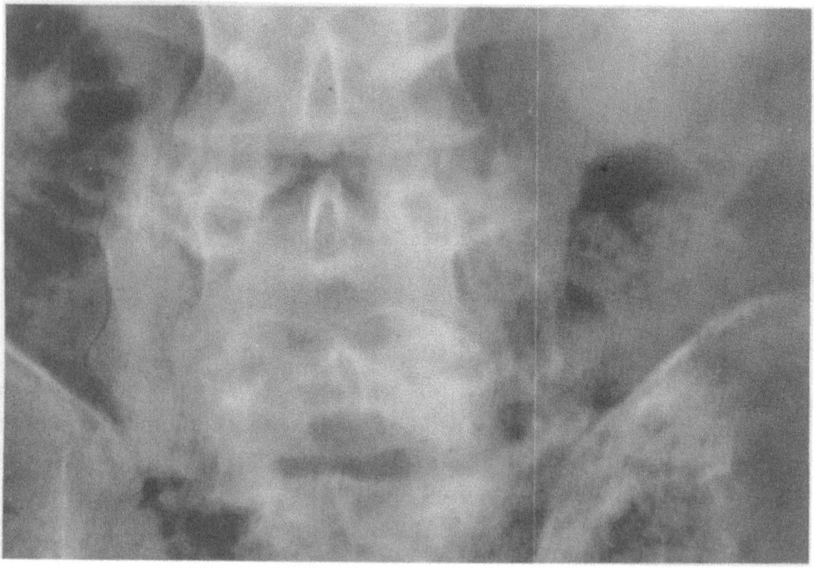

B

Figure 16.8. **A:** Lateral radiograph showing spondylolysis of the neural arch at L4 and disc space narrowing of L4-L5 and L5-S1. **B:** Lateral view postoperatively showing posterior in situ intertransverse fusion L4 to the sacrum.

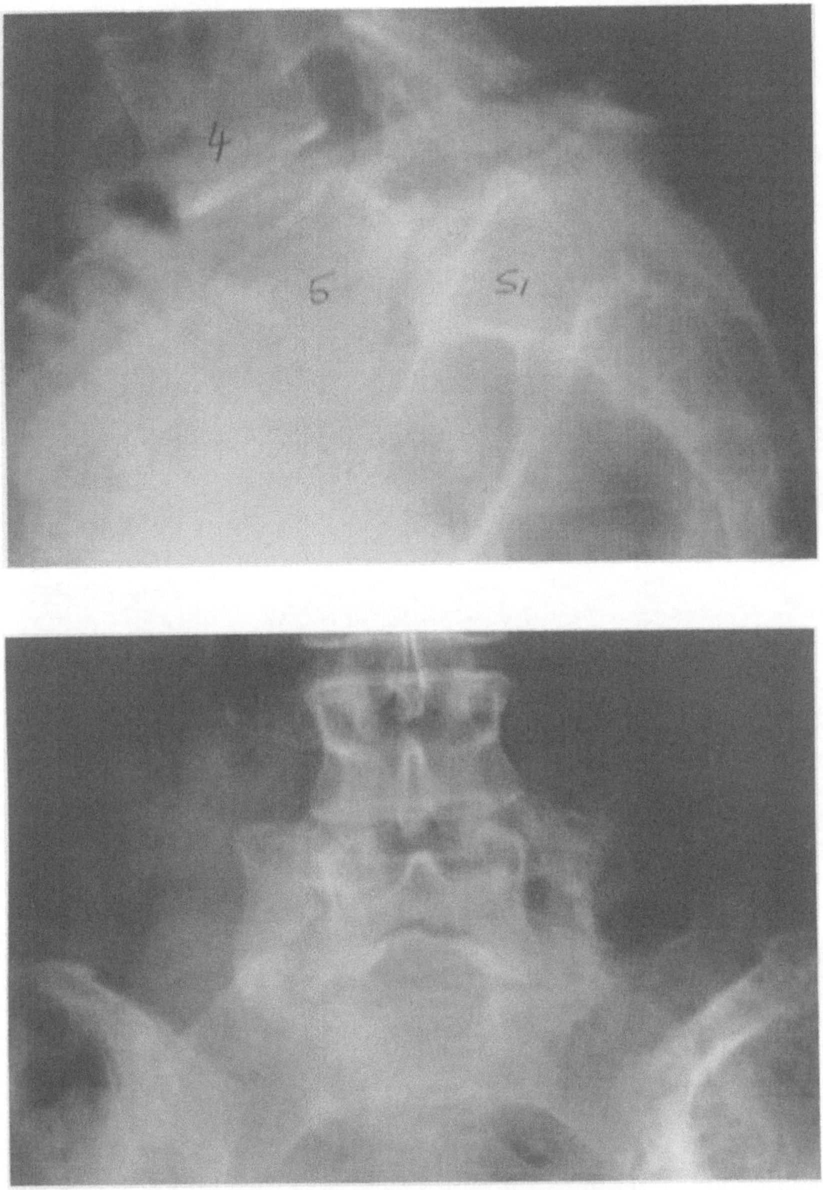

A

B

Figure 16.9. **A:** Lateral radiograph showing grade II spondylolisthesis L5-S1 with disc space degeneration showing the dome-shaped configuration of S1. **B:** Postoperative AP view showing the posterior in situ intertransverse fusion L4 to the sacrum.

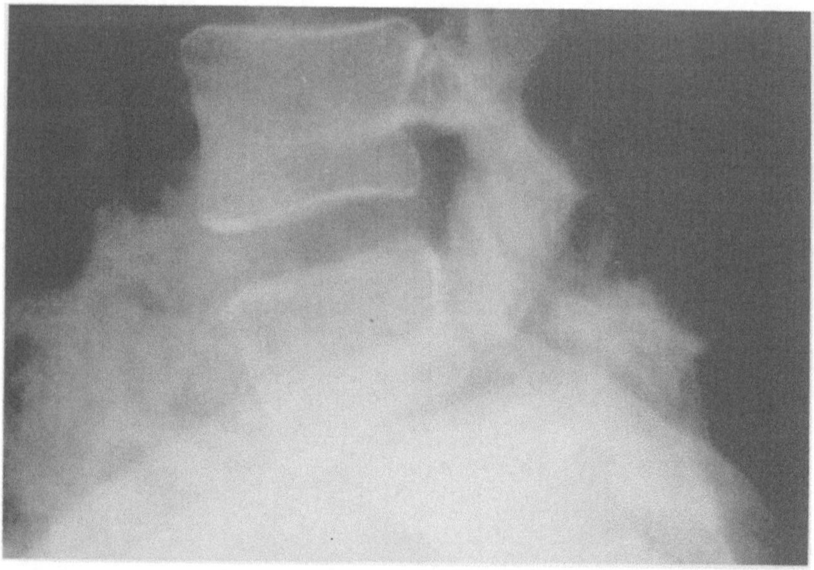

A

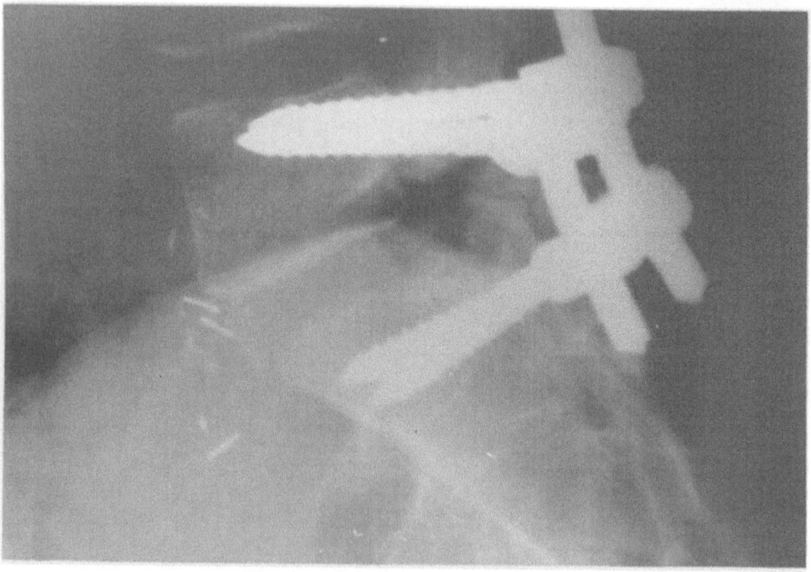

B

Figure 16.10. **A:** Postoperative lateral radiograph showing the in situ fusion with pseudarthrosis and instability. **B:** Lateral view postoperatively with reduction, interbody graft, CD pedicle fixation, and repeat intertransverse fusion L5-S1.

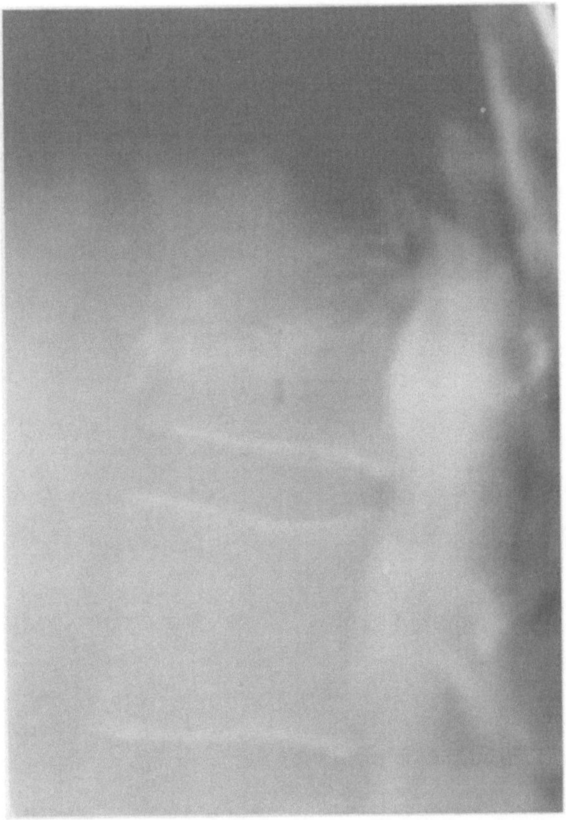

A

Figure 16.11. A: Lateral radiograph showing a wedge-shaped compression fracture of L1. **B:** Lateral view postoperatively showing anterior discectomy T12-L1, posterior pedicle fixation, and in situ fusion T12-L1.

underwent operative reduction of the deformity, anterior interbody fusion with bank bone graft, and a posterior fusion using the Harms (Moss) fixation system (Fig. 16.12B,C). The clinical outcome was good.

13. This 70-year-old woman developed progressive osteoporotic collapse of T12 with angular deformity and marked kyphosis. She suffered mechanical thoracolumbar pain, but had no radicular symptoms and no neurological deficits. Plain radiographs showed the marked col-

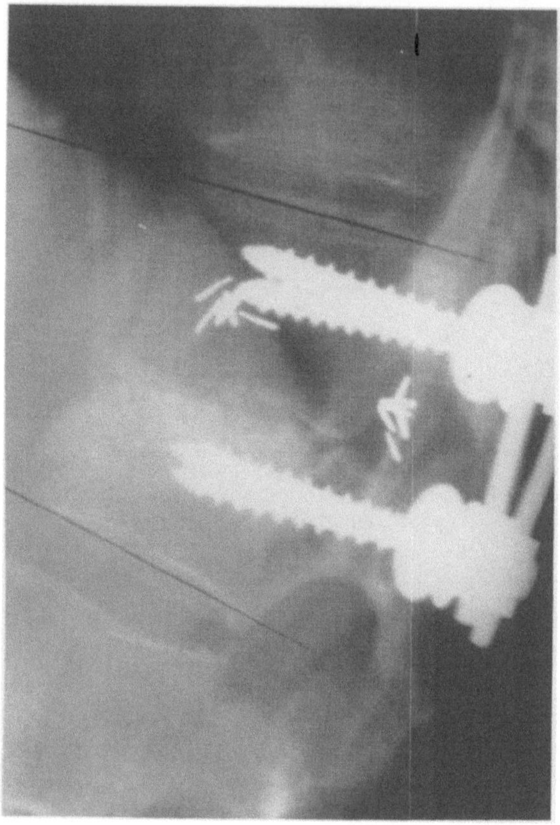

B

Figure 16.11. (*cont.*)

lapse of T12 and the accompanying angular deformity (Fig. 16.13A). She underwent reconstruction with vertebral body resection and application of Harms cage filled with autogenous iliac bone graft. In addition posterior pedicle fixation with the Harms (Moss) system was performed (Fig. 16.13B,C). The postoperative clinical outcome was good.

Rotational Instability

14. This 13-year-old girl presented with a progressive idiopathic scoliosis over a 4-year period. She had no focal mechanical pain and no radicular pain. Plain radiographs demonstrated 40° of thoracolumbar scoliosis over the T10-L3 levels (Fig. 16.14A). She was treated with short anterior segmental correction and fixation using the ventral derotation system (VDS) of Zielke (Fig. 16.14B).

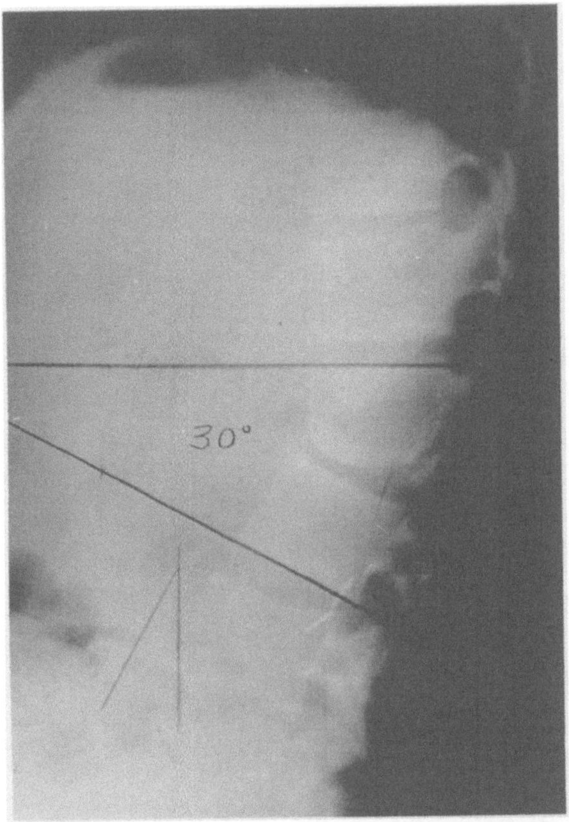

A

Figure 16.12. A: Lateral radiograph showing the kyphotic deformity and disc space collapse L2-L3. **B:** Lateral view postoperatively showing the reduction of the deformity, anterior interbody fusion, and posterior fixation using the Harms (Moss) fixation system. **C:** AP view of the same.

Complex Instability

15. This 60-year-old man presented with low back pain and symptoms of pseudoclaudication. There were no neurological deficits. Plain radiographs demonstrated the degenerative changes, scoliosis, lateral listhesis, and spinal stenosis. He underwent lumbar laminectomy L2-L5 coupled with in situ intertransverse fusion using autogenous iliac bone graft (Fig. 16.15) with a good clinical outcome.
16. This 60-year-old woman presented with low back pain and symptoms of pseudoclaudication. There were no neurological deficits. Plain radiographs showed degenerative disc disease, spinal stenosis, lateral listhesis, and spondylolisthesis at L4-L5. She was treated with lumbar

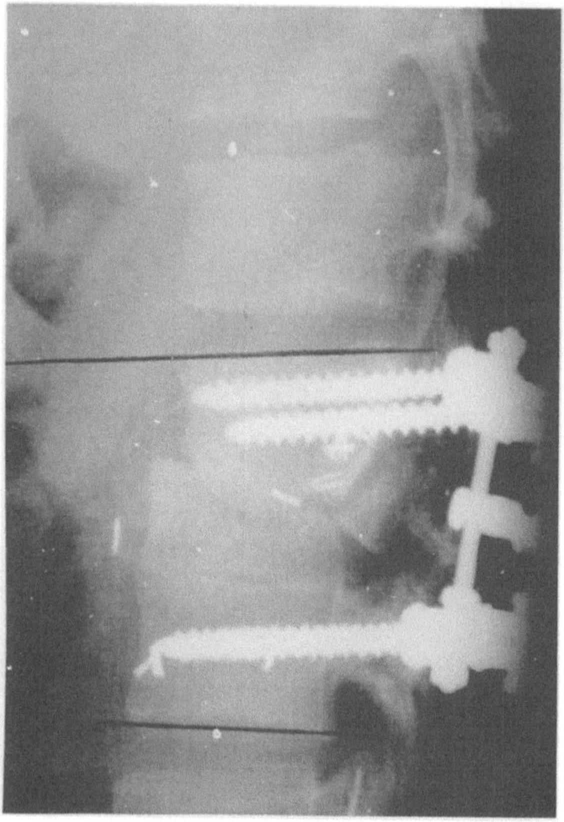

B

Figure 16.12. (*cont.*)

laminectomy L1 to L5 along with multilevel pedicle fixation using the CD system. In addition anterior interbody fusions from L1 to L5 using bank bone and intertransverse fusions from L1 to L5 using autogenous iliac graft were performed (Fig. 16.16). The clinical outcome was good.

17. This 65-year-old woman who had undergone previous laminectomy and fusion with instrumentation for lumbar spondylosis developed osteomyelitis at the L2-L3 level and around infection simultaneously presented to the author with severe back pain and neurogenic claudication. Plain radiographs showed a progressive mechanical collapse of L2-L3 (Fig. 16.17A). Percutaneous needle biopsy for diagnosis was negative. She underwent posterior segmental fixation and stabilization using the CD system. At 6 months, spontaneous interbody fusion appeared to be developing at L2-L3 (Fig. 16.17B).

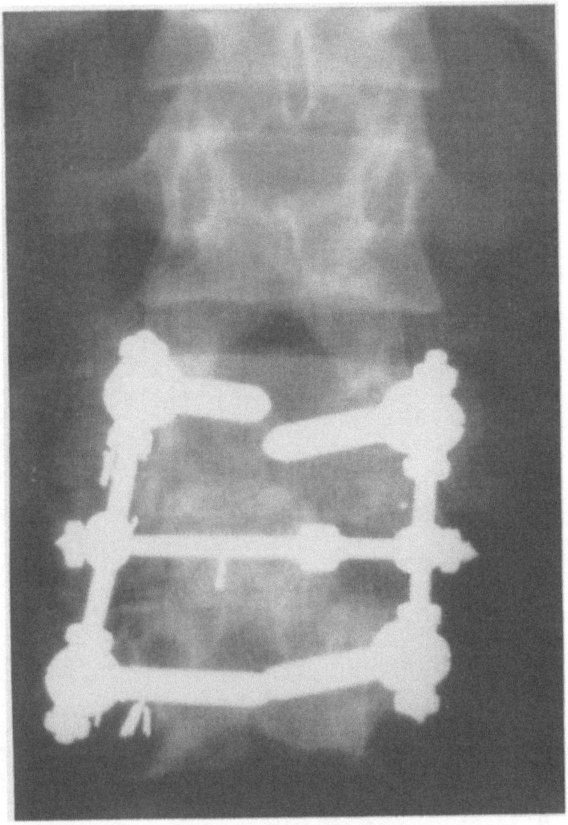

Figure 16.12. (*cont.*)

Anterior interbody fusion is to be contemplated if the spontaneous fusion process does not mature.

Discussion

Longitudinal instability (L) with disc space collapse, as in disc degeneration, the postdiscectomy syndrome, or discogenic sclerosis, is a cause of intractable low back pain in some cases and may require spinal fusion for the alleviation of mechanical symptoms without neurological features. Surgical options include (a) posterior in situ intertransverse fusion, which has a relatively high success rate in one level fusions at the L5-S1 segment; (b) internal fixation with facet screws plus intertransverse fusion; and (c) a more complex fusion including internal fixation using rods and

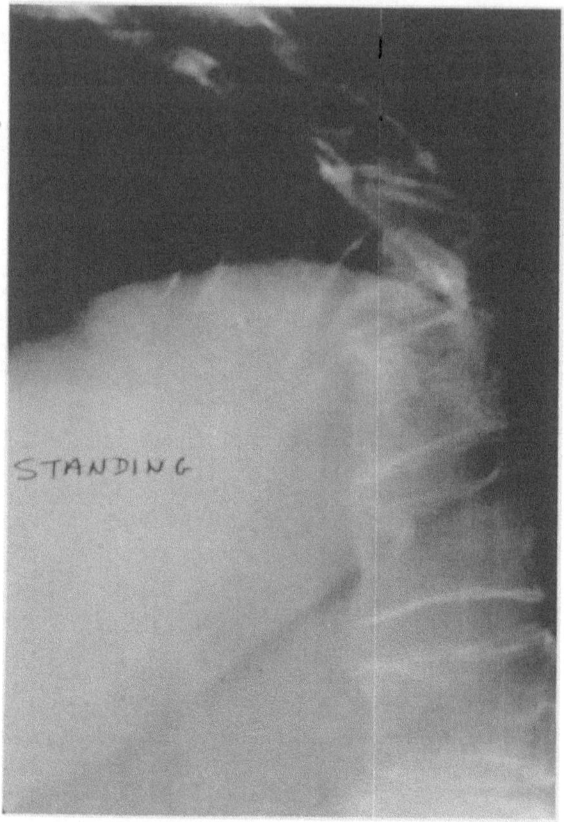

A

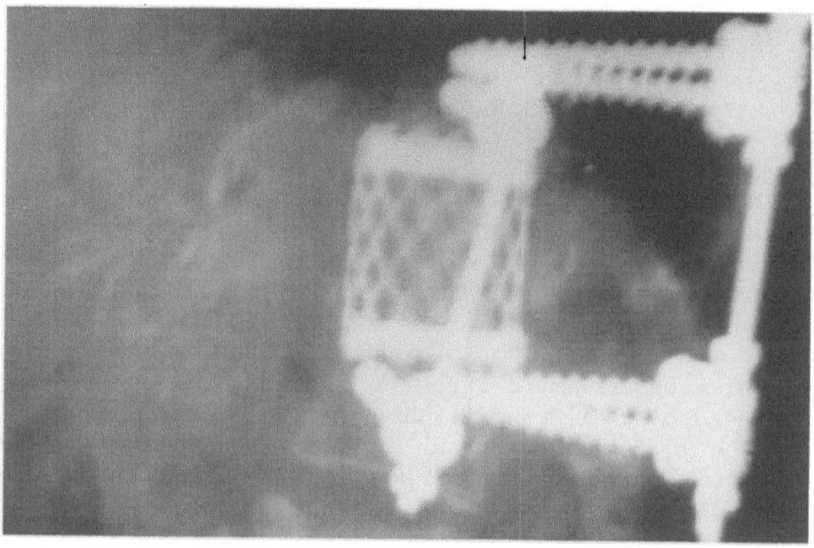

B

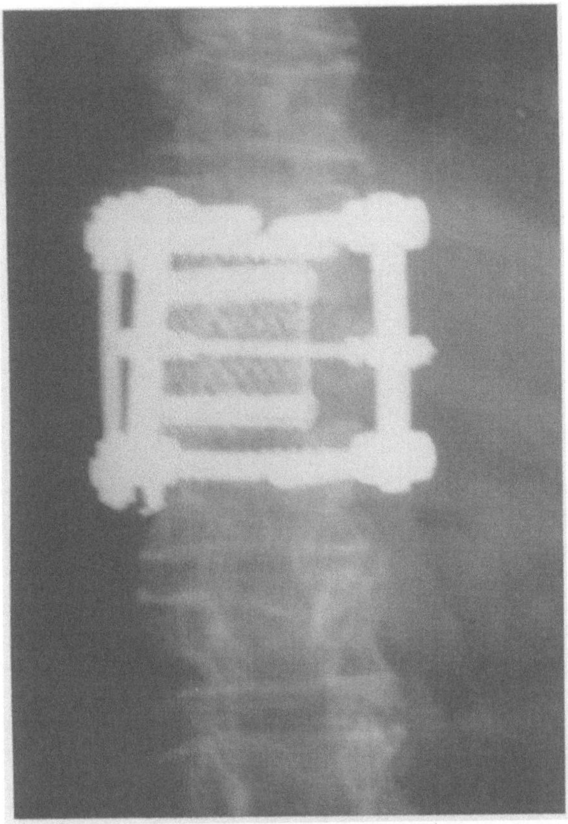

C

Figure 16.13. (*cont.*)

pedicle screws plus posterior fusion coupled with anterior interbody fusion.

The early experience suggests that when necessary this complex fusion technique gives the best results.

Translational instability (T) exemplified by spondylolisthesis is subject to the same principles outlined above with the exception of facet fixation in pars interarticularis defects. Certainly, in revision fusions for spondylolisthesis, posterior pedicle fixation and fusion coupled with anterior interbody fusion is my preferred method.

Figure 16.13. A: Lateral standing radiograph showing the marked collapse of T12 and angular deformity. **B:** Lateral postoperative view showing reconstruction with vertebral body resection, application of Harms cage filled with autogenous bone and Harms (Moss) posterior pedicle fixation system. **C:** AP view of the same.

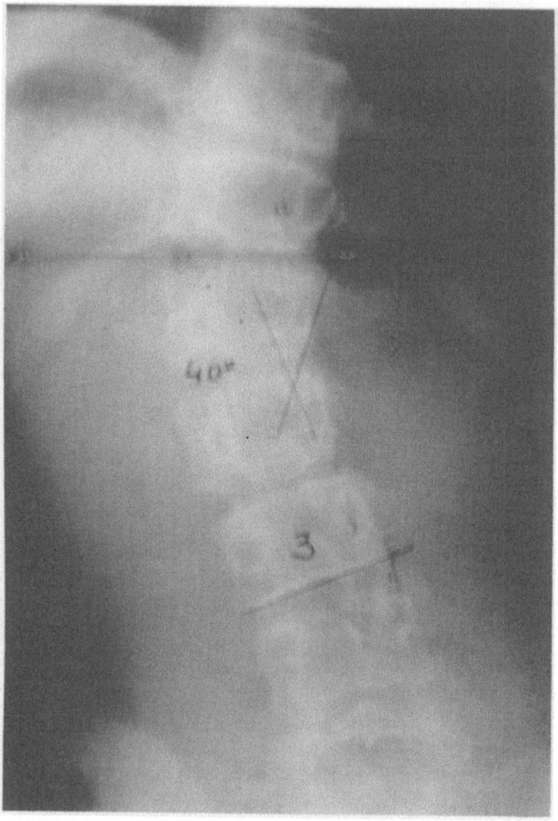

A

Figure 16.14. A: Lateral radiograph showing a 40° thoracolumbar scoliosis from T10-L3. **B:** Lateral view postoperatively showing short anterior segmental correction with the ventral derotation system (VDS) of Zielke.

Angular instability (A) exemplified by burst wedge fractures in osteoporotic women is best treated by combined anterior and posterior fusions with pedicle fixation one level above and one level below, using Harms cage or bank bone for anterior support.

Rotational instability (R) exemplified by thoracolumbar scoliosis is best treated by the anterior ventral derotation system of Zielke, fusing the minimum number of levels and using anterior bone graft to minimize kyphosis.

With respect to complex instabilities (C), (a) in pseudospondylolisthesis at L4-L5 with neurogenic claudication and disc space collapse in the older man, decompression alone may suffice. However, in the younger, more active woman with high disc spaces and pseudospondylolisthesis, decompression with pedicle fixation and posterior fusion coupled with anterior

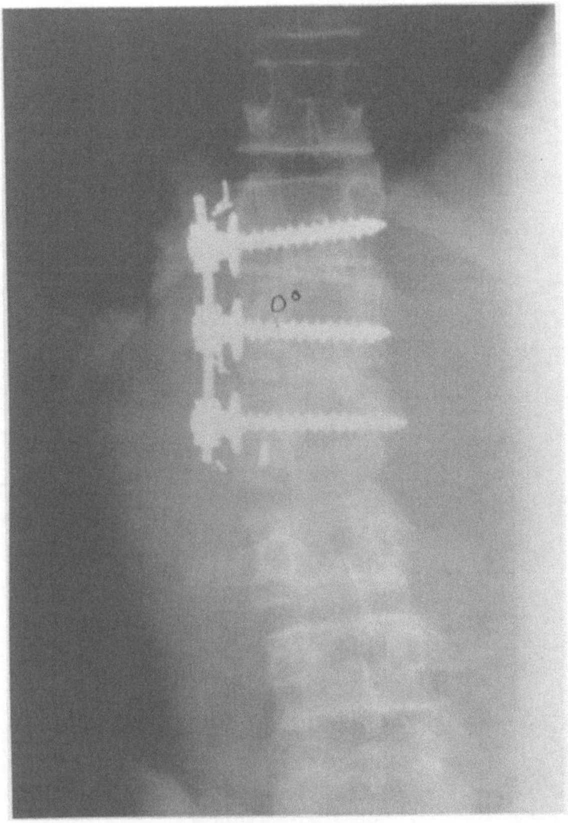

B

Figure 16.14. (*cont.*)

interbody fusion is likely to yield the best results. (b) In septic discitis, early antibiotic treatment after appropriate cultures yields excellent results, with many cases progressing to spontaneous interbody fusion. However, in some cases, progressive osteolysis with longitudinal collapse and angular deformity develops. In this latter situation, realignment of the spine using a posterior rod and pedicle system over the appropriate levels (usually two or three levels) coupled with anterior debridement and mechanical support such as strut graft or possibly Harms cage constitutes appropriate surgical care. (c) In burst fractures with canal compromise and instability, posterior fusion using long rods bridging the distance two to three levels above and one to two levels below is commonly utilized with or without anterior decompression. However, in this author's opinion, initial posterior distraction alignment coupled with posterior rod-pedicle fixation one level above and one level below supported by anterior interbody fusion plus or minus decompression offers the best re-

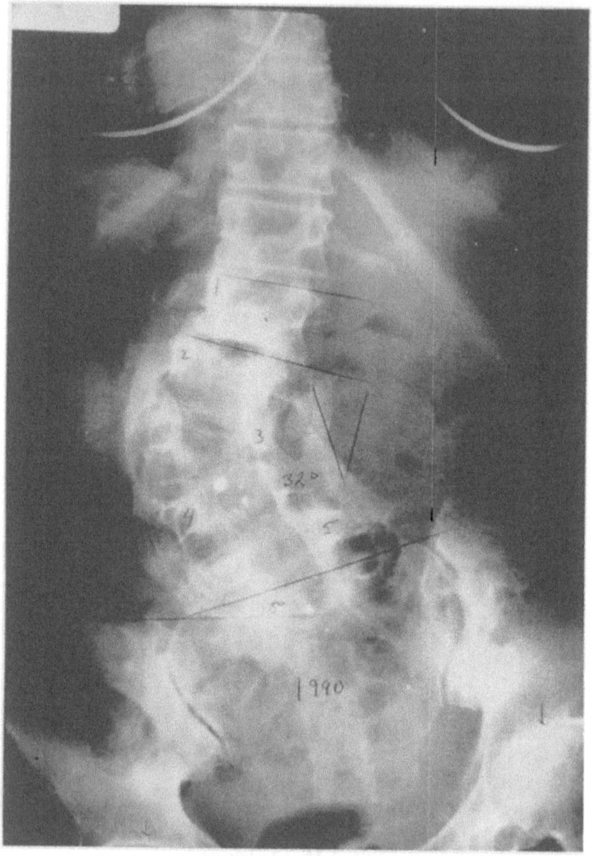

Figure 16.15. Lateral radiograph showing lumbar laminectomy L2-L5 coupled with in situ intertransverse fusion.

construction with the least risk of late problems associated with longer fusions. (d) Spinal stenosis with pseudospondylolisthesis at L4-L5 and lateral listhesis at L3-L4 and scoliosis (complex instability) is a pattern more commonly seen in the active female patient and is best treated by (i) decompression for the stenosis and (ii) a posterior pedicle fixation and fusion over the segments.

Failure to stabilize the above condition would likely lead to progressive deformity. Exceptions may include the older man who has associated ankylosing hyperostosis and the older woman with severe osteoporosis where internal fixation often fails.

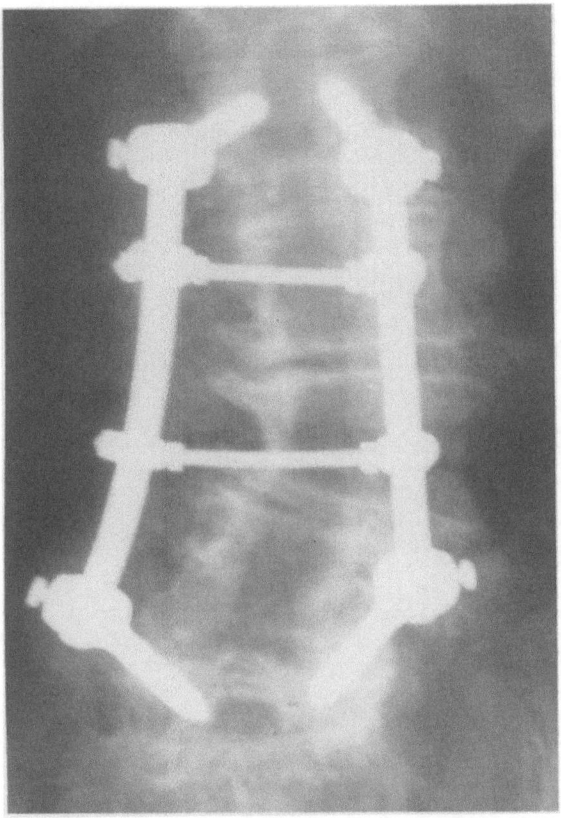

A

Figure 16.16. A: Lateral radiograph showing lumbar laminectomy, multilevel CD pedicle fixation L1-L5, intertransverse fusion L1-L5, and interbody fusions L1-L5. **B:** AP view of the same.

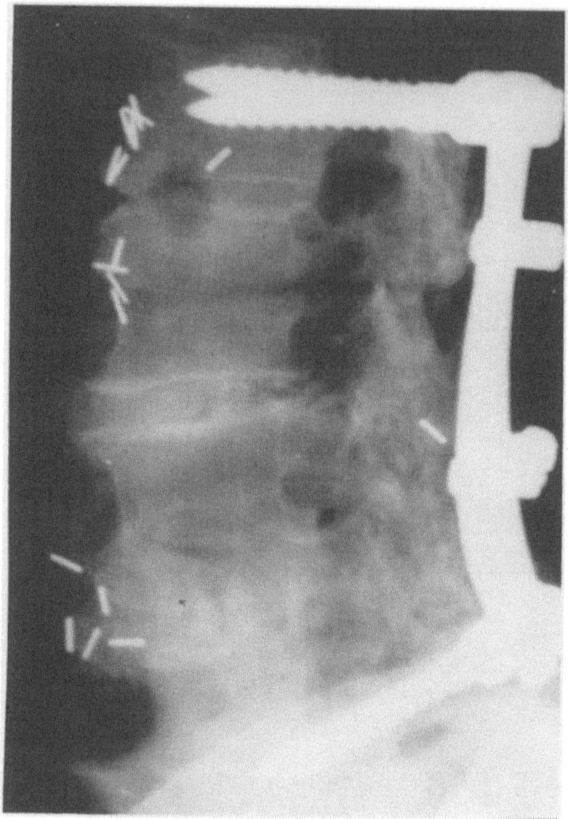

B

Figure 16.16. (*cont.*)

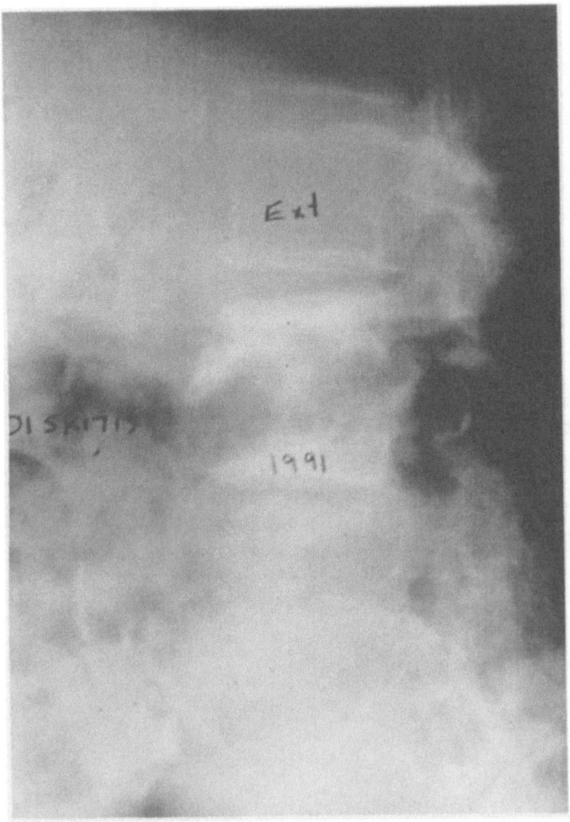

A

Figure 16.17. **A:** Lateral radiograph of L2-L3 osteomyelitis on presentation to the author. **B:** Lateral view 6 months postoperatively showing posterior segmental fixation and stabilization using the CD system with the appearance of a fusion beginning to develop at the L2-L3 level.

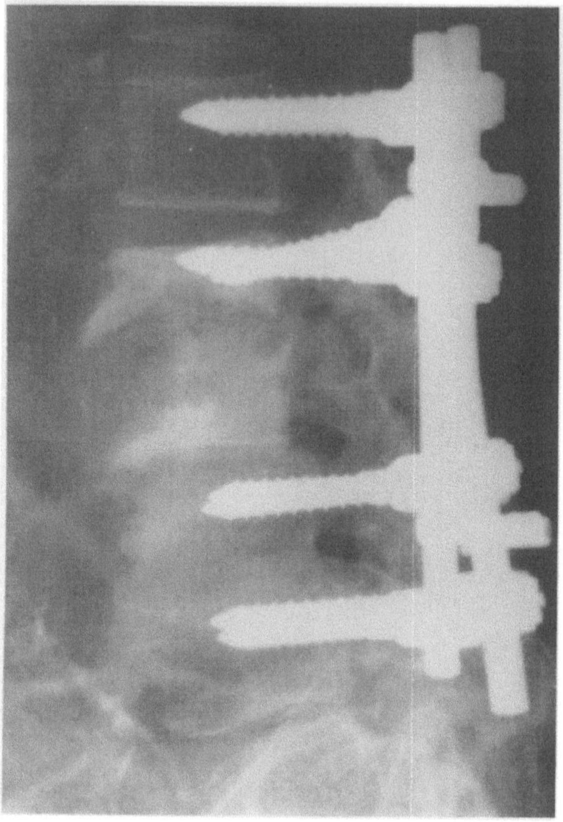

B

Figure 16.17. (*cont.*)

Summary

Suffice it to say that we do not as yet have the perfect methods for analyzing biomechanical instability or the potential for progressive instability nor do we have the final surgical solutions for these complex problems.

However, as we progress in our capacity to assess functional biomechanical patterns and as our knowledge of the biology of healing and repair increases, better fixation systems will be developed and a new era of spine surgery will be upon us.

Discussion

The Use of Cross-Linking in Fixation

Dr. Hughes inquired about the use of cross-linking in degenerative disease. It certainly makes for a stronger construct. Dr. Kostuik said: Biomechanically it would be stronger, but I don't use them since they are too expensive. Dr. White said: There is a lot of cross-linking going on especially in spondylolisthesis since many look stable postoperatively, but actually are not. Classic degenerative scoliosis is an unstable situation and will progress as will spondylolistheses. My associates are using cross-linking a lot and Wiltse will use double rods.

Dr. O'Leary said: I am not sure whether we can link this, but also I am not sure whether it is required. I have no problem doing it or not doing it. I have done it in some and not in others. If the internal fixation involves multiple levels I am more likely to use it than not.

Does Laminectomy Per Se Produce Instability?

Dr. Holtzman inquired does laminectomy per se produce instability? Dr. Farcy said: It depends on how far lateral you go. Prof. Louis added: We must respect the continuity of the posterior column. We have to decompress the medial anterior part of the posterior column, respecting the posterolateral compartment at least 6 mm in width at the pars interarticularis level and facet level. If that is the case fusion should not be required.

The second inquiry relates to the permissible degree of facetectomy that will preserve stability. Dr. Holtzman noted that patients with spinal stenosis and multiple osteophytes seem to have considerable stability even if there is an associated scoliosis. Partial facetectomy is necessary to afford nerve root decompression; to what extent is that destabilizing? Dr. Kostuik said: That is the problem. Many people have much more than a partial facetectomy and those are the people I see in consultation.

Dr. O'Leary said: I think when one makes a very narrow laminectomy in the center one can just undermine the opposite side, taking away a little bit of the superior facet and preserving the majority of the facet joint. If only 2 mm of the medial aspect of the facet is removed, the nerve root is given freedom. Dr. Holtzman added: Mostly the superior articulating process contributes to the nerve root compression. Prof. Louis said: A partial facetectomy is often not sufficient to expose the nerve root to the level of the foramen of exit, and Dr. White added that then you have removed more than a facet. I have done a good decompression and I showed you 10 of them yesterday. There is evidence that at least 10 of our cases without a facetectomy did go on to further slippage, further narrowing, and stenosis, requiring reoperation. I have an additional 10 cases that I have managed and that is the gist of my query. How do we answer that question? I feel that this signifies that laminectomy even without facetectomy is a potentially unstable situation. Dr. Kostuik added: Yes, I agree.

CHAPTER 17

The Mechanical Stability of Lumbosacral Spondylolisthesis

Yizhar Floman

Spondylolisthesis was first described in 1782 by Herbiniaux (16) who was an obstetrician. He described a case of a woman with a complicated delivery due to a marked lumbosacral slip, i.e., spondyloptosis. At the time of Herbiniaux, spondylolisthesis was thought to occur acutely. Kilian (19) in 1854 was the first to recognize the gradual chronic nature of the slip. He was also the one who proposed the name *spondylolisthesis*, which is comprised of two Greek words: *spondylos*, meaning vertebra, and *olisthesis*, meaning slip. Robert (31) in 1855, proposed that a pars defect is essential for the development of a slip and Lambl (21), in the same year, was the first to describe a pars defect in patients. However, some pathological studies, described cases of lumbosacral olisthesis without a pars defect, leading to a debate between investigators. Neugebauer (27), in a now classic publication in 1888, described two types of spondylolisthesis, with and without a pars defect.

Wiltse, et al. (40) classified the various forms of spondylolisthesis into five distinct types. To this now classic classification, Wiltse and Rothman (41) added a sixth type, the postsurgical spondylolisthesis.

Type I is characterized by dysplasia of the L5-S1 facets as well as the upper sacrum. As a result, resistance to anterior shear forces by the L5-S1 segment is reduced and may lead to forward translation of the cephalad vertebra, i.e., forward slip. Because the slippage in this type occurs with an intact neural ring, signs of cauda equina compression may be manifested early on, without significant displacement. On the other hand, as anterior shear forces increase, pars elongation or even pars breakage can occur as a secondary phenomenon.

Type I olisthesis is divided into two subtypes: in A, the dysplastic articular process is axially oriented, and in B, the articular process is sagittally oriented.

Type II olisthesis is the lytic, isthmic type due to stress fracture of the pars interarticularis (42). Spondylolysis, or pars interarticularis defect, occurs in about 6% of the general population (15), but there is a higher incidence of spondylolysis in certain racial and familial groups (15). The current school of thought about the etiology of spondylolysis hypothesizes that a genetically weakened posterior arch, under the influence of upright posture and repetitive microtrauma, finally gives in and a fracture occurs in the pars interarticularis. No case of spondylolysis has been found among cerebral palsy patients who never ambulated (32) except in athetoid patients in whom an increased incidence of spondylolysis has been described (11).

In children, the pars may be overloaded because of their hyperlordotic posture due to a physiologic hip flexion contracture. Likewise, a lumbosacral slip is more common in patients with Scheuermann's kyphosis and compensatory lumbar hyperlordosis (26). The pars is a pivotal center that connects the pedicle, transverse process, lamina, and facet joints. Stress analysis in polarized light clearly shows that there is stress concentration in the pars interarticularis (37). Spondylolysis is found in increased frequency in individuals engaged in various sports activities, especially in gymnasts and weight lifters, where the percentage of pars defect may reach up to 50% to 80% (17.33). Spondylolysis and olisthesis may occur under a long fusion mass, as after scoliosis surgery, and a pars fracture may heal following a successful fusion in mild olisthesis (28).

There are two subtypes in type II: A, a lytic lesion; and B, an elongated pars from repeated stress fractures that go on to heal and to refracture again. These lesions usually develop during early childhood, and slip progression occurs mainly during the adolescent growth spurt (8).

Type III is degenerative spondylolisthesis that occurs as a result of long-standing segmental instability and facet joint arthritis.

Type IV is a traumatic spondylolisthesis. It is a result of major trauma; the posterior defect occurs in other sites rather than in the pars itself.

Type V is a pathological fracture of the isthmus, secondary to the various bone disorders and, in the new type VI, the spondylolysis and olisthesis occur following surgery, such as after extensive posterior decompressions (41).

Biomechanics of Spondylolisthesis

The intervertebral discs and the posterior elements, including the facet joints and the spinal ligaments, all play a significant role in stabilizing the spinal motion segment. Although the intervertebral disc determines the extent of movement between the vertebral bodies, the facet joints determine the direction of movement. The facet joints also are essential in resisting anterior translatory motion between two adjacent vertebral bodies. The ligamentum flavum is prestressed, due to its high content of elastin, and compresses the two adjacent vertebral bodies and their posterior elements against each other.

A pars interarticularis defect significantly reduces the role of the posterior elements in stabilizing the spinal motion segment. When the pars defect is bilateral, it may lead to spondylolisthesis, which implies that anterior displacement of the vertebral body at the spondylolytic level occurs over the subjacent vertebral body. This displacement is the result of an anterior shear force acting parallel to the disc space between the two vertebrae. In the majority of adult cases, this anterior slip is in a "stable" equilibrium and shows no detectable progression of the olisthesis.

According to Troup (38), the forces that generate the slip arise from three main sources: gravity acting on the torso above the slip level, activity of the truncal muscles, and forces generated during motion. While the subject is standing erect with preservation of the normal lumbar lordosis, the L5-S1 disc is inclined anteriorly and downward. In this posture, both the disc and the zygapophyseal joints will be under axial and shear stress (38). Shear forces under the influence of gravity will be greatest when the trunk is flexed and the vertebral end plates are inclined almost vertically. The muscular influence on shear forces is more complex; depending on posture, the shear force will be directed either anteriorly or posteriorly. An exception is the iliopsoas muscle, which consistently generates a considerable anterior shear force (38). This anterior shear force can rise sharply while the subject is landing on his feet, as after a jump.

Trunk balance can be evaluated by rating the relationship of the second sacral vertebra to both the center of L5 body and the hip joints (39). If a horizontal line is traced from the center of S2, anteriorly, two perpendiculars will intersect this line, one dropped down from the center of L5 and the other traced from below starting at the center of the hip joint. If the sacrum moves to a more vertical position, the pelvis retroverts and pushes the hip joints anteriorly. This will increase the torque and anterior shear force on L5, and increase the slip (39).

The main resistance to all these anterior shear forces is the intervertebral disc. When a low-grade spondylolisthesis has already occurred, the stability of the spinal motion segment is mostly dependent on the intervertebral disc. As long as the disc retains its normal biochemical and biomechanical properties, the spinal motion segment will remain stable, despite the fact that a certain degree of forward displacement of the cephalad vertebra has occurred. Thus, a grade I or II isthmic lumbosacral spondylolisthesis should be considered to be mechanically stable in adults as long as the intervening disc maintains its structural and functional integrity.

Evidence that grade I to II isthmic lumbosacral spondylolisthesis is stable comes from several in vivo radiologic studies. Penning and Blickman (30) studied in vivo sagittal plane motion in individuals with lumbosacral spondylolisthesis. They x-rayed 24 individuals with spondylolisthesis but could not demonstrate abnormal sagittal translatory motion at the lumbosacral olisthetic level. On the other hand, increased motion was detected at spinal motion segments above the spondylolisthesis. At the olisthetic level itself, there was a wide scatter of axes of movement and hypermobility, but no translational motion abnormality (30).

Pearcy and Shepherd (29) studied symptomatic patients with grade I and II olisthesis by biplanar radiography. They found decreased motion at the lumbosacral level in flexion, extension, lateral bending, axial rotation, and in coupled motions as well. These investigators found no forward or backward translation greater than 2 mm, nor any trend for individuals with symptomatic lumbosacral olisthesis to have larger translations than a control group of healthy individuals (29). However, at the lumbosacral level, all olisthetic individuals had a significant decrease in flexion and extension as compared to normal controls ($p < .05$). Coupled movement at the L4-5 and L5-S1 levels was found to be comparable to those of normal subjects. At higher lumbar levels, coupled motion was larger in symptomatic spondylolisthesis.

Pearcy and Shepherd (29) concluded that the decreased motion at the level of symptomatic spondylolisthesis was due to muscle splinting. They questioned, therefore, the notion that mild lumbosacral spondylolisthesis, in adults, is mechanically unstable. If these motion characteristics are not unstable, they should not be accompanied by nociceptive stimulation. If so, fusion of the so-called unstable segment would not alleviate back pain in adult individuals with mild spondylolisthesis without evidence of disc degeneration. This latter conclusion concurs with Macnab (24), who stressed that in individuals older than 25 years with mild spondylolisthesis, back pain did not correlate with the slip. Although Pearcy and Shepherd (29) could not demonstrate increased forward or backward shear in patients with mild lumbosacral olisthesis, Lowe and associates (23) studied motion in grade III to IV spondylolisthesis. Increased slip was demonstrated on standing x-rays as compared to supine x-rays in this patient population. Similarly, Kessen et al. (18) were able to demonstrate increased anteroposterior translation in patients with spondylolisthesis by stressing or loading the spine.

In a normal motion segment, there is a fixed motion pattern between the vertebral bodies. This motion is defined by the location of the instant center of rotation and by the extent of motion. If a particular motion segment is unstable, either the instant center of rotation is abnormally located, excessive mobility is present, or both. Penning and Blickman (30) found that discs below an isthmic olisthetic defects showed a somewhat larger spread of the instant center of rotation. This finding may imply that the disc at the olisthetic level may be degenerated, as it is known that the location of axis of movement is widely spread in degenerated intervertebral discs (10). However, this abnormal shift of the instant center of rotation is not always associated with excessive intervertebral translatory motion.

Mild Lumbosacral Spondylolisthesis and Trauma

Attesting to the stability of mild lumbosacral spondylolisthesis is the fate of this lesion in individuals who sustained major trauma to the lumbar spine. The incidental occurrence of lumbar spine fractures in individuals with preexisting first-degree isthmic spondylolisthesis may be looked upon as a simulated in vivo biomechanical experiment, testing the stability of the lumbosacral subluxation.

Among 300 patients with thoracolumbar spine fractures managed at the author's institution during a 10-year period, seven such cases were collected (7). All seven patients had a grade I spondylolisthesis; five patients sustained a burst fracture of the lumbar spine and two a compression fracture of the lumbar spine (Figs. 17.1 and 17.2). In none of the cases was there radiologic evidence for disc degeneration at the lumbosacral level. In two patients, there was a previous history of low back pain and lumbosacral olisthesis. In five patients, the olisthesis was judged to be old by a "negative" 99m-Tc-MDP bone scan of the olisthetic level, whereas the fractured vertebra showed intense uptake. In two patients operated on, no signs of hematoma or injury were found at the lumbosacral level. Thus, in all patients, no evidence was found to indicate that olisthesis was affected by lumbar trauma.

The occurrence of major lumbar spine fractures above the slip in patients with preexisting spondylolisthesis sheds light on the in vivo mechanics of lumbosacral olisthesis. These seven cases further support the notion that mild lumbosacral olisthesis is mechanically stable and can absorb vertical compression forces as well as considerable anterior shear forces without any ascertainable evidence of damage. Bradford (3) stated that acute traumatic lumbosacral spondylolisthesis is not uncommon in patients with burst fractures of the thoracolumbar spine. Floman and co-investigators (7) disagree, and state that the vast majority of so-called acute traumatic lytic spondylolisthesis in patients with burst fractures are old and existed prior to the acute spinal trauma. Rarely, acute traumatic lumbosacral olisthesis occurs as a result of bilateral facet dislocation (25) (Fig. 17.3).

Floman and his co-investigators (7) drew several conclusions from their retrospective survey.

1. Whenever a spondylolisthesis and major spinal trauma are concomitantly diagnosed, a bone scan should be performed to date the olisthesis. A "negative" bone scan at the lumbosacral junction in addition to radiographic findings of a smooth, well-rounded pars defect, should lead to the conclusion that the spondylolisthesis is old and not related to recent trauma (Fig. 17.2).
2. If the olisthesis is found to be old and the lumbar fracture is to be sur-

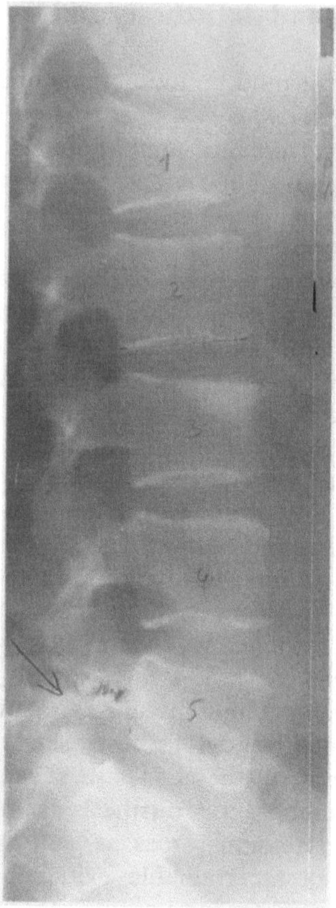

Figure 17.1. A 30-year-old man was involved in a motor vehicle accident. Lateral x-ray of the lumbosacral spine reveals compression fractures of L1 and L3 and a grade I lumbosacral isthmic spondylolisthesis.

Figure 17.2. **A:** Lateral radiograph of the lumbar spine in a 28-year-old male who sustained burst fractures at L2 and L4. In the past he sustained a L1 compression fracture. Note the first-degree lumbosacral slip. **B:** 99 m-Tc-MDP bone scan of the same individual. Note the intense isotope uptake at L2 and L4. There is normal uptake of the isotope at the lumbosacral level. **C:** Right oblique radiograph of the lumbar spine of the same individual. Note the smooth and well-rounded pars defect of L5. **D:** Axial CT of the same individual. Note the well-established pars defects. (Reprinted with permission from ref. 7)

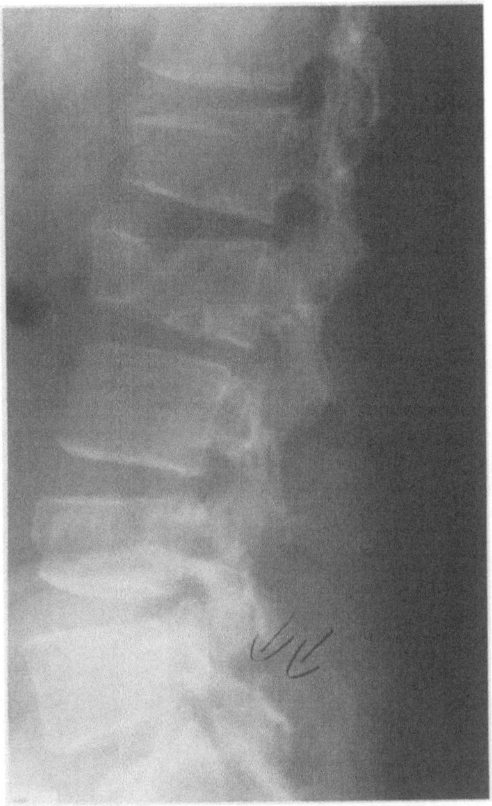

A

B

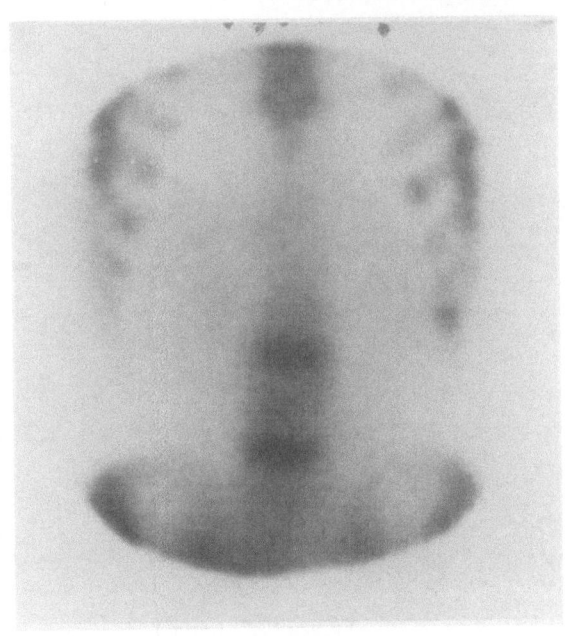

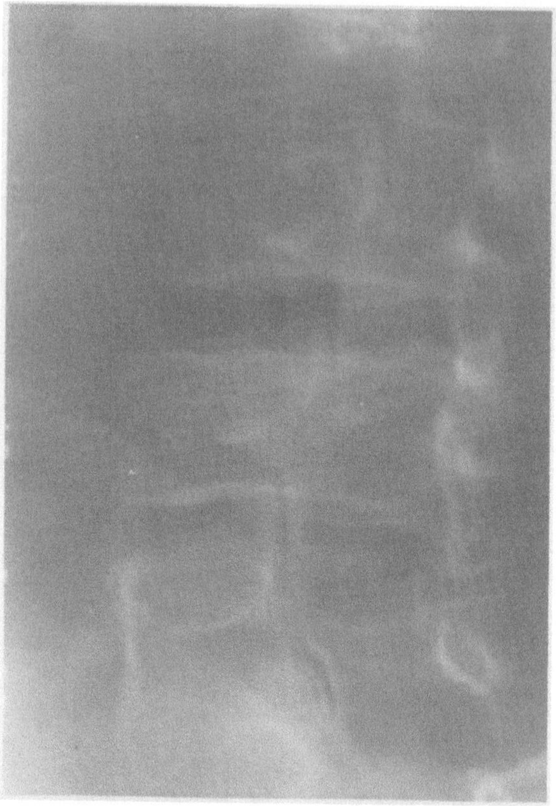

C

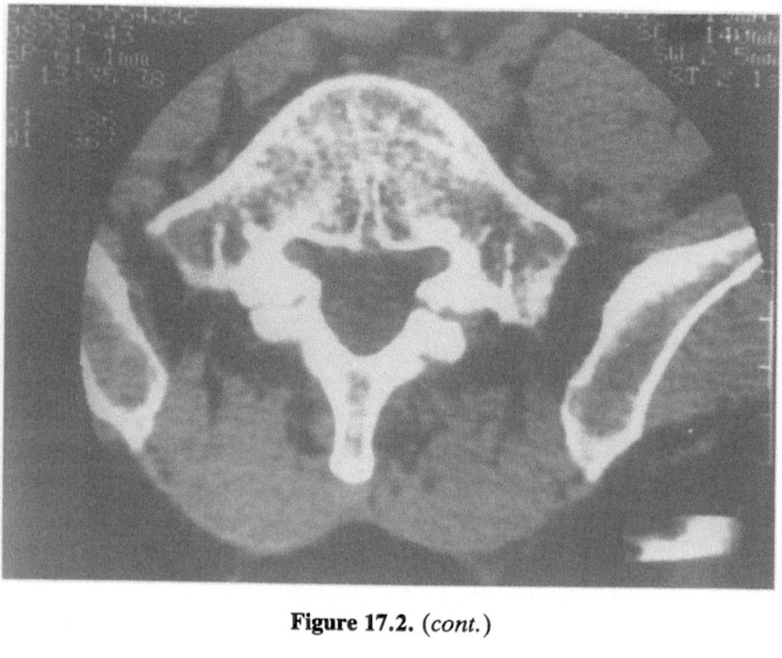

D

Figure 17.2. (*cont.*)

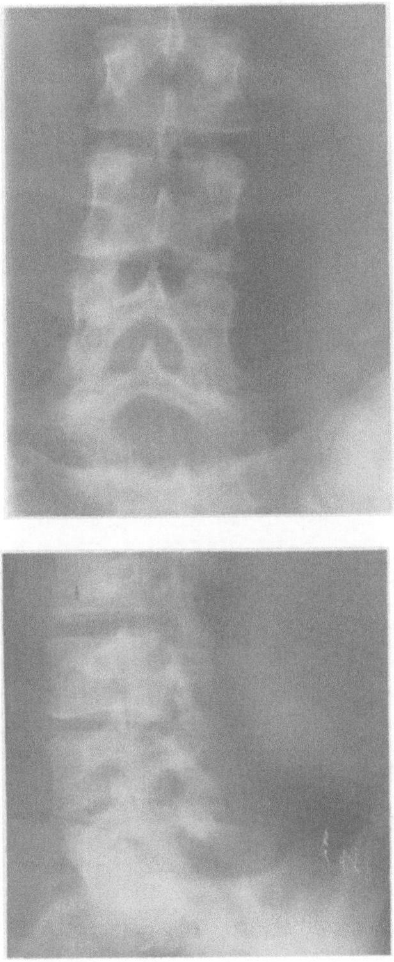

Figure 17.3. A 19-year-old man survived a light plane crash. He sustained a lumbosacral bilateral facet dislocation with a lumbosacral slip. **A:** AP x-ray. No pars defect is evident. **B:** An oblique view shows the pars interarticularis to be intact. **C:** Lateral x-ray shows the tilted L5 body. No pars defect is evident. **D:** Axial CT scan. Note the slip and the dislocated facets with secondary changes (CT was performed 4 months postinjury).

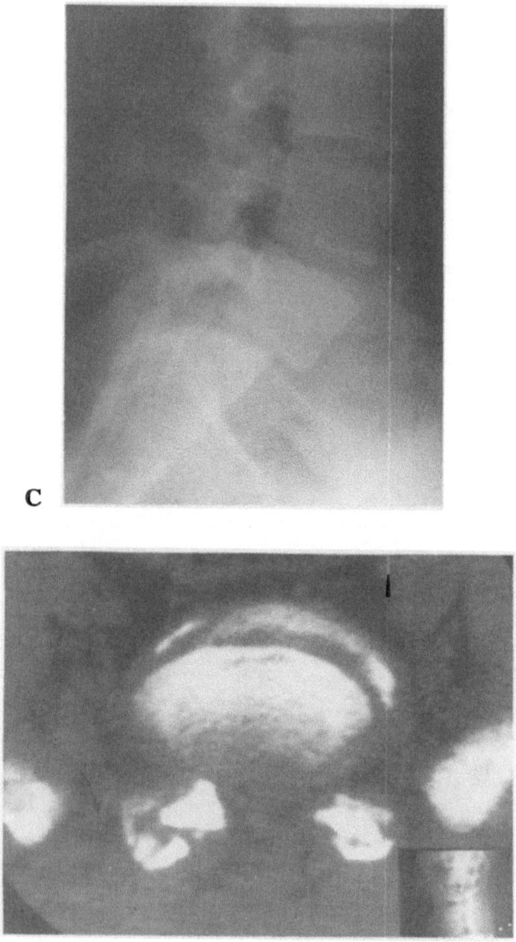

C

D

Figure 17.3. (*cont.*)

gically stabilized, the slipped vertebra should not be included in the fusion area. Only when an L4 burst fracture is to be surgically stabilized should the fusion extend down to the sacrum, preferably employing pedicle screw fixation.

3. A spondylolytic spondylolisthesis, unless otherwise proven, should not be considered to be caused by a single acute traumatic episode.
4. It may be assumed that grade I isthmic spondylolisthesis may have no less ability to absorb vertical compression and shear forces than the adjacent normal segments.
5. The incidence of lumbosacral spondylolisthesis in patients with thoracolumbar fractures is the same as that of the general population, not higher ($p < .213$).

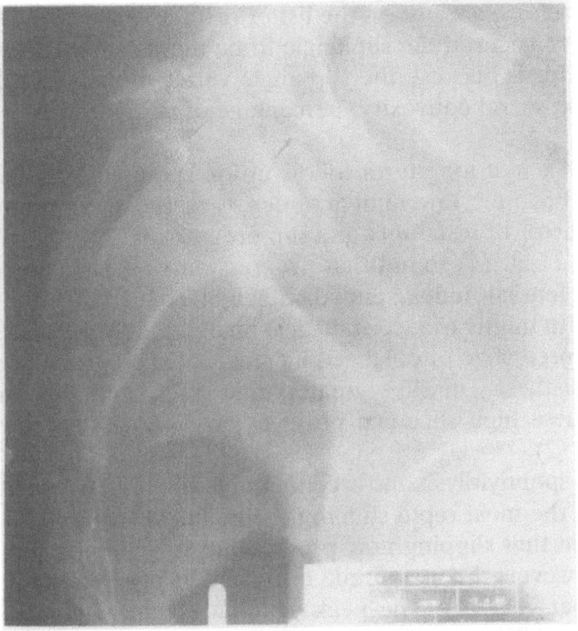

Figure 17.4. Lateral x-ray of the lumbosacral spine in a 21-year-old man. Note the lumbosacral slip, the dysplastic wedge-shaped L5, and the rounded sacrum. The patient underwent bilateral lateral spine fusion.

Radiographic Risk Factors of Slip Progression (2,43)

The body of S1 may be eroded anteriorly while the posterior aspect is convex. The hallmark of the radiographic deformity, or dysplasia, is the trapezoid shape of the body of L5 (Fig. 17.4). The percentage of slip is calculated according to the modified Taillard method. Sacral inclination is measured between a line parallel to the posterior aspect of S1 and a vertical line perpendicular to the floor, or to the bottom of a standing x-ray. A vertical sacrum will give a 0° reading. A normal sacral inclination is 42° to 43°. Slip angle is the measurement in degrees of the frontal tilt of L5 over S1 (parallel to the inferior aspect of the L5 body and perpendicular to the posterior aspect of the S1 body). A significant slip angle creates a lumbosacral kyphosis and a sagittal plane malalignment. The lumbar index is calculated by dividing the height of the posterior aspect of L5 by the height of the anterior aspect of L5.

Risk factors that cause slip to progress are a young age, female gender, high-grade slip, high slip angle, a low lumbar index, and a rounded top of the S1 body with a posterior arch defect (2).

Lordosis and a vertical sacrum are considered secondary to the high slip and, therefore, are not on the list of risk factors for progression. Boxall et al. (2) considered the slip angle to be the most sensitive indicator of instability. This is because the slip angle varies directly in relation to the lumbar index, sacral convexity, percentage of slip, lordosis, and sacral inclination.

Sarasta (34), in a long term follow up on spondylolisthesis, found that wedging of L5, i.e., low lumbar index, was the most important radiographic predictor of instability and slip progression.

Danielson et al. (4) found that progression was correlated to high slip angles, low lumbar index, and disc height reduction at the slip level. However, with multivariance statistical analysis, none of these factors was found to be predictive of olisthesis increase. Slip progression is greatest in dysplastic olisthesis, in slips greater than 50%, and slip angles greater than 45°. These high slips can progress even in the face of a seemingly solid fusion. (2).

Although spondylolysis most commonly occurs between the ages of 5 and 7 years, the most rapid slipping occurs between 9 and 15 years. Most authors agree that slipping may progress up to 25 years, but is rare after that (4). However, the magnitude of this adult progression is quite small, i.e., 0.6% per year (4). The peak of adult progression was found to be between 20 and 25 years of age (4). Ninety percent of the slip was present at the time of diagnosis. Seitsalo et al. (35) found that 23% of the patients exhibited some progression during almost 15 years of observation.

Vidal and Marnay (39) have put forward a biomechanical explanation of how a lumbosacral slip will relentlessly progress after it reaches a certain degree of olisthesis. They studied 200 cases of lumbosacral slip, with standing x-rays that included most of the spine, and the entire sacrum, pelvis, and femoral heads. They found that in advanced spondylolisthesis, there is a dramatic change in the anteroposterior equilibrium between the pelvis, sacrum, and hip joints. This change will influence the forward displacement of L5 on S1, and may perpetuate its downward progression. Although in normal subjects and in subjects with mild olisthesis the lumbosacral articulation is above the hip joint, in the same coronal and sagittal lines, this equilibrium changes in more severe forms of olisthesis, especially in the dysplastic one. The trunk weight acts on S1 and exerts a force that pushes the sacrum into a horizontal position, whereas the hip joints, through the reaction of the ground, tend to retrovert the pelvis. The pivot of this coupled motion is the second sacral vertebra (39). This is, however, a stable condition as all lumbopelvic ligaments are intact.

In certain types of spondylolisthesis, this equilibrium is disturbed, rotating the pelvis backward, and pushing the hip joints forward. As a result, the sacrum assumes a more vertical position. This allows L5 to plunge downward as the distance between the sacrum and the hip joints increases (39). It must be remembered that the slip increase is partly real and partly apparent. Most of the slip is a true posteroanterior sagittal translation, but part of it is apparent because of the pelvic retroversion and the sacrum moving into a more vertical position.

Symptomatology as Related to Instability

It is quite clear that when dealing with symptoms attributable to lumbosacral slip, children and adolescents should be viewed distinctly from adults.

Lafond (20) found that only 25% of children and adolescents with isthmic slips were symptomatic. Fredrickson et al. (8) reported similar data. Therefore, mild olisthesis should not be stabilized in asymptomatic teenagers. Olisthesis greater than grade II to III should be stabilized in symptomatic adolescents. A slip greater than grade III, or slip angle greater than 45°, should be stabilized even without symptoms in this age group.

On the other hand, the mere presence of spondylolysis or mild olisthesis in adults should not be considered as the source of either back or leg pain, per se. Macnab (24) has shown that the presence of spondylolysis in adults is not correlated with symptoms. The percentage of spondylolysis in adults older than 25 years, who have low back pain, was the same as in the general population. Sarasta (34) found that a slip greater than 25% was associated with increased back pain. Moreover, disc height reduction at the slip level and wedging of L5 increased the likelihood of back and leg pain. Apel et al. (1) found that patients with grade I olisthesis managed conservatively fared better than those managed by bilateral lateral L4-S1 fusion. They presented data on a small group of patients, but with a 40-year follow-up. Failure to achieve fusion correlated with poor results in the surgical group.

Therefore, stabilization of first or second grade isthmic slip in adults should not be attempted automatically. Attesting to this are the findings of Haraldsson and Wilner (13) that only 57% of adults with a lumbosacral slip who underwent bilateral lateral fusion had good results. This was in contrast to 95% good results obtained in individuals younger than 20 years who underwent fusion (13). In both groups the fusion rate approached 100%. Similar findings were reported by Hanley and Levy (12).

Slip Progression in Adults Due to Disc Degeneration

In the past, progression of spondylolisthesis has been recorded before skeletal maturity but has been doubted to occur in adults (22,34). Even a recent review on spondylolisthesis, published in a book entitled *The Adult Spine*, states that a progressive lumbosacral olisthesis is rare in

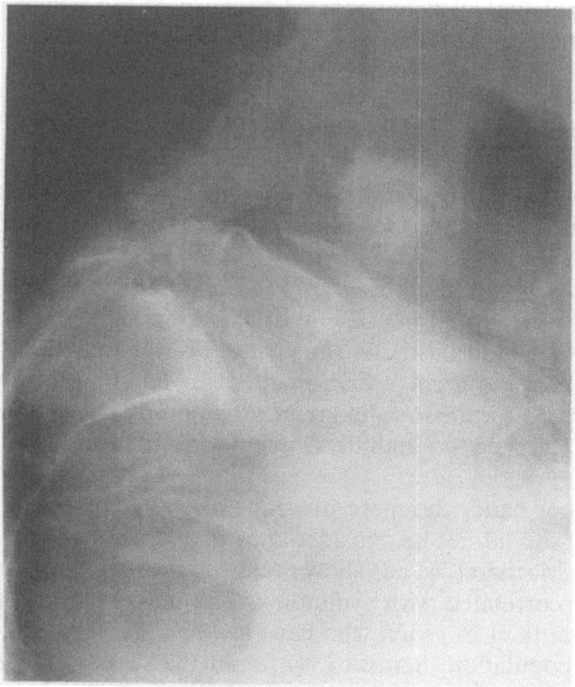

Figure 17.5. A 62-year-old woman with a triple-level isthmic spondylolisthesis ("ladder" or "cascading" spine) at L3-4, L4-5, and L5-S1. Note the severe disc degeneration at L3-4 and L5-S1. The disc at L4-5 is also mildly degenerated.

adults (11). At our institution, we have observed that this is not the case. It is not uncommon for middle-aged individuals to present with increasing low back and leg pain due to a "sudden" progression of a preexisting lumbosacral spondylolisthesis. The increased olisthesis is always the result of degeneration of the disc below the pars defect (Fig. 17.5). As the disc degenerates, it cannot resist the anterior shear forces, giving rise to the increased olisthesis. Some of these individuals will report that they were aware of their mild lumbosacral slip for years, but functioned in a normal fashion with occasional, mild backache. Others were asymptomatic and unaware that they had a lumbosacral olisthesis. In both groups, the increasing back pain is due to progression of the slip as a result of disc degeneration.

In the last 4 years, the author has seen seven patients with a progressing lumbosacral slip. There were five women and two men, and their age range was 40 to 58 years (average 48 years). Four of them were operated and instrumented with CD pedicular screw fixation and bilateral lateral fusion (Figs. 17.6 and 17.7).

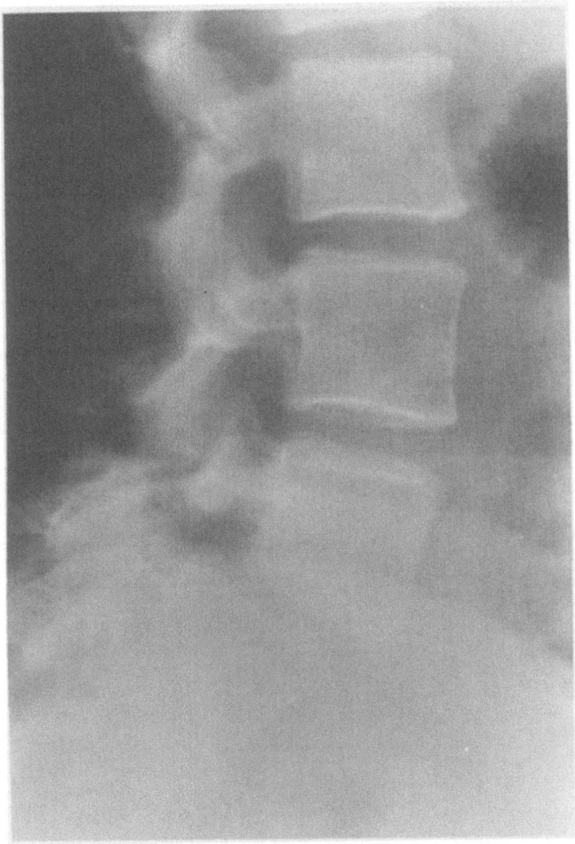

A

Figure 17.6. A 54 year-old woman presented with a history of increasing low back pain and bilateral leg pain during a 10 year period. The initial X-ray (**A**) shows a grade I isthmic lumbosacral spondylolisthesis with a "normal-looking" disc space. Subsequent lumbosacral x-ray (**B,C**) 4 and 6 years later reveal a progressing L5-S1 disc degeneration with increasing spondylolisthesis.

Similarly, five patients with progressing L4-5 isthmic slip were operated as well, with instrumentation and fusion (Figs. 17.8 and 17.9). Three had posterior CD instrumentation, one was operated via anterior approach, and one patient had a posterior lumbar interbody fusion with a metal block. Progression of L4-5 lytic olisthesis in adult life is better documented in the literature (11).

The stability of spondylolisthesis may be analyzed according to the three-column concept of spinal stability of thoracolumbar fractures, popularized by Denis (5). Denis considered a spine injury to be unstable if more than one spinal column was involved. In such a case, the deformity may progress and put the neurological structures at risk. In the

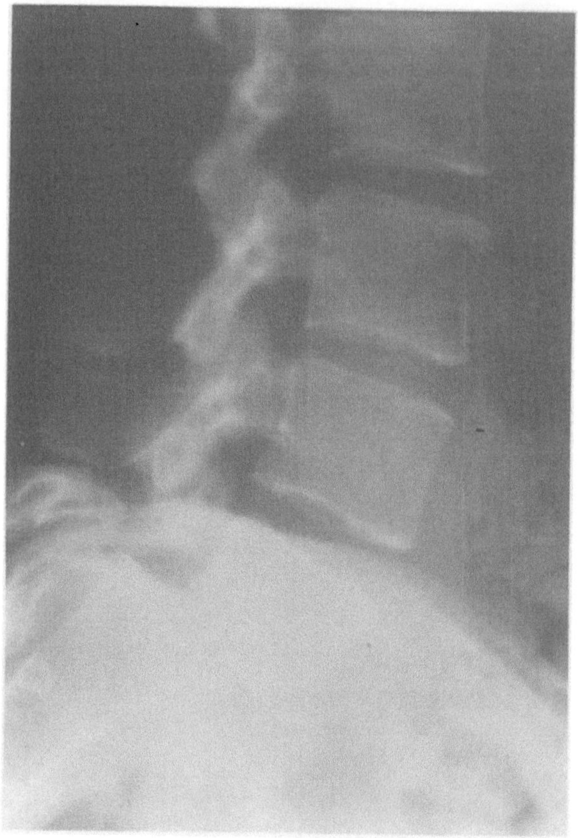

B

Figure 17.6. (*cont.*)

latter situation, the injured spine should be stabilized by either external or internal fixation. The same analogy can be applied to isthmic spondylolisthesis. In grade I or II lytic olisthesis, only the posterior column is involved (i.e., the pars interarticularis defect), whereas the anterior and middle columns are intact. The most important structure in these columns is the intervertebral disc, which provides the main resistance to the anteriorly directed shear forces. However, with disc degeneration at the lumbosacral level, all three columns of the spine are involved, leading to instability. Indeed, this is exactly the setup that permits progression of the slip, converting a stable, although not normal, motion segment into an unstable one.

There is ample evidence in the literature to suggest that disc degeneration is a key in converting a stable spondylolisthesis into an unstable, progressing slip. The classic teaching was that disc degeneration and her-

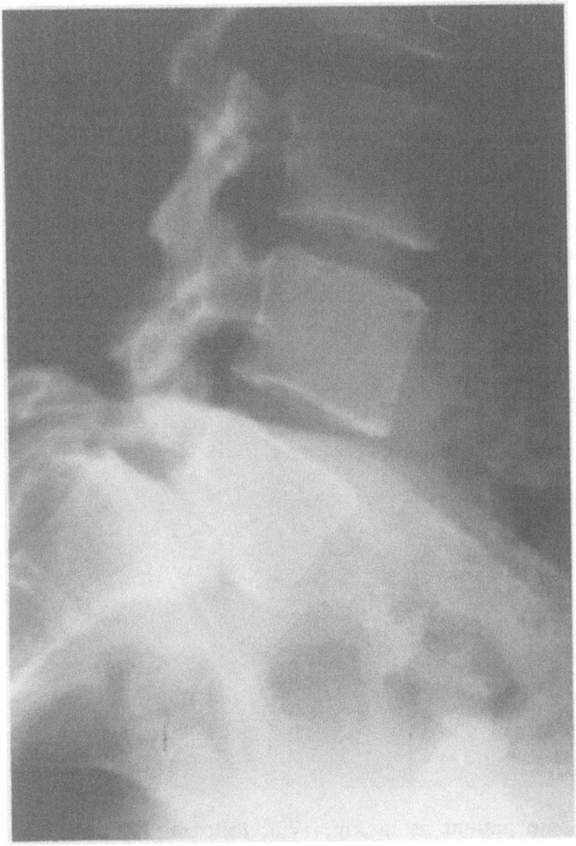

C

Figure 17.6. (*cont.*)

niation occur at the level above the slip and not at the level of the pars defect. Macnab (24) ascribed the pain in adults with spondylolisthesis to degeneration of the disc above the pars defect. Farafan et al. (6) stressed that disc degeneration below the pars defect occurred as a result of a rotatory and anteriorly directed shear forces. Farafan et al. observed an increased incidence of disc degeneration in patients with lumbosacral spondylolisthesis. Disc degeneration in spondylolisthesis may start at an early age. Haraldsson and Wilner (13) found evidence for this in 25% of adolescents admitted for surgical stabilization of spondylolisthesis. Sarasta (34) found progression of the slip to be highly correlated with disc degeneration. Disc degeneration was higher in patients with spondylolisthesis than in controls. The difference was statistically significant in the age group older than 40 years. Sarasta found that in slippage greater than 25%, the likelihood of low back ache was higher than in the general

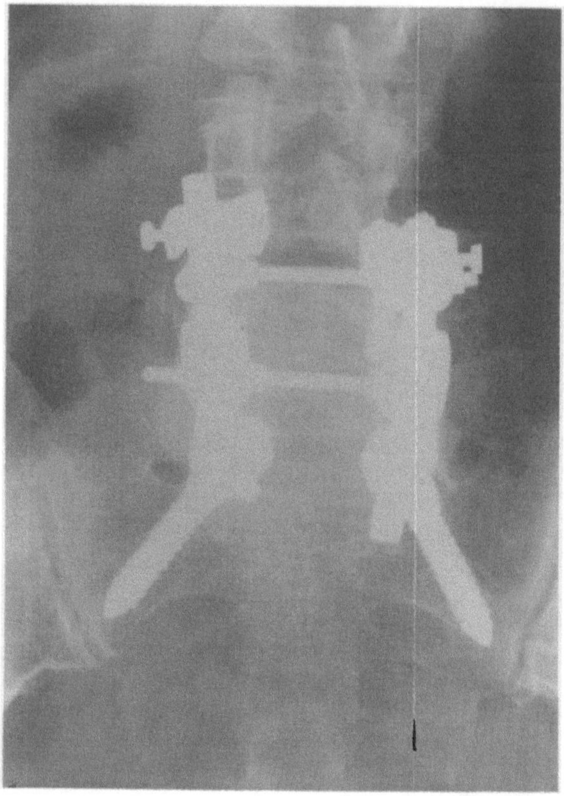

A

Figure 17.7. Same patient as in Fig. 17.6, following Cotrel-Dubousset pedicle screw instrumentation of the sacrum (S1 + S2) and L5 with complete reduction of the lumbosacral slip. The patient's sciatica resolved as well as her lower back pain. **A:** AP x-ray. **B:** Lateral x-ray.

population. A greater slip was also associated with earlier radiographic evidence of disc degeneration. The average slip progression in adults was 5 mm, and occurred at a period greater than 20 years. In a small percentage of cases (5%) slip progression was more than 10 mm (34).

Adult progression of the olisthesis occurs also in high-grade slips. Three of 11 nonoperated patients with high slip grades described by Harris and Weinstein (14) progressed.

Szypryt et al. (36), using magnetic resonance imaging (MRI), observed that in patients with spondylolisthesis, older than 25 years, there was a higher incidence of disc degeneration, whereas in younger patients the incidence of disc degeneration was the same as that of a control group. In-

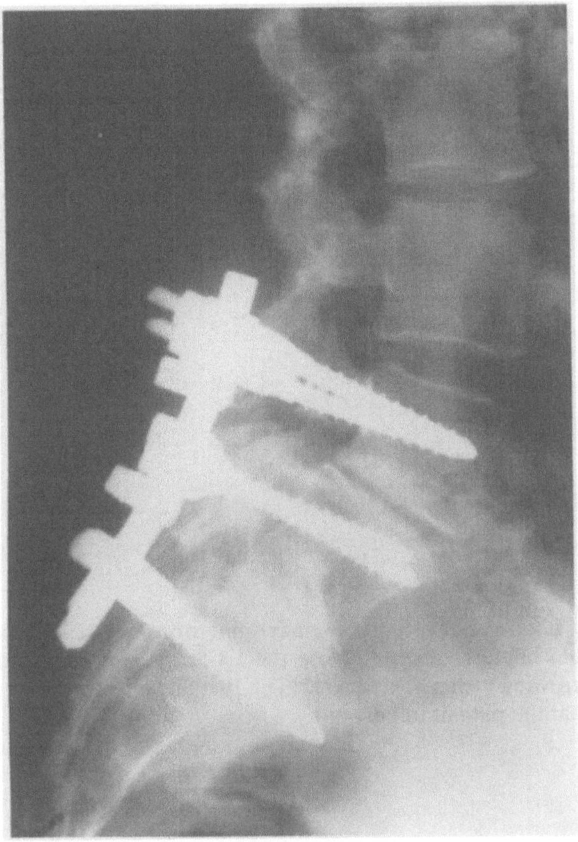

B

Figure 17.7. (*cont.*)

dividuals with spondylolisthesis who were between 25 and 45 years had a 70% incidence of disc degeneration. Fredrickson et al. (9) followed children with spondylolisthesis from age 5 to 40 years. They noted that, in some individuals, progression of the slip occurred with degeneration of the disc below the pars defect. Disc degeneration was evidenced by disc space narrowing. These investigators thought that disc narrowing and progression of the slip occurred concurrently.

Danielson et al. (4) noted in a large group of patients with spondylolisthesis that an increase in olisthesis occurred between 14 and 30 years of age, with a peak between the ages of 20 to 25 years. The increased slip, although real, was small, i.e., 0.6% per year. Recently Seitsalo et al. (35), in a long-term follow-up of 272 patients with spondylolis-

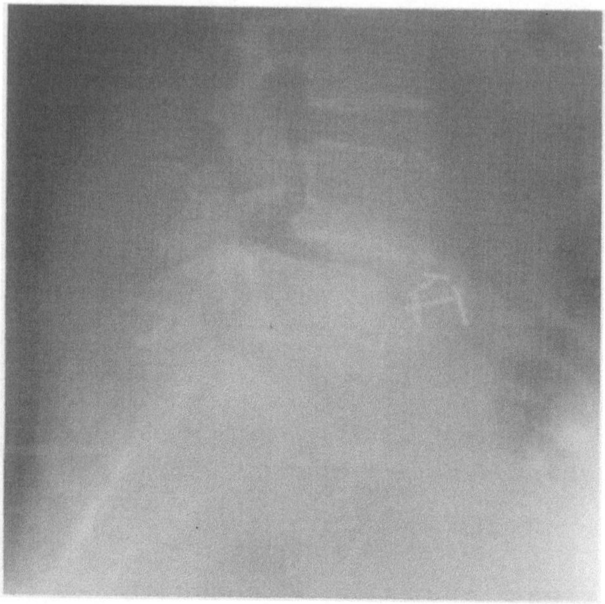

Figure 17.8. Lateral x-ray of the lumbar spine of a 45-year-old woman with low back pain and bilateral sciatica. Note the L4-5 grade II spondylolisthesis. Note also disc narrowing at the same level. (The metallic clips were used during a hysterectomy that the patient underwent.)

thesis, found that 23% of them progressed, although 90% of the slip had occurred at the time of diagnosis. They concluded that the role of the intervertebral disc in buffering the instability imposed by the pars defect and the anterior shear forces is essential.

Apel et al. (1) reported on a small group of individuals with low-grade lumbosacral slip and with ultralong follow-up. Of the five patients who were managed nonoperatively, one suffered from disabling low back pain due to slip progression as a result of disc degeneration.

Figure 17.9. Same patient as in Fig. 17.8, following total laminectomy of the loose lamina, with release of both L5 nerve roots, and implantation of pedicle screws at L4 and L5 with reduction of the slip and partial restoration of the disc height. The device used is the Malaga vertebral fixation system. **A:** AP x-ray. **B:** Lateral x-ray.

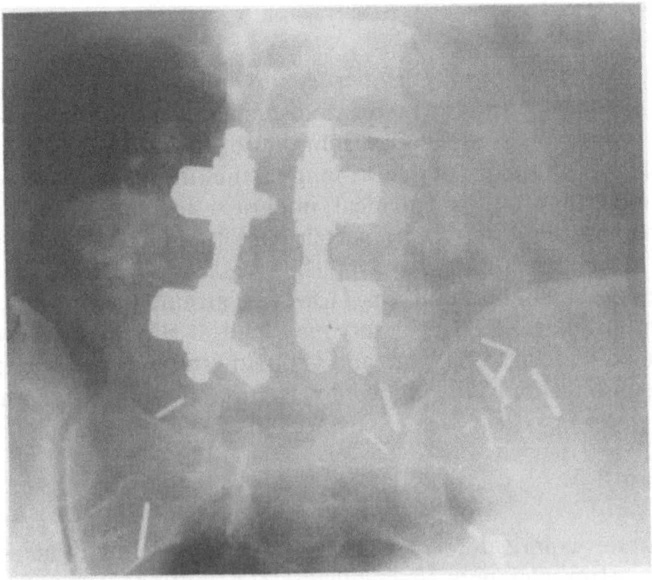

A

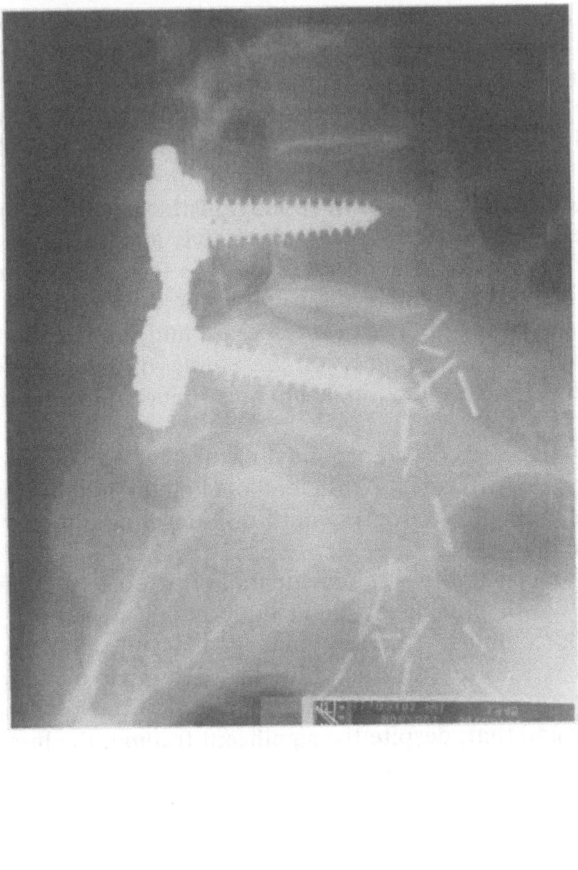

B

Conclusions

A bilateral pars defect may lead to spondylolisthesis. This anterior slip occurs as a result of anteriorly directed shear forces. The main resistance to these shear forces is the intervertebral disc. In adults, mild lumbosacral spondylolisthesis remains stable as long as the intervening disc maintains its biochemical and biomechanical integrity. Indeed, individuals with preexisting spondylolisthesis can sustain major trauma to their spines, resulting in a burst fracture (above the slip), without ascertainable evidence of damage to the lumbosacral slip. However, around the fifth decade, disc degeneration below the pars defect may lead to slip progression. This is accompanied by increasing back and leg pain, and may necessitate instrumentation and fusion of the involved vertebrae to relieve symptoms.

Summary

A pars interarticularis defect (spondylolysis) significantly reduces the role of the posterior elements in stabilizing the motion segment. Bilateral spondylolysis may lead to anterior displacement of the involved vertebra over the subjacent vertebra below (spondylolisthesis). Most often, spondylolisthesis occurs at the lumbosacral level. This displacement is the result of anterior shear forces acting parallel to the disc. The main resistance to this anteriorly directed shear forces is the intervertebral disc.

In normal subjects and in subjects with mild lumbosacral olisthesis, the lumbosacral articulation is above the hip joint in the same coronal and sagittal planes. In certain types of spondylolisthesis, the sacrum assumes a more vertical position, retroverting the pelvis and pushing the hip joint anteriorly. The pivot of this coupled motion is the second sacral vertebra; as a result, L5 is no longer in the same coronal and sagittal planes, and may plunge downward, between the sacrum and the hip joints. Risk factors associated with slip progression are young age, female gender, high-grade slip, low lumbar index, high slip angle, and rounding of the tope of the sacrum.

In most adults, lumbosacral spondylolisthesis is minimal, and does not exceed slip grades of I or II. At the end of skeletal growth, this is a stable lesion that is unlikely to progress until disc degeneration has occurred at the slip level.

Attesting to its stability is the incidental occurrence of lumbar fractures in individuals with preexisting, mild lumbosacral olisthesis. Among 300 cases of thoracolumbar fractures managed at the author's institution, seven such cases were detected. Five had a lumbar burst fracture, and two had a lumbar compression fracture in addition to the lumbosacral slip. It was found that, despite the significant trauma, the lumbosacral slip was able to withstand considerable axial and anterior shear forces without ascertainable evidence of damage.

On the other hand, once the biochemical and biomechanical integrity of the disc below the isthmic defect is lost, the lumbosacral slip will become unstable and will progress. This occurs most often in the fifth decade of life. Seven adult patients with a progressive isthmic lumbosacral slip due to disc degeneration were seen in the last 4 years. Similarly, seven patients with a progressive L4-5 isthmic slip due to disc degeneration were seen, as well. Once the lesion becomes unstable, instrumentation and fusion are indicated.

References

1. Apel DM, Lorentz MA, Zindrick MR. Symptomatic spondylolisthesis in adults four decades later. *Spine*. 1989;14:345–348.
2. Boxall D, Bradford DS, Winter RB, Moe JH. Management of severe spondylolisthesis of children and adolescents. *J Bone Joint Surg*. 1979;61A:479–495.
3. Bradford DS. Management of spondylolysis and spondylolisthesis. In: American Academy of Orthopaedic Surgeons. *Instructional Course Lectures*. CV Mosby; St. Louis: 1983;33:151–162.
4. Danielson B, Frennered K, Irstam L. Radiographic progression of isthmic lumbar spondylolisthesis in young patients. *Spine*. 1991;16:422–425.
5. Denis F. Spinal instability as defined by the three-column spine concept in acute spinal trauma. *Clin Orthop*. 1984;189:65–76.
6. Farafan HF, Osteria V, Lamy C. The mechanical etiology of spondylolysis and spondylolisthesis. *Clin Orthop*. 1976;117:40–55.
7. Floman Y, Margulies JY, Nyska M, Chisin R, Liebergall M. Effect of major axial skeleton trauma on preexisting lumbosacral spondylolisthesis. *J Spinal Dis*. 1991;4:353–358.
8. Fredrickson BE, Baker D, McHolick WJ, Yuan HA, Lubicky JP. The natural history of spondlylolysis and spondylolisthesis. *J Bone Joint Surg*. 1984;66A:669–707.
9. Fredrickson BE, Baker D, Murtland A, Yuan HA. Spondylolisthesis: the natural history age 5-40. Presented at the North American Spine Society Meeting in Monterey, CA, 1990.
10. Gertzbein SD, Seligman J, Holtby R, Chan KW, Ogston N, Kapasouri A, Tile M. Centrode characteristics of the lumbar spine as a function of segmental instability. *Clin Orthop*. 1986;208:48–51.
11. Grobler LJ, Wiltse LL. Classification, non-operative and operative treatment of spondylolisthesis. In Frymoyer JW, ed. *The Adult Spine, Principle and Practice* New York: Raven Press; 1991:1655.
12. Hanley EN, Levy JA. Surgical treatment of isthmic lumbosacral spondylolisthesis. Analysis of variables influencing results. *Spine*. 1989;14:48–50.
13. Haraldsson S, Wilner S. A comparative study of spondylolisthesis in operations on adolescents and adults. *Arch Orthop Trauma Surg*. 1983;101:101–105.

14. Harris IE, Weinstein SL. Long term follow up of patients with grade II and IV spondylolisthesis. Treatment with or without posterior spine fusion. *J Bone Joint Surg*. 1987;69A:960–969.
15. Hensinger RN. Spondylolysis and spondylolisthesis in children. In: *Disorders of the Lumbar Spine*. Floman Y, Rockville, MD: Aspen; 1990:553.
16. Herbiniaux G. *Traite sur Diverse Accouchemonts Laborieux et sur les Polypes de la Matirce*. Bruxelles: De Boubers, 1782.
17. Jackson DW, Wiltse LL, Cirincione RJ. Spondylolysis in female gymnasts. *Clin Orthop*. 1976;117:68–73.
18. Kessen W, During J, Beeker TW, Gondfrooij H, Crowe A. Recordings of movement of the intervertebral segment L5-S1. A technique for the determination of the movement at the L5-S1, spinal segment using three specified postural positions. *Spine*. 1984;9:83.
19. Kilian JF. *Schilderungen neuer Backenformen und ihrer Verhalten in Leben*. Mannheim: Bassermann und Mathy; 1854.
20. Lafond G. Surgical treatment of spondylolisthesis. *Clin Orthop*. 1962;22:175–179.
21. Lambl, D.L.: Zehn thesen ueber spondylolisthesis. *Zentralbl Gynakol Urol*. 1855;9:250.
22. Laurent LE, Einola S. Spondylolisthesis in children and adolescents. *Acta Orthop Scand*. 1964;31:45–64.
23. Lowe RW, Hayes TD, Kaye J, Bagg RJ, Luekens CA. Standing roentgenograms in spondylolisthesis. *Clin Orthop*. 1976;117:80–84.
24. Macnab I. *Backache*. Williams & Wilkins; Baltimore: 1977:51.
25. Macnab I. McCulloch J. *Backache* 2nd ed. Baltimore: Williams & Wilkins; 1990:100–101.
26. Neithard FB. Scheuermann's disease and spondylolysis. *Orthop Trans*. 1983;7:103.
27. Neugebauer FL. A new contribution to the history and etiology of spondylolisthesis. *New Sydenham Society Selected Monographs*. 1888;121:1–64.
28. O'Neill DB, Micheli LJ. Post operative radiographic evidence for fatigue fracture as the etiology in spondylolysis. *Spine*. 1989;14:1342–1355.
29. Pearcy M, Shepherd J. Is there instability in spondylolisthesis? *Spine*. 1985;10:175–177.
30. Penning L, Blickman JR. Instability in lumbar spondylolisthesis: A radiologic study of several concepts. *Am J Radiol*. 1980;134:293–301.
31. Robert K. Eine eigentuemliche angeborene lordose, wahrscheinlich bedingt durch eine verschiebung des Koerpers des letzen lindenwirbels auf die vordere flaeche des ersten kreuzeinwirbels. *Monat Geburtskunde Frauenkrank*. 1985;5:891–894.
32. Rosenberg NJ, Barger WL, Friedman B. The incidence of spondylolysis and spondylolisthesis in nonambulatory patients. *Spine*. 1981;6:35–38.
33. Rossi F. Spondylolysis, spondylolisthesis and sports. *J Sports Med Phys Fitness*. 1978;18:317–340.
34. Sarasta H. Long term clinical and radiological follow up of spondylolysis and spondylolisthesis. *J Pediatr Orthop*. 1987;7:631–638.
35. Seitsalo S, Osterman K, Hyvarinen H, Tallroth K, Schlenzka D, Poussa M. Progression of spondylolisthesis in children and adolescents. A long term follow up of 272 patients. *Spine*. 1991;16:417–421.

36. Szypryt EP, Twining P, Mulholland RC, Worthington BS. The prevalence of disc degeneration associated with neural arch defects of the lumbar spine assessed by magnetic resonance imaging. *Spine*. 1989;14:977–981.
37. Taillard WF. Etiology of spondylolisthesis. *Clin Orthop*. 1976;117:30–39.
38. Troup JDC. Mechanical factors in spondylolisthesis and spondylolysis. *Clin Orthop*. 1976;117:59–67.
39. Vidal J, Marnay T. La morphologie et l'equilibre corporel antero posterier dans le spondylolisthesis L5-S1. *Rev Chir Orthop*. 1983;69:17–28.
40. Wiltse LL, Newman PH, Mcnab I. Classification of spondylolysis and spondylolisthesis. *Clin Orthop*. 1976;117:23–29.
41. Wiltse LL, Rothman LG. Spondylolisthesis. Classification diagnosis and natural history. *Semin Spine Surg*. 1989;1:78–94.
42. Wiltse LL, Widell EH, Jackson DW. Fatigue fracture: The basic lesion in isthmic spondylolisthesis. *J Bone Joint Surg*. 1975;57A:17–22.
43. Wiltse LL, Winter RB. Terminology and measurement of spondylolisthesis. *J Bone Joint Surg*. 1983;65A:768–772.

Discussion

Measuring The Degree of Translation in Spondylolisthesis

Dr. O'Leary asked about the position of the patient in measuring the degree of translation in spondylolisthesis. Dr. Floman replied: On a standing lateral x-ray. Dr. O'Leary said: In my experience if you take the same patient and have him lie down supine in lumbar extension with a pillow supporting the lumbar region you would be surprised at the degree of reduction. I feel that the supine position with the lumbar spine in extension is the best method to assess the degree of translation. I similarly have seen reduction after positioning the patient in the operating room. Dr. Floman responded that they are then under general anesthesia. Dr. O'Leary continued: I do believe that there are muscular forces operative in the upright position that prevent reduction from taking place.

To Reduce Spondylolisthesis or Not?

Dr. Kostuik began by saying Dr. Floman, you showed some cases where you reduced the spondylolisthesis and some where you did not. Why and when should one reduce the slip?

Dr. Floman responded: The cases I showed that had been reduced were actually some of the first cases I did. After listening to other physicians and realizing that the neurological complications after reduction may reach 30% to 40% in very good centers I became concerned and decided to use instrumentation to change the slip angle and to correct somewhat the kyphotic deformity, but it was not aimed at slip reduction. Dr. Kostuik said: The slip angle is a measurement of kyphosis.

Dr. Kostuik asked Prof. Louis if he reduces grade III and IV slips? Prof. Louis responded that he performs reduction when it is reasonable to do so. The term "reasonable" applies to an adolescent without osteophyte formation and when the spondylolisthesis is mobile. Dr. Kostuik asked: How do you determine when it is mobile? Prof. Louis said: At the beginning of my operation my patient is committed to spinal traction of 15 kg and I can easily see on the image intensifier if a reduction can be achieved. If reduction of one-third is seen I know that full reduction is reasonably possible without problems. If, on the other hand, the spondylolisthesis is fixed, then it is not reasonably reducible. Dr. Kostuik asked: Do you sometimes examine the patients under general anesthesia? Prof. Louis said: No. Dr. Kostuik continued: There are some reports of iatrogenic nerve problems in hyperextension under general anethesia in North America. Dr. Bollini said: There are some risk factors in adolescents. One is the dome-shaped S1 and the other is the duration of the lesion.

Dr. Kostiuk continued: This represents a tremendous change in approach. Both Dr. Bollini and Prof. Louis have a large surgical experience, yet in many centers in Europe spondylolistheses are just reduced without regard to the slip angle. This has provoked considerable controversy. If you have mobility in an adolescent my opinion is that it is fair enough to go ahead, but adults should not be reduced. Prof. Louis said: I agree with "some adults." Dr. Kostuik said: Some adults are young. Prof. Louis noted that individuals who are 45 without osteophytes may be considered young.

Dr. White said: The big question is why reduce at all. The champion of not reducing has been Dr. Wiltse. He and one of my current partners, Dr. Jim Reynolds, reviewed their cases over a 10- to 20-year period and videotaped them. For the most part I thought they looked pretty good. There were still a few gawky kids and adults, but most were normal and all had grade III and IV slips and demonstrated normal ranges of motion.

The Etiology of the Neurological Deficit Occasioned by Reduction

Dr. White asked: Is the neurological deficit due to a traction injury of the L5 nerve root or the ventral ramus? Dr. Kostuik said: I think the L5 root is the one that gets affected most often. As you know there are large and fairly tough ligaments that extend from the transverse processes onto the ilium and in spondylolisthesis it is speculated that the ligaments may be thicker and the ventral rami may be adherent to them. Dr. Farcy said that Bradford described a lesion at L3 or L2 in one of his reductions. Dr. O'Leary said that the question may also relate to traction on the lumbosacral plexus. Dr. Holtzman added that one of the problems with the L5 nerve root is the frequent association of the artery of Lazorthes that may nourish both the nerve root and the conus medullaris. No efforts are made to document this vessel preoperatively, as one would document the artery of Adamkiewicz. Dr. Kostuik concurred that the L5 root is the most sensitive in the cauda equina and that it was his impression that the increasing trend worldwide was to change the slip angle rather than to reduce.

CHAPTER 18

The Surgical Treatment of Failures of Laminectomy and Spinal Fusion

John P. Kostuik

The two major areas of surgery of the spine consist of either decompressive procedures and/or fusion procedures. This chapter deals with the failures of either or both. In order to expedite and simplify this for the reader it is the author's intention to divide the chapter into two parts: first, failures of laminectomy or decompressive procedures, and second, failures of fusion.

Failure to alleviate signs and symptoms and subsequent deterioration following a fusion or decompression procedure presents as a difficult problem for both the surgeon and patient. Failures following decompressive surgery vary from 5% to over 50% with a general average of about 15% (122). This variation is due to the different forms of procedures, the pathology of the population analyzed, as well as different criteria used to measure success (48). It is well recognized that patients receiving third-party funds, i.e., workers compensation, have a lesser success rate than patients whose economic outcome is dependent on their own efforts (89). Because of the development of the special physician patient relationship, the surgeon performing the initial operative procedure often cannot objectively arrive at a decision with reference to further surgery in his own patient. The treating surgeon to some extent frequently buries his head in the sand and denies a problem.

Causes of Failure

The three W's have been described as encompassing the failures of spinal surgery. These are the wrong patient, the wrong diagnosis, and the wrong surgery. Included in this is improper preoperative diagnosis and improper indications.

It is simple to eliminate the wrong surgeon Jones (54) reviewed 180 residency training programs of which 88% believed spinal surgery was an important component of clinical practice. However, only 74% provided what was deemed to be adequate training. Today, spinal surgery is about to enter the 21st century. The current state of the art in this field is approximately comparable to joint replacement surgery 15 to 20 years ago. Because of the increasing complexity of spinal surgery, and the increasingly sophisticated techniques and instrumentation, we believe a spinal surgeon of tomorrow will need to have completed a fellowship and devote the majority of his time to spinal problems for these complex techniques to be mastered.

The wrong patient is a more complex problem, and can be divided into two general categories: the patient was chosen for treatment by fusion or decompression when the pathology at hand could not be expected to benefit from that operation, or the patient's psychosocial circumstances and expectations simply precluded success. An example of the former is the utilization of spinal fusions for a patient with nonspecific, chronic, disabling low back pain, where history, physical examination, and imaging studies indicate no definite pathology. In these circumstances, failure rates as high as 80% are recorded, leading most authorities to conclude spinal fusion has no role in the management of nonspecific spinal pain. Similarly, the psychosocial determinants of success and failure in spine disease and surgery require emphasis, as they relate to spinal surgery and its indications. The wrong operation is an even more complex issue, and ranges in cause from inadequate imaging studies, which led to misdiagnosis, all the way to a poor choice of surgical technique from the large menu of alternatives that currently are available to the spinal surgeon.

An inadequate preoperative assessment combined with the failure to understand the objectives of the patient together with the failure to understand the impact of psychosocial problems on outcome can result in disaster.

An increasing emphasis today has been placed upon the use of sophisticated imaging techniques. It should be remembered that a careful analysis of subjective pain complaints, namely history taking, forms more than 90% of the basis of decision making to proceed to surgery. Objective physical findings and confirmatory imaging studies help to localize the source of the subjects complaints.

Though some failures can be described as being a result of the three W's, some complications occur that are beyond the surgeon's control including such things as arachnoiditis or extradural scarring.

Surgery is but one aspect in the total care of the patient (70). Although surgery plays a major role it is not the only event leading to a successful outcome. The role of rehabilitation and postoperative care is almost equally important. This is particularly true in surgery for a previous, failed procedure. The ultimate goal is pain relief and restoration of function and patient satisfaction. Surgery is one of the steps in the rehabilitative process.

This chapter not only deals with the causes of failures (Table 18.1) for patients who have had decompressive procedures or fusion of the lumbar

Table 18.1. A: Classification of failures.

1. No impovement immediately following surgery with outright failure to improve mono- or polyradiculopathy
   - A. Wrong preoperative diagnosis
     1. Tumor
     2. Infection
     3. Metabolic disease
     4. Psychosocial
     5. Discogenic pain
     6. Decompression done too late for disc sequestration (>6 months)
   - B. Technical error
     1. Missed level or levels
     2. Failures to perform adequate decompression
        - a. Missed fragment including foraminal disc
        - b. Failure to recognize spinal stenosis as part of lumbar disc herniation
        - c. Conjoined nerve root
2. Temporary relief but recurrence of pain
   - A. Early recurrence of symptoms (within weeks)
     1. Infection
     2. Meningeal cyst
   - B. Midterm (within weeks to months)
     1. Recurrent disc prolapse
     2. Battered root
     3. Arachnoiditis
     4. Patient expectation
   - C. Longer-term failure (within months to years)
     1. Recurrent stenosis of development of lateral stenosis from disc space collapse
     2. Instability

spine and reviews solutions (107), but additionally an analysis is made of what should be done initially in order to possibly avoid a second operative intervention. Finally, presentations of patients with surgical failures and treatment alternatives are presented.

Although the three W's account for many failures this approach does not account for the problems that follow a properly performed procedure in the correct patient for the right diagnosis. Such failures are represented by unavoidable complications or can result from ongoing degenerative disease.

Classifications of Failures of Decompressive Surgery

Failures of decompressive surgery can be divided into two main types (Table 18.2): first, those in which radiculopathy predominates, and second, those in which low back pain is a major problem. Both of course may coexist. In addition the classification of complications is included (Table 18.1B).

Table 18.1. B: Other complications.

Local	General
Posterior	
Early:	
Hemorrhage	Blood transfusion reactions
Ecchymoses	Hemolysis
Wound dehiscence	Anemia
Neurological	Urinary retention
Laminar fracture	Sepsis
Pedicle fracture	Metabolic disorders
Sepsis	Psychosis
Vascular (anterior)	Drug overdose
Iliac crest	Hypotension
Anterior	
Early:	
Hemorrhage	Cholycystitis
Vascular (vessel)	Pancreatitis + All listed under Posterior
Ureteric damage	
Renal damage	
Splenic damage	
Bowel damage	
Sympathetic disruption	
Iliac crest hemorrhage	
Iliac crest fracture	
Wound dehiscence	
Sepsis	
Graft extrusion	
Anterior and posterior	
Intermediate:	
Wound sepsis	
Fracture at fixation points	
Instrumentation failure	
Vascular aneurysm (anterior only)	
Retroperitoneal fractures	
Ureteric obstruction (anterior only)	
Hydronephrosis	
Incisional hernia	
Iliac crest fracture	
Nerve irritation secondary to donor site	
Late:	
Late sepsis	
Instrumentation failure	
Donor site problems	
Retroperitoneal fibrosis	
Ureteric obstruction (anterior only)	
Hydronephrosis (anterior only)	
Vascular aneurysm (anterior only)	
Incisional hernia	

Table 18.2. Causes of failure classified by the dominant symptom.

Radiculopathy predominant	Low back pain predominant
Neural tumors	Osseous tumors
Infections—epidural abscess	Infections
Inadequate decompression	Discitis
Missed fragment	Osteomyelitis
Foraminal disc	Discogenic pain
Conjoined nerve root	Segmental instability
Recurrent disc prolapse	
Peridural fibrosis	
Meningeal cyst	
Arachnoiditis	

Approaches to the Patient with a Failed Spinal Decompression

History and Physical Examination

Clinical history is the most significant factor in assessing probable causation of continuing symptoms. Finnegan et al. (29) identified three typical pain syndromes:

1. The patient has no initial relief of symptoms or his symptoms are worse. It is likely that the wrong diagnosis was made or the wrong operation was performed.
2. The patient has initial relief, sometimes accompanied by increased numbness or even weakness, followed by gradual onset of recurrent radiculopathy over weeks to months, It is likely that nerve root injury has occurred with subsequent scarring.
3. The patient has complete relief of symptoms but later, over months to years, develops recurrent radiculopathy—often suddenly. It is likely that recurrent disc has occurred.

Frymoyer et al. (36) also emphasized the importance of long-term failures, which they felt were usually the manifestation of an ongoing degenerative process. In patients who had undergone decompression for radiculopathy, low back pain as a continuing problem may be a major factor regardless of whether or not an arthrodesis has been performed. The patient may have expected complete relief of all back symptoms, an expectation that is probably in most cases ill-founded. The ability to differentiate between the usual expected continuum of back pain from those with severe back pain for which an anatomic cause can be established is difficult.

In addition to the factors outlined above other important things in the history are the presence or absence of systemic symptoms, work, psychosocial history, and the status of compensation or legal proceedings. Efforts must be made to obtain prior records of other interventions.

Physical examination, although not as important as history taking, does have a role. This role may not be particularly rewarding if low back pain is a predominant complaint. If residual deficits from prior surgery or neurological problems are present, interpretation of the neurological examination may be difficult. It is recognized that 40% to 50% of patients who have had previous discotomy have residual alterations in reflexes and sensation corresponding to the level of previous root involvement (36,85). Nerve tension signs are useful when indications of failure when positive, since these are usually alleviated after successful surgery. The physical findings may be confused as a result of the pathology. Patients with recurrent stenosis may have minimal physical findings or misleading findings (114). The presence of nonorganic physical findings as described by Waddell et al. (115) may help to identify patients who have an inappropriate pain pattern.

Imaging Assessment

Imaging studies are the confirmatory basis for diagnosis. The most likely cause for continuing symptoms should be established on the basis of history and physical examination. The various imaging techniques are emphasized in greater detail in the section on failed fusions. In the author's opinion the use of computed tomography (CT)-enhanced myelography has proven to be more effective to date than enhanced magnetic resonance imaging (MRI). CT myelography is capable of diagnosing arachnoiditis and although MRI is more effective for soft tissue analysis, I feel that CT myelography is of added value as it more clearly demonstrates bony problems. This is particularly true in cases of possible spinal stenosis.

CT discography may be of value in assessing far out lateral syndromes as well as assessing annular tears.

Facet blocks are not of much value as a diagnostic tool in case of failed surgery because of dorsal scarring, if that is present (28).

Selected nerve root blocks have proven to be extremely valuable in differentiating various aspects of root pain. They are by no means infallible. An injection of 1 to 2 cc in the base of a nerve root may anesthetize an adjacent root. Moreover, they do not differentiate extrinsic from intrinsic compression or scarring (62,75).

The failures of decompressive surgery can also be classified as to immediate early recurrence of symptoms, midterm failures, as well as long-term failures.

Immediate Failure

Wrong Diagnosis. Radiculopathy has a variety of causes including lumbar disc herniation and spinal stenosis. Most other causes are rare and include such things as infections and tumors Wiesel et al. (123) found that only 109 of 5,362 were ultimately found to have an underlying cause. Schofferman et al. (102) emphasized occult infections as an important cause of symptoms in patients with low back pain and radiculopathy. The incidence of spinal infections including epidural abscesses is 0.037/1,000, disc space infection 0.037/1,000, and multiple myeloma 0.07/1,000 (22). Other causes include neural tumors (72), retroperitoneal tumors including endometriosis, viral plexopathies, and peripheral neuropathies of metabolic, viral, or traumatic etiology. Other causes to be ruled out are vascular disease, metastatic neoplasms, and arthritic conditions of the hip (1,42,67).

Treatment. Treatment, especially surgery, should be tailored to the specific pathology.

Psychosocial Causes. Psychosocial causes have been found to be a major factor in many surveys of failure of decompressive surgery (29,70,89,105). Important factors in predicting failure are workman's compensation, job dissatisfaction, low education, low income, heavy job requirements, cigarette smoking, psychological disturbances, and litigation (25,44,107,122).

In assessing the patient with prior failure of decompressive surgery, these factors must be clearly understood and may require a multidisciplinary approach (70). It is particularly important in the presence of psychosocial factors to identify a specific anatomic cause if any surgery is to be contemplated, indeed even in a primary case or exploratory surgery.

Surgical intervention is inappropriate unless a specific anatomic cause is clearly defined. Prolonged rest is inappropriate (23). The use of aggressive rehabilitation programs (78), pain clinics (83), progressive exercise programs (79), and work hardening programs must be considered and have proven to be successful in many patients with underlying psychosocial factors.

Discogenic Pain. Discogenic pain per se has been difficult to understand. Crock (16) has described internal disc disruption. This has been proven on discography with reproduction of the patient's symptoms in the presence of varying degrees of morphological degeneration. In the author's opinion, degenerative disease of the disc results in a cascade of problems including facet pain as well as pain of discogenic origin. Walsh et al. (116) have shown that discography bears a high degree of sensitivity and specificity in patients without prior surgery. Conversely, Nachemson (84) disputes this evidence. Esses et al. (27) have shown that rigid external skeletal fixation applied percutaneously is a better predictor of outcome for fusion than either radiography, discography, or facet blocks. One of the problems many surgeons have failed to comprehend is that discography has a relatively high incidence of false negatives in the lumbar spine, primarily in those cases that show extensive degeneration but where pain is not reproduced. Because of the significant annular tears it is impossible to increase the intranuclear pressure sufficient upon injection to reproduce the patients symptoms, in the author's opinion.

In the patient who has undergone previous discotomy and has persistent symptoms, discography may be of little value at that level, unless there is a positive reproduction of pain on disc distention. Some authors have found discography CT scanning of value in such cases.

Crock (16), Norton (89), and Pilgaard (95) have reported surgical success in 95% of primary cases of discogenic pain. O'Brien et al. (90) suggest that these primary results may be duplicated in patients with prior surgical failures.

Treatment. If surgery is considered in cases of disc disruption, the alternatives include anterior interbody fusion (17,18) and posterior anterior/posterior surgery (90). In the author's opinion posterior interbody fusion after prior decompression is exceedingly difficult because of preexisting postoperative scarring, which may be enhanced by posterior interbody fusion and which places the patient at greater neurological risk.

Missed Levels. Factors that may lead to surgery being done at the inappropriate level in cases of primary disc herniation include (a) abnormalities of segmentation, (b) mislabeling of imaging studies, (c) failure to verify the patient's side of complaints, (d) obesity, and (e) microsurgical approaches. There has been an increase in frequency of the wrong level being operated on with the development of microsurgical approaches. Intraoperative x-rays may be difficult to obtain particularly in obese people.

Treatment. Since the patient's pathology has not been alleviated, it is felt that surgical intervention is warranted. If this diagnosis is made early, i.e., within a day or two, the patient should be returned to the operating room at that time. More frequently, persistence of symptoms beyond a few weeks is the common scenario. The patient should be reevaluated bearing in mind the possibility of the wrong level or side having been operated upon. The surgeon should be frank with the patient, admit that he has erred, and deal with the patient as expeditiously as possible.

Delayed Decompression. Although Weber (119) has shown that the outcome of the patient with a disc herniation and sciatica is the same at 1 year whether he is operated upon or not, frequently the patient who is operated upon 6 months or later from the onset of sciatica, together with evidence of root tension as exhibited by limited straight leg raising, and perhaps impaired nerve root conduction as exhibited by a degree of motor and sensory change, does not do as well with surgery as those patients who have had surgery performed prior to this time. This is especially the case in the presence of a sequestered disc. Sequestration results in root scarring. Many patients have undergone decompression where there has been a preexistent long-standing history of back pain with a more recent history of sciatica. Discotomy or decompression is undertaken with the idea that this will alleviate both the sciatica and back pain. This is a major error and the removal of a disc or decompression of the contents of the epidural canal will do little to relieve long-standing back pain, which in my opinion often occurs as a result of instability. Although the sciatica may be helped, back pain may be aggravated or persist. In such conditions, following appropriate assessment including discography and facet blocks, fusion should be considered.

Inadequate Decompression. Negative exploration has a high correlation with failure (106). Macnab (75) emphasized the importance of causes other than disc herniation as a cause of sciatica and recommended a thorough examination in patients with continued nerve root compression. He included such causes as facet impingement, pedicular kinking, foraminal migration of disc material, spinal stenosis, and extraforaminal disc herniation (Table 18.3). In 18 of 68 cases no cause could be found. O'Connell (91) as well as Macnab (75) have described variations in neurological presentation, other than the classical presentation. They described L4-5 disc herniations producing generally L5 pain, and similarly an L5-S1 disc herniations producing S1 pain. Such a far lateral herniated nucleus pulposus or two-level disc herniations may occur as frequently as 10% (91). Further, a central disc herniation can produce compromise of more than one root or even a cauda equina syndrome. Conjoined roots that in some series occur as often as 11% may be another cause for variation in signs and symptoms. The far out lateral syndrome disc herniation can affect the more proximal root rather than the root at the level of herniation. This explains how an L4-5 far out disc herniation produces L4 symptoms

Table 18.3. Causes of failure after spinal fusion.

Time	Back pain predominant	Leg symptoms
Early (weeks)	Infection	Nerve impingment by fixation device or cement
	Wrong level fused	
	Insufficient levels fused	
	Psychosocial distress	
Midterm (months)	Pseudarthrosis	Fixation loose
	Disc disruption	
	Early adjacent disc degeneration	Early adjacent disc degeneration
	Inadequate reconditioning	
	Graft donor site	Graft donor site
Long-term (years)	Late pseudarthrosis	Disc with pseudarthrosis
	Adjacent level instability	Adjacent level stenosis
	Acquired spondylolysis	Adjacent level disc
	Abutment syndrome	Stenosis above fusion
	Compression fracture above fusion	

(117). Modern imaging techniques are more successful in identifying these variations. As a consequence negative explorations should become rare occurrences.

Operative failure occurs as a result of inadequate technique, which does not permit a complete decompression. The surgery must be tailored to the pathology including the use if necessary of extraforaminal stenosis as part of the patient's radiculopathy in association with the disc herniation, which may also be a cause for continued radioculopathy if the stenosis is not recognized. This has been emphasized by Burton et al. (10) and Macnab (75).

Macnab (75) has suggested that in the presence of multilevel stenoses it is important to identify the root or roots that require decompression rather than doing wide, extensive decompressive procedures. He feels that on the basis of nerve root injection studies the positive root or roots may be more readily identified, thus allowing for a less extensive decompression. The decision as to how many levels to decompress in the presence of multilevel stenoses is often an enigma. The use of nerve root injection studies and more recently the use of somatosensory evoked potentials done pre- and intraoperatively may be of value.

Other causes of inadequate decompression are found in cases of degenerative spondylolisthesis and isthmic spondylolisthesis. In degenerative spondylolisthesis decompression is usually done for L5 radioculopathy; however, the L4 root may be entrapped in the lateral recess. In the case of an L5 isthmic spondylolisthesis the L5 root is most commonly affected by bony cartilaginous material. The S1 roots may be affected as well, although less commonly, and in a case of spondylogenic spondylolisthesis of L5 and S1 the L4-5 disc proximal to the listhesis may also be herniated.

Treatment. Repeat decompression following accurate localization is recommended. Because of the previous surgery scarring may be extensive. At the time of surgery it is recommended that the surgeon proceed from areas of normal tissue, i.e., bone, to the edges of scar overlying the previous decompression. Using fine dissection, a plane can usually be developed between the edge of the bone and the soft tissue without exposing the underlying dura. Bone is then removed, proceeding to the more normal epidural contents of the canal. Following this as much bone or soft tissue as necessary should be removed. A commonly used criterion for adequacy of decompression is the fact that the root can be retracted immediately a minimum of 5 mm and when the root is free a probe can be easily passed into the foramina. The disc space need not be approached unless there is evidence of the presence of residual significant disc material based on preoperative radiological images.

Motion segment stability may be affected if considerable bone has been sacrificed and/or the facet joint is destroyed. In these patients fusion may be necessary in addition to the decompressive procedure.

Inadequate Nerve Root Decompression. This is most commonly seen as a result of midline decompression without adequate nerve root decompression. In patients with lateral or foraminal stenosis decompression should include foramenotomy or resection of part of the inferior facet or undercutting of the facet.

Conjoined Nerve Root. Although various studies have indicated an incidence of conjoined nerve root of between 2% and 14% it is more likely that the true incidence represents closer to the latter figure. As a result of failure to recognize the possibility at the time of surgery the nerve root may become excessively scarred due to surgical trauma or the actual root may be cut or evulsed or may be overlooked. The CT myelography provides perhaps the most accurate diagnosis of a conjoined root. Frequently the misinterpretation is with a disc herniation. The surgical approach is similar to that for lateral recess stenosis.

Temporary Relief Followed by Early Recurrence (Days to Weeks)

Infection. The incidence of wound infection following decompression varies from 0.5% to a high of 4% (40,47,106). This higher figure is more commonly encountered today with the use of microdiscectomy when the microscope is used. Infections vary from mild wound infection to discitis to frank osteomyelitis and on to epidural abscess.

Discitis. Discitis may present in its classical form with significant uncontrollable back pain and extreme discomfort; not infrequently, however, cases of discitis are not recognized and are diagnosed only in retrospect when sclerosis of the end plates is seen with significant settling of the disc space following discotomy. The erythrocyte sedimentation rate remains elevated and bone scanning at 10 days and MRI may be positive. The most common organism is *Staphylococcus aureus*. Though spontaneous fusion may occur in as many as 50%, this has not generally been this author's experience.

Cultures, including wound aspirates, often remain negative particularly if any form of antibiotic has been used, even for a short period (31). Blood cultures, urine cultures, wound cultures, and if necessary culture biopsy from the disc space may be necessary in order to isolate an organism. Although in the past immobilization and spica cast has been recommended, in our experience bed rest with bathroom privileges associated with intravenous antibiotics for 10 days followed by oral antibiotics is usually sufficient.

Pilgaard (95) noted that the nonoperative treatment was usually sufficient and most patients went on to spontaneous fusion in from 6 months to 1 year. Postinfection discitis in contrast to osteomyelitis rarely requires surgical intervention.

Postoperative Osteomyelitis. Although the initial presentation is similar to discitis, the latter becomes more chronic, as symptoms persist and indeed may be increased. Osteomyelitis may also be associated with systemic problems including anorexia, failure to thrive, and in some cases cachexia. The sedimentation rate remains elevated. In not all cases, however, are systemic symptoms present. The pathological picture is one of disease progression starting with disc space narrowing, and subsequently plate erosion, leading to vertebral body collapse. In contrast to discitis, cultures are more likely to be positive.

Treatment. If diagnosed early enough the response to antibiotics is satisfactory. For most cases, 6 weeks of antibiotics treatment intravenously has been recommended, suggesting that intravenous antibiotics for a period of 10 days to 2 weeks followed by oral antibiotics may suffice, provided that the sedimentation rate is closely monitored.

Surgery is indicated if there is progressive vertebral body collapse associated with instability and/or the development of neurological signs and symptoms. Treatment usually consists of anterior debridement and bone grafting associated with appropriate antibiotics. Infection is rarely posterior and is more likely to be associated with an epidural abscess. Epidural abscesses are often associated with vertebral body osteomyelitis.

Epidural Abscess. An epidural abscess is extremely rare following surgery. Neurological symptoms and signs may be rapid and confused with those seen as a result of hematoma. Surgical treatment is indicated with appropriate decompression and antibiotics.

Meningeal Cyst. A meningeal cyst is usually a result of unrecognized durotomy with the development of a ball valve phenomenon (53,81). The nerve root or roots become part of the cyst. Radicular pain may present. A diagnosis can be made with the use of myelography with or without CT scanning or MRI scanning. Meningeal cysts are uncommon and occur in less than 1% of patients and are more common following decompression for spinal stenosis than for disc excision.

Treatment. Not all cysts are in need of treatment. Treatment consists of surgical excision of the cyst and closure of the dural opening. Care must be taken to see the cyst does not contain nerve roots and if it does, these should be dissected free of the cyst before closing the defect. If the defect is large, a graft may be necessary for closure.

Midterm Failures (Weeks to Months)

Recurrent Disc Prolapse. This is the most common cause for failure. In some series (33,34,38) the recurrent herniation may occur at the same level, at the same side, at the opposite side, or at new level (38).

Patients initially do well but may present as early as a few days but more typically a few weeks following surgery with recurrent symptoms. The history and physical examination is compatible with disc herniation, but because of residual deficits from the initial herniation physical examination may be difficult.

The incomplete removal of the disc does not influence the risk of recurrence. Spengler (107) found that excision of only the herniation results in no increased incidence of recurrence in comparison with more radical evacuation of the disc space. The past practice of excising a second disc based on myelographic findings in order to prevent herniation at this level should not be done (91).

Treatment. The treatment approach should be similar to that of a primary disc herniation. Consecutive measures are first attempted. These include a few days of bed rest, analgesics, nonsteroidal anti-inflammatory drugs, and graduated mobilization.

Because of the natural reluctance for repeat surgery on the part of the surgeon and perhaps the patient, many of these patients are treated nonoperatively, whereas if their presentation had been de novo, surgery would have been undertaken. Studies (43,119) have shown that most patients do well without surgery. This is based on the natural history of disc herniation where it is recognized that most patients followed long-term, whether treated surgically or nonoperatively, have approximately the same outcome (119). Some surgeons have felt that the outcome is poor with recurrent disc herniation because of increased scarring with or without intervention.

The alternative to nonoperative care is repeat surgery. It is recommended at this time that a conventional incision should be used rather than microdiscotomy. Frymoyer et al. (38) felt that the outcome of repeat surgery is similar to that of a primary disc excision.

In a consecutive series of 500 discotomies for disc herniation, the author has experienced two recurrences. These were both encountered early in my experience. In both cases this disc space was curetted rather than doing a simple removal of the loose fragment.

Differential diagnosis include failure to recognize sequestrated fragments. These patients usually do not do well in the immediate postoperative period. Failure to recognize sequestrated fragments is usually a failure to recognize the possible migration of disc fragments, which mostly occurs proximally from the midpoint of the vertebral body.

Perineural Scarring. The incidence of perineural scarring resulting in postoperative symptoms as a result of the so-called battered root has been reported to occur in as low as 1% to 2% (106) to as high as 12% (36). Burton et al. (10) quoted an 8% cause of failure due to this pathology. The most common cause in my experience is iatrogenic. Perineural scarring is frequently associated with the presence of conjoint roots. Another factor is excessive bleeding, and Hoyland et al. (49) have implicated the use of cottonoid patties.

The patient usually does well in the immediate postoperative period but then develops a recurrence of sciatica, often with no increased neurological deficit. The patient's symptoms may initially be helped by nonsteroidal anti-inflammatory drugs, but symptoms may persist and increase for a number of months.

The differential diagnosis is obviously one of recurrent disc herniation. The most extreme form of the battered root is direct nerve injury to one or more roots, including the cauda equina syndrome. The incidence of the latter varies from 0.4% to 4%. Spangfort (106) has reported on caudal injury with disturbance of bowel and bladder function. He noted only 5 out of 2,504 cases following disc excision. More recently the addition of free fat grafts to prevent epidural scarring may produce cauda equina syndromes as well.

Prevention includes the use of proper surgical technique and proper identification of pathology. Whether the use of fat grafts prevents epidural scarring is controversial. In the author's opinion they probably do not. Vascularized fat grafts may however be preferable, but often are technically difficult to perform.

Surgical treatment is controversial and includes the application of various materials including silicone to prevent scarring, dural sleeve splitting, the removal of scar, and spinal fusion. As well, more recently the use of a electrical stimulator has been advocated. None of these modalities has been shown to be of any particular value over any other.

Epidural Fibrosis. Epidural fibrosis is the normal outcome following any decompressive procedure. Epidural fibrosis itself without the presence of direct trauma to roots is unlikely to be a cause for symptoms, in the author's opinion. The use of enhanced CT or MRI may differentiate fibrosis from other causes of extrinsic neural compression. Attempts at prevention with the use of fat grafts remains controversial. The use of laminoplasty (restoration of the posterior elements) in the author's opinion has been more valuable than plain fat grafts in the prevention of epidural fibrosis.

Arachnoiditis. The most common cause for arachnoiditis has been the use of oil-based radiopaque contrast media for myelography. Other causes are bleeding during myelography, intrathecal injection of corticoid steroids, and surgical trauma. Arachnoiditis is a nontreatable condition. Fortunately there does not seem to be continued deterioration.

The long-term follow-up by Guyer et al. (41) showed no increase in symptoms with the passage of time ranging from 10 to 21 years. The use of oil-based contrast media was the most common cause in their series. Pain was a major reason for dysfunction with no increasing neurological deficits noted.

Long-Term Failures (Months to Years)

A definition of long-term failure is difficult. The causes include recurrent disc herniation, which has been seen by this author as late as 10 years following previous discectomy. Other causes were recurrent stenosis including the development of lateral stenosis, foraminal stenosis due to progressive degeneration and disc narrowing, and instability following either discectomy or decompression.

Failure to recognize associated disease processes that may go on to increased morbidity may be one cause. Prevention of this is difficult. It has been well shown that the addition of spinal fusion is not preventative in may cases of discectomy and the routine decompression at multiple levels as practiced in two decades following the Second World War based on the presence of myelographic bulges is not recommended (34).

Recurrent Stenosis Including Lateral Stenosis Secondary to Disc Space Collapse. The incidence of disc space collapse following disc excision varies from 16% to 100% (36,40,44,85,86). As a result of disc space narrowing and the development of changes in the facets, recess stenosis may develop. The incidence is similar in respect to sex and occupation (36,86). Some authors (114) have related recurrent stenosis to original canal size or other structural problems (103). Some patients develop symptoms of spinal stenosis that may be related to one or more roots. This usually occurs after a long period of relief of symptoms following their initial surgery. Patients are more likely to develop a lateral recess stenosis rather than a central or mixed stenosis. Frequently the cause is the excision of disc material in the presence of lateral stenosis. The latter may be recognized or not recognized. If a disc herniation is removed in the presence of lateral recess stenosis the patient should be forewarned that there is a possibility of recurrence of symptoms later. If the majority of the patient's symptoms are a result of a disc herniation rather than the presence of associated stenosis, then in the author's opinion only the herniation should be dealt with.

Treatment. Treatment should as far as possible be nonoperative including the use of nonsteroidal anti-inflammatory drugs, epidural blocks, and modification of activities. With failure of nonoperative treatment decompression is advocated.

Instability After Disc Excision. Back pain symptoms resulting from postoperative instability is said to occur in as many as 10% of patients following disc excision (27,93,109). The patients usually develop gradual onset of back pain following surgery, and it may occur months to years later. In the author's opinion this tends to be more common in patients who have had some degree of back pain prior to disc excision, which was not initially recognized by the treating surgeon and therefore not dealt with properly using appropriate postoperative care. Malcolm et al. (77) have reported an increased problem of instability following disc excision at the L4-5 level. In the author's opinion these patients are best dealt with by a prolonged conservative care program. The indications for spinal fusion are those for spinal fusion in general; localized documented instability as evidenced by the use of discography, facet blocks, and those of external skeletal fixation (27,92,93).

Instability After Lumbar Decompression. The controversy over whether or not to add a fusion to a decompression for spinal stenosis still exists. The sacrifice of 50% of both facets or complete sacrifice of a single facet significantly alters the motion segments kinematics. It is felt by this author that decompression involving partial destruction of the facets on both sides at a single-level decompression should be accompanied by fusion. If facets on one side are affected at two or more levels, then a fusion should also be added.

There is no doubt that postmenopausal women with some degree of osteoporosis are at greater risk of developing late instability. The patient in whom the disc heights are reasonably maintained, i.e., the younger patient, is also at greater risk of developing late instability following extensive lumbar decompression (52). Levels proximal to L5-S1 are more susceptible to later instability. The narrower the disc spaces, the greater the degree of degenerative changes, i.e., osteophytes, and the less the chance of developing late instability. Patients who have a degenerative spondylolisthesis and are only decompressed are at greater risk of developing late instability.

Treatment. If instability has been demonstrated and confirmed by studies such as facet blocks, discography, and/or the use of external fixators or dynamic motion x-rays, then spinal fusion may be indicated. The ability to perform a spinal fusion in the presence of a previous, extensive decompression may be difficult. The advent of pedicle fixation has in the author's hands improved the incidence of successful arthrodesis. If there have been multiple previous procedures then an anterior fusion is preferred (98).

Surgical Failures After Spinal Fusion: Causes, Surgical Treatment and Results

The early enthusiasm for lumbar spinal fusion as a treatment for low back pain with or without sciatica has decreased considerably because of the poor results. In the past 5 years, enthusiasm is again increasing for a variety of reasons: the causes of failure have become better understood; new operative techniques, such as rigid internal fixation, have allowed fusions to be performed more predictably, and demonstrated that more difficult adult deformities can be corrected. New diagnostic tests such as MRI and discography have led to a better understanding of the causes of lumbar pain, particularly those associated with degenerative conditions. Although some of the diagnoses are still debated, for example "disk disruption," surgeons are treating them aggressively, and are demonstrating good results.

Table 18.4. Causes of failure after spinal fusion.

Time	Back pain predominant	Leg symptoms
Early (weeks)	Infection	Nerve impingment by fixation devices or cement
	Wrong level fused	
	Insufficient levels fused	
	Psychosocial distress	
Midterm (months)	Pseudarthrosis	Fixation loose
	Disc disruption	
	Early adjacent disc degeneration	Early adjacent disc degeneration
	Inadequate reconditioning	
	Graft donor site	Graft donor site
Long-term (years)	Late pseudarthrosis	Disc with pseudarthrosis
	Adjacent level instability	Adjacent level stenosis
	Acquired spondylolysis	Adjacent level disc
	Abutment syndrome	Stenosis above fusion
	Compression fracture above fusion	

In other instances, surgeons now are dealing with the late consequences of prior fusion, whose treatment may require further stabilization. With these developments there is an even greater need to understand the sources of failure that accompany spinal fusion, and how these problems can be managed when they appear.

In this part of the chapter I will consider an overview of the causes of failure after lumbar fusion, and discuss the general approach to the patient with respect to history and useful physical and imaging information. I will then detail the causes of failure in terms of how often they occur, how they are recognized, and how they are treated. Finally, an overview will be given as to which results may be obtained. Although spinal fusion is employed for a variety of pathologic conditions, this chapter focuses on failures that follow fusion for degenerative conditions.

A more specific classification for the failures of spinal fusion are shown in Table 18.4. Here we have divided these failures by the time of appearance, as well as by the predominant symptom. The importance of a temporal division was emphasized by Finnegan et al. (29) in the analysis of failures of both decompression and fusion. When the patient had no immediate relief, the wrong diagnosis on the wrong operation should be suspected. When the patient has immediate relief and then has recurrent symptoms within weeks to months following the operation, new pathology or a complication of the operation should be suspected. When the patient has good relief, and months to years later has recurrent symptoms, new pathology or ongoing degeneration should be suspected. Table 18.4 shows the relative distribution of failures as a function of time after surgery.

It should be emphasized that we are not referring to leg symptoms that relate to an original decompression performed in conjunction with a fusion, since this topic has been covered earlier. Rather, we are referring to leg symptoms independent of the original pathology, which in the case of prior fusion are more likely to suggest spinal stenosis, rather than a single-level radiculopathy.

In addition to these general sources of failure, there are also specific systemic and local complications that follow spinal fusion. In some instances these complications may cause symptoms that are at times more devastating to the patient than the condition for which treatment was initially sought. These complications will be detailed later in this chapter.

Approach to a Patient with a Failure Following Fusion

A complete history and physical examination is essential, and all prior historical records, operative reports, and imaging studies need to be reviewed. A history of never having pain relief from a previous operation strongly suggests the wrong preoperative diagnosis or the wrong operation, whereas a long interval of relief and return to function, followed by insidious onset of symptoms, suggests a late degenerative lesion. Obviously if the patient did not have relief, never returned to function, and had a long preoperative interval of disability, the possibility of psychosocial dysfunction should be strongly entertained. The physical examination rarely gives a precise diagnosis, particularly if the original surgery included a decompression. Limitation of spinal motion is a nonspecific symptom of failure rather than an observation identifying its causes (36). Similarly, limitation of motion is frequently associated with psychosocial dysfunction, particularly in the patient who appears to have had the right operation and achieved a solid fusion. Leg symptoms should be carefully analyzed. If the patient had no leg symptoms and a normal neurologic examination prior to the first operation, and the current examination shows deficits, this is of major importance and suggests a high probability there is new pathology or a complication due to a fixation device. If the patient had preoperative leg symptoms before the first operation, the neurologic findings are most likely residual, unless an entirely new set of objective deficits are present. If the patient has diffuse leg symptoms as part of the overall pain complaint, it is common for these to be localized to the graft donor site. However, the usual graft donor complaints seem to be highly associated with overall failure of symptomatic relief rather than due to a specific complication at the donor site (37).

Psychosocial Issues

The psychosocial issues are of major importance in evaluating patients with failed fusion who have not had a pain free interval and have not returned to normal function as opposed to those who have had a pain free interval prior to the new onset of symptoms (21,108).

Plane Radiography

The plane radiographs must be interpreted with care. In postoperative patients it is common to identify disc space narrowing and even excessive motion at the adjacent functional spinal segment. For example, a positive Knuttsen's sign is identified in 20% of patients at the L3-4 level above an L4 to the sacrum fusion, but few have symptoms (36). However, a number of radiographic signs are particularly useful: (a) the unequivocal presence of a pseudarthrosis; (b) a pars defect above a midline fusion, most commonly at the L3 lamina; (c) an obvious failure of instrumentation with cutting out of devices attached to the lamina, or breakage of screws—a more subtle sign may be a halo around a pedicle screw, indicating motion in an apparently solid fusion.

The addition of motion radiography is an important test in the identification of pseudarthrosis, as originally stressed by Bosworth and Cleveland (11). Because some motion is common, particularly in a solid midline fusion, it is important to identify at least four degrees of motion before a pseudarthrosis can be suspected with confidence (36). The major difficulty lies in accurate centering and positioning of the patient for the flexion and extension view. Translation of 3 to 4 mm is also diagnostic of abnormal motion.

Bone scintigraphy is rarely indicated, but is helpful on occasion in a patient suspected of having an infection, or occasionally when a pseudarthrosis is suspected and is confirmed by flexion-extension films and tomography. Most spinal fusions show increased uptake up to 2 years following fusion, and significant "hot spots" within the general area of increased uptake or a localized area 2 years or more following fusion may be indicative of a pseudarthrosis.

CT Scans

The CT scan is invaluable in assessing the bony canal and in one series is reported to demonstrate the cause of failures in 13% of cases, most of which were secondary to improper diagnoses prior to the first operation (94). The test is particularly enhanced by the addition of myelographic dye, which remains the most sensitive mechanism to identify spinal stenosis. In patients with apparent instability and stenotic symptoms, it is important to obtain a flexion and extension view with the dye in place before proceeding to the CT scan. CT scans, especially if enhanced by myelographic dye, are valuable postsurgically for the assessment of canal content, but may easily miss a transverse pseudarthrosis if the cut is not at the appropriate level. These deficits may be overcome by three-dimensional CT or magnetic resonance imaging reconstructions, which may prove to be of great value in the assessment of fusion mass integrity. For example, Laasonen and Soini (64) studied 48 patients with a painful lumbosacral fusion by careful CT scanning. Sixteen had unsuspected fragmented grafts, and nine had hairline pseudarthroses, which may have caused their symptoms. Similarly, hypocycloidal frontal plane tomography was investigated by Dawson et al. (19) and revealed unsuspected pseudarthrosis in patients who had previous fusions for scoliosis. The imaging evidence for pseudarthrosis was later confirmed by surgical exploration. Pseudarthroses occur in two modes: (a) transverse or (b) plate. The former is the traditional well known form of pseudarthrosis. The latter is a failure of the graft material to unite with the underlying laminae and/or transverse processes despite the fact that the fusion mass, derived from the graft material, is solid.

Myeloscopy

Myeloscopy was initially felt to provide the answer to many of the problems of continued radicular pain following surgery. This, however, has not met universal enthusiasm. In the country of its origin, the originator remains the only person participating in clinical trials. Its value may lie in the assessment of arachnoiditis.

Facet Blocks

The problem with facet blocks in a failed surgical case (82) is that the presence of scarring frequently inhibits an accurate infiltration and hence in the failed case this may be of limited value. It is of value in assessing levels proximal to a previous fusion, however. As well, the local infiltration of anesthesia into a pseudarthrosis may help determine whether or not the pseudarthrosis is the cause of the patient's pain. Infiltration may be done into both anterior or posterior pseudarthroses. As well, the infiltration of local anesthesia around internal fixation devices may help determine whether these may be a cause of postoperative pain. However, the sensitivity and specificity of these techniques is unknown.

Discography

Discography can be used in two fashions, one to assess disc degeneration and the other as a pain-provocative test. As a method of assessing disc degeneration, magnetic resonance imaging is at least as valuable and is noninvasive.

Discography may be used to diagnose painful levels within an area of obvious disc degeneration as is noted on plain radiographs or magnetic resonance imaging and is perhaps more reliably used as an assessment of discs proximal to obvious degenerative levels both as an assessment of minor degrees of degeneration and/or as part of the pain-provocative study.

Macnab (75) has stated that discography is valuable in proving whether posterior pseudarthrosis is a painful source or not. He felt that reproduction of pain on discography at the suspected level of pseudarthrosis proved that the pseudarthrosis was the source of pain. We have not been fully convinced of his belief. Technically to perform discography in the presence of a previously performed posterolateral fusion with or without pseudarthrosis may be difficult. We prefer to do discography from a posterolateral rather than a transdural approach.

In patients with previous surgery the use of discography may be of great value in differentiation of pain. The patient with a previous fusion

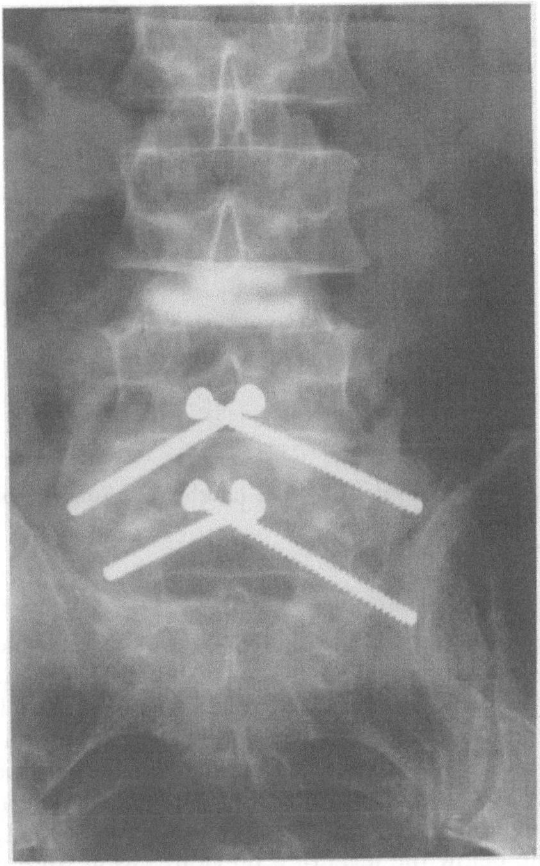

Figure 18.1. A 53-year-old man, operated on for segmental instability of L4-S1; AO translaminar screws were used. Preoperative discography at L4-S1, L5-S1 reproduced his pain. Postoperatively, pain persisted despite a solid fusion. Repeat discography at L4-5 reproduced his pain despite the solid fusion. L3-4 discogram was normal.

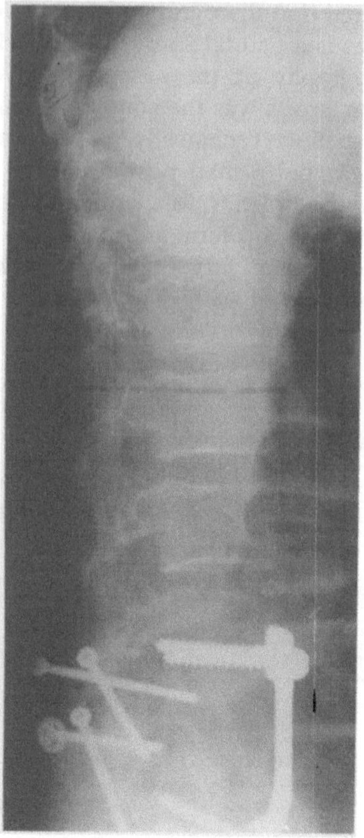

Figure 18.2. Lateral view. Anterior L4-S1 interbody fusion ("I" plate was added for fixation), which relieved the pain.

who continues to have pain but otherwise shows no evidence of psychosocial problems may have two sources of pain that can be diagnosed with the aid of discography. First, levels proximal to a fusion can be evaluated. When the patient has had a previous L4 to the sacrum fusion and presents with pain some time postoperatively or many years postoperatively, the use of discography at levels above the fusion may help determine whether these are a source of subsequent or continuing pain. Second, discography may be of value below the level of a previous fusion. In a small number of patients with continuing pain without psychosocial problems who radiographically on plain x-rays, dynamic x-rays, and tomography show no evidence of pseudarthroses, subsequent pain was reproduced on discography (118). Subsequent anterior procedures with disc excision and fusion and addition of bone graft despite the solid posterior fusion has resulted in relief of pain. We feel that these cases are examples of what Crock (18) described as internal disc derangement (Figs. 18.1 and 18.2).

Nachemson (84) has recently criticized discography. The reasons given are that the outer part of the annulus has a multilevel nerve supply as does the dorsal longitudinal ligament. This may result in difficult and false interpretations. The criticism that previously normal pain-free people may have pain from a discogram is not valid, since the point is whether or not the discogram reproduced the patient's typical pain in the same area and of the same quality. As well, in a significantly degenerative disc, the application of pressure at the time of discography may not occur, since there are so many annular tears that it is impossible to raise the intradiscal pressure to a sufficient degree to reproduce pain. In these instances the fluid medium used to inject and raise pressure escapes too rapidly. There is no doubt that the injection of irritants at different sites of the motion segments can elicit back pain and leg pain.

Discography has, in our hands, helped us to differentiate the painful from nonpainful levels and thus aided in the assessment of the number of levels requiring fusion. It has been of particular value in the failed back patient.

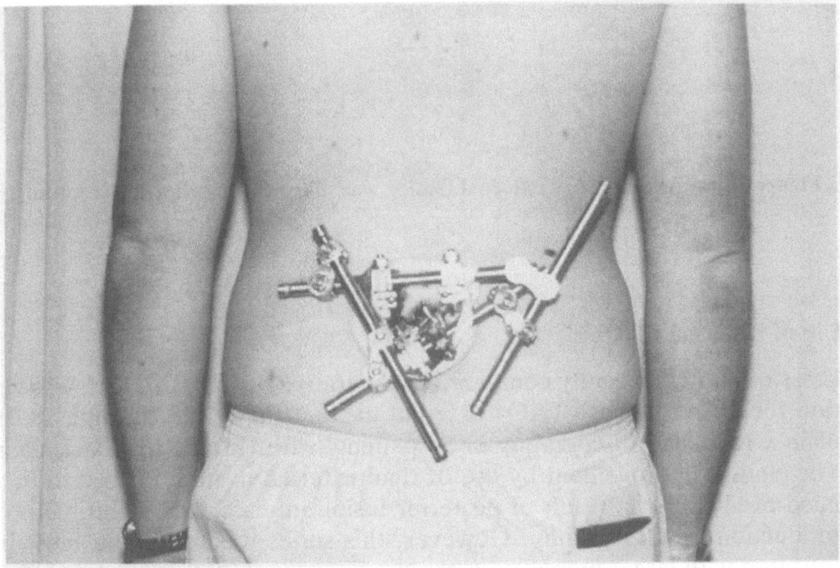

Figure 18.3. A 39-year-old man presented with a 2-year history of disabling low back pain. Plane films were unremarkable (except for a small traction spur). L4-5 was unstable on flexion-extension radiographs. Discograms were done. L3-4 was normal. L4-5 and L5-S1 were degenerate and pain was reproduced on disc distention.

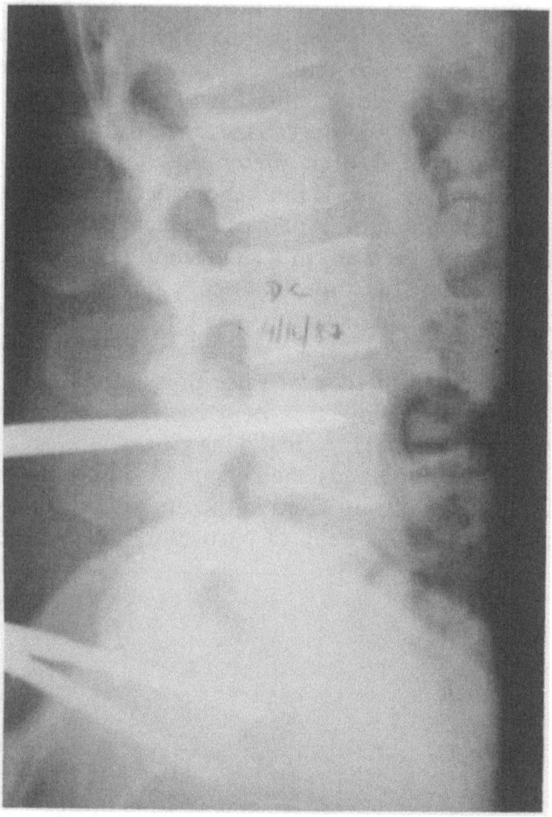

Figure 18.4. A temporary external fixator was placed with relief of symptoms.

Use of External Fixator

Esses et al. (27) recently compared preoperative testing with the Association for Osteosynthesis (AO) external fixator (Figs. 18.3 through 18.7), plain x-rays, and discography in 30 patients with chronic low back pain. The clinical improvement by use of rigid external fixation proved to be a good predictor of a result of posterior fusion in discography and pain reproduction by discography. However, this series was small and must be repeated with larger numbers. Although Esses et al. (27) have shown that external fixation may be a good predictor of outcome following spinal fusion, a similar study by Olerud et al. (92,93) did not come to the same conclusion. After initial reporting of Olerud et al. of success similar to that of Esses et al., further evaluation was less successful. This physical modality as a method of prediction of the outcome of a spinal fusion requires further evaluation.

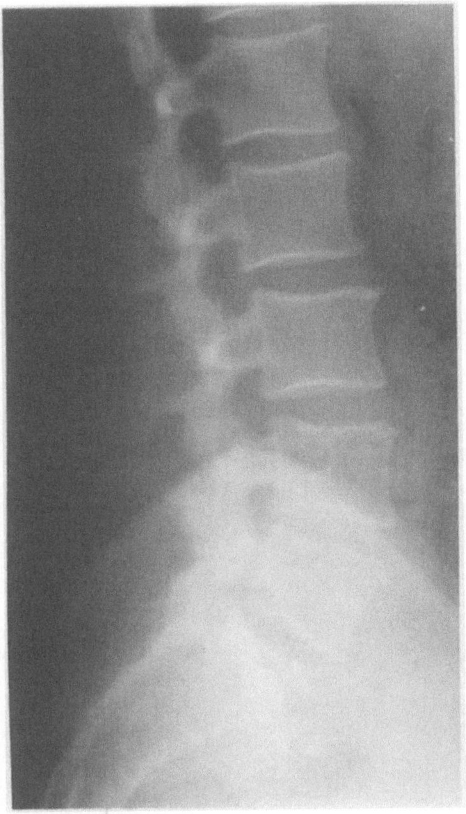

Figure 18.5. A temporary external fixator was placed with relief of symptoms.

Let us now look at the specific causes of failure that occurs after lumbar spinal arthrodesis.

Causes of Early Failure

Infection

The rate of infection following lumbar surgery is variable; it depends on the era in which the operation was performed, operative time, history of prior surgery, the approach used, and the use of prophylactic antibiotics and instrumentation. Incidence rates ranging from less than 1% to greater than 10% have been reported. In general, the lower figures have been reported in the past decade. In 1966, Prothero et al. (96) reviewed 1,000 cases of midline and intertransverse process fusion and compared patient cohorts treated a decade apart. The operative indications were multiple; the overall infection rate of 3.4% was no different for the two time intervals. At about the same time, Freebody et al. (32) reported an incidence

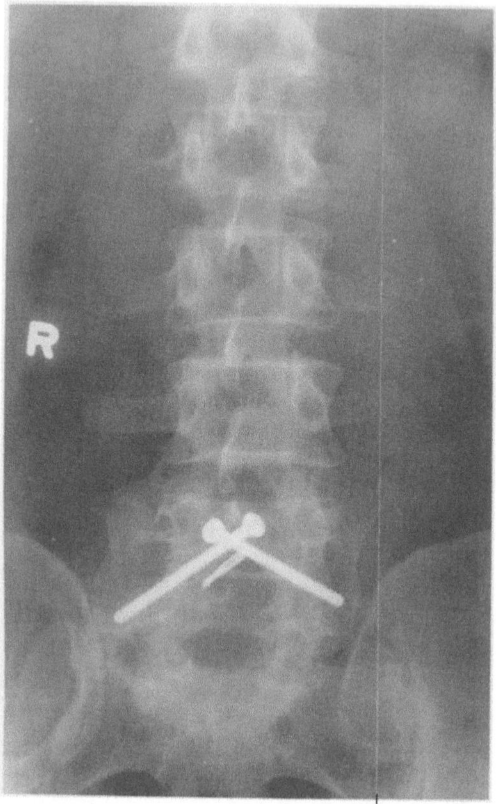

Figure 18.6. The patient then underwent a two-level fusion of L4-S1. Despite a solid fusion, pain persisted.

of wound infection of 3.0%. The highest rate of recently reported infection was that of 18% (125) in patients treated with pedicle fixation, which was attributed to the long operative time that resulted from a steep learning curve, rather than to the use of instrumentation per se. Others have noted a similar association and reached the same conclusion. Although there is no certain proof, Kostuik and Hall (61) thought that anterior fusion had a lower rate of infection than the posterior approach. In 100 anterior fusions performed for burst fractures together with decompression and instrumentation, Kostuik et al. (58,59) noted one deep infection. In 67 cases of anterior fusion and instrumentation performed for degenerative disease or previously failed posterior surgery, no deep infections occurred. One deep infection occurred in 108 cases of anterior instrumentation and fusion for scoliosis. No infections occurred in 205 cases of kyphosis instrumented and fused anteriorly.

Whether this infection rate can be reduced by antibiotics is debatable.

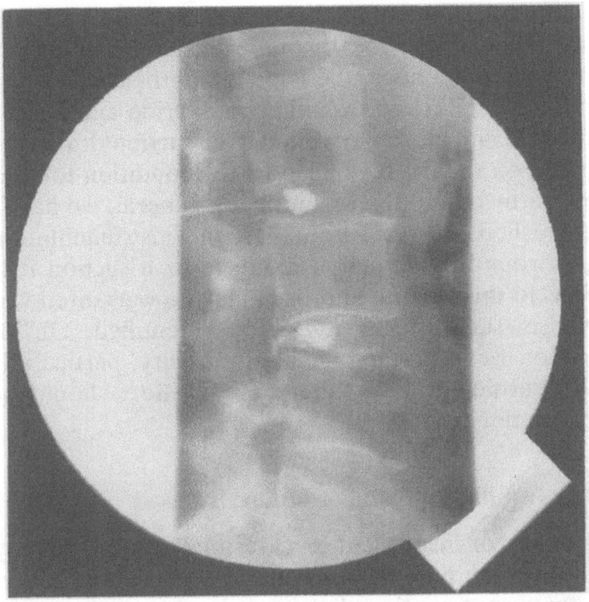

Figure 18.7. Discograms done at L3-4 revealed a degenerative painful disc. L2-3 was normal. The fusion was extended one level and the pain was relieved.

A generally accepted but not proven belief is that antibiotics are warranted with fusions, particularly if metallic devices are implanted. In an early retrospective and uncontrolled study, Fogelberg et al. (30) reported lower infection rates in both spine and hip surgery with the use of postoperative penicillin. In a similar uncontrolled study, Lonstein et al. (71) reported infection rates respectively of 2.8% with and 9.3% without antibiotics, in patients treated for scoliosis with and without Harrington instrumentation. If antibiotics are employed for prophylaxis, a general body of basic and clinical research supports the drug being given preoperatively, intraoperatively, and for as little as 24 hours postoperatively. This teaching is opposed to the historic belief that antibiotics should be administered for longer postoperative intervals.

Presentation. The classic presentation of deep wound infection is 5 to 7 days postoperatively. Rarely, infections are clinically observed in the first 24 hours. We have encountered one such patient with a streptococcal infection. The clue was a rapidly developing sore throat and a watery hematoma, suggesting bacteriologic fibrinolysis. Dependent on host immunologic competency and the virulence of the organism, the presentation ranges from high grade fever and severe pain, to an indolent course, often accompanied by delay in diagnosis. Superficial signs may be notably absent in a large, muscular, or obese patient.

Treatment. A superficial wound infection can be appropriately treated by antibiotics and relief of any local wound tension, including drainage to the fascia. In deeper infections, the issue is whether or not to remove instrumentation and/or graft, and whether to debride and leave the wound open, or to debride and close the wound over suction drainage. This decision is dependent on the degree of sepsis, the condition for which the operation was performed, and the organism. In general, we have performed debridement, washed the bone graft, left the instrumentation in place, and closed the wound over suction drainage or a suction irrigation system. Exceptions to this general approach may be warranted when a gram-negative organism such as *Pseudomonas* is identified. Obviously if the original indication was for severe spinal instability, particularly when associated with neurologic involvement, every effort should be made to retain the fixation device.

Wrong Level or Insufficient Number of Levels Fused

Patients with wrong or insufficient level fusions usually are only identified when a significant time interval has elapsed after the operation, although their failure for symptomatic relief is noticeable early on. Often their postoperative symptoms are attributed to wound healing, and later, pseudarthrosis is often suspected. The most apparent source of failure of this type is when a surgeon fails to perform a fusion over the area of obvious pathology, equivalent to failure to decompress a known disc herniation. In the older literature, a common cause of failure was thought to occur when the surgeon overlooked two-level lumbar disc herniations when combined decompression and fusion was performed. It will be remembered that some clinical reviews indicate that two-level lesions occurred in up to 10% of patients (86). For that reason, many reports stressed the importance of two-level decompressions, and fusion in all patients with suspected L5-S1 or L4-L5 disc herniations. Today's sophisticated imaging techniques make these earlier recommendations obsolete. However, this issue is more difficult when subtle pathologic conditions are being treated, such as disc disruption or degenerative scoliosis. Recommendation is made for performing discography at all lumbar levels, until a morphologically normal disc is identified and the patient has no pain reproduction. This is a controversial view. The use of the MRI image is also controversial in this regard; Zuckerman et al. (125) and Kornberg (57) each report a small group of patients with normal MRIs later shown to have an unequivocally positive discogram.

In the older literature, the extent of the fusion was often based on the plain radiographic findings, such as disc space narrowing and osteophyte. When the primary indication was "lumbar disc disease," more than two-level degeneration was used as a contraindication to L4 to the sacrum fusions. For this reason, many authorities believed a floating fusion at L4-5 should never be done. Fusion that involved L4-5 was thought to necessitate an L5-S1 fusion as well. However, Brodsky et al. (6) has shown satisfactory results can be obtained with the floating fusion, providing the L5-S1 level is carefully analyzed. We have advocated that the extent of a fusion in complex degenerative conditions should be determined by preoperative facet blocks and discography, although the precise sensitivity and specificity of these tests has yet to be established. At this time there is no certain data that tells us how often missed levels cause failures of spinal fusion.

Presentation. As previously noted, fusion at the wrong level is suspected only after a significant time delay in all but the most gross and obvious omissions. Back pain that fails to improve during the first 3 months would suggest this diagnosis, but frequently, it is only when the fusion is solid that this type of failure is suspected. In these instances the differential diagnosis typically is pseudarthrosis, or the wrong patient was chosen. In the latter instance, the patient falsely may be assumed to have psychosocial or compensation issues that are the cause of symptoms.

Treatment. The treatment is based on establishing that the fusion was inadequate in its extent, or that the wrong levels have been fused. This decision necessitates the use of all of the preoperative analytic techniques outlined earlier in this chapter (Figs. 18.3 through 18.7).

Representative Cases

Psychosocial Distress. The issues of psychosocial distress, compensation, and their effects on the incidence of later surgical failures is emphasized. The important time to identify these factors is before the operation, not after it. Finnegan et al. (29) have stressed the importance of this. The analysis of entrants into rehabilitation programs also emphasizes the commonality of psychosocial distress, and compensation in the etiology of fusion failures (2). How commonly this failure occurs is uncertain. In one series where fusion was performed in conjunction with disc excision, 15% of patients had no obvious causation for their continued pain and disability (36).

Early Failures: Nerve Root Impingement

We are not including here early failures due to preoperative misdiagnosis, intraoperative errors, or nerve root complications, such as scarring, that follow decompression. These are detailed earlier in this chapter. The major cause of nerve root impingement that directly relates to fusion today is usually a result of internal fixation devices, particularly those involving the pedicle. The most important insight on this problem is derived from Weinstein et. al.'s (119) study of screw misplacement, when experienced and inexperienced surgeons performed the operation in cadaver specimens set up to simulate a real procedure including C-arm radiographic control. Misplacement of the screws occurred in 21% of all pedicles, many of which were in close proximity to the nerve. The addition of methylmethacrylate to increase holding strength is an additive risk factor for nerve damage, since thermal and mechanical damage can result.

This cause of failure also is observed in devices that depend on laminar fixation, and is usually due to a jumped hook. A particularly high rate of nerve root complications are noted with the Knodt rod. The problem usually occurs in the lumbosacral area, and necessitates rod removal in 20% to 50% of patients. In general, nerve root symptoms, when they occur with this device, are a late rather than early complication. Causation of nerve root impingement, specific to one or another fusion technique, includes nerve root traction injury, or graft extrusion. The incidence of graft extrusion with posterior lumbar interbody fusion varies, and was reported in one of Cloward's (12) 321 cases four of Lin's (68) 500 cases, and four of Collis's (14) 750 cases. Lin (69) suggests the overall rate is 0.3% to 2.4%, but for inexperienced operators, the rate is a "disturbing" 9%. The rate of nerve root damage is less certain, although Lin (69) noted a temporary dropped foot in 25 of 5,000 patients (0.005%), of whom all but three recovered in 6 months. With posterior fusion techniques, neurologic deficit or pain may occasionally result from graft material becoming dislodged, or from an unrecognized fracture of a facet, producing a fragment that causes nerve impingement. How often this occurs is unknown, but it is probably rare.

Presentation

The diagnosis is most suspect particularly in patients who have had no preoperative nerve root symptoms, but who early after their surgery have neurologic deficit or radicular pain. More difficult is a patient who had nerve involvement, a decompression in combination with the fusion, and in whom the postoperative picture is that of increased deficit or pain. In these instances, a large differential diagnosis is necessary as detailed earlier in this chapter. The diagnosis is also complicated because of the presence of metal, which may make imaging techniques such as MRI impossible, or CT scans difficult to interpret because of image scatter. In these cases, it may be necessary to resort to polytonal tomography, with or without myelographic enhancement, although when the screw misplacement or fixation displacement is obvious, plane radiographs will suffice (Figs. 18.8 and 18.9).

These same diagnostic issues also come into play when later nerve root symptoms occur. Assuming the nerve root compression is within the area encompassed by the fusion, fixation device displacement should be considered. Usually when this occurs, there may be obvious clues from plain

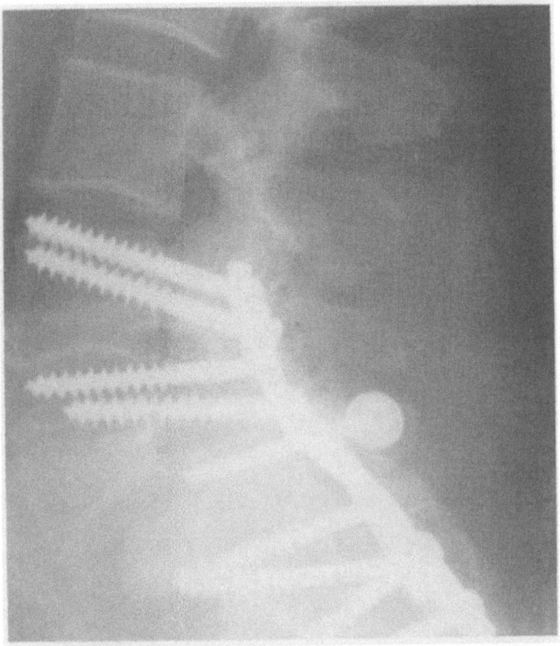

Figure 18.8. A 42-year-old woman with grade II L5-S1 spondylolisthesis. Discography revealed a typically painful L4-5 disc. Facet blocks at L4-S1 relieved her of pain. Arthrodesis was done using contoured AO-DCP plates and screws. One screw missed the L5 pedicle resulting in root pain, while two screws appear to be in the disc space of L4-5. The screw with the washer is a translaminar screw used to hold the lamina in place following laminoplasty.

radiography, i.e., jumped hook, or the diagnosis may be suspected by the presence of a radiolucent "halo" around one or more portions of the device.

Treatment

Dependent on the magnitude of symptoms and neurologic deficits, the option ranges from doing nothing until the fusion is mature, to immediate removal in more severe cases, and replacement of the screw or an alternative fixation device.

Midterm Failures: Back Pain Predominant

Pseudarthrosis

Pseudarthrosis is the most common cause of failure in spinal fusion. It is also the most difficult to establish as the source of failure, because many

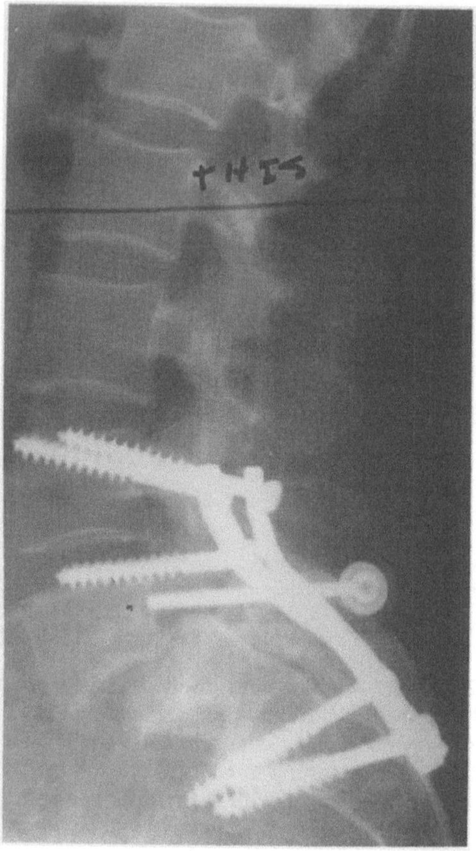

Figure 18.9. The screw was removed and symptoms abated. A solid fusion was obtained. The sacral screws are in the ala and thus appear too long in the lateral projection, while one L4-5 screw remains in the disc space.

patients will have radiographic evidence of fusion failure with no symptoms (20,36). Conversely, repair of a pseudarthrosis often will not result in symptomatic relief. For example, one long-term follow-up study of patients who had undergone refusion demonstrated satisfactory results in only 60% of the patients who had repair of a pseudarthrosis (38). It is, however, anticipated that today with better means of internal fixation this will be improved upon. The calculation of the rate of pseudarthrosis is highly variable and dependent on the following factors: (a) the number of levels fused; (b) the fusion technique, including both the type (i.e., anterior interbody, midline posterior, etc.), as well as the presence or absence of internal fixation; (c) the source of bone graft; (d) the underlying pathology for which the fusion was performed; (e) constitutional and

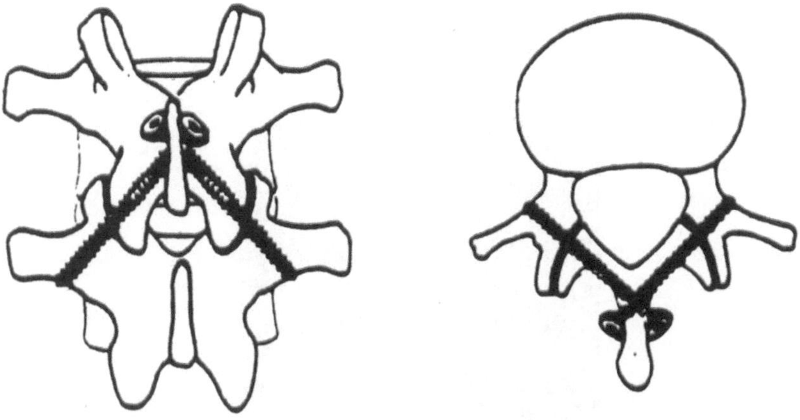

Figure 18.10. AO translaminar screw technique; 4.5-mm cortical screws are used. Facets are denuded with a burr of curet of articular cartilage, and packed with cancellous bone graft. The laminae and transverse processes are decorticated with a burr. The screws aim for the base of the transverse process (see Fig. 18.1 also).

other factors such as age and possibly sex of the patients, and smoking; (f) the type of external protection afforded the patient; and (g) the radiographic criterion utilized to assess the presence or absence of pseudarthrosis. These issues are mentioned to emphasize that the rate of pseudarthrosis cannot be calculated unless one has full knowledge of the relevant variables that influence its occurrence. In posterior surgery a one-level fusion usually bears an incidence of pseudarthrosis of 5%. For two levels, this may increase to as high as 20%, and for three or more levels, 40% or greater in fusions performed to the sacrum (74).

In anterior surgery, the incidence of pseudarthrosis for one- or two-level anterior fusions is in the area of 20%. Given the current state of internal fixation devices, no clear statistics are available as to the incidence of pseudarthroses. This is particularly true for failed back surgery. Jacobs et al. (51) have recently shown that with the use of AO translaminar screw fixation (Figs. 18.7 through 18.10), the incidence of pseudarthrosis is approximately 5%. These were in previously unfused patients. Kostuik and Errico (60), in a review of operations with internal fixation devices used to treat various etiologies of low back pain, have shown that with the use of Luque sublaminar wires and $\frac{1}{4}$ Luque rods, the incidence of pseudarthrosis in three or more levels lumbosacral fusion was about 15% (Fig. 18.11). This study was done prospectively in a consecutive series. This was a significant decrease from 40% without internal fixation.

Kostuik et al. (58) reported an 18% incidence of pseudarthrosis in a series of 56 patients who had previously undergone posterior spinal fusion but had failed when anterior fusion was used with the aid of internal fixa-

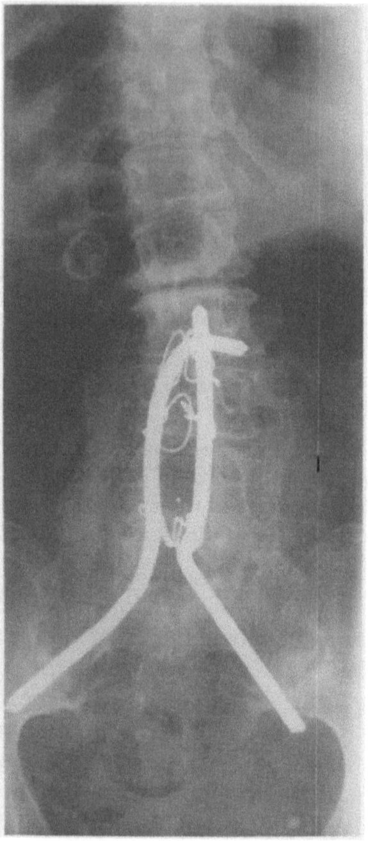

Figure 18.11. A 48-year-old woman underwent an L3-S1 fusion using Luque rods and sublaminar wires. She did well for 10 years but developed mild back pain and degenerative changes above her fusion at L2-3.

tion devices. The fixation devices initially including the use of single-cable Dwyer or single-rod Zielke systems, which were subsequently replaced by double-rod Zielke systems. When double-rod systems alone are analyzed, the incidence of pseudarthrosis decreased to 9%. Current, improved methods of anterior fixation should decrease this even more.

Clinical Presentation. The clinical presentation of pseudarthrosis is highly variable, and ranges from no symptoms to significant persisting and disabling back pain (20,36). Rarely should pain be ascribed to a pseudarthrosis until a 6-month interval has elapsed, and even then, continued motion may not necessarily indicate that the fusion is a failure. For that reason, we usually do not consider a fusion failure to be present until the patient has a 1-year interval. Exceptions are when there are obvious reasons to make that conclusion, such as graft dislodgment, or an obvious failure of fixation. Frequently a pseudarthrosis may remain undetectable for years. In our opinion, no fusion is solid until 2 years have elapsed. Because pseudarthrosis can be asymptomatic, it is important to evaluate the patients for other sources of continued symptoms or recurrent symptoms. The strategies that have been used to determine a symptomatic pseudarthrosis were presented earlier in this chapter.

Treatment. Because pseudarthrosis frequently accompanies other causes of failure, we will consider treatment of this condition later in this chapter.

Midterm Failures: Disc Disruption

This issue has been discussed in general under the heading of wrong diagnosis. However, there is a small subset of patients who achieve a solid arthrodesis, yet have continuing symptoms. This usually occurs when the first operation has been a posterior fusion and the continuance or onset of new symptoms occurs in the face of a solid fusion. Biomechanical studies have suggested an apparently continuous graft may nevertheless allow continued deflections of a magnitude sufficient to cause symptoms (65,99,124). In these instances, discography may be employed to determine the diagnosis, although this technically may be difficult because of obstructing bone between the transverse processes.

Treatment

If a solid posterior fusion is present, the obvious solution is an anterior interbody technique. If "disc disruption" is part of the presentation of a pseudarthrosis, then anterior fusion or circumferential fusion, with or without instrumentation, may be considered (Fig. 18.12).

Representative Case Example

Midterm Failures: Early Adjacent Degeneration

Rarely does degeneration cause symptoms in the months that follow spinal fusion in a segment that was normal prior to the operation. The exception may be in cases where rigid internal fixation or possible circumferential fusion has been performed. Hsu et al. (50) have reported accelerated degeneration with internal fixation, whereas Dewar (21) reported this complication occurred with circumferential fusion. This led him to abandon the technique.

Presentation. The typical presentation of degeneration adjacent to a fusion will be detailed later in this chapter, but it is important to stress here that the single most unequivocal indication of accelerated degeneration is

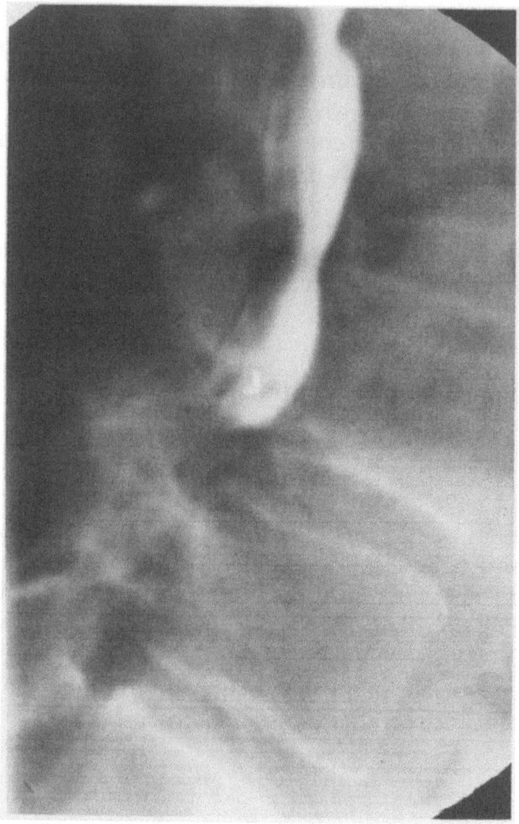

Figure 18.12. L5-S1 fusion performed 2 years previously. The patient developed a degenerative slip 18 months later. An acute disc sequestration was found in addition to the spondylolisthesis at L4-5. The fusion was extended to L4 with internal fixation following decompression.

a new disc herniation at the level adjacent to the fusion (Fig. 18.8). More common is the development of disc degeneration, without herniation, resulting in instability (Figs. 18.13 and 18.14) or spinal stenosis.

Treatment. The treatment is identical to that for later degeneration and will be presented there.

Graft Donor Site Problems

This issue will be discussed later in this chapter.

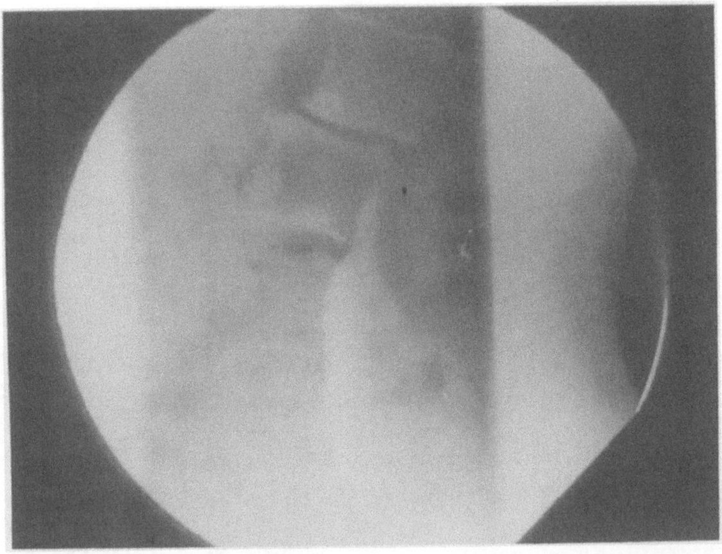

Figure 18.13. A 58-year-old woman had spinal fusion 18 years previously. Myelogram demonstrates flow defects proximal to the fusion (L2-3) with retrolisthesis at L2-3 and L1-2.

Midterm Failures: Inadequate Reconditioning

There is very little data that can establish how often patients are inadequately reconditioned. However, it must be a common problem, based on our clinical experience. Very often patients are referred either because they are thought to have an anatomic failure of fusion, or because they are thought to have psychosocial or compensation factors interfering with their recovery. Where those problems leave off and inadequate conditioning enters in is less relevant than the knowledge that the two often go hand in hand. Frequently, the patients have had a long period of disability and deconditioning prior to the first operation, complicated by the fact that posterior fusion techniques enervate the paraspinal muscles.

Clinical Presentation

Continued back pain, particularly that which increases with physical activity (i.e., mechanical pain), must be suspected in all patients as a source of failure, unless the causation is obvious and anatomic. Thus, pseudarthrosis cannot be considered the source of symptoms until adequate physical rehabilitation has occurred without successful resolution of symptoms.

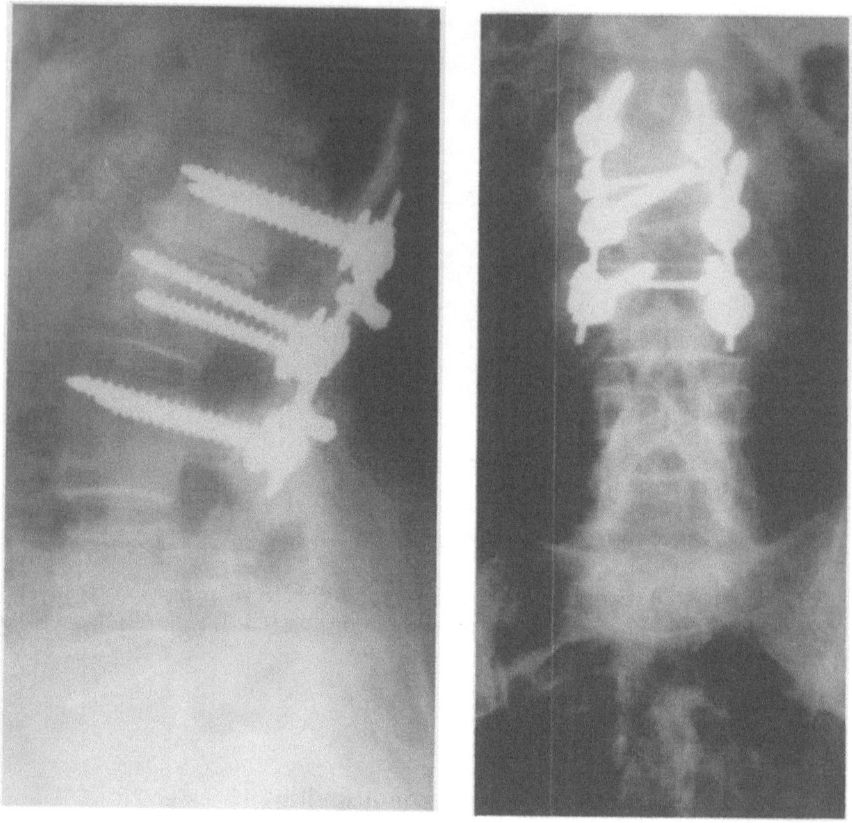

A B

Figure 18.14. A,B: The fusion was extended to L1 with instrumentation (Zielke); symptoms were relieved.

Treatment

It can be argued that a chronically debilitated patient can be returned to function solely by outpatient physical therapy or by a work-hardening program. If these methods are chosen, the operating surgeon must take an active role in monitoring the program, and establishing a time-limited goal. Too often, a patient will continue month after month with a combination of inadequate reconditioning and emphasis on modalities. General principles would suggest that a more intensive, multidisciplinary rehabilitation is appropriate in those patients who fail to respond to less-structured programs. The surgeon constantly finds himself in the dilemma of when to repeat all studies, and when to consider reoperation, versus continuing the rehabilitation program. There is no certain guideline, other than the general principle that the more certain the anatomic causation for pain, the more reasonable is surgical intervention; the less certain, the greater the reason to continue a nonoperative approach.

Long-Term Failures: Late Pseudarthrosis

The general issues in pseudarthrosis have already been presented. It is uncommon for a patient who has previously had symptomatic relief to present after 1 year with pain due to a pseudarthrosis. There are two general exceptions: The first is a disc herniation under a fusion. In a follow-up study of a minimum 10-year duration and an average follow-up of 13.7 years, Frymoyer et al. (35) found that no patient with a solid fusion had a disc herniation. Of 23 patients who required a second operation, 13 required fusion for back pain only, four for a recurrent disc herniation at the same level as their pervious surgery, and one had a new herniation at a new level, under the fusion. All patients with new or recurrent herniation had a pseudarthrosis. Thus, a patient presenting with a disc herniation under a fusion must be highly suspect of having an accompanying pseudarthrosis. A less certain source of failure is in a patient who had spine fusion, and later presents with symptoms and findings indicative of arachnoiditis. In this situation, it is less certain that the increasing symptoms can be alleviated by repair of the pseudarthrosis.

Treatment

The principles are the same as for the previously detailed treatment of pseudarthrosis. Obviously, if a disc herniation accompanies the pseudarthrosis the disc must be decompressed.

Long-Term Failures: Adjacent Motion Segment Degeneration

Segments adjacent to a previously performed lumbar fusion are at risk for the later development of a variety of degenerative changes; these may be either asymptomatic or symptomatic, and may include the clinical and radiographic features of segmental instability, degenerative spinal stenosis, or lumbar disc herniation (5.66). These changes are four times more likely to occur at L4-5 (20%) when the original fusion was performed at L5-S1 for a degenerative condition, than at L3-4 when the original fusion spanned from L4 to the sacrum, where the rate is 4% to 5% (36). Similarly, when the fusion was performed for thoracolumbar deformities, the magnitude of symptomatic degeneration increases, the lower into the lumbar spine the original fusion was extended (13,46,73,80).

The dominant reason for these degenerative changes are mechanical. Fusions cause increased stresses on adjacent segments, as measured experimentally and in humans with biplanar radiography (65,99,110). Inadvertent damage to facets or enervation may be contributory.

Table 18.5. Comparison of radiographic findings in fusion and nonfusion patients.

Variable	Fusion patients (%)	Nonfusion patients (%)	Significance
Traction spurs L3–L4	14.3	14.3	$0.01 > p < 0.025$
Traction spurs L4–L5	8.1	19.4	$0.01 > p < 0.025$
Traction spurs L3–L4	50.0	22.5	$p = 0.005$
Facet subluxation L1–L2	70.8	45.0	$0.01 > p < 0.025$
Facet subluxation L3–L4	82.8	84.0	$p = 0.005$

Asymptomatic Degeneration

Asymptomatic degenerative changes may include osteophyte, disc space narrowing, hypermobility with or without translation (i.e., a positive Knuttsen's sign), and spinal stenosis. A comparison of plain radiographic findings in patients treated with and without fusion 10 or more years after their operation are shown in Table 18.5. This table demonstrates the high rate of degenerative changes, which were unrelated to symptoms. In particular, claw spurs were more common in heavy-laboring males above the fusion. Hypermobility was also more common. A subsequent study by Lehmann, et al. (66) in 1987 analyzed patients 30 or more years after fusion, and included CT studies as part of the radiologic evaluation. Almost 50% of patients had radiographic evidence of segmental instability and/or spinal stenosis. Again, these radiographic findings in general were unrelated to symptoms. They found, however, that 85% of patients were satisfied with their outcome 30 or more years after their spinal fusion.

Because there is a high incidence of radiographic changes, the most difficult clinical task is to determine if the level above the fusion is causing symptoms in a patient who has back pain alone. In these instances, discography is the procedure of choice, in our opinion. If segmental instability is present, without an actual fixed deformity such as a new degenerative spondylolisthesis, the problem is also complex. In these instances discography, and possibly facet blocks, may again be useful to determine if the lesion is symptomatic.

Spinal Stenosis

The diagnostic problem becomes significantly easier if the patient has peripheral symptoms of claudication. Brodsky (5) in particular has stressed that this is the most common cause of recurrent symptoms after a fusion. Although he reported a large number of cases, it was impossible from his study to determine the actual incidence of this late cause of failure (Fig. 18.15).

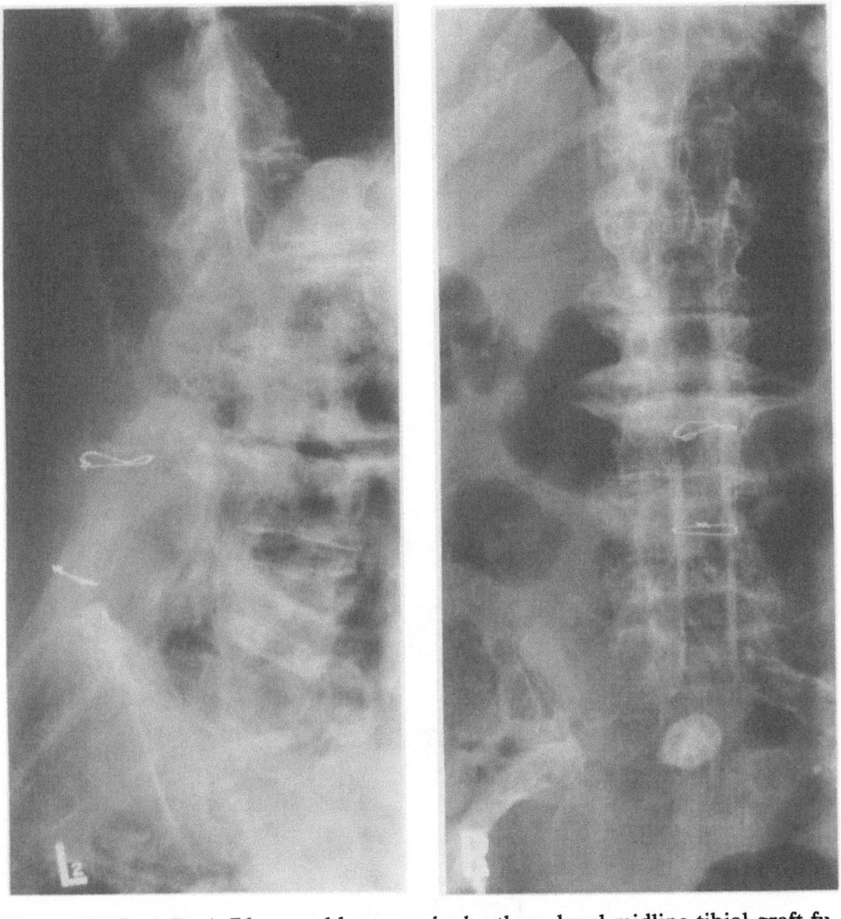

A B

Figure 18.15. A,B: A 76-year-old woman had a three-level midline tibial graft fusion 35 years previously with an excellent result. **C,D,E:** Preoperative CT demonstrates a complete block with very severe spinal stenosis at the level immediately proximal to the fusion. She became paraparetic with grade I-II power and loss of bowel and bladder control. One year following decompression, she walks with one cane and has complete bowel and bladder control.

C

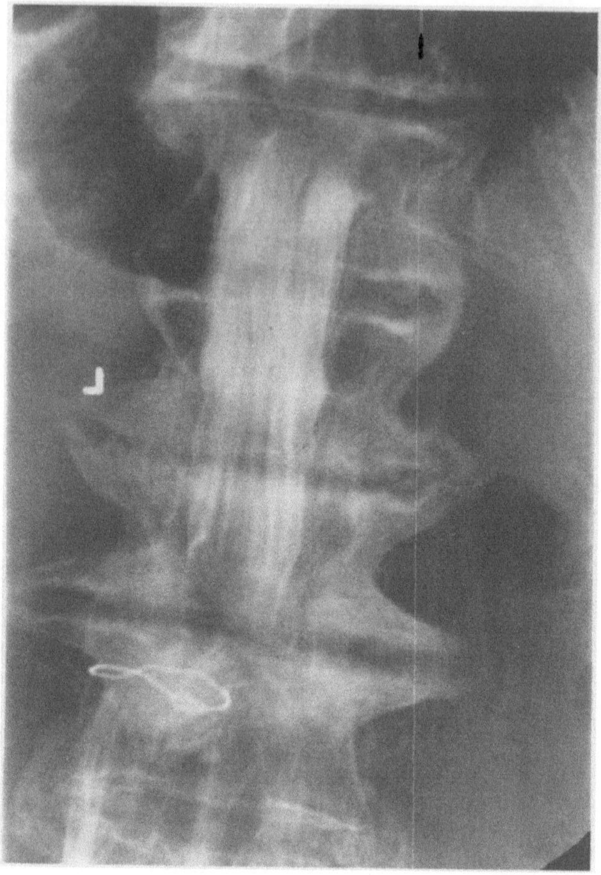

Figure 18.15. (*cont.*)

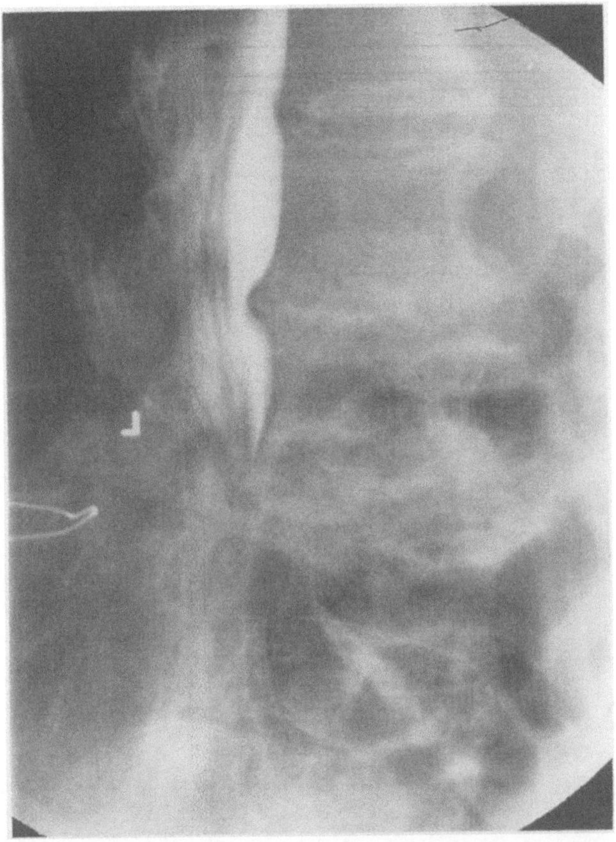

D

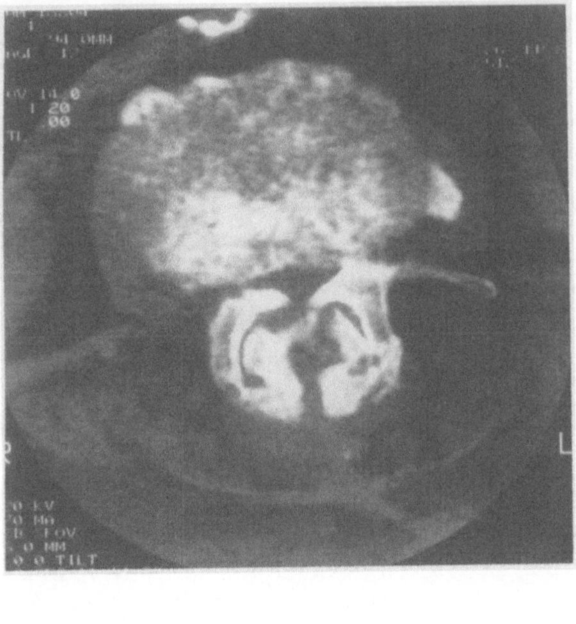

E

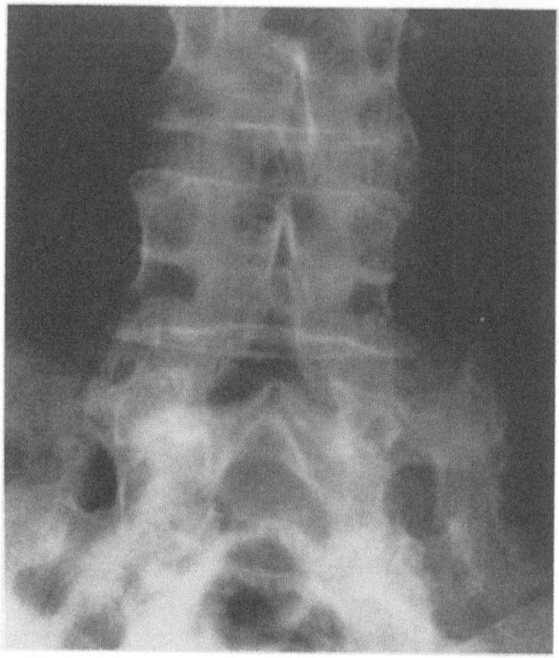

A

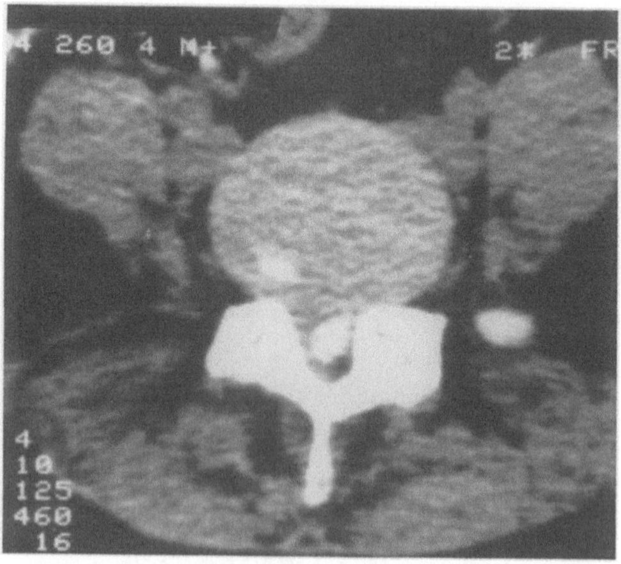

B

Figure 18.16. **A:** A 67-year-old woman had prior decompression of L4-5 and L5-S1. She presented with a solid arthrodesis, and recurrent back and leg pain. **B,C:** Myelographically enhanced CT scan demonstrates a disc herniation at L3-4. The level below demonstrates well-placed pedicle screws and a normal canal.

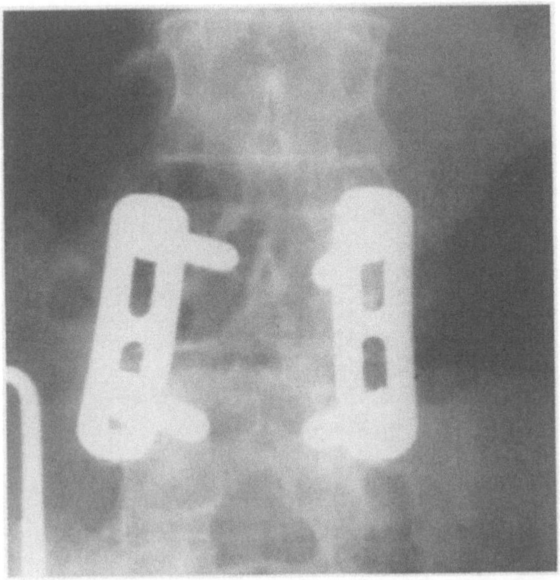

C

Figure 18.16. (*cont.*)

Disc Herniation

This is the easiest problem to diagnose with certainty, because the clinical symptoms, physical findings, and confirmatory images are typical. How often true disc herniation occurs varies widely. In the 10-year study by Frymoyer (35), a 4% rate at L3-4 was found in fusions from L4 to the sacrum, which is similar to that reported by DePalma and Rothman (20).

Treatment. The treatment of failures above a fusion is largely based on the pathology, but in our opinion should usually include an extension of the spinal fusion, combined with appropriate decompression based on the preoperative symptoms, physical findings, and radiologic images. In general, the accompanying fusion should include instrumentation, particularly when the segment is unstable. However, selected cases may be appropriately treated by posterior fusion techniques, or anterior interbody fusions with instrumentation (Fig. 18.16).

Long-Term Failures: Spinal Stenosis Under a Fusion

This problem is almost exclusively a problem with posterior midline fusions. Macnab (75) thought it occurred in 20% of all patients treated pre-

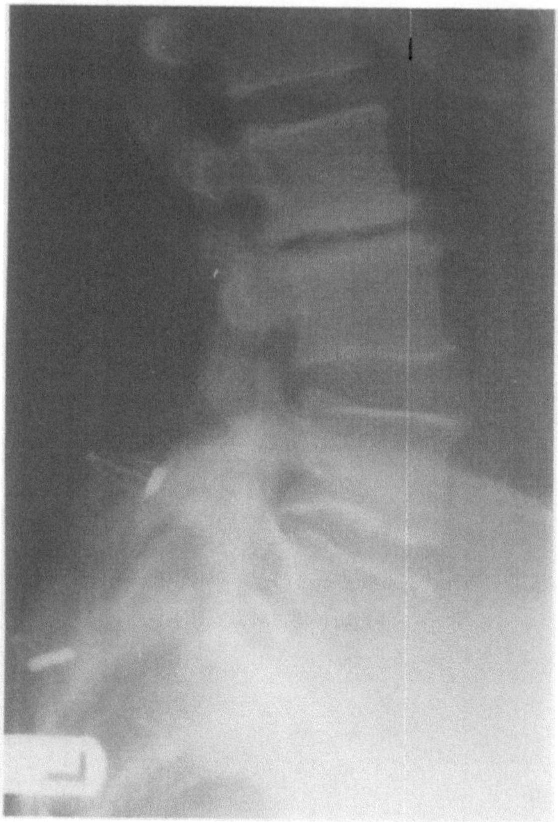

A

Figure 18.17. A,B,C,D: A 51-year-old man had undergone a two-level fusion 21 years previously. He later developed symptoms of spinal stenosis. A myelogram CT from L2-L4 was done and demonstrates stenosis. He underwent decompression L3-4 with only partial relief of his symptoms. A repeat myelographically enhanced CT scan shows full decompression at L2-4 but at L4-L5 spinal stenosis persists. A further decompression was done with improvement. It is anticipated that the instability at L2-3, L3-4 may increase and require stabilization, which ideally should have been done at the time of the L2-L4 decompression.

viously with that technique, but later Brodsky's (5) clinical experience suggested this was a significant overestimate of the problem. His opinion is supported by Lehmann's et al.'s (66) finding that a stenotic appearance was common under a midline fusion many years after the operation, but rarely were symptoms of spinal stenosis present. The presumed etiology is hypertrophy of the graft over time in response to Wolff's law. Stenosis has never been reported as occurring beneath a fusion performed in adolescence or adult life for scoliosis. The majority of cases reported by

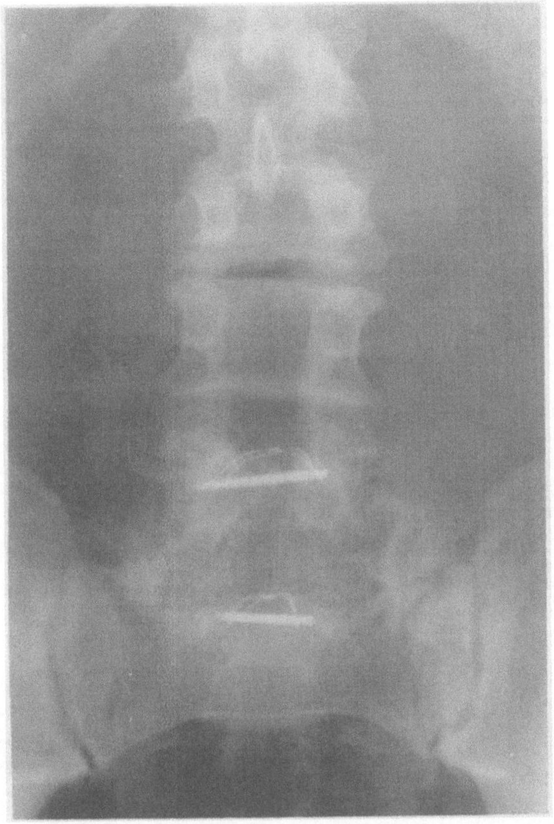

B

Figure 18.17. (*cont.*)

Macnab (75) had their fusions done prior to the common recognition of the spinal stenosis syndrome. Thus, it is quite possible that they had spinal stenosis prior to their fusion (Fig. 18.17).

Clinical Presentation

The condition is suspected in a patient with long-standing midline posterior fusion, insidious and progressive onset of symptoms of spinal stenosis, and imaging studies that demonstrate the absence of significant stenosis above the fusion, and a significant stenosis beneath it.

Treatment

The treatment is decompression. This is made difficult by the massive amount of bone that overlies the lamina, the inability to identify the old

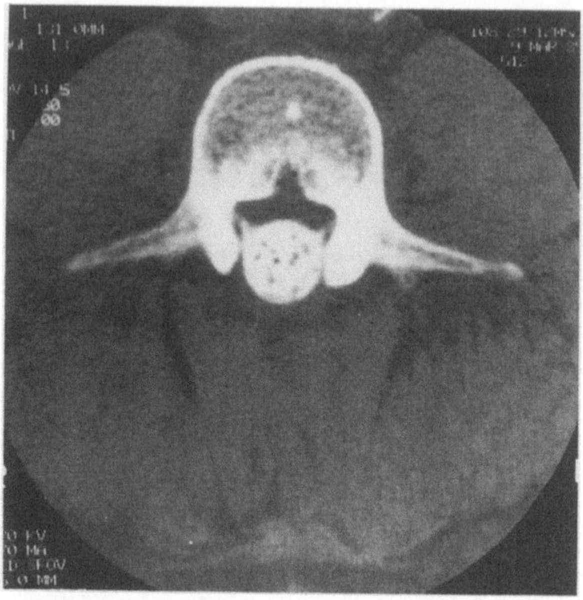

C

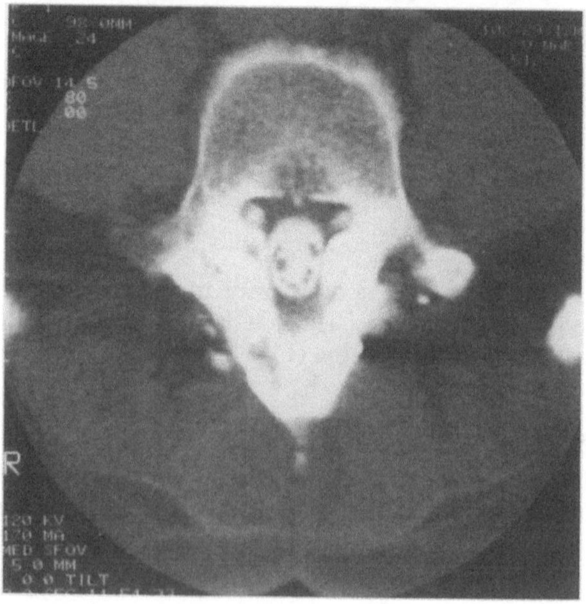

D

Figure 18.17. (*cont.*)

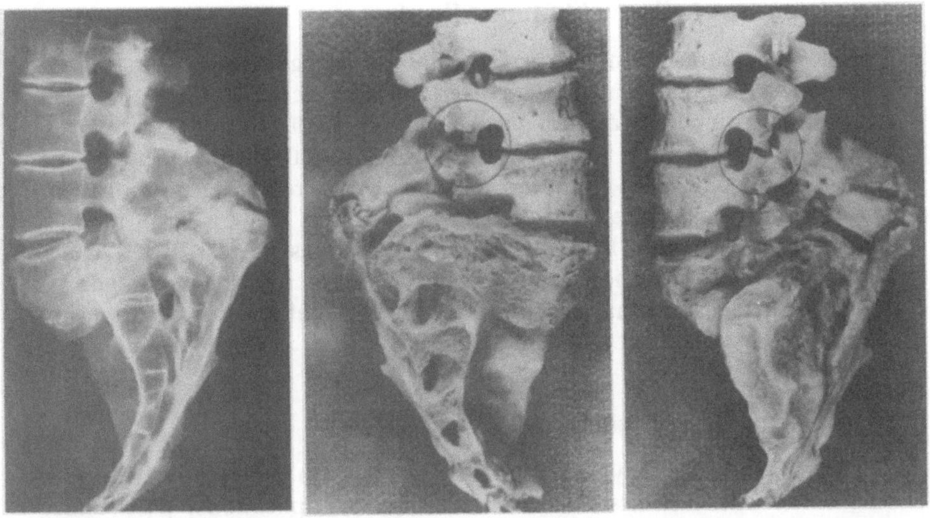

Figure 18.18. Acquired spondylolysis above a fusion (from the collection of the late Dr. R.I. Harris). This patient underwent an L4-S1 fusion for a severe spondylolisthesis when she was a young woman. She did well but later in life developed breast cancer and died. At autopsy the spine was harvested. A pseudarthrosis at L4-5 was found plus an acquired spondylolisthesis L3-4, which was not present initially.

lamina, and by frequently associated scar. In very difficult cases, it may be necessary to go to the next level to identify tissue planes, and move back from that level. In that event, the fusion should be extended, unless the level is anatomically normal, and minimal bone sacrifice is necessary.

Late Causes of Failure: Acquired Spondylolysis

This is almost exclusively a later cause of failure in posterior midline fusion and is reported on 0% to 2.5% of patients treated by that technique (8,36,45,97,100,113) (Fig. 18.18). The causation is thought to be secondary to repetitive mechanical forces, and can be produced in the laboratory, after simulated posterior midline fusions (99). Weakening of the neural arch by overzealous decortication, or possibly interference with the blood supply have also been suggested (76). It has been rarely reported with transverse process fusion (3).

Treatment

The treatment is stabilization and fusion by anterior interbody or posterior intertransverse process fusion, with or without instrumentation.

Late Causes of Failure: Abutment Syndrome

This complication was noted in early literature regarding posterior midline fusions (11), and has been reported in more recent literature to be an overlooked source of failure, particularly when the facets are involved (17,111). The etiology is either overzealous initial graft placement, or later hypertrophy. The condition may be considered when motion pain occurs, particularly in extension, and radiographs show a large midline fusion mass, usually at L4, abutting on the spinous process of L3. Diagnostic anesthetic injections can be employed to confirm the diagnosis. Surgical management may include excision of the abutment, or extension of the fusion to the next adjacent level.

Graft Donor Site Problems

The graft donor site may be a source of problems in general, whereas specific donor sites are associated with unique complications, particularly nerve entrapments.

Pain

Graft donor site pain is a common complaint of all patients particularly in the early postoperative phase. How long the pain persists is debatable. Kurz et al. (63) state it is common in up to 15% in the first 3 months. However, a long term study (37) reported that 37% of the patients had donor site pain 10 or more years after their operation. Statistical analysis made it uncertain if the pain was actually related to the donor site or part of a general pain syndrome. When donor site pain was present, it was more common if the graft had been taken from the same side as the original sciatica, and there is a high association between persisting back pain, leg pain, and donor site pain. These complaints occurred independent of any radiographic changes, such as degeneration, which occurred at the donor site. A positive Trendelenburg sign was seen in 18% but appeared to be independent of the donor site.

Specific Complications

Specific complications can occur, however, which are painful and require later treatment. These include sacroiliac disruption, when the graft is from the posterior iliac crest, hernias in both anterior and posterior grafts, and fracture at the graft donor site, typically when the graft is taken from the anterior ileum. Heterotopic bone formation has also been thought to occasionally cause local pain, although in a long-term study, the presence of heterotopic bone bore little relationship to symptoms (37). Sacroiliac instability occurs rarely, and is rarely included in large series as a significant complication. Fractures are usually an avulsion of the anterior wing of the ileum, and may necessitate internal fixation. Fractures extending into the acetabulum have been alluded to in the literature (15).

Similarly, hernias are an infrequent complication and usually related to full-thickness grafts. Bosworth (4) described this complication in posterior iliac graft donor sites, as well as technique for its repair.

Infection

The donor site as a local source of infection is reported by Kurz et al. (63) to be less than 1%.

Nerve Pain

Bone graft incisions may cause peripheral nerve injury, or later nerve symptoms may result from entrapments secondary to scar or occasionally heterotopic bone formation. The classic site is in the anterior iliac, where involvement of the lateral femorocutaneous nerve produces meralgia paresthetica. This complication is reported in 1% to 14% of patients (120). Even more rarely other cutaneous nerves such as the ilioinguinal, genitofemoral, or the femoral nerve may become involved (15,63,105).

In posterior grafting, the clunial nerves are most commonly involved (Fig. 18.19). We advocate not using an incision over the crest that extends more than one hand's breadth to help avoid this problem. The use of a hockey stick incision, tunneling procedure, or longitudinal incision are methods to avoid this problem. Drury (24) suggested the diagnosis of clunial nerve neuroma could be made by local anesthetic injections, and that resection of the neuroma could relieve that symptom.

In addition, a variety of more dramatic complications may include hemorrhage, particularly from gluteal arteries in posterior iliac grafts, and even visceral injuries.

General Complications

Table 18.1B lists the array of complications that have been associated with lumbar spinal fusions, some of which are specific to a particular technique, and others of which are generic.

Surgical Treatment

Because there are so many different causes for failure after spinal fusion, the operative choices are numerous and must be carefully selected. Again, the general principle applies: the more certain the history, physical examination, and imaging studies, the more likely success will occur. In general, the most predictable results will occur in patients with leg symptoms, rather than with low back pain alone. Alternatively, uncertainty about diagnosis will predictably lead to less certain results, particularly

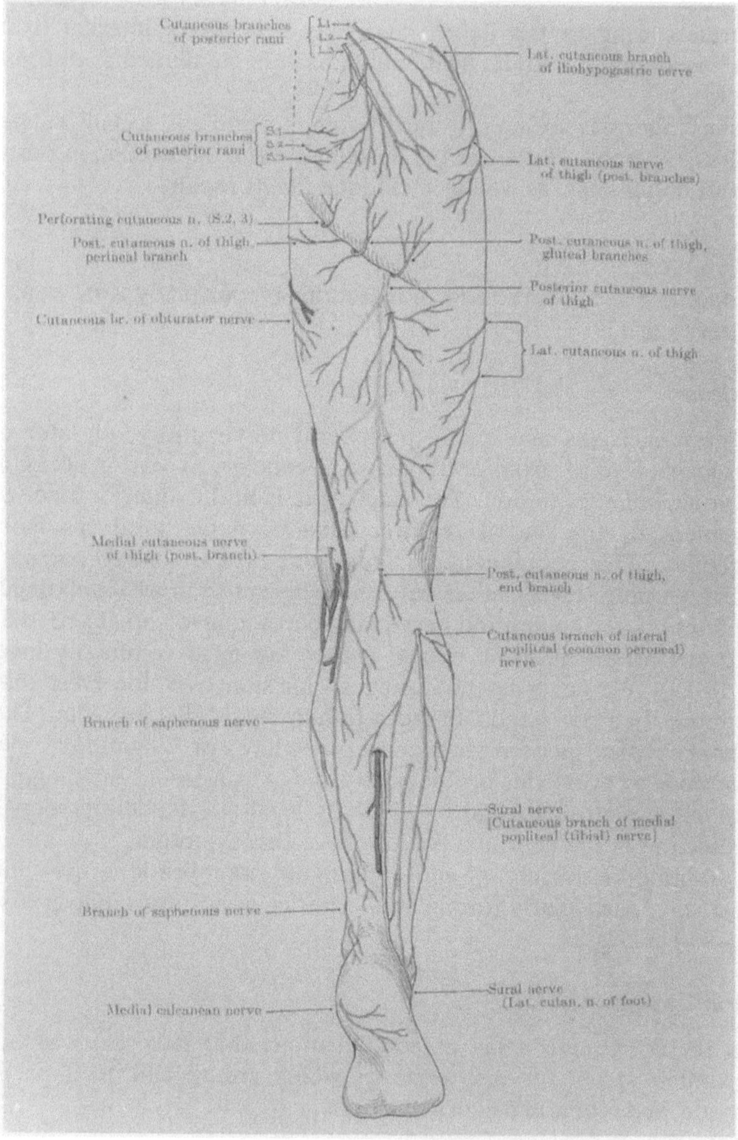

Figure 18.19. Clunial nerves pass over the iliac crest approximately 8 cm from the posterior iliac spine.

in patients with long-standing disability, and psychosocial dysfunction. In this regard, pseudarthrosis is one of the most difficult conditions to assess as a source of symptoms, and not surprisingly the outcome from repair of pseudarthrosis is the most difficult to predict.

It should also be evident that the second, third, or even fourth operation introduces additional risks, including higher rates of infection, lower rates of successful fusion, as well as specific problems related to scarring and to devascularization of bone and soft tissues.

A few general principles of surgical treatment are useful, as one approaches these complex patients, who are categorized by the type of surgery previously performed.

Failed Previous Posterior Surgery. When adequate bone stock is present, the patient may again be approached posteriorly, particularly when a new

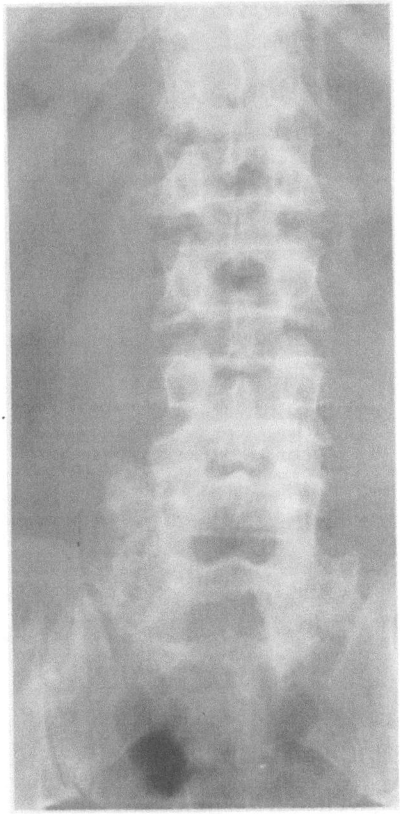

Figure 18.20. A 42-year-old man underwent an L4-S1 intertransverse fusion without instrumentation 2 years previously. A pseudarthrosis at L4-5 was felt to account for persistent pain.

level of pathology is present that necessitates decompression and new or refusion. We believe the fusion in general should be accompanied by the use of internal fixation, of which pedicle screw devices seem most useful (Figs. 18.20 and 18.21). If the decompression required is wide, and involves additional facet sacrifice, serious consideration should be given to a second stage anterior procedure. This need is particularly evident if there is inadequate bone stock for fusion, or rigid posterior fixation cannot be obtained (Fig. 18.22).

Failed Previous Posterior Surgery with Wide Laminectomy. If decompression is not necessary, and stabilization is the major object, this is best obtained with an anterior fusion. The presence of a wide laminectomy usually leaves inadequate bone stock for posterior refusion, particularly

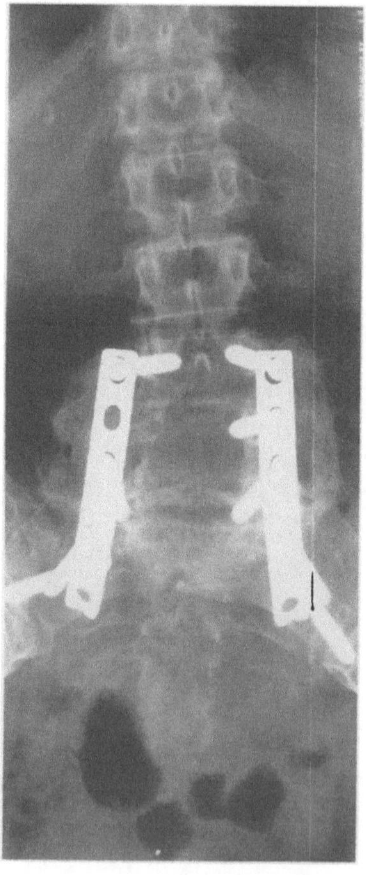

Figure 18.21. A fusion at L3-S1 was performed using AO plates. Preoperatively a discogram also revealed problems at L3-4. Pseudarthroses were found at L4-5 and L5-S1. The patient had good posterior bone stock and has gone on to solid fusion.

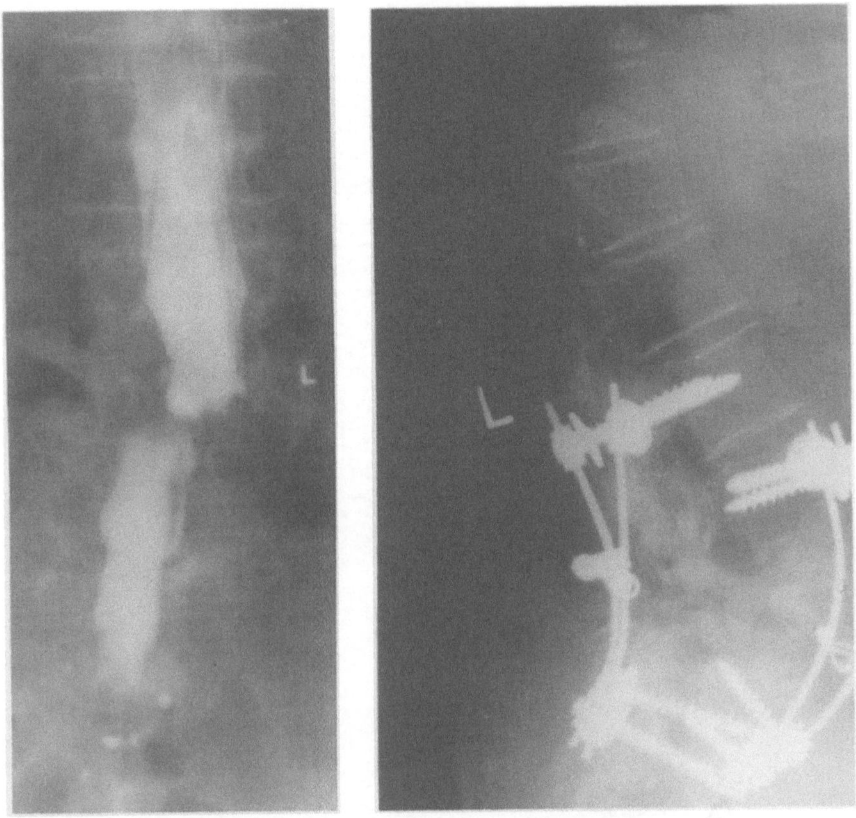

A B

Figure 18.22. A: A 68-year-old woman. Six previous procedures had been performed including attempts at instrumentation using Harrington rods. Severe sepsis had occurred on one occasion. The patient was paraparetic, in a wheelchair. Note the translation of the dye column on myelography. **B:** A two-stage procedure was necessary. First a posterior approach to decompress and realign the cauda equina. The stubs of the pedicles were used to provide some fixation because of inadequate area for a fusion. As a result of the previous surgery, the laminectomies, and extensive scarring, the second procedure was done via the anterior approach and consisted of interbody grafts. The internal fixation screws (Zielke) were reinforced with methylmethacrylate bone cement for the severe osteoporosis. The patient walks with canes and has regained bowel and bladder control.

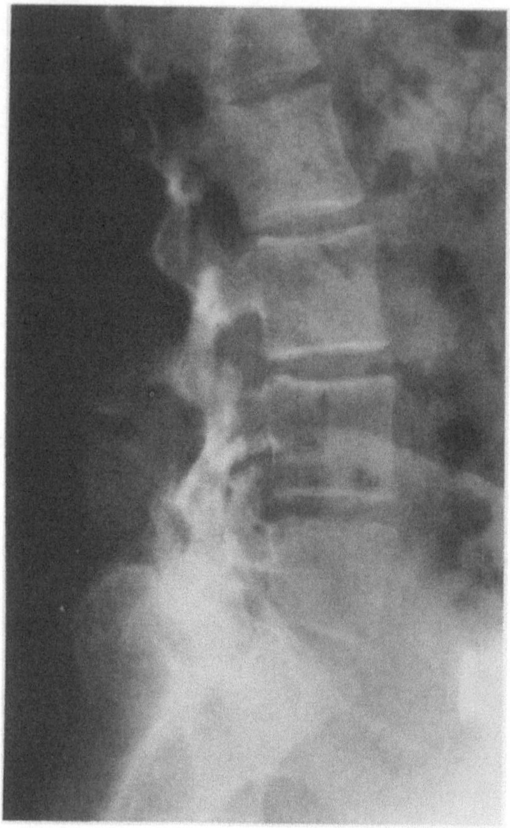

A

Figure 18.23. A: A 36-year-old woman who had undergone two previous attempts at fusions. Pseudarthroses were located at L4-5 and L5-S1 on plane radiography and tomography. **B:** An anterior interbody fusion of L4-S1 was performed. An I-beam plate was used to enhance fusion. The plate was contoured to the sacral prominatory. The patient is pain-free and has returned to work.

when there is extensive scarring and poor blood supply (Figs. 18.23 through 18.25).

Failure of Two or More Previous Posterior Fusions. Under these circumstances an anterior fusion is beneficial to achieve stability. Whether this is accompanied by anterior instrumentation will depend on the number of levels, as well as the specific levels, and the assessment of which stability might be achieved without instrumentation (Fig. 18.26).

Failure of Previous Anterior Surgery. If there has been previous anterior surgery, and a resultant pseudarthrosis, a posterior approach with internal fixation is the method of choice. However, patients who have had

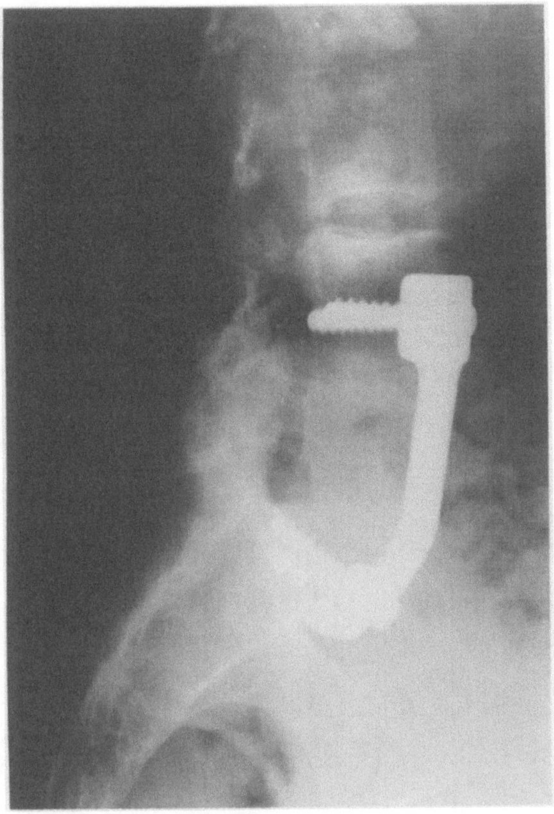

B

Figure 18.23. (*cont.*)

both prior anterior and posterior surgery are again better approached anteriorly. In either event, it is advisable to insert stents up both ureters to prevent inadvertent cutting of these structures, which are at risk because of retroperitoneal scarring. Even though the ureters still may be cut, the complication is easier to recognize and repair with the stints in place.

It is also important to realize that the additional retroperitoneal scarring caused by additional procedures may result in urinary tract obstruction. Fortunately, this complication is rare; however, repeat anterior surgery in the lumbosacral area in particular, has a definite risk of vascular complication, involving both venous and arterial structures. The surgeon must be prepared to deal with the consequences of the injuries. It is also prudent to consider postoperative anticoagulation therapy, because of an increased risk of thromboembolism.

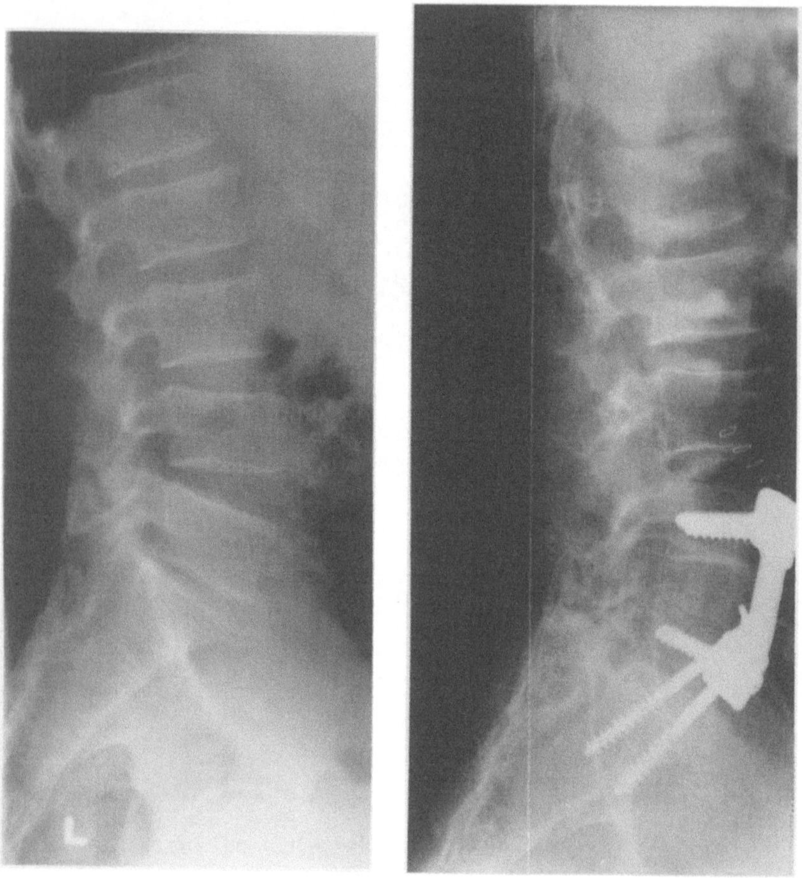

A

B

Figure 18.24. **A:** A 42-year-old man had undergone three previous decompression attempts and fusion plus decompression. Pseudarthroses were noted at L4-5, L5-S1. **B:** An anterior interbody fusion of L4-S1 was successfully done. An I-beam plate was used from L4-5, and two 6.5-mm AO cancellous screws from L5 into the sacrum. If the promontory (L5-S1 angle) is very prominent this screw placement is preferred to contouring the plate.

Who Should Have Combined Procedures, i.e., Anterior and Posterior Surgery. The issue of who should have a combined procedure is of increasing interest. As already noted, this approach is indicated when a posterior approach is mandated for decompression, but prior decompression and fusion have left inadequate bone stock either for a fusion bed, and/or for the insertion of posterior fixation devices. The stumps of the pedicles, if they remain, are a possible site for the insertion of a pedicle screw.

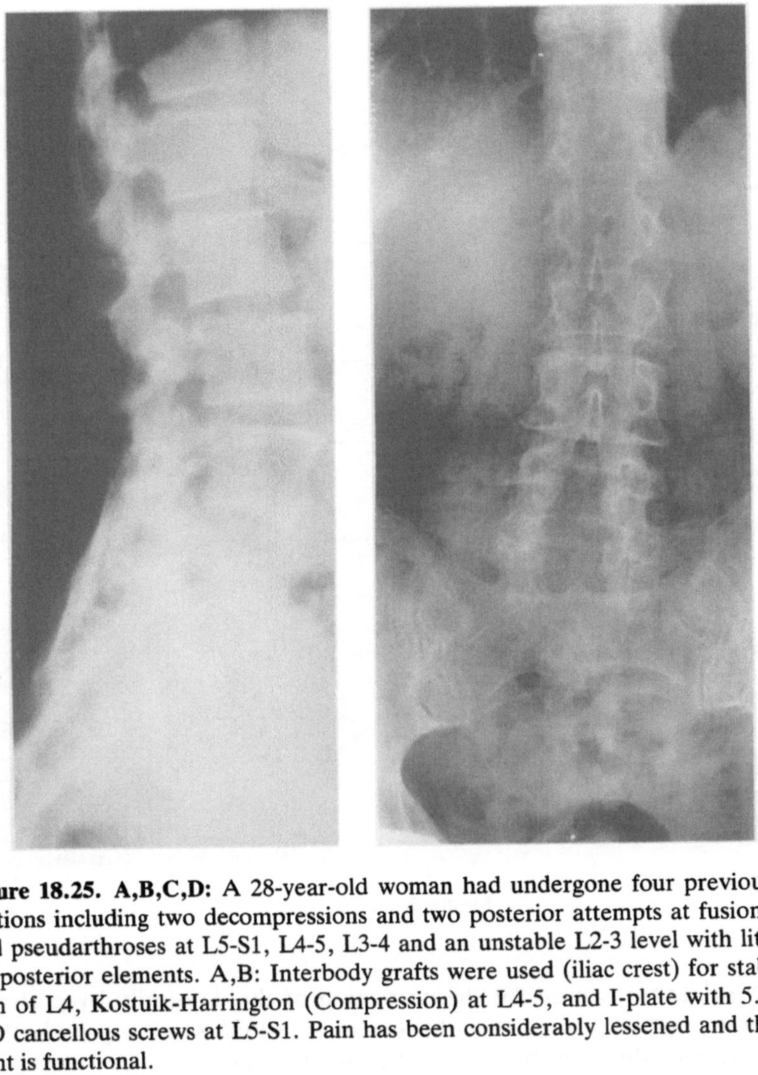

A B

Figure 18.25. A,B,C,D: A 28-year-old woman had undergone four previous operations including two decompressions and two posterior attempts at fusion. She had pseudarthroses at L5-S1, L4-5, L3-4 and an unstable L2-3 level with little or no posterior elements. A,B: Interbody grafts were used (iliac crest) for stabilization of L4, Kostuik-Harrington (Compression) at L4-5, and I-plate with 5.5-mm AO cancellous screws at L5-S1. Pain has been considerably lessened and the patient is functional.

Frequently, the extensive scarring and devascularization make the posterior fusion alone unlikely to succeed, and the combined anterior posterior approach is utilized (Figs. 18.22, 18.26, 18.27, and 18.28).

A second indication is in cases where there is significant loss of lumbar lordosis from previous surgery. The problems of the iatrogenic flat back deformity must be considered; under this circumstance, the anterior procedure is used to mobilize the disc spaces, which are then filled with morcellized bone. Internal fixation is contraindicated. A second stage pos-

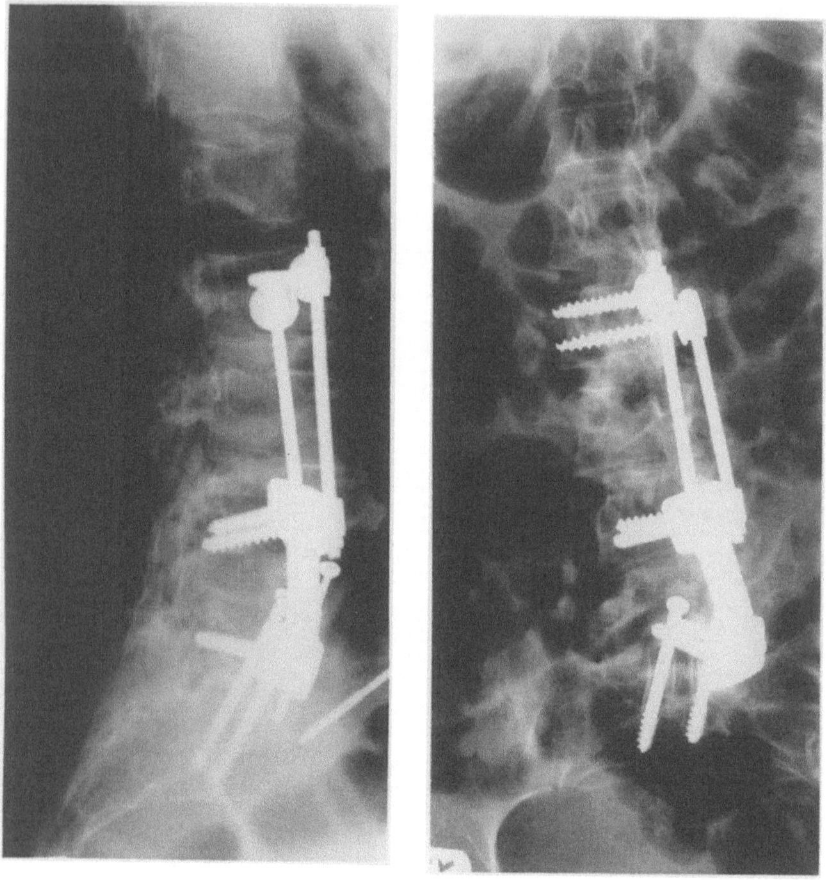

C D

Figure 18.25. (*cont.*)

terior procedure is used for the correction of the deformity by posterior osteotomy and instrumentation to recreate the lordosis. If a pseudarthrosis is present, this may be used in lieu of the osteotomy, but usually requires widening to achieve the necessary correction.

We do not feel that circumferential fusion is indicated for primary, unoperated patients. This is with the possible exception of some cases of degenerative spondylolisthesis or in patients requiring four or more levels of fusion to the sacrum, as noted in surgery for adult scoliosis (61).

Who Should Have a Posterior Lumbar Interbody Fusion

The use of posterior lumbar interbody fusion in itself is controversial because of a high risk of neurologic injury, graft extrusion, and the inability

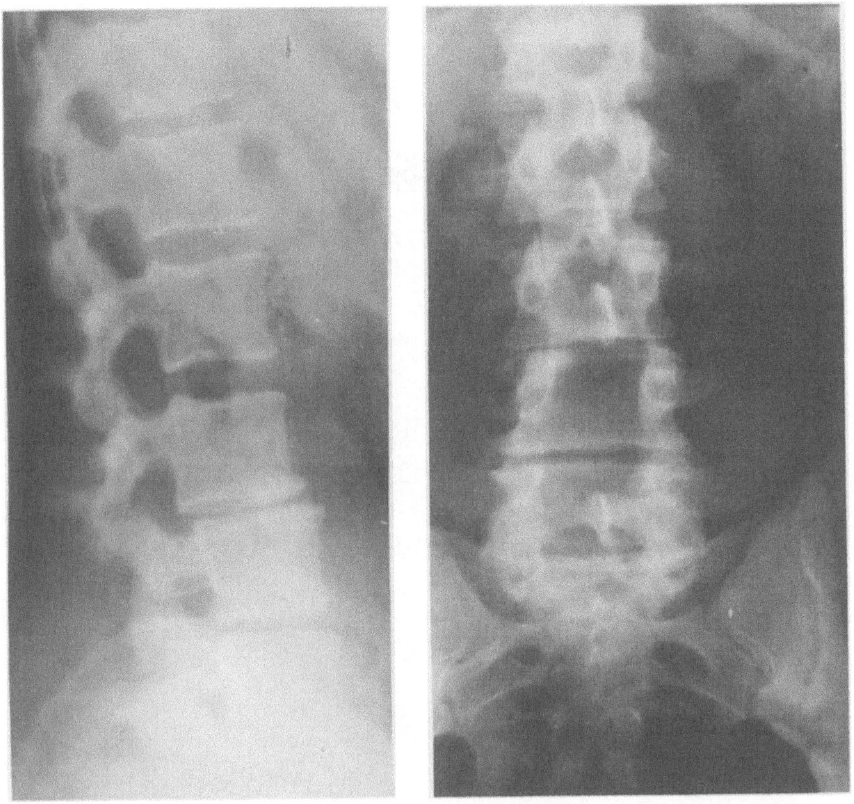

A B

Figure 18.26. **A,B:** A 51-year-old woman who had undergone five previous procedures including multiple decompression and attempts at posterolateral fusion. L2-3 was unstable as well. **C,D:** Interbody fusion (iliac crest) with double Zielke instrumentation L2-S1. Patient returned to work as a pharmacist assistant after being off work for 7 years. Double rods are necessary for rotational control.

to obtain an adequate rate of fusion even in primary cases. The major problem is the wide exposure necessary to obtain placement of the grafts, which the detractors of the procedure feel results in unusual scarring. However, the proponents of the procedure feel this complication is avoidable (104).

We feel that in previous failed fusion, the role of posterior lumbar interbody fusion is extremely limited on the basis of technical problems that are encountered as one approaches the dense scar that often is present. If an interbody fusion is felt to be necessary, we feel that the anterior route is preferable, but not everybody agrees.

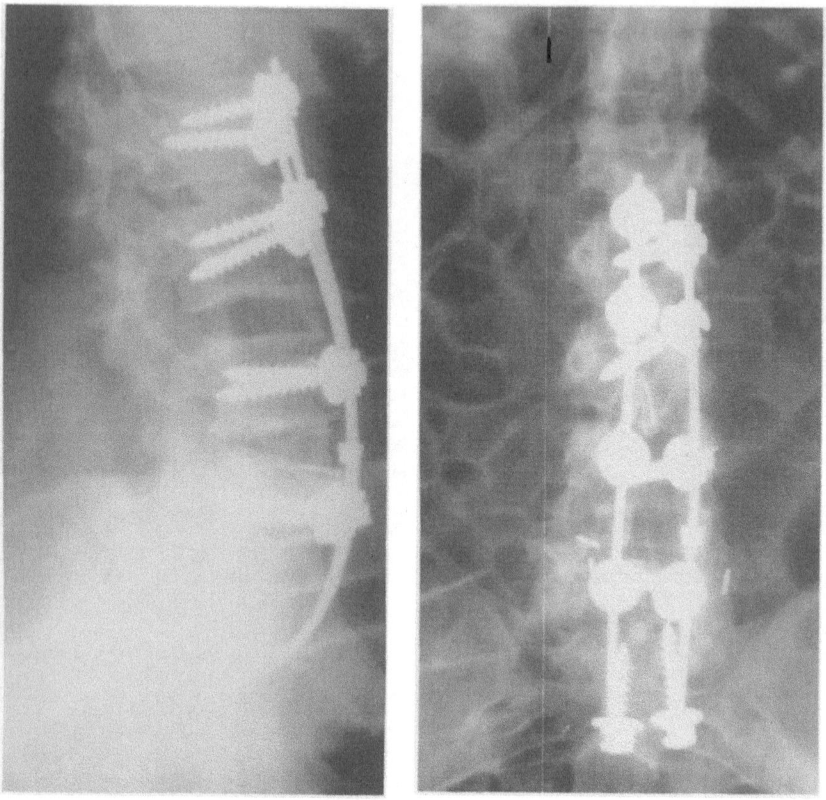

C D

Figure 18.26. (*cont.*)

Technical Details

Depending on the specific condition being treated, and the history of prior surgery, certain technical details are useful to keep in mind. First we will look at the general issue of posterior refusion.

Fixation. As noted, we prefer pedicle devices whenever possible, if posterior internal fixation is deemed necessary. In failed prior posterior fusion, the anatomic landmarks of the pedicle may be difficult to define, and radiologic control is essential. If there is a large amount of old bone graft present, the screws may be attached into the graft without involving the pedicle. More often this is not the case, or osteoporosis is an additional source of concern. Under these circumstances the pedicle should be defined. Time can be saved by estimating the anatomic point of insertion, and making a drill hole. A K-wire is placed in the hole, and fluoroscopic confirmation then obtained. If they are not, slight alterations in level can

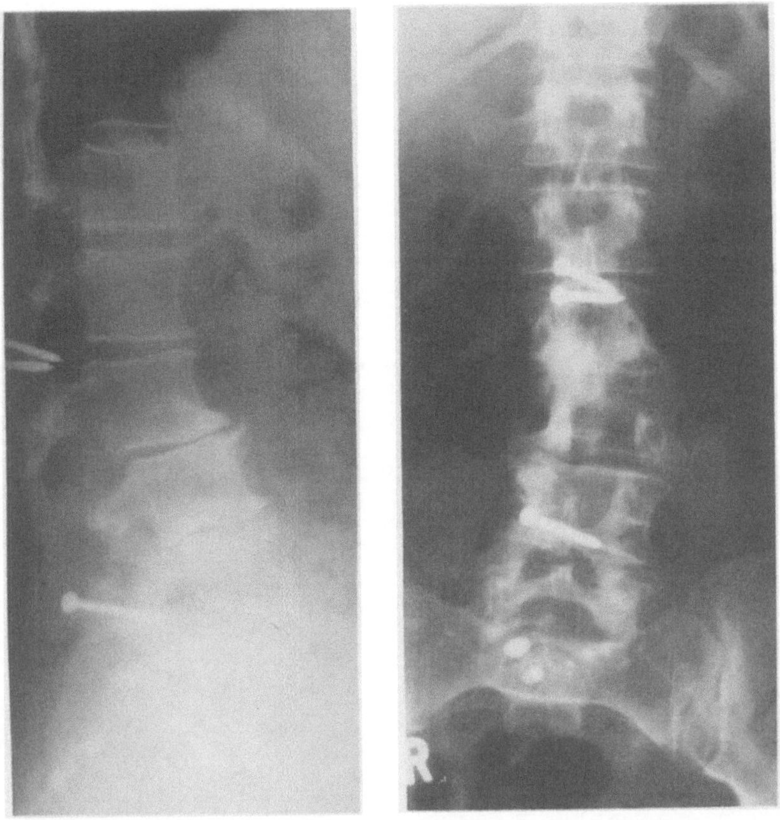

A B

Figure 18.27. A,B: A 62-year-old woman. Six previous procedures had been attempted with resultant severe instability, neurological pain, and back pain. **C,D:** A two-stage procedure was performed including posterior decompression. The pedicle stumps were used for stabilization posteriorly but because of inadequate bone stock an anterior fusion was done using interbody grafts and double Zielke rods. The patient is remarkably improved 5 years later and drives from Toronto to Florida annually for holidays.

succeed in achieving the proper entry point, which is then completed with an awl or tap drill.

Once a pedicle fixation system is placed, the linkage must be carefully selected. Plates appear to be more rigid, but are less adaptable. Although they may be contoured for lordosis, it is difficult to adapt them to a rotatory or lateral deviation deformity. Conversely, rods can be easily contoured three-dimensionally, but many of the devices are less rigid than a plate device. Ultimately, the choice of device rests with the surgeon's experience, and the preoperative assessment of which system will deal best with the complexities of the individual patient.

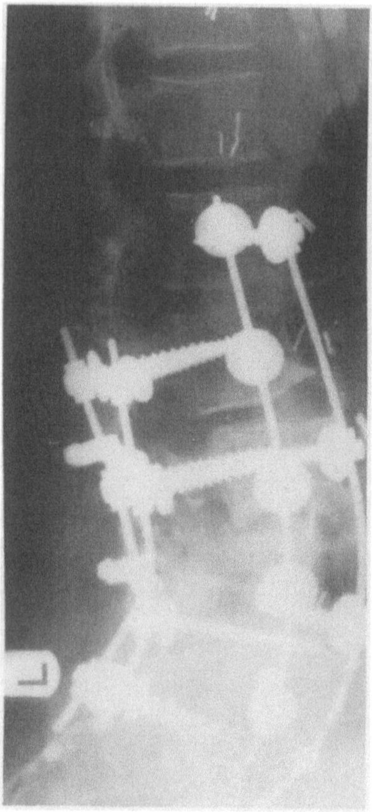

C

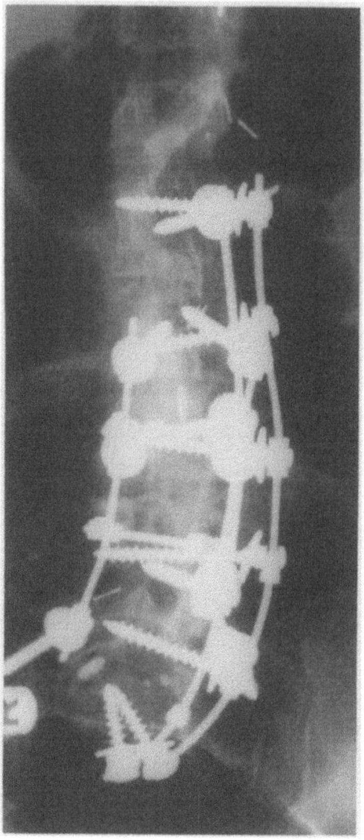

D

Figure 18.27. (*cont.*)

Figure 18.28. A: A 63-year-old woman had undergone a two-level L4-S1 fusion 12 years previously. She developed symptoms of spinal stenosis and segmental instability proximal at L3-4 and L2-3. **B:** Her surgeon extended the fusion following posterior decompression at L2-3, L3-4, to T10. One year later the hooks disengaged. The rods were removed but the pseudarthroses were not repaired. **C,D,E:** Her deformity progressed, together with increased instability and pain. The L3 vertebral body appears to be avascular. She developed marked lateral quadriceps weakness and could not stand. A postmyelographic CT shows her residual block. **F,G:** Posterior decompression was performed together with Cotrel-Dubousset instrumentation and fusion using pedicle screws distally. The L4-S1 fusion was solid but all other levels had pseudarthroses. Because of the long fusion extending to the fixed sacrum and poor posterior bone stock (**E**) (small amount—extensive scarring) an anterior fusion was done.

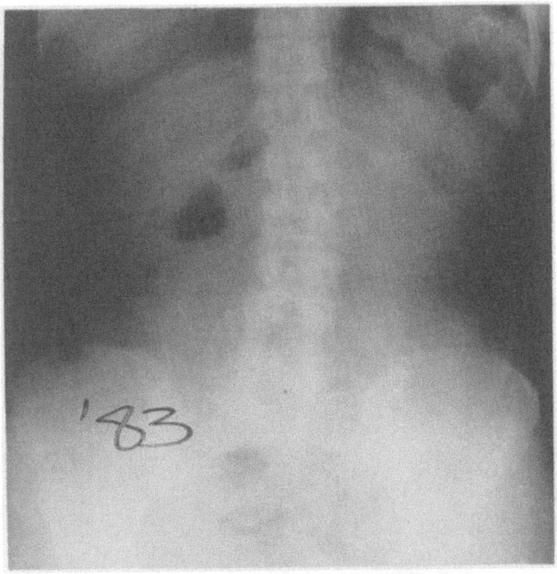

A

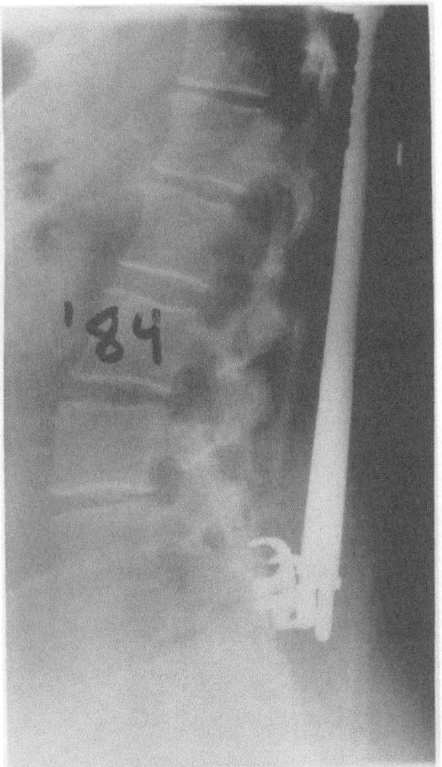

B

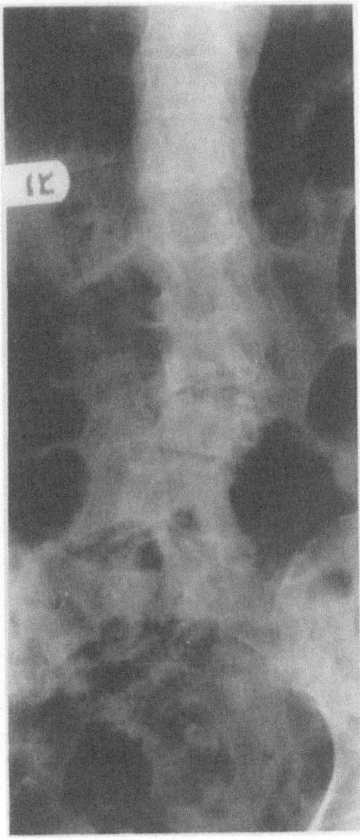

C

D

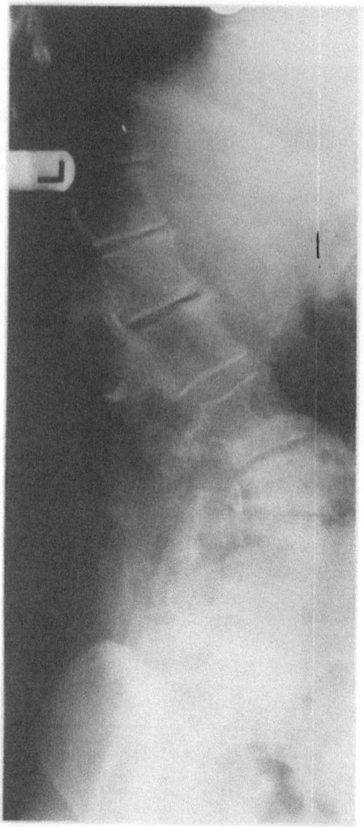

E

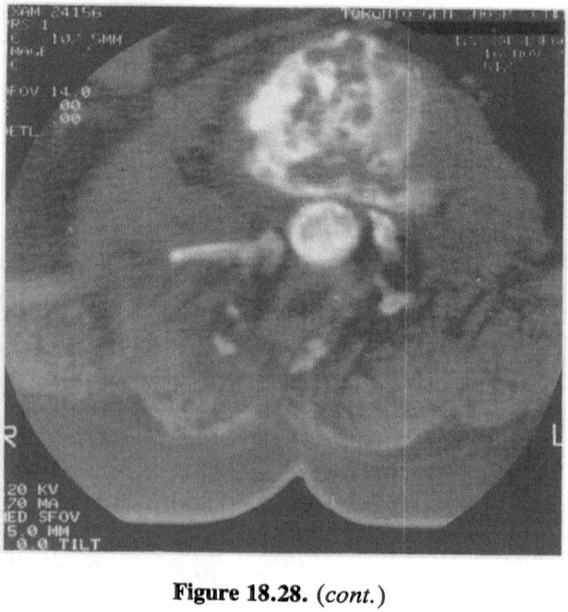

Figure 18.28. (*cont.*)

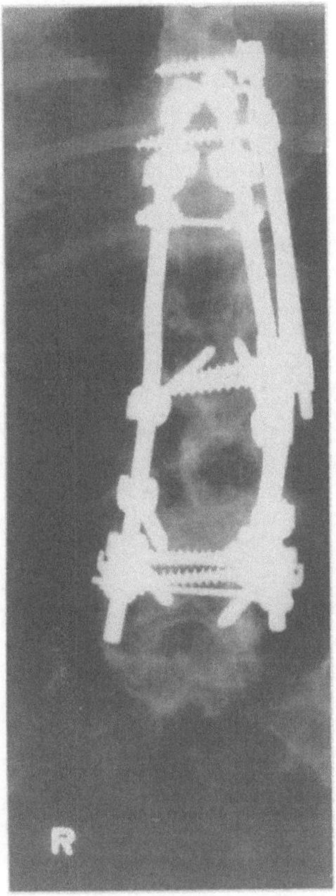

F

Figure 18.28. (*cont.*)

Regardless of the type of device used, it is important to obtain at least two points of fixation, proximal and distal to the pseudarthrosis, such that there are a total of eight points (Fig. 18.21). The inclusion of the sacrum also raises a number of technical difficulties. The main problems are screw orientation, and the number of screws that can be employed. In our experience, the use of single screws at each side of the sacrum is insufficient, although others have not had that concern (Fig. 18.29). In general, we try to introduce four screws, two on each side. The point for entry is usually at the base of the first sacral pedicle (Fig. 18.30). In the female access to the sacral promontory from this point of entry is not difficult, but in the narrow male pelvis, the challenge is greater. Thus in males, we have used a similar point of entry but have directed the screw to the thickest part of the ala, aiming distally and laterally at about 30°. A second screw is then introduced into the second sacral pedicle, going directly laterally (Fig. 18.31). Because of the close proximity of the sac-

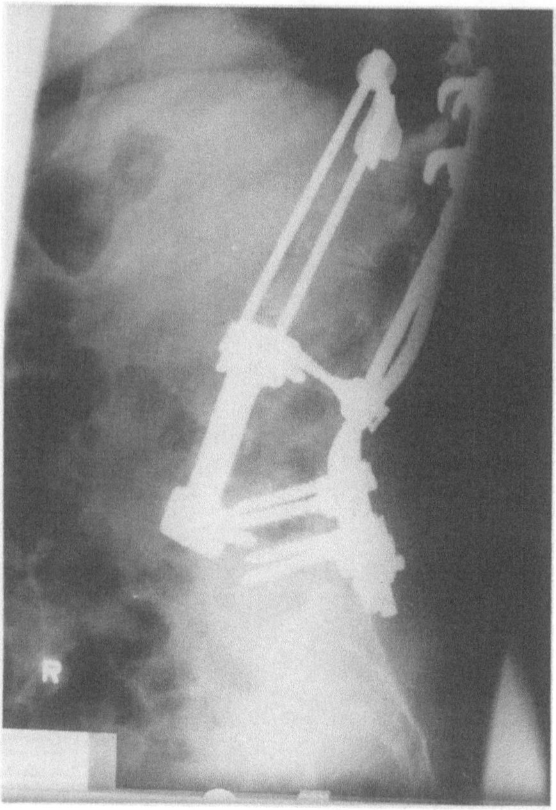

G

Figure 18.28. (*cont.*)

rim to the overlying skin, the use of a bulky fixation device should, if at all possible, be avoided.

More recently, particularly with the Cotrel-Dubousset form of instrumentation, introduction of two screws both at the base of the first sacral pedicle has resulted in more easy alignment and introduction of the device rod. The first screw is angled into the promontory and the second laterally directed into the ala.

Posterior Decortication. In the presence of a preexisting pseudarthrosis, or when a new laminectomy is required that involves the old fusion, a wide exposure is necessary. Although most pseudarthroses are at right angles to the longitudinal axis of the spine, this is not always the case, and the defect may not be easily identifiable. All too frequently, an exploratory operation fails to identify the pseudarthrosis, even when it was suspected preoperatively. As already note one cause is termed a "plate pseudarthrosis," where the bone graft has consolidated into a solid plate

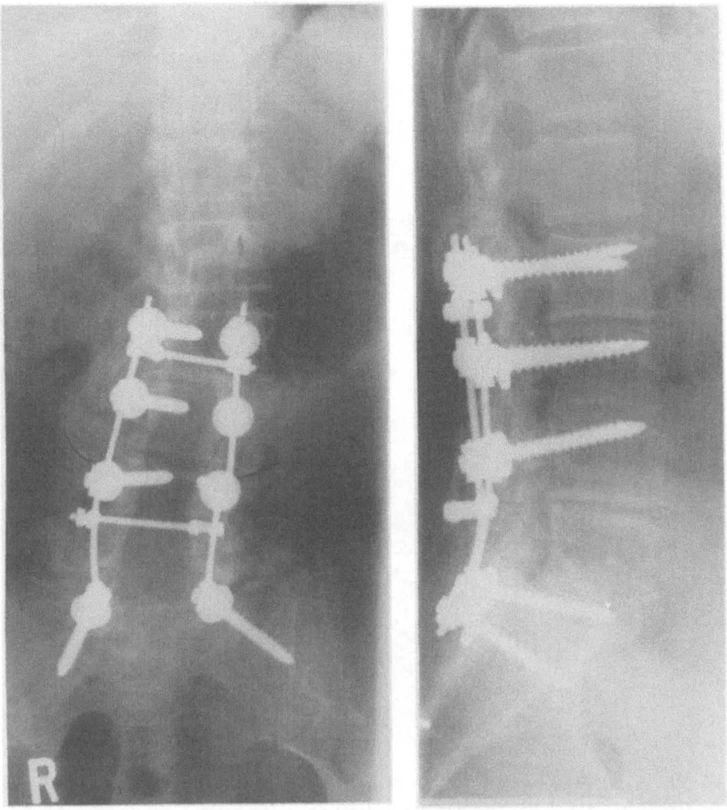

A B

Figure 18.29. A,B: A 63-year-old woman underwent four-level decompression fusion and Zielke instrumentation for severe spinal stenosis 4.5 years previously. Only one screw was used on each side of the sacrum at S1 directed into the arch. She developed pseudarthrosis.

of bone, which has not adhered to the underlying lamina or transverse processes. Failure to recognize this condition is usually due to inadequate preoperative imaging, including lateral, AP, and axial tomograms, and also including three-dimensional reconstructions.

Sources of Bone Graft. Although it is tempting to use local bone graft obtained from the old fusion, we feel in most cases it is important to supplement the fusion with autogenous graft. Usually sufficient bone can be harvested from one or the other iliac crest, or both. An alternative is to obtain anterior iliac crest graft, before starting the posterior approach.

When the approach is again anterior, the decision as to the bone graft source is somewhat more debatable. Although autogenous bone is preferable, allograft may help in this situation.

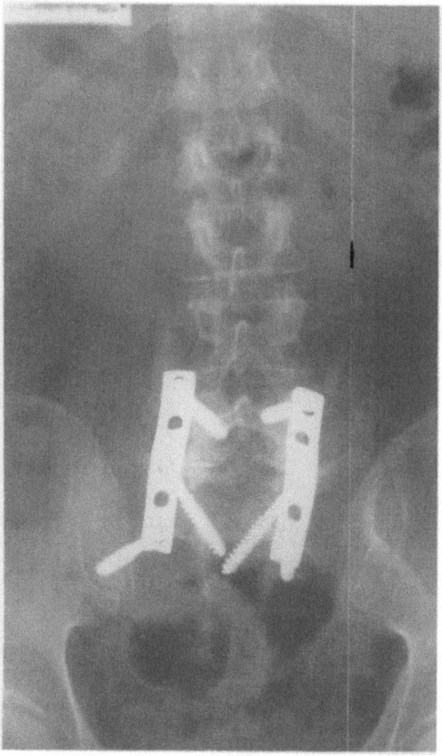

A

Figure 18.30. A,B: A 42-year-old woman underwent decompression, fusion and AO plate fixation at L4-S1 for spondylolisthesis. The S1 screws are directed toward the promontory; the S2 screws appear to penetrate too far anteriorly but are really in the ala of the sacrum.

Management of Osteoporosis. This situation presents a number of major challenges. First, the radiographic determination of fusion after a primary intervention is often difficult. Second, fixation devices may be more difficult to apply. As previously noted, we do not advocate the use of methylmethacrylate in the pedicles, with the exception of the first sacral pedicle. However, methylmethacrylate can be injected into the vertebral body to enhance fixation, with minimal risk.

Let us now consider the technical issues in the anterior approach to refusion.

Fixation Devices. The role of anterior fixation remains more controversial, particularly because of the increased inherent risks of the procedure, and in general, the less biomechanically favorable devices.

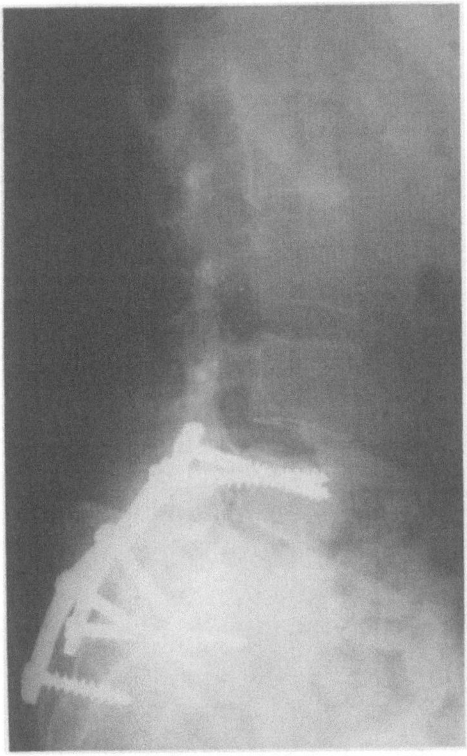

B

Figure 18.30. (*cont.*)

Approaches. For a single simple approach to L5-S1 a transverse suprapubic incision may be used, and is cosmetically more acceptable. A transperitoneal or retroperitoneal approach can then be developed. We prefer the retroperitoneal approach because the bowel contents are well contained, and retraction is easier.

For a two-level approach, a left paramedian incision, and retroperitoneal approach is utilized. If fixation devices are affixed to the sacrum, and pass beneath the left common iliac system (Fig. 18.32), we prefer to lay down a thin sheet of silicone rubber. This prevents direct adherence of the vessels to the scar, and if later surgery is required, the dissection is facilitated.

For approaches to three levels or more, we prefer a flank approach, but when the fusion is to be extended to the sacrum, the bed of the 12th rib is used. Incision is carried to the rectus sheath, which is then split, and the incision carried down as a paramedian incision, followed by a retroperitoneal approach.

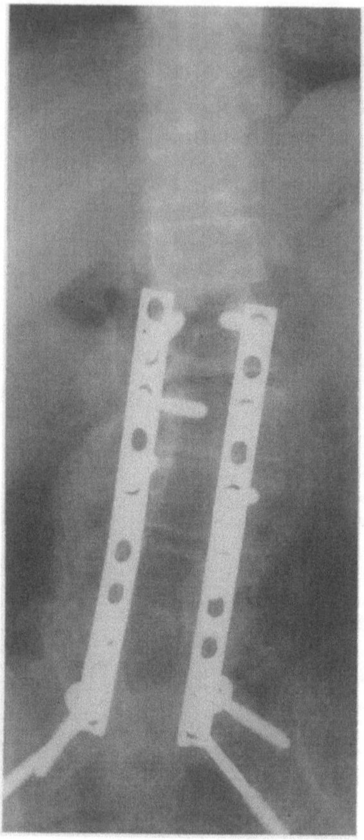

Figure 18.31. In the male patient the sacral screws are directed laterally into the thickest part of the ala of the sacrum penetrating both cortices in over 300 cases. We have had no vascular problems. This patient has had two previous procedures and required repeat and proximal decompression to L1, with stabilization. His result was satisfactory.

In all patients rehabilitation of the abdominal musculature is necessary, but in the elderly patient, this may be difficult. Not uncommonly, an incisional hernia is the consequence.

Surgical Results of Repeat Fusion

As noted previously, the results of a second operation are less predictable. In a simple group of patients treated for pseudarthrosis, where the previous surgery was simple posterior fusion, a success rate of only 60% was obtained, often despite a subsequent solid arthrodesis (23). This analytic problem becomes even more difficult when the published series are

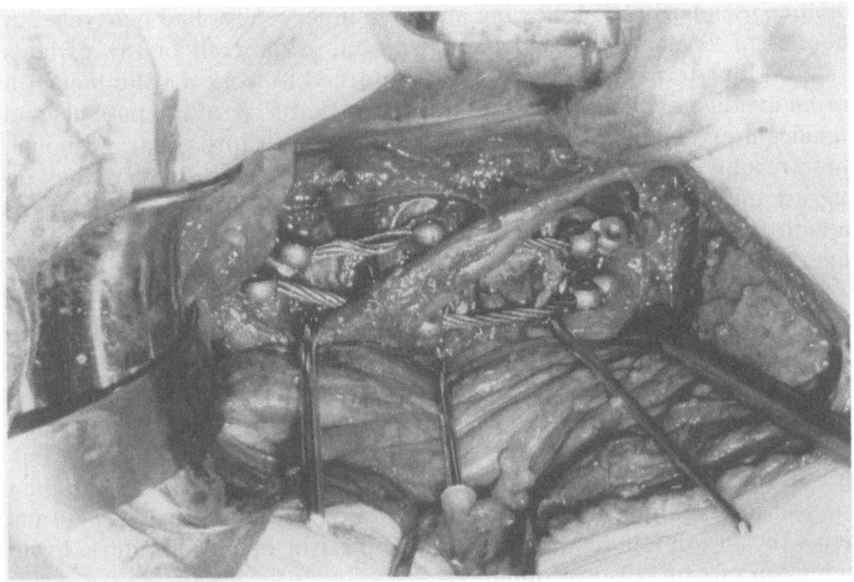

Figure 18.32. The left common iliac vessels have been dissected out. In this example Dwyer cables go from L4-L5 to S1 passing beneath the vessels. The screws pass anterior to posterior. The vessels have been modified by tying off and sectioning the iliolumbar vessels.

a mixed population with respect to original pathology, when numerous sources of failures are included, and when a variety of surgical techniques have been used. However, a number of studies are instructional, and give some broad indication of the results that can be achieved.

The first lesson is that patients properly selected can achieve reasonable, but by no means perfect, results, even when the problems are complex. The author (60) has treated 35 patients with fusion and sublaminar wiring. All the 35 patients had been off work for an average of 9 years since their last operation. Thirteen returned to work. Satisfactory results were obtained in an additional nine patients who had significant decrease in pain, but did not return to work. Pain persisted in 13 patients despite a solid arthrodesis being achieved. A subsequent clinical series was performed between 1984 and 1988 (58,59) and involved 246 patients treated by a variety of posterior pedicle fixation. At 2 years, the pseudarthrosis rate was 8%. During the same period, 51 patients underwent anterior salvage surgery with fusion and instrumentation. The most instructive part of this series was the 38 patients who were treated by anterior salvage surgery for a posterior pseudarthrosis, while an additional group included six patients with degenerative disease above or below the previous fusion. The incidence of pseudarthrosis was 9%. Of those who had developed yet another pseudarthrosis following anterior surgery, 50% had pain relief at more than 2 years following the operation. Almost all of the patients were on long-term disability, yet 43% returned to work despite being off for an average of 4 years. Also of interest is that 57% of the patients had significant psychological problems, yet had a satisfactory result. Although these results do not compare to those of primary spine surgery, they do suggest there are a group of patients who can benefit. The challenge is how to further the selection technique and surgical approach to improve upon these results.

Other series, in general, give somewhat similar results with respect to the later incidence of pseudarthrosis following refusion. Fujimaki et al. (39) reported on 38 salvage cases treated by anterior interbody fusion without instrumentation. Only one pseudarthrosis occurred.

Thalgott et al. (112) reported on the use of AO (Swiss) dynamic compression plates (DCP) for internal fixation in 31 patients with prior failures of fusion; 17 of these 31 had failed interbody fusions. Following their surgical intervention, a pseudarthrosis rate of 24% was noted. In 14 patients the fusion failure was for a prior posterior operation, and a lower nonunion rate of 14% was obtained.

Zuckerman et al. (125) have used the Steffee system, but their failures included a variety of patients who had not been subjected to previous fusion. Of note was their high rate of screw breakage and infection.

Alternative Nonsurgical Treatment

As noted earlier in this chapter, an alternative for many patients is a vigorous rehabilitation program, particularly in the postoperative course, when the fusion is deemed solid. Additional therapy that may be considered is the use of electrical stimulation in patients with pseudarthrosis. This technique was first proposed by Dwyer (26) and has been used by Kane (56), in a controlled study of both primary fusion and repair of pseudarthrosis. A large amount of basic research has been done in the peripheral skeleton, as has some experimental work in animals. Kahanovitz and Arnoczky (55) have suggested electrical stimulation enhances bone formation. In primary fusion, Kane (56) has observed a rate of fusion of 91.5%. The comparison group achieved success in 81%. In secondary fusions, less certain data is available, but Kane recommends the procedure be accompanied by bone grafting. In a randomized prospective study of "difficult" patients, 15 of 28 controls (54%) achieved fusion compared with 25 of 31 stimulated controls (81%) who gained solid arthrodesis.

As an alternative, the use of pulsating electromagnetic coils, applied externally, has been advocated by Simmons (104). In a preliminary study, 13 patients with failures of posterior interbody fusion were analyzed, 10 of whom showed increased bone formation, and 77% of whom went on to solid arthrodesis. His results have not been replicated by Brodsky and Kahlic (7), who demonstrated only a 36% success rate in patients with posterior fusion and pseudarthrosis.

References

1. Baker AS, Ojemann RG, Swartz MN, Richardson EP Jr. Spinal epidural abscess. *N Engl J Med*. 1975;293:463–468.
2. Beals RK, Hickman NW. Industrial injuries of the back and extremities: Comprehensive evaluation—an aid in prognosis and management; a study of one hundred and eighty patients. *J Bone Joint Surg*. 1972;54A:1593–1611.
3. Blasier RD, Munson RC. Acquired spondylolysis after postero-lateral spinal fusion. *J Pediatr Orthop*. 1987;7:215–217.
4. Bosworth DM. Repair of hernia through iliac-crest defects. *J Bone Joint Surg*. 1955;37A:1071.
5. Brodsky AE. Post-laminectomy and post-fusion stenosis of the lumbar spine. *Clin Orthop*. 1976;115–130.
6. Brodsky AE, Hendricks FL, Khalil MA, Darden BV, Brotzman TT. Segmental ("floating") lumbar spine fusions. *Spine*. 1989;14:447–450.
7. Brodsky AE, Kahlic MA. Efficacy of electrical bone growth stimulation among 97 patients with pseudarthrosis of the lumbar spine. Presentation pre-annual North American Spine Society Meeting, Colorado Springs, June 1988.
8. Brunet JA, Wiley JJ. Acquired spondylolysis after spinal fusion. *J Bone Joint Surg*. 1984;66B:720–724.
9. Burton C. The role of spine fusion: Question 4. *Spine*. 1981;6:291.
10. Burton CV, Kirkaidy-Willis WH, Yong-Hing K, Heitoff KB. Causes of failure of surgery on the lumbar spine. *Clin. Orthop*. 1981;157:191–199.
11. Cleveland M, Bosworth DM, Thompson FR. Pseudarthrosis in the lumbosacral spine. *J Bone Joint Surg*. 1948;30A:302–312.
12. Cloward RB. The treatment of ruptured lumbar intervertebral discs by vertebral body fusion: Indications. Operative technique, after-care. *J Neurosurg*. 1953;10:154–168.
13. Cochran T, Irstam L, Nachemson A. Long-term anatomic and functional changes in patients with adolescent idiopathic scoliosis treated by Harrington rod fusion. *Spine*. 1983;8:576–584.
14. Collis JS. Total disc replacement: A modified posterior lumbar interbody fusion. Report of 750 cases. *Clin Orthop*. 1985;193:640–667.
15. Cotler JM, Star AM. Complications of spinal fusions. In: Cotler JM, Cotler HB, eds. *Spinal Fusion, Science and Technique*. New York: Springer-Verlag; 1990.
16. Crock HV. A reappraisal of intervertebral disc lesions. *Med J Aust*. 1970;1:983–989.
17. Crock HV. Observations on the management of failed spinal operations. *J Bone Joint Surg*. 1976;58B:193–199.
18. Crock HV. Internal disc disruption: A challenge to disc prolapse fifty years on. *Spine*. 1986;11:650–653.

19. Dawson EG, Clader TJ, Bassett LW. A comparison of different methods used to diagnose pseudarthrosis following posterior spinal fusion for scoliosis. *J Bone Joint Surg*. 1985;67A:1153–1159.
20. DePalma A, Rothman R. The nature of pseudarthrosis. *Clin Orthop*. 1968;59:113–118.
21. Dewar FP. Circumferential fusion for degenerative disc disease. Toronto, Unpublished data, 1963.
22. Deyo RA. Reducing work absenteeism and diagnostic costs for backache. In: Hadler NM, ed. *Clinical Concepts in Regional Musculoskeletal Illness*. Orlando: Grune & Stratton; 1987:25–50.
23. Deyo RA, Diehl AK, Rosenthal M. How many days of bedrest for acute low back pain? A randomized clinical trial. *N Engl J Med*. 1986;315:1064–1070.
24. Drury BJ. Clinical evaluation of back and leg pain due to irritation of the superior cluneal nerve. *J Bone Joint Surg*. 1967;49A:199.
25. Dvorak J, Valach L, Fuhrimann P, Heim E. The outcome of surgery for lumbar disc herniation. II. A 4-17 years follow-up with emphasis on psychosocial aspects. *Spine*. 1988;13:1423–1427.
26. Dwyer AF. Experience of anterior correction of scoliosis. *Clin Orthop*. 1973;93:191–206.
27. Esses SI, Botsford DJ, Kostuik JP. The role of external spinal skeletal fixation in the assessment of low-back disorders. *Spine*. 1989;14(6):594–601.
28. Fairbank JC, Park WM, McCall IW, et al. Apophysial injection of local anaesthetic as a diagnostic aid in primary low-back pain syndromes. *Spine*. 1981;6:598–605.
29. Finnegan W, Fenlin JM, Marvel JP, Nardini RJ, Rothman RH. Results of surgical intervention in the symptomatic multiple-operated back patient. Analysis of 67 cases followed for 3-7 years. *J Bone Joint Surg*. 1979;61A:1077–1082.
30. Fogelberg RB, Zittmann EK, Stinchfield FE. Prophylactic penicillin in orthopaedic surgery. *J Bone Joint Surg*. 1970;52A:95–98.
31. Fraser RD, Osti OL, Vernon-Roberts B: Discitis following chemonucleolysis; An experimental study. *Spine*. 1986;1:679-687.
32. Freebody D, Bendall R, Taylor RD. Anterior transperitoneal lumbar fusion. *J Bone Joint Surg*. 1971;53B:617–627.
33. Frymoyer JW. The role of spine fusion. Question 3. *Spine*. 1981;6:284–290.
34. Frymoyer JW. Back pain and sciatica. *N Engl J Med*. 1988;318:291–300.
35. Frymoyer JW, Hanley E, Howe J, Kuhlmann D, Matteri R. Disc excision and spine fusion in the management of lumbar disc disease; a minimum ten-year follow-up. *Spine*. 1978;3:1–6.
36. Frymoyer JW, Hanley EN, Howe J, Kuhlmann D, Matteri RE. A comparison of radiographic findings in fusion and nonfusion patients ten or more years following lumbar disc surgery. *Spine*. 1979;4:435–440.
37. Frymoyer JW, Howe J, Kuhlmann D. The long-term effects of spinal fusion on the sacroiliac joints and ilium. *Clin Orthop*. 1978;134:196.
38. Frymoyer JW, Matteri RE, Hanley EN, Kuhlmann D, Howe J. Failed lumbar disc surgery requiring second operation. A long term follow-up study. *Spine*. 1978;3:7–11.
39. Fujimaki A, Crock HV, Bedbrook GM. The results of 150 anterior lumbar

interbody fusion operations performed by two surgeons in Australia. *Clin Orthop*. 1982;165:164–167.

40. Gurdjian ES, Webster JE, Ostrowski AZ, et al. Herniated lumbar intervertebral discs—An analysis of 1176 operated cases. *J Trauma*. 1961;1:158–176.
41. Guyer DW, Wiltse LL, Eskay ML, Guyer BH. The long-range prognosis of archnoiditis. *Spine*. 1989;14(12):1321–1341.
42. Hadler NM. Regional back pain (editorial). *N Engl J Med*. 1986;315:1090–1092.
43. Hakelius A. Prognosis in sciatica. A clinical follow-up of surgical and nonsurgical treatment. *Acta Orthop Scand Suppl*. 1970;129:1–76.
44. Hanley EN Jr, Shapiro DE. The development of low-back pain after excision of a lumbar disc. *J Bone Joint Surg*. 1989;71:719–721.
45. Harris RI, Wiley JJ. Acquired spondylosysis as a sequel to spine fusion. *J Bone Joint Surg*. 1963;45A:1159–1170.
46. Hayes MA, et al. Clinical and radiological evaluation of lumbosacral motion below fusion levels in idiopathic scoliosis. *Spine*. 1988;10:1161–1167.
47. Hirsch C, Nachemson A. The reliability of lumbar disk surgery. *Clin Orthop*. 1963;29:189–194.
48. Howe J, Frymoyer JW. The effects of questionnaire design on the determination of end results in lumbar spinal surgery. *Spine*. 1985;10:804–805.
49. Hoyland JA, Freemont AJ, Denton J, Thomas AM, McMillan JJ, Jayson MIV. Retained surgical swab debris in post-laminectomy arachnoiditis and peridural fibrosis. *J Bone Joint Surg*. 1988;70B:659–662.
50. Hsu KY, Zucherman J, White A, Wynne G, Reynolds J, Goldthwaite N, Schofferman J. Deterioration of motion segments adjacent to lumbar fusion. Proceedings of the North American Spine Society Annual Mtg, Colorado Springs, Colorado, 1988.
51. Jacobs RR, Montesano PX, Jackson RP. Enhancement of lumbar spine fusion by use of translaminar facet joint screws. *Spine*. 1989;14:12–15.
52. Johnsson KE, Redlund-Johnell I, Uden A, Willner S. Preoperative and postoperative instability in lumbar spinal stenosis. *Spine*. 1989;14:591–593.
53. Jones AA, Stambough JL, Balderston RA, Rothman RH, Booth RE Jr. Long-term results of lumbar spine surgery complicated by unintended incidental durotomy. *Spine*. 1989;14:443–446.
54. Jones JB. The training of orthopaedic surgery residents in lumbar disc surgery. *Clin Orthop*. 1971;81:88–92.
55. Kahanovitz N, Arnoczky SP. The efficacy of direct current electrical stimulation to enhance canine spinal fusions. *Clin Orthop. Rel Res*. 1990;251:295–299.
56. Kane WJ. Direct current electrical bone stimulation for spinal fusion. *Spine*. 1988;13:763.
57. Kornberg M. Discography and magnetic resonance imaging in the diagnosis of lumbar disc disruption. *Spine*. 1989;12:1368–1369.
58. Kostuik JP, Carl A, Ferron S. Anterior interbody fusion and instrumentation for lumbar degenerative disc disease. Unpublished data, 1986.
59. Kostuik JP, Carl A, Ferron S, Dowling T, Errico T, Abbitbol JJ. Results of instrumentation and fusion for salvage surgery in degenerative disc disease. Canadian Orthopaedic Association, Vancouver, 1990.

60. Kostuik JP, Errico T. Luque instrumentation in degenerative conditions of the lumbar spine. *Spine*. 1990;15(4):318–321.
61. Kostuik JP, Hall BB. Spinal fusions to the sacrum in adults with scoliosis. *Spine*. 1983;8:489–500.
62. Krempen JF, Smith BS. Nerve root injection: A method for evaluating the etiology of sciatica. *J Bone Joint Surg*. 1974;56A:1435–1444.
63. Kurz LT, Garfin SR, Booth RE. Harvesting autogenous iliac bone grafts. A review of complications and techniques. *Spine*. 1989;14:1324–1331.
64. Laasonen EM, Soini J. Low-back pain after lumbar fusion: Surgical and computed tomographic analysis. *Spine*. 1989;14:210–231.
65. Lee CK, Lagranda NA. Lumbosacral spinal fusion: A biomechanical study. *Spine*. 1984;9:574–581.
66. Lehmann TR, Spratt KF, Tozzi JE. Long-term follow-up of lower lumbar fusion patients. *Spine*. 1987;12:97–104.
67. Liang M, Kormaroff AL. Roentgenograms in primary care patients with acute low back pain; A cost-effectiveness analysis. *Arch Intern Med*. 1982;142:1108–1112.
68. Lin PM. PLIF complications and pitfalls. *Clin Orthop*. 1985;193:90–102.
69. Lin PM. Technique and complications of posterior lumbar interbody fusion. In: *Lumbar Interbody Fusion, Principles and Techniques in Spine Surgery*. Linn PM, Gill K, eds. Rockville, MD: Aspen Press; 1989.
70. Long DM, Filtzer DL, BenDebba M, Hendler NH: Clinical features of the failed-back syndrome. *J Neurosurg*. 1988;69:61–71.
71. Lonstein J, Winter R, Moe J, Gaines D. Wound infection with Harrington instrumentation and spine fusion for scoliosis. *Clin Orthop*. 1973;96:222.
72. Love JG, Rivers MH. Spinal cord tumors simulating protruded intervertebral discs. *JAMA*. 1962;179:878–881.
73. Luk KD, et al. The effect on the lumbosacral spine of long spinal fusion for idiopathic scoliosis. A minimum 10 year follow-up. *Spine*. 1987;12:996–1000.
74. Macdonald G, Pennel G. Lumbar spine fusion. Presented at the Workman's Compensation Course, Toronto, 1966.
75. Macnab I. Negative disc exploration: An analysis of the causes of nerve-root involvement in 68 patients. *J Bone Joint Surg*. 1971;53A:891–903.
76. Macnab I, Dali D. The blood supply of the lumbar spine and its application to the technique of intertransverse lumbar fusion. *J Bone Joint Surg*. 1971;53B:628–638.
77. Malcolm B, Vaughan PA, Maistrelli G. The results of L4-5 disc excision alone versus disc excision and fusion. *Spine*. 1988;13:690–695.
78. Mayer TG, Gatchel RJ, Kishino N, Keeley J, Capra P, Mayer H, Barnett J, Mooney V. Objective assessment of spine function following industrial injury: A prospective study with comparison group and one-year follow-up. *Spine*. 1985;10:482–493.
79. McKenzie RA. *The Lumbar Spine, Mechanical Diagnosis and Therapy*. New Zealand: Spinal Publications; 1981.
80. Michel CR, LaLain JJ. Late result of Harrington's operation. Long-term evolution of the lumbar spine below the fused segments. *Spine*. 1985;10:414–420.
81. Miller PR, Elder FW Jr. Meningeal pseudocysts (meningocci Spurtus) following laminectomy. *J Bone Joint Surg*. [*Am*]. 1968;50P:268–276.

82. Mooney V. The failed back—an orthopaedic view. *Int Disabil Stud.* 1988;10:32–36.
83. Mooney V, Cairns D, robertson J. A system for evaluating and treating chronic back disability. *West J Med.* 1976;124:370–376.
84. Nachemson A. Editorial comments: Lumbar discography—where are we today? *Spine.* 1989;14(6):555–557.
85. Nashold BA Jr, Blaine S, Hrubec A. *Lumbar disc disease: A twenty-year clinical follow-up study.* St. Louis: CV Mosby; 1971.
86. Naylor A. Late results of laminectomy for lumbar disc prolapse: A review after ten to twenty-five years. *J Bone Joint Surg.* 1974;56B:17–29.
87. Naylor A, Shentall RD, Micklethwaite B: An electron microscopic study of the segment long spacing collagen from the intervertebral disc. *Orthop Clin North Am.* 1977;8:217–223.
88. Nerubay J, Marganit B, Bubis JJ, Tadmor A, Katznelson A: Stimulation of bone formation by electrical current on spinal fusion. *Spine.* 1986;11:167–169.
89. Norton WL. Chemonucleolysis versus surgical discectomy: Comparison of costs and results in workers compensation claimants. *Spine.* 1987;11:440–443.
90. O'Brien JP, Dawson MH, Heard CW, Momberger B, Speck G. Simultaneous combined anterior and posterior fusion. A solution for failed spinal surgery with a brief review of first 150 patients. *Clin Orthop.* 1986;203:191–195.
91. O'Connell JEA. Protrusions of the lumbar intervertebral discs. A clinical review based on five hundred cases treated by excision of the protrusion. *J Bone Joint Surg.* 1951;338:8–30.
92. Olerud S, Hamberg M. External fixation as a test for instability after spinal fusion L4-S1. A case report. *Orthopaedics.* 1986;9(4):547–549.
93. Olerud S, Sjostrom L, Karlstrom G, Hamberg M. Spontaneous effect of increased stability of the lower lumbar spine in cases of severe chronic back pain: The answer of an external transpeduncular fixation test. *Clin Orthop.* 1986;203:67–74.
94. Phytinen J, Lahde S, Tanska EL, Laitinen J: Computed tomography after lumbar myelography in lower back and extremity pain syndromes. *Diagn Imag.* 1983;52:1922.
95. Pilgaard S. Discitis (closed space infection) following removal of lumbar intervertebral disc. *J Bone Joint Surg.* 1969;51A:713–716.
96. Prothero SR, Parkes JC, Stinchfield EE. Complications of low-back fusion in 1000 patients. *J Bone Joint Surg.* 1966;48A:57–65.
97. Quinnell RC, Stockdale HR. Some experimental observations on the influence of a single lumbar floating fusion on the remaining lumbar spine. *Spine.* 1981;6:263–267.
98. Raugstad TS, Harbo K, Hogberg A, Skeie S. Anterior interbody fusion of the lumbar spine. *Acta Orthop Scand.* 1982;53:561–565.
99. Rolander SD. Motion of the lumbar spine with special reference to the stability effect of posterior fusion. *Acta Orthop Scand Suppl.* 1966;90:1–143.
100. Rombold C. Spondylolysis: A complication of spine fusion. *J Bond Joint Surg.* 1965;47AM:1237–1242.
101. Sage FP. Post-operative fracture in the lumbar facets following lumbar disc surgery. *J Bone Joint Surg.* 1975;57A:1173.

102. Schofferman L, Schofferman J, Zucherman J, Gunthorpe H, Hsu K, Picetti G, Goldthwaite N, White A. Occult infections causing persistent low-back pain. *Spine*. 1989;14:417–419.
103. Schonstrom N. The narrow lumbar spinal canal and the size of the cauda equina in man. Department of Orthopaedics, Gothenburg University, Sahigren Hospital, Goteborg, Sweden.
104. Simmons JW. Treatment of failed posterior lumbar interbody fusion on the spine with pulsing electromagnetic fields. *Clin Orthop*. 1985;193:127–132.
105. Smith SE, DeLee JC, Rammamurthy S. Ilioinguinal neuralgia following iliac bone-grafting. Report of two cases and review of the literature. *J Bone Joint Surg*. 1984;66A:1306–1308.
106. Spangfort EV. The lumbar disc herniation: A computer-aided analysis of 2,504 operations. *Acta Orthop Scand Suppl*. 1972;142:1–95.
107. Spengler DM. Lumbar discectomy: Results with limited disc excision and selective foraminotomy. *Spine*. 1982;7:604–706.
108. Spengler DM, Freeman C, Westbrook R, Miller JW: Low back pain following multiple lumbar spine procedures. Failure of initial selection. *Spine*. 1980;5:356–360.
109. Stokes IA, Counts DF, Frymoyer JW. Experimental instability in the rabbit lumbar spine. *Spine*. 1989;14:68–72.
110. Stokes IAF, Wilder DG, Frymoyer JW, Pope MH. Assessment of patients with low back pain by biplanar radiographic measurement of intervertebral motion. *Spine*. 1981;6:233–239.
111. Terry A, McCall IW, O'Brien JP, Park WM. Graft impingement following posterolateral fusion. Proceedings of the International Society for the study of the lumbar spine, 1981.
112. Thalgott JS, LaRocca H, Aebi M, Dwyer AP, Razza BE. Reconstruction of the lumbar spine using AO DCP plate fixation. *Spine*. 1980;14:91–95.
113. Unander-Scharin L. Case of spondylolisthesis lumbalis acquisita. *Acta Orthop Scand*. 1950;19:536–544.
114. van Akkerveeken PF. Lateral stenosis of the lumbar spine. Libertas Drukwerkservice by, Utrecht, The Netherlands, 1989.
115. Waddell G, McCulloch JA, Kummel E, Venner RM. Non-organic physical signs in low-back pain. *Spine*. 1980;5:117–125.
116. Walsh TR, Weinstein JN, Spratt KF, Lehmann TR, Aprill CN, Sayre H, Found E. Lumbar discography: A controlled prospective study of normal volunteers to determine the false-positive rate. Presented to the International Society for the Study of the Lumbar Spine.
117. Watkins RG. Summary of etiologies of postlaminectomy syndrome. In: Watkins RG, Collis JS, eds. *Lumbar Discectomy and Laminectomy*. Rockville, MD: Aspen Publishers; 1987;267–269.
118. Weatherley CR, et al. Discogenic pain persisting despite solid posterior fusion. *J Bone Joint Surg*. 1986;38B:143.
119. Weber H. Lumbar disc herniation. A controlled, prospective study with ten years of observation. *Spine*. 1983;8:131–140.
120. Weikel AM, Habal MB. Meralgia paresthetica: A complication of iliac bone procurement. *Plast Reconstr Surg*. 1977;60:572–574.
121. Weinstein JN, Spratt KF, Spengler D, Crick C. Spinal pedicle fixation: re-

liability and validity of roentgenogram based assessment and surgical factors on successful screw placement. *Spine*. 1988;13:1012–1018.

122. Weisel SW. The multiply operated lumbar spine. *Instr. Course Lect.* 1985;34:68–77.
123. Wiesel SV, Feffer HL, Borenstein DG. Evaluation and outcome of low-back pain of unknown etiology. *Spine*. 1988;13:679–680.
124. Yang SW, Langrana NA, Lee CK. Biomechanics of lumbosacral spinal fusion in combined compression-torsion loads. *Spine*. 1986;11:937–941.
125. Zuckerman J, Hsu K, White A, Wynne G. Early results of spinal fusion using variable spine plating system. *Spine*. 1988;13:570–579.

Discussion

Method of Application of Methylmethacrylate

Dr. McCormick inquired as to the method of application of methylmethacrylate? Dr. Kostuik replied: Anteriorly we drill a hole or use an awl to start a hole. I then take a curet, enlarge the hole, and then if you have only one or two holes just take ordinary methylmethacrylate, put it in a 20-cc syringe, drill the end of the syringe open to accommodate a 3.2–drill point, and inject directly into the hole. Finally, impact the acrylic with your finger. I try to use methylmethacrylate without barium to show a better postoperative picture. The methylmethacrylate we use is in semiliquid form and it is cold. That should be fine for one or two holes. If there are more holes and you want to cut down on your costs, you do not want to keep going back to use more packages, then simply take it out of the refrigerator; it works quite well. It may take a bit longer to settle, but that should not be a problem.

Screws and Plates

Our screw heads are flat. We try to avoid putting any screw underneath the vessels, in the event that they back up. The screw heads we use have a cold well and they are very, very tight. The last five or six turns require a great deal of force. The outer diameter of the shank of the screw is wider than the outer diameter of the thread so that it abuts against the plate in a very tight fit. We have not had much of a problem with these.

Fat Grafts to the Epidural Space

Dr. Rydevik asked about the possible risks of fat grafts. I have heard of instances of cauda equina syndrome associated with their use. Dr. Kostuik said: I believe those have been instances where surgeons have tried to put fat back into the disc space or way around the front of the thecal sac. That may also be associated with epidural bleeding. In some cases the use of fat grafts does prevent hematoma expansion externally. Dr. Sonntag said: In some cases following laminectomy for lumbar spinal stenosis surgeons have used extensive fat grafts over the dorsal surface of the dura. I am not anti–fat graft, but I think it has only minimal use in a microdiscectomy procedure. Dr. Kostuik agreed and said that in reoperations on people who were said to have fat grafts he often only saw a few globules. Prof. Louis emphasized that he does not use fat grafts.

CHAPTER 19

Revision Surgery in Late Spine Instability, Including Sacral Stabilization

Jean-Pierre C. Farcy

The Concept of Spine Stability

Introducing the concept of spine stability offers the challenge to deal with two mechanical requirements that seem to be opposed: rigidity and plasticity.

As a matter of comparison, the single part of a ship that is a rigid beam is the mast of the ship. The mast supports the sails and carries all the strain. However, there is plasticity, provided by the stays that are symmetrically installed on the hull. Connective tissues, ligaments, and muscles can be compared to the complex system of stays, distributed evenly on each side to provide equilibrium and alignment. The cervical spine is the mast of a sailboat, the hull of which is represented by the scapular girdle, and the thoracolumbar spine is the mast of a second sailboat, the hull of which is the pelvis.

As compared to a mast, the spine is a construct made of rigid elements bound one to the other by discs and ligaments (23). The stays are represented by the muscles, which adapt automatically to maintain equilibrium by active contraction under the control of the extrapyramidal system. To meet the challenges of being mobile and carrying heavy loads, the spine is composed of bony elements. The shape of these elements differs in order to form a construct that provides constant protection to the nervous system as well as a flexible, solid axis for the body.

The spine, straight in the frontal plane, is curved in the sagittal plane, where there are four opposed curvatures. One balances the other to increase the strength of the spine when axial loads are applied. Any injury that causes disruption of bones, discs, or ligaments can result in drastic changes of contour, disrupting the alignment of the spine; a further result can be decreased diameter of the spinal canal. Any variation of the inside diameter of the spinal canal will subsequently create compression of the neural elements inside the spinal canal. Spine instability is defined by White et al. (37) as follows: "Clinical instability is the loss of the ability of the spinal elements to maintain a relationship between the vertebral segments under physiologic loads."

Instability results from acute or progressive disruption of one or more of the essential elements. Acute instability caused by fractures became a concern after World War II. In 1949, Nicoll classified thoracolumbar injuries into stable and unstable. Since then, Whitesides has raised the issue of spontaneous healing of fractures and expressed concern about residual instability. A multicolumn concept has been described by Rene Louis in France, and Dennis (8) recently offered a simplified classification of unstable fractures.

However, stability as addressed by all of these authors is related to the biomechanics of the spine, and this very theoretical picture really does not take into account the potential healing of the different elements involved in spine stability. The bone, when restored to its anatomic shape, is extremely well supplied by blood and generally heals pretty well. Bone healing is definitely more constant as one progresses cranially along the vertebral column.

When a vertebral body has been submitted to a combination of hyperflexion and axial loading, as happens in high-velocity injuries, the vertebral body "bursts." The cancellous bone is blasted away by the intrusion of disc material through the end plate (15), and the remaining vertebral body is like a crushed egg shell (13,19). When appropriate reduction has been obtained and anatomic contours restored, the vertebral body no longer contains the cancellous bone stock necessary for good bone healing. A clear understanding of this reality has modified the indications for burst fracture treatment.

Ligaments have poor healing potential (33) and, when healing occurs, fibrous and scar tissues replace the original, ligamentous tissues. The fibrous tissue is more bulky, offers less strength, and has very poor elastic qualities. The spinal disc, when transected, has no tendency to heal; rather, it degenerates.

More often, real instability appears insidiously, and is responsible for progressive development of undesired movement. Initially, the undesired movement is microscopic, but it increases progressively, and deformity develops or gets worse. The nerves are compressed progressively or damaged by repeated, small injuries and repeated impingement.

It is extremely difficult to obtain documentation of this type of instability. Only repeated, careful clinical evaluation can appreciate the development of symptoms and loss of function. Late instability is always a clinical instability; this diagnosis must be made according to clinical criteria.

Instability in the Cervical Spine

Among the anterior structures of the cervical spine, the annulus fibrosus of the disc represents the most important structure (1). Since the cervical spine facets are almost horizontal, the bonds provided by the discs between the vertebrae are more crucial. Part of this stability is provided by the posterior longitudinal ligament and the capsules of the facet joints, which are responsible for rotational stability. The cervical spine construct depends upon the systems of ligaments and discs for its extreme mobility as well as its stability (33,37). Ligament disruption in the cervical segments is part of all injuries and, since ligament integrity is not easy to evaluate, stress x-rays must be performed after complete immobilization to assess stability before removing a Halo-Vest or other, similar immobilization device.

When this concept is recognized, it can be understood that the Chance-like fracture or flexion-distraction fracture/subluxation are both shear fractures, which can be seen undisplaced or reduced with an almost normal x-ray but, nevertheless, also can be the most unstable. Facet dislocations and facet fractures, unilateral or bilateral, are often associated with neurologic damage and are unstable. The burst fracture will present with retropulsed fragments compressing the cord in the canal. However, they are least unstable at the level of the cervical spine because most of the posterior column is intact.

The fracture-dislocation most often accompanied by major cord injury is unstable while acute. However, bony healing will take place and not often becomes late instability. Although cervical fractures have been, in general, treated with extra caution and immobilized in Halo-Vests for a long period of time or fixed internally with internal fixation and bone graft, they have a high percentage of bony healing and, therefore, have resulted in satisfactory stability at treatment's end.

At the opposite end of the spectrum, a multiple level laminectomy, with or without resection of the facets, may be responsible for instability. Fusion and immobilization after laminectomy have not been the rule in the past. The classical syndrome, called "swan neck," is the type of late instability that requires treatment (14).

The "swan neck" deformity is a kyphotic deformity of the cervical spine with 50% subluxation of the facet joints, cervical canal narrowing, and cord compression.

Unfortunately, when instability has reached the point of inducing long tract signs and cord compression, the element of myelopathy with cord atrophy is a hazardous factor that is introduced when correction of deformity and stabilization are contemplated. It is mandatory to avoid any attempt at distraction to correct the deformity. If tempted to correct the kyphosis, the surgeon must contemplate anterior distraction, since the posterior column is not compressible and there is no "give" at the level of the facets. The hazards of endangering an already atrophic cord are very high, with the most serious possible complication being tetraplegia. Conducted with utmost caution and under Halo-Vest protection, staged procedures with multiple level posterior releases can be followed by anterior releases, correction of deformity, and bone graft. Decompression is obtained by correcting the kyphotic deformity and does not require direct vision of the cord, or even entering the cervical canal (14).

The advantages are rapid healing and rare failure of fusion at the level of the cervical spine. But the technique is extremely demanding, and the risks of staged procedures are extremely high. The surgeon must explain to the patient that, even with the most successful outcome, it is unlikely that a dramatic improvement of neurologic function will be obtained. At best, a stabilization of function can be offered at the levels assessed preoperatively. For the patient, it is always extraordinarily frustrating to undergo multiple surgeries for this unique rationale: to prevent any progression of neurologic symptoms rather than to obtain substantial improvement. However, this reality must be addressed and developed before performing any corrective surgery on cervical instability.

The techniques described have been modified with the development of hardware for internal fixation. The less rigid wires have been replaced by a more rigid combination of Roy-Camille plates and/or rods, and anterior plates described by AO, Caspar, Senegas, and others are part of the armamentarium for achievement of immediate cervical spine fixation. Biomechanical studies were conducted with specimens; hardware was compared for the ability to provide the most rigid construct, and multiple test results were obtained by Coe et al. (6).

Nonetheless, there is no hardware that will sustain long-term stress and strain without breaking or loosening if bone healing does not take place within a "normal" period of time. Ultimate success is obtained only if the anatomic alignment is restored and, therefore, the load is evenly distributed.

Instability of the Thoracic Spine

In the thoracic spine, since each vertebra is connected on each side to a rib, which is an element of stability against the rotational moment, instability takes place in the sagittal plane rather than in the transverse plane. When the anterior column, composed of discs and bodies, is disrupted, deformity develops in kyphosis. A subsequent subluxation of the facet joints will facilitate an increase of the already physiologic kyphosis, creating more rapid development of sagittal deformity.

If the disc is involved in shear stress, as can happen after thoracic laminectomies, the disc will fail and degenerate, and multiple spondylolistheses will develop, with increased instability and cord compression. The compression will cause permanent cord damage, and progressive myelopathy will develop with cord atrophy. When this type of instability is encountered, no matter how obvious the compression appears to be, there is no way to achieve improvement other than to stabilize the spine by providing a solid fusion. Any attempt at decompression carries the hazard of disrupting the few tenuous connections inside the atrophic cord, thus precipitating a paraplegia. We feel that multiple laminectomies for decompression are not indicated. When necessary to gain access to a tumor of the neural elements, they must be followed by a formal fixation and bone graft to obtain a solid arthrodesis.

Instability of the Thoracolumbar Junction and the Lumbar Spine

At the thoracolumbar spine, where fractures with a higher degree of deformity are most frequently encountered, the burst fracture is the most common. (Burst fracture instability was described previously.) These fractures do not always heal well, and their tendency to get worse is well known. Thoracolumbar injuries often involve the conus, so bowel or bladder dysfunction may occur even in the absence of other neurologic signs or symptoms. Cystometrics and urodynamics can prove useful adjuncts in the evolution of acute or chronic injury of the conus at the thoracolumbar level.

Instability can occur in both planes, but segmental kyphosis remains the most classic deformity. Often neither deformity nor instability, even subjectively, is perceived by the patient. However, pain and neurologic symptoms are usually the first symptoms that will bring the patient to the physician. We can encounter, besides kyphosis, associated deformities that include scoliosis, lateral translation, spondylolisthesis, or rotational malalignment. Each of these deformities may be indicative of the nature of the original injury. Rotational malalignment, lateral translation, and spondylolisthesis are more suggestive of an unstable type deformity.

All these symptoms can be found with simple radiologic evaluation, which is more likely to provide useful information than more complex imaging. This should be reserved for analysis of canal diameter [computed tomography (CT) scan], medullary damage [magnetic resonance imaging (MRI)], and dramatic canal narrowing (myelogram). Tomography is extremely helpful in the assessment of a deformity centered on a remodeling callus in which a pseudarthrosis can be identified. If the degree of ligamentous involvement is at issue, flexion and extension radiographs can provide additional information. Discs and ligaments are well visualized on MRI scans, which can provide precious information on the degree of degeneration of the disc material. The evaluation of canal compromise and nerve compression is well accomplished by CT scan, which is accurate in imaging the bony anatomy. These imaging methods complement each other to assess "real" problems in this transitional area of the spine.

It is essential to perform decompression because functional improvement has been documented even 2 years after root or cauda equina compression. It is even more critical to make a complete assessment of bone stock, angles of deformity, canal diameter, and nerve compression because there are possibilities for recovery in this area of the spine (17). Yet, the thoracolumbar segments are the part of the spine that is submitted to the largest flexion/extension, lateral bending, and rotational moments and, therefore, they are at risk for pseudarthrosis, increased deformity, late instability, and conus or cauda equina compression.

Late deformity can occur following brace, cast, or surgical treatment. The role of brace treatment has been reviewed extensively, and both good and bad results have been reported (16,21,22,31,37).

In terms of surgical intervention, isolated laminectomy has been clearly identified as a source of iatrogenic deformity (4,32). Late deformity, however, may develop despite instrumentation and fusion if biomechanical stability has not been reestablished (13,27). In our experience, we have noted that, short of frontal and sagittal corrections to restore anatomic alignment, there is no valid treatment option. Regardless of treatment modality, realistic expectations in terms of pain improvement and stabilization of neurologic deficits depend on complete decompression, correction of deformity, and permanency of correction made possible by solid, mature arthrodesis.

The deformities at the level of the thoracolumbar spine are the most pronounced, and it is a complex problem to pursue anatomic reduction. It is possible to address both the anterior and posterior aspects of the spine simultaneously. Even though technical improvements have made single stage anterior instrumentation and fusion a viable alternative for Kostuik in Canada, in our experience, it appears that posterior instrumentation in combination with anterior releases and bone grafting afforded significantly greater immediate stability than anterior bone grafting alone. When the deformities are rigid, a combination of anterior releases and posterior osteotomies for reduction is often necessary. In this respect, keeping the spine alignment under visual control while the anterior releases are performed and the posterior osteotomies are done simultaneously allows alignment without losing stability at any time.

If one wants to use the CD instrumentation, the construct can be made and, inasmuch as distraction is applied to the front, compression can be applied to the back and anterior strut graft can be inserted. We have found the CD system with pedicular screws, both double threaded and simple, to be efficient in conjunction with the rod construct to achieve tridimensional stable constructs (11–13). Final compression applied to the back or supplementation of fixation in the front can provide immediate stability and anterior and posterior bone graft with circumferential bone graft in view of a circumferential arthrodesis (17). The margin of safety is optimized if care is taken to avoid any lengthening of the neural elements; it is always better to shorten than to try to correct by lengthening a spine.

Technical expertise, experience, and comprehensive spinal cord monitoring are critical to a successful outcome. Simultaneous procedures require two experienced surgical teams, and have proven safe and successful in our late experience in the last 3 years. The principle of the technique has been explained more as a philosophy than as a specific technique. Many instrumentations are available, and all have "pros and cons." Certainly, it is more a question of personal training and experience that make a surgeon select a given instrumentation. Our preferred instrumentation is a combination of hooks, screws, and rods from the CD instrumentation. There are difficulties inherent to the CD system, but when the difficulties are overcome, it definitely provides a very versatile system that allows us to "play with" distraction and compression as necessary. It also allows the desired correction, and provides an extremely rigid construct that guarantees a solid fixation. Obviously, if the same philosophy and approach are respected, any anterior and/or posterior instrumentation will be able to achieve the same goal.

Lumbosacral and Sacral Spine

The sacrum is a block composed of the last five vertebrae, through which pass the sacral nerve roots. The sacrum presents two lines of weakness, at either side of the midline of the vertebral bodies at the level of the foramina. They create a situation like a perforated line that is ready to be disrupted by an injury. This disruption occurs in high-velocity injuries and, very often, presents a large displacement. Stabilization of these fractures is difficult and dangerous. When the fractures happen, they are rarely isolated but are found among multiple injuries. The patients usually are extremely unstable and require immediate lifesaving treatment. Immediate fixation and reduction of sacral fractures is not attempted but, rather, skeletal traction or external fixation is used to immobilize the fragments and obtain blood tamponade.

Delayed union and pseudarthrosis are often the outcome of sacral fractures. The instability of a fibrous union or pseudarthrosis creates a permanent shear at the level of the pseudarthrosis, stretching nerves and creating pain and discomfort.

Secondary fixation of the sacrum can be obtained with use of plates and screws from the ilium to the sacrum, or from one ilium to the other ilium, compressing the ilia together posteriorly to realign and compress the sacral fragments.

Iliosacral screws inserted from the posterior iliac crest through the lateral aspect of the posterior iliac crest, reentering the sacrum through the sacroiliac joint or posterior to the joint, provide both solid fixation for the sacrum and a lag effect on the fragments, allowing fracture reduction.

This technique offers successful fixation with almost constant fracture healing.

A similar screw has been used to provide sacral fixation when arthrodesis between the lumbar spine and the sacrum is indicated. The iliosacral screws, placed on either side of the sacrum, provide anchorage for hooks or connectors and allow compression or distraction by CD instrumentation between the sacrum and the lumbar spine. The screws provide safe, solid purchase into the sacral bone at the level of the first sacral vertebra, allow reduction of kyphotic deformities, and give a solid, long-term fixation by enhancing the success rate of the lumbosacral arthrodesis.

The technique of insertion of the iliosacral screws is difficult, and depends upon obtaining anteroposterior (AP) and lateral roentgenograms during surgery. Cannulated screws are used; a K-wire guide is inserted from lateral to medial, entering through the lateral aspect of the posterior iliac crest, reappearing on the back of the sacroiliac joint, and reentering the sacrum lateral to the first sacral facet joint. The K-wire guide stops at the midline, at the level of the sacral promontory.

On the AP roentgenogram, the K-wire tip should not cross the midline; the perfectly inserted K-wire will be parallel to the sacral end plate, immediately caudal to the end plate. On the lateral roentgenogram, the K-wire tip must end in the middle third of the first sacral vertebral body, in the sacral promontory. The K-wire also should be roughly parallel to the end plate of the first sacral vertebra. Using the K-wire as a guide, cannulated screws will be inserted to provide sacral fixation, which, in our experience, has proven its efficiency and attained successful lumbosacral fusion. One second screw can be placed parallel to the first screw, aiming at the second sacral vertebra (10).

To reduce displaced Malgaigne fracture-dislocations, cannulated lag screws were used. A plate (AO type) was placed on the posterior iliac crest, and the lag screws were placed through the plate to optimize the lagging effect to achieve a better reduction. When reduction is obtained and the fixation of the sacroiliac is in place, fixation of the symphysis pubis in reduced anatomic position is necessary to complete the reduction and obtain a stable situation.

The other types of sacral fractures can create nerve injuries. These fractures are described as a type of transverse fracture of the sacrum, but they do not create instability. The rare isolated fracture/dislocation of L5-S1 due to a rupture of the L5-S1 facet joints requires the same protocol, i.e., decompression, realignment, fixation, and bone graft, as explained for the lumbar fractures.

It is commonly accepted that any sagittal plane deformity that increases at the level of an injury or tumor means *instability*. More complex are the problems of chronic instability that develop late as a consequence of fracture (25,35), tumor, infection, systemic disease, or surgical treatment.

The patient who presents with progressive deformity also presents pain and neurologic symptoms. The number of these patients has increased because a more aggressive attitude toward spine problems is widespread, and the number of years of follow-up for fractures and spine surgery has increased. In an aging population, there is also an increased number of patients who present with degenerative instability showing as spondylolisthesis in the lumbosacral spine. In the elderly, the consequence of this instability is spinal stenosis, pain, and accompanying loss of quality of life.

At each level of the spine, instability is likely to create a different type of neurologic compromise: compressive myelopathy and quadriparesia will develop at the level of the cervical spine, paraplegia at the thoracic spine, conus compression at the thoracolumbar junction, and, below the conus, at the level of the lumbar spine and the lumbosacral junction, cauda equina compression and radiculopathies.

The Patient with Spine Instability

It is always a challenge to arrive at the diagnosis of instability. Patients who had neither previous acute spine problems nor surgery can present with pain, only, and the pain history (pain relieved by bed rest and increased by motion) can be helpful in predicting the mechanical etiology of instability. Other patients have a history of spine problems, accident, general systemic disease, or previous surgery.

All patients were reviewed, and many attempts were made to document the instability. In a few cases of pseudarthrosis or disc instability, it was possible to document loss of alignment on stress test images. The most common instability was documented by a progression of symptoms both neurologic and radiologic over a period of time. The clinical assessment showed decreased functions, decreased sensitivity, irritation of the long tract, and loss of function with quantification by motor index score. Roentgenograms and other types of imaging offered progressive documentation of deformities, malalignment, canal stenosis, and increased volume of syrinx or increased cord atrophy, well documented by MRI.

The cause of primary instability is very rarely a long-standing deformity such as idiopathic scoliosis, but can be the result of a segmental kyphosis, such as congenital angular scoliosis. Most primary instabilities are related to degenerative joint disease on adults, and it is interesting to note that a spine with idiopathic scoliosis is no more prone to have degenerative instability than a nonscoliotic spine. On the contrary, many spines with degenerative osteoarthritis present an increasing deformity in kyphoscoliosis due to instability.

The causes of secondary instability were large laminectomies, with or without attempted fusion, old fractures and fracture/dislocations in which bone and ligaments failed to heal, failed fusions, and a group of miscellaneous pathologies such as Charcot spine, benign tumors, and progressive infections and osteomyelitis.

Materials

We have reviewed a group of 179 patients who were followed in our institution after they were referred for problems that were not necessarily related to their accidents. All these patients were victims of spine fractures; the accidents had happened 29 months to 27 years prior to the time they were first seen.

Of this group, 114 patients, (64%) were seen either routinely or for unrelated problems; they presented neither neurologic symptoms nor pain. In the group of 32 patients with relatively recent accident dates, we were able to evaluate the x-rays obtained after initial treatment and to compare them with x-rays taken in the last 29 months. In addition, 22 other patients were evaluated upon referral for complications such as nerve compromise and pain. These complications were all related to instability and deformities in the sagittal plane.

The deformities in both the sagittal and frontal planes were measured, and percentage of deformity was evaluated. We regarded a correction as ideal (100%) when it had restored the anatomic contour. The 65 patients who were symptomatic showed sagittal malalignment. The malalignment was 75% to 95% in 35 patients, and 75% or less in 32 patients. In the last group, which fell short of alignment by 25% or more, the patients were all symptomatic, with nerve compromise.

The percentage to which we refer is not measured as a comparison to the absolute Cobb angle. Rather, it is calculated with regard to the anatomic contour of a given individual and was discussed as the sagittal index (13).

In comparison, the patients whose sagittal contours were restored to the best biomechanical advantage, closest to anatomic perfection, presented an excellent long-term result. The analysis of the symptomatic patients' histories, physical examinations, and the results of multiple tests and imaging always revealed compression and/or instability.

The treatment, which had been either conservative or surgical, always accepted a compromise. The accepted compromises were:

approximate correction
incomplete decompression
laminectomies with no fixation
suboptimal fixation.

The various treatments that we now call suboptimal were state of the art when they were performed. In retrospect, these treatments failed to accomplish complete decompression, anatomic correction, and successful, stable arthrodesis.

We have revised 54 patients with late deformities and late neural compression. Our approach, at the beginning, consisted of staged procedures to obtain anterior releases, posterior osteotomies, circumferential bone grafts, and internal fixation in the anatomic position.

The patients' deformities were corrected and solid anterior and posterior arthrodeses developed, bridging the vertebrae in both the front and back. The patients showed improvement in level of pain and functional amelioration. In addition, all patients who presented neurologic improvement and signs of motor and sensory recovery were those who had complete decompression with restoration of frontal and sagittal alignments, maintained by a solid fusion.

The surgical techniques are demanding, and require planning and trained teams working together, sometimes simultaneously. The complications we encountered were major in the last 54 patients who underwent surgery. They were definitely outnumbered by the number of patients who improved.

As stated before, the complications were:

one cerebrospinal fluid (CSF) leak
one deep infection
one pulmonary embolus
one paraplegia
two hardware failures.

If deep infection and pulmonary embolus are part of the most difficult complications to deter, the others were related to technical difficulties that we recognized and addressed. As a result, we have decided to double-team the cases of localized nerve compression and localized deformities, such as malunion and pseudarthrosis following fractures, operating simultaneously.

It appears that this collaboration optimizes a few points:

1. It eliminates instability between procedures.
2. It eliminates dislodging of the anterior strut graft.
3. It allows osteotomies with visual control of reduction and decompression.
4. It offers the possibility to use fixation to maintain the most adequate reduction.

With this improvement, our results have improved dramatically, and complications were reduced to three minor incidents in the last 27 cases.

The last advantage in these debilitated patients is the possibility of saving time and blood, enabling us to operate without nonautologous transfusion.

Summary

Stability of the spine depends upon the integrity of multiple rigid bony elements, the vertebrae, superimposed on one another and bound together by ligaments and discs. Such a construct optimizes the ability to bend in all directions while carrying a load.

A host of problems can affect one or more elements of this construct and disrupt the mechanical integrity of a component, creating a condition called instability. According to the extent of the disruption, which can affect one or more mobile segments and one or more components, different types of instability will result.

We addressed acute instability as encountered in spinal fractures and dislocations, chronic instability as a result of degenerative joint disease, and failure of treatment, such as failed fusions and instability following extensive laminectomies.

In our institution, patients with histories of spine fractures ranging from 29 months to 27 years were evaluated for residual pain, spine deformity in both the frontal and sagittal planes, and neurologic compromise after spine fractures. We found 114 patients (64%) who had neither complaints, increased deformity, nor nerve compromise; all of them were treated for their spine injuries by either conservative or surgical management. Alignment in both frontal and sagittal planes fell short of perfection by 2% to 7%. There were 32 patients (18%) with late deformities who had increasing angular deformities and nerve compromise that necessitated surgery. These 32 symptomatic patients presented a sagittal contour that was greater than 25% from perfect anatomic alignment. Thirty-three patients presented some pain but no nerve involvement. Their alignment lacked 5% to 25% of correct anatomic alignment. Considering that any deformity can be corrected to anatomic alignment, we evaluated correction in percentage of correction, considering individual anatomic alignment as 100%.

In reviewing the data, it appears that correction of sagittal deformity is among the criteria for successful long-term treatment. There are a host of techniques described that are excellent for achieving correction and fixation to enable a successful fusion. We attempted to describe the principle of circumferential arthrodesis.

In addition, 22 patients were referred to our care for late complications of spine fractures. They were without previous records, making it impossible to assess the results of the initial treatment. We elected not to add them to the data above, even though they all presented increased sagittal deformity, pain, and neurologic compromise. They were treated with the same protocol as the above 32 patients, and we have followed up on 54 patients treated for late deformities and late instability with pain and neurologic compromise. Decompression of the neural elements and realignment of the spine were achieved, and circumferential arthrodesis was performed.

Seven complications were encountered. Four patients were neurologically worse after surgery: motor index score loss was 20% to 25%. Forty-one patients showed pain improvement and stabilization. Nine patients improved dramatically: motor index score gain was 10% to 30%.

In summary, the restoration of anatomic alignment is essential to obtain a solid arthrodesis and clinical improvement. Spine instability must be recognized and treated.

Bibliography

1. Argenson C, Dintimille H. Lesions traumatiques experimentales du rachis chez le singe. *Rev Chir Orthop*. 1977;63:430–431.
2. Benson DR. Unstable thoracolumbar fractures, with emphasis on the burst fracture. *Clin Orthop Rel Res*. 1988;230:14–29.
3. Bernhardt M, Bridwell KH. Segmental analysis of the sagittal plane alignment of the normal thoracic and lumbar spines and thoracolumbar junction. *Orthop Trans*. 1989;13:106.
4. Bradford DS. Deformities of the thoracic and lumbar spine secondary to spinal injury. In: Bradford DS, Lonstein JE, Moe JH, Ogilvie JW, Winter RB, eds. *Moe's Textbook of Scoliosis*. 2nd ed. Philadelphia: WB Saunders; 1987:435–463.
5. Caspar W. Advances in cervical spine surgery. First Experiences with the trapezial osteosynthetic plate and a new surgical instrumentation for anterior interbody stabilization. *Orthop News USA*. 1982.
6. Coe JD, Warden KE, Sutterlin CE, McAfee PC. Biomechanical evaluation of cervical spinal stabilization methods in a human cadaveric model. *Spine*. 1989;14:1122–1131.
7. Dennis F. The three column concept and its significance in the classification of acute thoracolumbar spinal injuries. *Spine*. 1983;8:817–831.
8. Dennis F. Spinal instability as defined by the three column concept in acute spinal trauma. *Clin Orthop Rel Res*. 1984;189:65–67.
9. DeWald RL. Burst fractures of the thoracic and lumbar spine. *Clin Orthop Rel Res*. 1984;189:150–161.
10. Farcy JPC, Roye DP, Weidenbaum M. Cotrel-Dubousset instrumentation technique for revision of failed lumbosacral fusion. *Bull Hosp Jt Dis Orthop Inst*. 1987;47:1–12.
11. Farcy JPC, Weidenbaum M. A preliminary review of the use of Cotrel-Dubousset instrumentation for spinal injuries. *Bull Hosp Jt Dis Orthop Inst*. 1988;48(1):44–51.
12. Farcy JPC, Weidenbaum M. Pitfalls in fracture fixation with Cotrel-Dubousset instrumentation. *Proceedings of the 5th International Congress on Cotrel-Dubousset Instrumentation*. Montpellier: Sauramps Medical; 1989:103–110.

13. Farcy JPC, Weidenbaum M, Glassman SD. *The Sagittal Index in the Management of Thoracolumbar Burst Fractures*. Amsterdam: SRS; 1989.
14. Farcy JPC, Weidenbaum M, Sola C. Surgical management of severe cervical kyphosis following extensive laminectomies. *Spine*. 1990;15(1):41–45.
15. Ferguson RL, Allen BL. A mechanistic classification of thoracolumbar spine fractures. *Clin Orthop Rel Res*. 1983;189:77–88.
16. Frankel HL, Hancock DO, Hyslop G, Melzak J, Michaelis LS, Ungar GH, Vernon JDS, Walsh JJ. The value of postural reduction in the initial management of closed injuries of the spine with paraplegia and tetraplegia. Part I. *Paraplegia*. 1969;7:179–192.
17. Gertzbein SD, Court-Brown CM, Jacobs RR, Marks P, Martin C. Neurological outcome following surgery for spinal fractures. *Orthop Trans*. 1989;13:49.
18. Gertzbein SD, Court-Brown CM, Jacobs RR, Marks P, Martin C, Stoll J, Fazl M, Schwartz M, Rowed D. Decompression and circumferential stabilization of unstable spinal fractures. *Spine*. 1988;13:892–895.
19. Goutallier D, Louis R. Indications teraputiques dans les fractures instables du rachis. *Rev Chir Orthop*. 1977;63:475–481.
20. Gurr KR, McAfee PC, Shih CM. Biomechanical analysis of anterior and posterior instrumentation systems after corpectomy. *J Bone Joint Surg*. 1988;70A:1182–1191.
21. Guttman L. *Spinal Cord Injuries: Comprehensive Management and Research*. Oxford: Blackwell Scientific; 1957.
22. Jacobs RR, Asher MA, Sniker RK. Thoracolumbar spine injuries: A comparative study of recumbent and operative treatment in one hundred patients. *Spine*. 1980;5:463-477.
23. Kapandji IA: *The Physiology of the Joints. Vol. 3: The Trunk and the Vertebral Column*. Edinburgh: Churchill Livingstone; 1988.
24. Kostuik JP. Anterior fixation for fractures of the thoracic and lumbar spine with or without neurologic involvement. *Clin Orthop Rel Res*. 1984;189:103–115.
25. Leidholt J, Young J, Hahan H, Jackson R. Evaluation of late spinal deformities with fracture-dislocations of the dorsal and lumbar spine in paraplegics. *Paraplegia*. 1970;7:16.
26. Louis R, Maresca C, Sorbier J. Le double abord en deux temps rachis. *Rev Chir Orthop*. 1977;63:472–474.
27. Malcolm BW, Bradford DS, Winter RB, Chou SN. Posttraumatic kyphosis. *J Bone Joint Surg*. 1981;63A:891–899.
28. McAfee PC, Bohlman HH. Complications following Harrington instrumentation for fractures of the thoracolumbar spine. *J Bone Joint Surg*. 1985;56A:672–686.
29. McAfee PC, Bohlman HH. One stage anterior cervical decompression and posterior stabilization with circumferential arthrodesis. A study of twenty-four patients who had a traumatic or a neoplastic lesion. *J Bone Joint Surg*. 1989;71A:78–88.
30. McAfee PC, Bohlman HH, Ducker T, Eismont FJ. Failure of stabilization of the spine with methyl methacrylate. A retrospective analysis of 24 cases. *J Bone Joint Surg*. 1986;68A:1145–1157.

31. Reid DC, Hu R, Davis LA, Saboe LA. The nonoperative treatment of burst fractures of the thoracolumbar junction. *J Trauma*. 1988;18:1188–1194.
32. Roberts S, Manage J, Urban JPG. Biochemical and structural properties of the cartilage end plate and its relation to the intervertebral disc. *Spine*. 1989;14:166–174.
33. Roy-Camille R, Saillant G, Mazel C. Internal fixation of the unstable cervical spine by posterior osteosynthesis with plates and screws. In: Sherk HH, ed. *The Cervical Spine*. Philadelphia: JB Lippincott; 1989.
34. Stagnara P, DeMauroy JC, Dran G, Gonon GP, Costanzo G, Dimnet J, Pasquet A. Reciprocal angulation of vertebral bodies in a sagittal plane: approach to references for the evaluation of kyphosis and lordosis. *Spine*. 1982;7:335–342.
35. Sutherland CJ, Miller F, Wang GJ. Early progressive kyphosis following compression fractures. *Clin Orthop Rel Res*. 1983;173:216–220.
36. Weinstein JN, Spratt KF, Spengler D, Brick C, Reid S. Spinal pedicle fixation: Reliability and validity of roentgenogram-based assessment and surgical factors on successful screw placement. *Orthop Trans*. 1989;13:117–118.
37. White AA, Johnson RM, Panjabi M, Southwick WO. Biomechanical analysis of clinical stability in the cervical spine. *Clin Orthop Rel Res*. 1975;109.
38. Whitesides TE, Shah SG. On the management of unstable fractures of the thoracolumbar spine. *Spine*. 1976;1:99–107.

Discussion

The Need for Major Spinal Centers

Dr. Kostuik said: Thank you, Jean-Pierre. Of course, I think the goal of any group such as this is to try to avoid having cases such as Jean-Pierre has shown arrive on our doorstep. Unfortunately, this is an increasing problem not only in North America, but worldwide. The reason for it in part is the increasing number of people who are interested in spinal surgery and whose training has been based on disc excisions and simple fusions and who then take on something too complex. It is important for us as teachers to try to teach not only the technique of how to do these cases, but which cases should be selected for care in major spinal centers. As I said yesterday, I feel very strongly about this. I will discuss this further in the section on training of the spine surgeon.

Segmental Instability Related to Kyphotic Deformities from Previous Surgery

Dr. Farcy was asked: Why did the patient with lymphoma become paraparetic? The cement construct popped out of place and she became unstable. Since reoperation her neurological status has improved and she can walk, but not completely normally. Dr. Kostuik asked: How long after the insertion of the cement did it become loose? Dr. Farcy said: About 4 years. Dr. Kostuik said: That appears to me to be the source of the error. If a patient with myeloma or lymphona under the care of an oncologist is in good control with tumor remission my feeling is to take them back in 1 year and do a posterior fusion.

Dr. Sonntag asked about the methods of achieving reduction and the time frame involved. Dr. Farcy said: Our principle is not to initiate traction primarily. We advocate first performing osteotomies or vertebrectomies both front and back and place the patient in a halo and try to align the spine. The patient is placed in the halo before surgery begins. After readjustment of the halo or Gardner-Wells tongs the patient is put at bed rest and several days later a fusion is performed. To emphasize, we do the osteotomy first and then attempt the alignment very slowly on a conscious patient who helps me and understands what I am doing.

Dr. Kostuik added: Most of them that I have done have been aligned at the same time. I have put the patients on their side, placed the halo, and operated anteriorly and posteriorly to correct the deformity. Dr. Farcy added: In some cases I have been reluctant to proceed with the alignment because the spinal cord was so small.

Prof. Louis said: I appreciate the work of Dr. Farcy and in my practice I sometime perform correction of a malalignment of the cervical spine by a combined approach in one stage putting the patient on his side. I do, however, feel that it is safer to use the halo and I prefer it. On the other hand when you are accustomed to the technique of osteotomy it is a feasible option. I do not use two teams. I do the operation myself, performing both osteotomies and then reduction by gentle manipulation.

Dr. Kostuik said: I am sure Dr. Farcy uses two teams for the approach, but is managing the anterior and posterior osteotomies himself. Dr. Farcy concurred.

Prof. Louis said: For the malunion of the thoracolumbar spine I have for the past 8 years used the new technique of posterior osteotomy. I perform both anterior and posterior osteotomies with one approach. I make a wedge osteotomy of the spine, but not a common one. The common one uses a hinge at the level of the posterior aspect of the vertebral body, whereas I use a hinge just 3 mm before the anterior cortex of the vertebral body. This operation is accomplished within 3 hours. I do both approaches with only one incision.

Dr. Kostuik said: What you are describing here Master described 25 years ago for ankylosing spondylitis, where you take more bone, remove the back of the vertebral body and hinge it more anteriorly. The other alternative is to do a so-called eggshell procedure where you pin down the lamina posteriorly, remove whatever bone you need, and go through the pedicle to take out the vertebral body and the pedicles. I must emphasize that I never do an osteotomy in the thoracic spine since one of my patients became paraplegic. In the lumbar spine I generally do multiple osteotomies.

CHAPTER 20

Training the Future Spinal Surgeon

John P. Kostuik

The Need

This past decade has seen an explosion in the need for spinal surgeons. It is currently estimated that there is a growth in the field of spinal disability of approximately 10% a year. The incidence of spinal surgery has paralleled this growth of disability. Currently there are approximately 325,000 spinal procedures done per year in the United States. There are numerous geographic variations, with twice the amount of surgery being done on the West Coast as on the East Coast, and even within certain counties there are differences. This has been borne out in small group analysis studies. There have been no specific answers to why this growth has occurred. The problems and answers lie within the realm of economics, Spinal pain that occurs in the course of employment is considered disability under workers' compensation acts throughout the industrialized world. It is estimated that by the year 2010 disability from low back pain could bankrupt the country of Sweden. This suggests that the answer to this problem may be to take pain and disability as a result of back problems out of workers' compensation and replace them within the disabilities not encountered in the workplace.

There is going to be an increased need for spinal surgeons in the near future. One has only to look in the back of such journals as *The Journal of Bone and Joint Surgery (American)*, *Spine*, and *The Journal of Spinal Disorders* to see numerous want ads for spinal surgeons. However, this is due not only to the increased disability as a result of low back problems but to the medical-legal issue. In a group practice, rather than everyone paying the highest possible premium to allow all to do some degree of spinal surgery, it is more efficacious, based on a medical-legal point of view, cost, and patient perspective, and not necessarily in that order, to have within the group practice a subspecialist in spinal surgery.

The purpose of this chapter is not to describe the ergonomics and epidemiology, but rather to describe how to provide the training for the future spinal surgeon. This chapter does not purport to have all the answers to this problem, but simply perhaps to provide a guideline for future reference.

Following graduation from an accredited medical school and entrance into residency program, training in spinal surgery commences. There are two streams from which an exposure to the spine in a residency program might occur, one from the field of neurosurgery and the other from orthopedics. Following completion of residency, an accredited fellowship must be completed. This will lead to a certification of added qualification. The process of recertification at some later date yet to be defined should subsequently take place.

Before expanding on residency, fellowship certification, and recertification, it is important that we have a common definition of a spinal surgeon. At the present time in North America this is confusing. There are spinal surgeons who enter from the fields of either neurosurgery or orthopedic surgery. There are few highly qualified, exclusive, spinal surgeons. There are very few fellowships that offer complete exposure to the spine. There are numerous fellowships in low back surgery, deformity surgery, trauma surgery, and indeed fellowships only in cervical spine surgery. As a result there is a need for a definition of a spinal surgeon. Generally it is excepted that this is a person who subspecializes and spends more than 50% of his time in spinal surgery and who has had a fellowship. This embodies the majority of spinal surgeons, although many of those people age 40 or over who do 50% or more spinal surgery did not have a fellowship per se in spinal surgery.

There are no set criteria at the present time as to who is or is not a spinal surgeon. The fellowship directors provide a certificate upon completion of a fellowship. At the present time in the spine field, fellowships are not accredited to any governing association or by the Residency Review Committee, although following considerable efforts, particularly on the part of the American Academy of Orthopaedic Surgeons and the Committee on Musculoskeletal Specialty Societies, the spine field is close to developing its own fellowship criteria.

It is obvious that the definition of a spinal surgeon in the future will remain fairly general, although it is anticipated that there will be an increasing number of spinal surgeons devoting their full time to this subspecialty and who are capable of dealing with all aspects of disease or deformity related to the spine.

Certainly the Japanese example of a spinal surgeon should be considered. Currently the vast majority of spinal surgeons in Japan emanate from orthopedic surgery. These surgeons deal with all problems related to the spine from the occipital cervical joint, distally, including intradural problems. This definition is obviously an ideal one because of the large numbers of surgeons from both neurosurgery and orthopedics. Although this may present the ideal definition, it is unlikely to come about.

At the present time the majority come from the field of orthopedic surgery. Specialty societies, an example is the North American Spine Society, although multidisciplinary in nature, encourage membership from other fields including neurosurgery, but they currently form only 10% of these societies' numbers. A great deal of difficulty in attracting neurosurgeons to these societies has been encountered. Other examples are the International Society for the Study of the Lumbar Spine and to a lesser degree the Cervical Spine Research Society. More on the role of the spinal societies is to be discussed later.

Residency Training

Currently there are two streams in residency training from which the spinal surgeon may come. These are the neurosurgical stream and the orthopedic stream. Both of these subspecialties have little exposure to nonoperative methods of care, although this is much more likely to occur within the orthopedic setting.

Questions to be Asked

Should training remain as it is with exposure to other aspects of surgery in general, such as intensive care, plastic and reconstructive surgery, vascular surgery, and abdominal surgery?

Should the residency program be significantly altered, particularly for those people who decide early on that they wish to become spinal surgeons?

With the ultimate aim of a single certification in spinal surgery in the future, it is my feeling that an altered residency should be optionally provided. A basic exposure to surgery in general for approximately 18 months, and then a year exposure to neurosurgery or orthopedics, followed by a year of spinal surgery, might offer a complete of residency training. This is likely, however, to meet considerable resistance. In all likelihood the traditional residency programs will survive with minimal exposure to the spine. In such programs, the need for subsequent fellowships will be mandatory. Should the residency be altered? Then, ideally, 1 year of residency devoted to spinal surgery would be necessary. At the present time the governing bodies of neurosurgery generally feel that a fellowship in spinal surgery is not necessary. It is felt there is sufficient exposure during residency to spinal surgery. This may well be for the incomplete spinal surgeon who restricts himself to disc excision and to a few procedures in the cervical spine. It is not sufficient for the surgeon dedicated to spinal surgery.

Currently, most North American most neurosurgeons derive 90% of their income from spinal procedures, yet only 5% of the neurosurgery publications are on subjects related to the spine, and many of these are related to the dura and its contents. Obviously there is a significant educational lack in current training programs in neurosurgery related to the spine.

Can the same be said for orthopedic residents? There has been an increasing emphasis and exposure to spinal problems, particularly with the advent of improved forms of internal fixation of the spine in recent years. At the present time most orthopedic programs have a reasonable exposure to spinal disease, injury, and deformity, with adequate operative care exposure. However, there are still some programs where this is not satisfactory. It is felt that these programs can hardly be accredited for orthopedic residency, let alone for any spinal care program. Currently, spine within the field of orthopedic surgery rates number three in terms of the number of applicants for fellowship programs and job demand. It is the most rapidly increasing field in the musculoskeletal sciences.

Currently, during the residency it is felt that neurosurgeons in training should be exposed to a minimum of 6 months of orthopedics, preferably most of this related to the spine, and, vice versa, orthopedic residents should be exposed to 6 months of neurosurgery and in particular to work related to the dural sac and its contents.

In no case does this render a resident a competent spinal surgeon following completion of his residency under the traditional format.

Fellowships

There is considerable confusion in the field of fellowship programs. Most of these lie under the aegis of orthopedic surgery. The number of neurosurgical residents attempting to obtain fellowships under the tutelage of an orthopedic surgeon or in an orthopedic program is increasing.

Most fellowships have been in the past preceptorship-type programs, and often with little academic input. Fellows have been slaves to their preceptors, who helped them go through a great volume of clinical material but with little critical assessment or education.

Fellowships are extremely varied and currently involve total spine, low back only, injury only, cervical spine only, or deformity; the latter is particularly true in the field of pediatric spine.

We have not yet defined the role of the pediatric spine surgeon. Should the general spinal surgeon be cognizant of all the problems related to he pediatric spine or should this remain in the realm of the pediatric spinal surgeon? Certainly if we were to train total spinal surgeons then they must be cognizant and capable of dealing with pediatric problems.

In the author's estimation the fellowships offered should be university affiliated with a distinct academic focus, including such fields as anatomy, biomechanics, biochemistry as it relates to the disc, pathophysiology, and radiology including access to invasive radiology, i.e., discography, facet blocks, nerve root injection blocks, etc. The course content should have scheduled formal lectures covering all aspects of spinal problems, operative and nonoperative. The fellowship must have access to other subspecialties for consultation and exposure, including vascular surgery, urology, and rehabilitation and to nonoperative care. There must be access to anatomical specimens with the capability of autopsy dissections where necessary. The fellowship must be in a environment that conducts clinical research at the very least so that either one major or two minor papers per year are published by the fellow. Ideally the exposure to basic laboratory research related to the spine either of a biomechanical, biochemical, or neurophysiological nature should be available.

Clinical content has been discussed by many with no consensus being arrived at among the various spinal societies. Ideally, there should be exposure to 200 operative cases each year, preferably with the fellow being the leading surgeon in 50 of them. The total surgeon would require exposure to 50 or more trauma cases a year and 50 or more deformity cases, with the remainder consisting of low back and cervical spine surgery, with some exposure to tumor, preferably 10 to 20 cases, and infectious diseases, 10 cases per year.

The fellowship must consist of exposure to metabolic bone disease with an understanding of bone metabolism and physiology and muscle metabolism and physiology, together with the neurological control mechanisms. A comprehensive knowledge of neuroanatomy of the spinal cord and the peripheral nerves and the role of chemical mediators within these, i.e., dorsal root ganglion, must be provided.

Most of all, any fellowship must be inquisitive and questioning.

Considerable debate as to the duration of the fellowship has ensued with an increasing interest in 2-year fellowships. One year would relate to clinical and or basic research with attendance at clinics. The second year would be fully clinical. Considering the increasing complexity of spinal surgery and the inadequate exposure at the residency level this represents the ideal aim. Currently practicality in terms of funding preclude, with rare exceptions, a fellowship duration beyond 1 year. A 6-month fellowship for someone who has been practicing or who has had considerable exposure to spine in his residency at a high-level institute may suffice, but this is the rare exception and requires the mature surgeon.

Certification

Following completion of fellowship it is the current practice of most program directors to provide a certificate of added qualification. As previously mentioned, this is nonspecific and generic and under no review. The Residency Review Committee in orthopedics at least is planning accreditation of fellowship based upon the criteria above. Upon following completion of an accredited fellowship, a certificate may be issued.

Ideally this should involve an examination process. At this time none is available. This would entail considerable forethought particularly because of the variation of fellowships and the various anatomical areas of the spine.

Certificate of Limited Qualification

Since at the present time there is a tremendous variation of the definition of spinal surgeon, it will be some time before the total spine surgeon can be accepted as the only surgical answer to the problems of the spine. Certificates of limited qualification should be issued, such as spinal surgeon–scoliosis, or spinal surgeon–low back, or spinal surgeon–trauma.

Governing Bodies

Still to be decided is who is to issue the certificates. Currently, as previously stated, these are provided by the fellowship directors, if they are provided at all. At the present time the fellow might make a certificate, put it on his wall, and claim to be a spinal surgeon despite the fact that he may never do any surgery in practice or only a very limited amount. It is this author's feeling that there should be a governing body issuing the examination process. This could be issued by the boards of either neurosurgery or orthopedics. Because the ultimate aim of this chapter is the development of the total spinal surgeon I feel that there should be a separate governing body. This would necessitate the development of a board of spinal surgery. Perhaps the governing bodies could be the American Board of Orthopaedic Surgeons and the American Board of Neurosurgery.

This then brings into question the nonoperative needs of the spinal patient, which is currently poorly taught to surgeons. There are beginning to be a few fellowships in nonoperative spinal care. There is an increasing emphasis being fostered in particular by the North American Spine Society and its ad hoc committee on nonoperative care. Surgical candidates should have a minimum exposure in a 2-year fellowship of 3 months to rehabilitation techniques. In all likelihood, this would significantly decrease the incidence of surgery and provide the surgical candidate with the proper exposure to epidemiology and ergonomics, and the proper evaluation of physiotherapy, back education, work hardening, and the psychological aspects of back problems.

The Role of Spine Societies

Should spinal societies such as the North American Spine Society, the Cervical Spine Research Society, the International Society for the Study of the Lumbar Spine, and the Scoliosis Research Society play a leading role in the education of the future spinal surgeon? Their current role is one of continuing education. Perhaps the societies, at least in North America, could be merged into one, with a common board that could act as the governing body for certification and recertification of spinal surgeons. It has been mentioned that these societies are self-serving; however, this is rarely true, and such societies provided more benefit to the populace, within the subspecialty, than the larger, more all-encompassing groups such as the academies. It is currently this author's feeling that the North American Spine Society, which encompasses all aspects of spinal surgery and nonoperative care including radiology, psychology, and rehabilitation, should assume the predominant role providing guidelines for the future of spinal care; hence, the development of spinal surgeons. Such societies as mentioned above will encompass and embrace the burgeoning young spinal surgeons and, it is hoped, lead them along an enlightened path rather than the narrow tunnel that so often exists. This brings up the final question of recertification.

Recertification

Recertification remains even more controversial than accreditation. Currently within the musculoskeletal societies only one has a recertification process. The American Academy of Orthopaedic Surgeons has issued a limited license requiring recertification in the future and in 6 to 7 years the first group will have to be recertified in orthopedic surgery. The process for this has not been established. Recertification in my estimation is such a difficult field with potential problems in spinal surgery, but it is a necessity. Recertification would have to be issued by the governing body. The process by which the recertification would take place will require considerable forethought and should include such things as practice review, continuing medical education, exposure to peer review, and a knowledge update, and should be required every 7 to 10 years.

By virtue of practice review, continuing competency can be exhibited as well as knowledge and sufficient patient and operative exposure. A knowledge update questionnaire, sufficient exposure, and continuing education are self-explanatory.

In conclusion, one can ask if the total spinal surgeon can be trained. It is my feeling that it is possible, following a residency either through neurosurgery or orthopedic surgery with a fellowship of probably 2 years and with the subsequent recertification process. Such a surgeon can be developed. This will require a number of hurdles and it is likely to be 15 or more years away. Meanwhile, certificates of limited qualification should be provided under the auspice of a governing body, preferably a national society or a body established through the joint efforts of the American Academy of Orthopaedic Surgeons and the Academy of Neurosurgeons.

Society will demand it, hospital boards will demand it, and although this may be viewed as fragmentation of parental organizations, ultimately the boards and academies of both orthopedic surgery and neurosurgery will demand it. The result will be a better qualified person capable of caring for the patient with spinal problems regardless of source and etiology, and will result in a closer association between neurosurgery and orthopedics than is currently seen in many centers in North America. The ultimate result is a better surgeon who would provide better care and would continue to advance the frontiers of science.

Closing Remarks

Harold M. Dick

The collegial atmosphere of our major universities can engender collaboration between the specialties and subspecialties. This type of collaboration, if successful, can give rise to entirely new fields in both medicine and surgery. Such an event is imminent, namely, the creation of the specialty of the spine surgeon and it is our obligation to oversee and nurture its growth.

Columbia University's College of Physicians and Surgeons and the Columbia Presbyterian Medical Center historically have provided for such developments. Our predecessors in orthopedics, Dr. Frank Stinchfield and Dr. Alexander Garcia, worked closely with Dr. Lester Mount and Dr. Edward Schlesinger, neurosurgeons at the New York Neurological Institute on spine problems, combining their expertise on neural tissue dissection and decompression with the bilateral intertransverse iliac graft fusions that were developed at the New York Orthopedic Hospital. It was a common, everyday occurrence to have these teams care for the spine patients.

At that time they knew far less about the term "spinal instability" and the issues of disc removal and facet resection than about their impact upon the stability of the spine, but they brought together in the 25 years of their collaboration a series of over 1,000 consecutive cases of discectomy and fusion. Concomitantly, the concept of spinal stenosis was evolving and beginning to impact upon the approaches to degenerative spinal disease, which we now deal with on a regular basis.

This bridging of the territorial imperatives, which frequently exists between departments, was critical for our institution and represented a frontier that is now being furthered by conferences such as the Stonwin Medical Conference. This gives me a reason to feel a great sense of pride and also optimism for the future.

We look forward to the input of bioengineers, neurologists, and rehabilitation experts to accomplish the ultimate goal of offering the patient, child or adult, neurologically intact or seriously paralyzed, the possibility of achieving the best possible outcome.

Index

T